Syringomyelia

Graham Flint • Clare Rusbridge

Editors

Syringomyelia

A Disorder of CSF Circulation

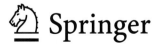 Springer

Editors
Graham Flint
Department of Neurosurgery
Queen Elizabeth Hospital
University Hospitals Birmingham
Birmingham
UK

Clare Rusbridge
Fitzpatrick Referrals
Eashing
Godalming
Surrey
UK

Faculty of Health and Medical Sciences
School of Veterinary Medicine
University of Surrey
Guildford
Surrey
UK

ISBN 978-3-540-72484-1   ISBN 978-3-642-13706-8   (eBook)
DOI 10.1007/978-3-642-13706-8
Springer Heidelberg New York Dordrecht London

Library of Congress Control Number: 2014931381

Printed on acid-free paper

Springer is part of Springer Science+Business Media (www.springer.com)

Those of us who are able-bodied and who treat people affected by neurological conditions can only admire their capacity to live and cope with physical disability. During my career, I have been privileged to meet many such people and their families, but my exposure to this fortitude of the human spirit goes back to my earliest childhood, having a father who lost his sight as a young man. My mother stood by him, despite this major setback in their lives and, amongst the many people with disabilities who I have since met, my parents remain the 'original and best'. I duly dedicate my contribution to this monograph to the family that has always supported me. To my parents, Tom and Rita Flint, who first gave me my values in life; to my wife, Marian, who continues to support me in all that I do; and to my daughter Alicia, who provides my inspiration for the future.

Graham Flint

I have worked on Chiari malformation and syringomyelia since 1997 when I documented my first canine case. My passion and obsession with this disease would not have been possible without the support of my soul mate and husband. I am grateful that he encouraged me to complete a PhD and for his many sacrifices to minimise the impact of my working on our family life. Like Graham, I also owe much to my parents. My father, a naturalist and scientist, gave me a rich childhood experience, nurturing my love of animals and inspiring me to become a vet. My mother has worked tirelessly (and unpaid) as my research assistant for over a decade, and much of our understanding of canine Chiari malformation is due to her. Therefore, I dedicate my contribution to John and Penny Knowler, Mark Rusbridge and my children Jillian and Thomas.

Clare Rusbridge

Foreword

This monograph provides a much needed, up-to-date reference work for medical professionals who have an interest in this field. It is an extensive and comprehensive collection of informative contributions, covering all aspects of syringomyelia, from basic sciences through to present-day clinical practice. Additional interest and information is provided by chapters on topics such as art and mythology.

The editors, consultant neurosurgeon Graham Flint and veterinary neurologist Clare Rusbridge, are both leaders in this field, and they have invited, from around the world, 18 other authors, themselves experts in the different aspects of this disease, to contribute to this volume.

The knowledge and expertise contained in this book will, undoubtedly, help advance the understanding and treatment of this condition. It will be essential reading for health professionals and others interested in increasing their knowledge about this enigmatic condition.

As the former chairman of a syringomyelia patient support charity, I would like, on behalf of sufferers and their families, to express our gratitude to all the authors who have contributed to the production of this most inclusive and instructive monograph and to the other health professionals, who do such wonderful work in the treatment of syringomyelia and Chiari.

Rugby, UK   Anthony A. Kember

Preface

Five monographs on the subject of syringomyelia have been published over the past 40 years, and these remain invaluable reference sources for those who have an interest in this and related conditions (see below). In addition, international symposia have been organised in Kobe (2001), Rugby (2007), Berlin (2010) and Sydney (2013), events which reflect the continuing interest in this field. The editors therefore felt that it was now timely to pull together, in a single volume, the current state of knowledge and understanding about this most enigmatic of neurological conditions. We hope that it will provide a basis for future research and innovation in this field.

The title of this book reflects our belief that syringomyelia should be regarded not simply as a disorder affecting the spinal cord but rather as a pathological process which involves the cerebrospinal fluid pathways as a whole and of water movement in the central nervous system in general. Our authors offer expertise in a variety of fields, ranging from basic sciences through to living with the effects of syringomyelia or Chiari malformation. They are distinguished by their research, publications or long clinical experience and often all three.

The book looks again at many of the topics covered in previous monographs but brings us up to date with present-day thinking about molecular and developmental biology, as well as the ever present question as to why, exactly, syringomyelia cavities develop in the first place. In addition, we have introduced some additional topics, including mathematical modelling and the biochemistry of syringomyelia. The book also deals with some practical issues, including the impact of syringomyelia and Chiari on pregnancy and what it is like to be a patient living with these conditions. Medicolegal aspects of these disorders are also considered.

Readers will notice some overlap or repetition of material between chapters. We have permitted this in order that authors can present their material in context and so that individual chapters can, to some extent, stand alone. It also allows the reader to appreciate where there are differences of opinion or varying interpretations of available data.

The book is aimed at any health-care professional who has an interest in syringomyelia and related disorders but will be of particular interest to a recently qualified specialist, who wishes to take an interest in the management of these most challenging conditions.

Birmingham, UK   Graham Flint
Surrey, UK   Clare Rusbridge
January 2014

Previous Monographs

Anson JA, Benzel EC, Awad IA (1997) Syringomyelia and the Chiari malformations. Neurosurgical topics. AANS Publications Committee. The American Association of Neurological Surgeons. Park Ridge, Illinois, p 202

Barnett HJM, Foster JB, Hudgson P (1973) Syringomyelia. Major problems in neurology. W B Saunders, London, p 318

Batzdorf U (1991) Syringomyelia: current concepts in diagnosis and treatment. In: Wilson C (ed) Current neurosurgical practice. Williams & Wilkins, Baltimore, p 208

Klekamp J, Samii M (2002) Syringomyelia: diagnosis and treatment. Springer, Berlin, p 195

Tamaki N, Batzdorf U, Nagashima T (2001) Syringomyelia. Current concepts in pathogenesis and management. Springer, Tokyo, p 263

Acknowledgements

The editors wish to express their gratitude to the many people involved in the preparation of this monograph. Individual authors have given their time and effort freely and with enthusiasm. Thanks are also due to Keith Kushner, Wagih El Masri, Holger Volk and Fernando Constantino-Casas for proofreading the authors' own chapters and to Richard West for reviewing appendix 3. All of these colleagues have made very helpful suggestions. We are grateful to Sue Line, Susan Kember, Rebecca Dodwell-Pitt and Lynn Burton for providing accounts of their personal experiences, as patients. We are also grateful to Debbie Gordon for her invaluable work in checking all of the references in the book. The staff at Springer have been supportive from the outset and tolerant of delays and postponements. Our partners, Marian Flint and Mark Rusbridge, have lived as monograph 'widow and widower' for many months, and to both of them we owe our sincere thanks. The project itself was accomplished under the direction of the Ann Conroy Trust and our thanks in particular go to Barbara Winward and to Susan and Tony Kember, without whose support this monograph would not have been completed. Finally we wish to thank our many patients, who have taught us and continue to teach us about this enigmatic disease.

Contents

Contributors

The editors have assembled a team of international authorities, in the fields of syringomyelia, Chiari malformations and CSF circulation, to contribute to this book. Several of these authors have in turn invited colleagues to assist in the preparation of their compositions. The names of these collaborators are acknowledged in individual chapters. The following statements identify the principal authors.

Ulrich Batzdorf
Professor, Department of Neurosurgery,
University of California,
Los Angeles (UCLA), CA, USA

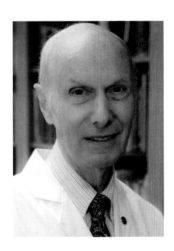

Ulrich Batzdorf received his medical education at New York Medical College, where he also served as instructor in the Department of Biochemistry. His postgraduate training included 2 years of general surgery at the University of Maryland; neurology training at the National Hospital, Queen Square, London; a neuropathology fellowship at the University of California, San Francisco; and neurosurgical training at the University of California, Los Angeles (UCLA). He has been on the faculty at UCLA since 1966, where he currently is a professor in the Department of Neurosurgery. Past interests have included tissue culture of brain tumours and cervical spondylotic myelopathy. Interest in syringomyelia, Chiari malformations and related disorders dates back over 30 years and has included clinical research resulting in numerous publications, book chapters as well as editing of a book on syringomyelia.

Enver Bogdanov
Head of Neurology and Rehabilitation
Department,
Kazan State Medical University
and Republican Clinical Hospital
of Republic of Tatarstan,
Kazan, Russia

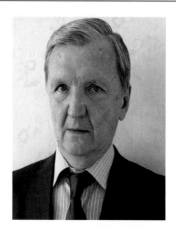

Enver Bogdanov graduated and completed his neurological residency in
Kazan State Medical University. He subsequently visited and studied at a
number of institutions, including the Institute of Neurology, Queen Square,
London, and the Institute Neurological Disorders and Stroke of NIH,
Bethesda, USA. His research interests include the epidemiology and natural
history of syringomyelia.

Andrew Brodbelt
Consultant Neurosurgeon,
The Walton Centre NHS Trust, Liverpool,
UK

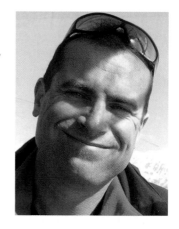

Andrew Brodbelt is a consultant neurosurgeon at the Walton Centre in
Liverpool, UK. He trained in neurosurgery in Liverpool and completed his
PhD entitled 'Investigations in post traumatic syringomyelia' under Marcus
Stoodley in Sydney, Australia, in 2004. His research interests include the
biochemical, fluid dynamic and biomechanical processes involved in syrinx
formation and propagation. He is an author on thirteen peer-reviewed publications and two book chapters on syringomyelia and CSF dynamics.

Novak Elliott
Lecturer of Biofluid Mechanics,
Fluid Dynamics Research Group,
Department of Mechanical Engineering,
Curtin University, Perth, WA, Australia

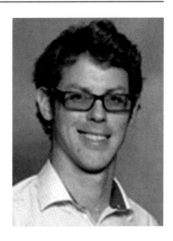

Novak Elliott qualified initially in information technology at the University of Western Australia in 2000 and subsequently in mechanical engineering and biomedical engineering at the University of New South Wales, Australia, in 2004, before further studying mechanical engineering at the University of Warwick, UK, in 2009. He has since worked in the software, mechanical and biomedical engineering industries and is presently a lecturer in biofluid mechanics at the Department of Mechanical Engineering, Curtin University, Australia. His research interests are in the interaction of fluid and solid mechanics and the part they play in biological phenomena.

Graham Flint
Consultant Neurosurgeon,
Department of Neurosurgery, Queen
Elizabeth Hospital, University Hospitals
Birmingham, Birmingham, UK

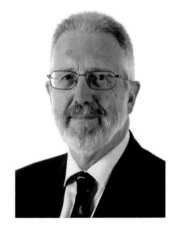

Graham Flint trained in Birmingham, UK, where he has been a consultant neurosurgeon at the Queen Elizabeth Hospital for over 20 years. A large part of his practice consists of treating patients with Chiari malformations and syringomyelia. For many years he has worked with the Ann Conroy Trust, developing services for patients and organising educational events for colleagues. He founded British Syringomyelia Group and was instrumental in setting up the international symposium, Syringomyelia 2007, held in Rugby, UK. As co-editor of this monograph, he aims to disseminate medical knowledge and understanding about syringomyelia and related disorders, to the benefit of patients with these conditions.

Anton Haass
Neurological Department,
University of the Saarland,
Homburg/Saar, Germany

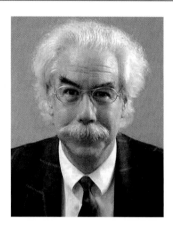

Anton Haass's interest in syringomyelia was evoked by his cooperation and friendship with Professor Bogdanov in Kazan, Tatarstan, where he had the opportunity to see many patients with the condition. He also admires the early neuropathologists, who created the name for this disease instead of 'tubular spinal cord'. Use of this name led him to take an interest in the depiction of syrinx in art and then inspired him to study the history of representation of the female form, from the first figurines about 40,000 years ago up until the time of Rubens.

John Heiss
National Institute of Neurological Disorders
and Stroke (NINDS),
National Institutes of Health in Bethesda,
MD, USA

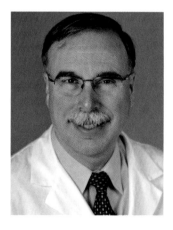

John Heiss is the Chair and Residency Program Director of the Surgical Neurology Branch, National Institute of Neurological Disorders and Stroke (NINDS), at the National Institutes of Health in Bethesda, Maryland, USA. He has extensive experience in treating patients with syringomyelia and Chiari I malformation and in conducting clinical research. He has lectured extensively and has published numerous original research papers, review articles and abstracts based on his research. He is vice-chair of the Combined Neurosciences Institutional Review Board and has served on many grant review panels and medical and scientific advisory boards.

Jan Keppel Hesselink
Professor of Molecular Pharmacology at the
University of Witten/Herdecke,
Witten, Germany

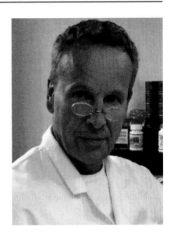

Jan Keppel Hesselink is a fellow of the Pharmaceutical Faculty in Medicine (FFPM) in the UK. He worked for several years at Bayer AG in Germany and has been an advisor for research and development and business strategies to the Dutch Royal Academy of Science. Currently he is a consultant for life science companies and investors. He was founder of the Chronic Pain Coalition and of the Institute for Neuropathic Pain. His research focus is in the development of topical analgesic creams and the use of endocannabinoids as analgesics.

Jörg Klekamp
Associate Professor of Neurosurgery,
Hanover Medical School,
Hanover, Germany

Neurosurgeon, Christliches Krankenhaus
Quakenbrück, Quakenbrück, Germany

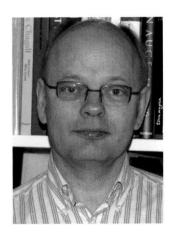

Jörg Klekamp received his neurosurgical training at Nordstadt Hospital, Hanover, Germany, under the supervision of Madjid Samii. He became a certified neurosurgeon in 1994. Since 1991 he has undertaken clinical and experimental studies on spinal cord pathologies, including syringomyelia. In 1992 and 1995 he continued his study on syringomyelia at the University of California in Los Angeles, Department of Neurosurgery, in collaboration with Ulrich Batzdorf. In 1995 he received the Wilhelm-Tönnis Award 1995 of the German Society of Neurosurgery, for clinical and experimental studies on syringomyelia. Since 2002 he has been Associate Professor of Neurosurgery at the Hanover Medical School and, since 2004, a neurosurgeon at Christliches Krankenhaus Quakenbrück, Germany.

Sid Marks
Consultant Neurosurgeon,
James Cooke University Hospital,
Middlesbrough, England, UK

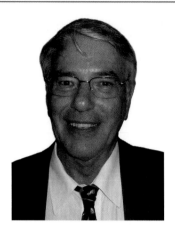

Sid Marks qualified as a doctor in Rhodesia, in 1974, as a graduate of the medical school in Birmingham, UK. He moved, in 1976, to England where he qualified first as a physician before, in 1980, beginning training and then qualifying as a neurosurgeon. He took on the duties of consultant neurosurgeon in 1987. His interest in hindbrain hernia began soon after this. From its beginning, he has been an active core member of the British Syringomyelia Group.

Jerry Oakes
Pediatric Neurosurgeon,
Children's Hospital of Alabama,
AL, USA

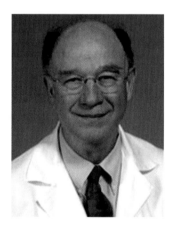

Dr. Oakes has been interested in the Chiari malformations and syringomyelia in his entire practicing career and has authored more than 80 peer-reviewed papers and 35 book chapters devoted to some aspect of the subject. In 2009 he published his experience with 600 operated patients showing surgical decompression is safe and highly effective in relieving strain-induced occipital pain and control or ablation of the syrinx cavity. He is currently most interested in developing clear guidelines for selecting surgical patients who would benefit from surgical intervention.

Panagiotis Papanagiotou
Director of the Clinic for Diagnostic
and Interventional Neuroradiology,
Klinikum Bremen, Bremen, Germany

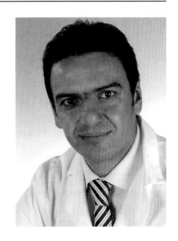

Panagiotis Papanagiotou is the director of the Clinic for Diagnostic and Interventional Neuroradiology in Klinikum Bremen. He was senior consultant in the Clinic for Diagnostic and Interventional Neuroradiology of the Saarland University Hospital in Homburg, Germany. He received his medical degree from University of Thessaly, Greece, in 2002. He is a specialist in radiology and neuroradiology. His research interests include the interventional treatment of acute ischemic stroke as well as in the imaging of syringomyelia. His clinical work focuses on MRI and in the minimal invasive neurointerventional treatment.

Guy Rouleau
Director, CHU Sainte-Justine Research
Center, Montreal, QC, Canada

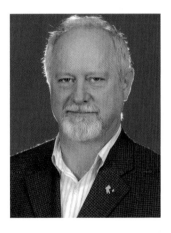

Over the last 20 years, Guy Rouleau has focused on identifying the genes causing several neurological and psychiatric diseases, including autism, amyotrophic lateral sclerosis, hereditary neuropathies, epilepsy and schizophrenia, as well as providing a better understanding of the molecular mechanisms that lead to these disease symptoms. Amongst his main achievements are his contribution to the identification of over 20 disease-causing genes and his discovery of new mutational mechanisms. He has published over 500 articles in peer-reviewed journals. He has supervised nearly a 100 students at the master's, PhD and postdoctoral levels. He has received numerous awards for his contribution to science and society.

Anil Roy
Department of Neurosurgery,
Emory University School of Medicine,
Atlanta, GA, USA

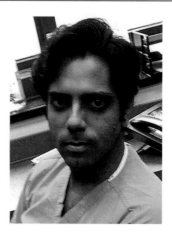

Anil Roy is a resident in neurosurgery at Emory University in Atlanta, Georgia. He completed his college education at Northwestern University in Evanston, USA, majoring in Communication Sciences and Disorders, with a focus on cognitive neuroscience. His medical schooling was at Northwestern University, Chicago, where his previous interest in neuroscience led him into neurosurgery. He has studied a variety of basic and clinical neuroscience topics, including music perception, sonic hedgehog signalling, spinal fusion complications, arachnoid cysts and syringomyelia. Other interests include functional and cerebrovascular neurosurgery.

Clare Rusbridge
Fitzpatrick Referrals,
Eashing, Godalming,
Surrey, UK

Faculty of Health and Medical Sciences,
School of Veterinary Medicine,
University of Surrey,
Guildford, Surrey, UK

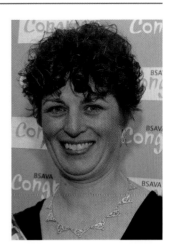

Dr Clare Rusbridge graduated from the University of Glasgow in 1991 and following an internship at the University of Pennsylvania and general practice in Cambridgeshire, she completed a BSAVA/Petsavers Residency and was Staff Clinician in Neurology at the Royal Veterinary College. She became a Diplomate of the European College of Veterinary Neurology in 1996 and a RCVS Specialist in 1999. In 2007 she was awarded a PhD from Utrecht University for her thesis on Chiari-like malformation and Syringomyelia. For 16 years she operated a neurology and neurosurgery referral service at the Stone Lion Veterinary Hospital in Wimbledon. In September 2013 Dr Rusbridge joined Fitzpatrick Referrals and the University of Surrey where she is continuing her clinical and research work. Her professional interests include neuropathic pain, inherited diseases, epilepsy and rehabilitation following spinal injury. She treats many animals with painful and/or distressing inherited disease which motivates her research aiming to find a better way of diagnosing, treating and preventing these conditions. In 2011 she was awarded the J. A. Wright (a.k.a. James Herriot) Memorial Award by The Blue Cross Animal Welfare Charity for her work with the Cavalier King Charles spaniel society with regard to syringomyelia. Dr Rusbridge is an Honorary Friend of the Ann Conroy Trust and a member of the British Syringomyelia Group. She is a frequently invited international lecturer in the veterinary and human medicine fields and has authored or co-authored many journal articles and book chapters, and acts as a reviewer for a number of journals.

Gurish Solanki
Consultant Neurosurgeon,
The Children's Hospital, Birmingham,
England, UK

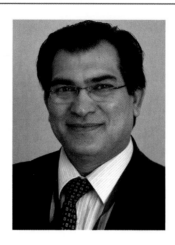

Guirish Solanki is a consultant neurosurgeon at Birmingham Children's Hospital and honorary senior clinical lecturer at University of Birmingham, UK. His neurosurgery training included periods at the National Hospital for Neurology and Neurosurgery and Great Ormond Street Hospital for Children, in London, UK. He is a keen educator and is a regional training programme director. He lectures regularly at national and international courses and convenes the European Paediatric Neuro-oncology Hands-On Workshop. He is chair of the Liaison Committees of the European Society of Paediatric Neurosurgeons and the International Society of Paediatric Neurosurgeons. He has published on the subjects of craniofacial surgery, neuro-oncology and spinal surgery. He has a particular interest in craniocervical junction/foramen magnum disorders and syringomyelia.

Marcus Stoodley
Professor of Neurosurgery,
Australian School of Advanced Medicine,
Macquarie University, Sydney, NSW,
Australia

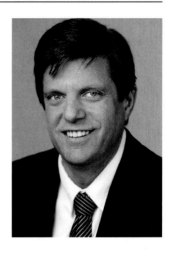

Marcus Stoodley graduated from medical school at the University of Queensland. After completing neurosurgery training in Australia, he undertook further subspecialty training in vascular neurosurgery at Stanford University and the University of Chicago, USA. In 1997, he was awarded a doctorate for his research on the pathophysiology of syringomyelia. On returning to Australia in 1999, he worked at the University of New South Wales and the Prince of Wales Hospital, where he established a neurosurgery research laboratory. In 2008 he joined Macquarie University, where he now directs the neurosurgery laboratory at the Australian School of Advanced Medicine and where he continues research on syringomyelia, as well as developing new biological treatments for brain arteriovenous malformations. He has produced more than 100 publications and has supervised over 15 research students.

Dominic Thompson
Department of Neurosurgery,
Great Ormond Street Hospital
for Children, London, England, UK

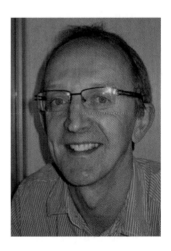

Dominic Thompson has been a full-time paediatric neurosurgeon in the department of neurosurgery at the Great Ormond Street Hospital for Children in London, UK, since 1998. He is a regular faculty member at international conferences and training courses and is a member of the editorial boards of Child's Nervous System and Acta Neurochirurgica. He has a specialist interest in congenital and acquired anomalies of the paediatric spine and has extensive experience in the management of craniovertebral anomalies and spinal dysraphism in childhood. He has published a number of original papers, review articles and book chapters, on a wide range of paediatric neurosurgical topics.

James van Dellen
Consultant Neurosurgeon,
Queen Elizabeth Hospital, Birmingham,
UK, and BUPA Cromwell Hospital,
London, UK

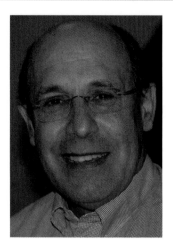

James van Dellen was formerly head of the Department of Neurosurgery and dean of the Faculty of Medicine, in Durban, South Africa, from 1980 to 1986 and again from 1989 to 1998. From 1986 to 1987 he was chief of Neurosurgical Service, Harbor Hospital, and associate professor at the University of California, Los Angeles (UCLA). Between 2000 and 2009 he was professor of Neurosurgery at Charing Cross and Imperial College Healthcare NHS Trust, London, UK. He is a past president of the Society of Neurosurgeons of South Africa. His research interests have included discogenic disease, shunt infections, dural substitutes, CNS neurocysticercosis infections, pyogenic cerebral infections and aspects of cerebral trauma, and his current areas of interest include adult hydrocephalus, syringomyelia and Chiari malformations.

Roy Weller
Emeritus Professor of Neuropathology,
Southampton University
School of Medicine, Southampton,
England, UK

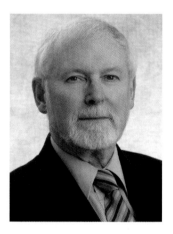

Roy Weller was professor of Neuropathology in the University of Southampton, where he was responsible for the clinical neuropathology service for the Wessex Regional Neurological Centre. He taught neuropathology and organised research projects for students in the Faculty of Medicine at Southampton University. He has attended many international conferences and held visiting professorships in Europe, Africa and Asia. His major research interests have been in hydrocephalus, neuroimmunology and Alzheimer's disease. He has identified the theme that connects these disorders, being the unique systems by which fluid and solutes drain from the CNS, and how restricted perivascular drainage of interstitial fluid from the CNS fails in conditions as diverse as Alzheimer's disease, hydrocephalus and syringomyelia.

Historical Aspects

1

Ulrich Batzdorf

Contents

U. Batzdorf
Department of Neurosurgery,
University of California, Los Angeles (UCLA),
Los Angeles, CA, USA
e-mail: ubatzdorf@mednet.ucla.edu

1.1 Early Observations

1.1.1 First Descriptions of Syringomyelia

Stephanus, also known as Estienne, Stephano and Stevens, is credited with providing the first description of what we now call syringomyelia, in 1545 (Fig. 1.1). The relevant description reads "Moreover, as for the interior substance of the marrow of the back, one finds, in the middle of it, stretched and standing out from the right edge, an obvious cavity which appears to be a ventricle of the marrow. Compressed and contained in this cavity is a special reddish-brown aqueous humour, a little more liquid, that is, not the same, as that of the anterior ventricles of the brain. And such is the substance, origins and discourse of the marrow contained in the spine, which for long enough has been improperly labelled marrow, expecting that it [the reddish humour] was more solid and more cavity inside the marrow of the back".[1] This strongly suggests that Stephanus described a post-traumatic cavity. A spinal cord cystic cavity associated with hydrocephalus was first reported in 1688 (Brunner 1688).

---

[1] Translation courtesy Caroline Batzdorf.

G. Flint, C. Rusbridge (eds.), *Syringomyelia*,
DOI 10.1007/978-3-642-13706-8_1, © Springer-Verlag Berlin Heidelberg 2014

De diſſectione partium corporis humani libri tres, à Carolo Stephano, doctore Medico, editi. Vnà cum figuris, & incisionum declarationibus, à Stephano Riuerio Chirurgo cõpositis.

Cum priuilegio.

PARISIIS.

Apud Simonem Colinæum.

1545.

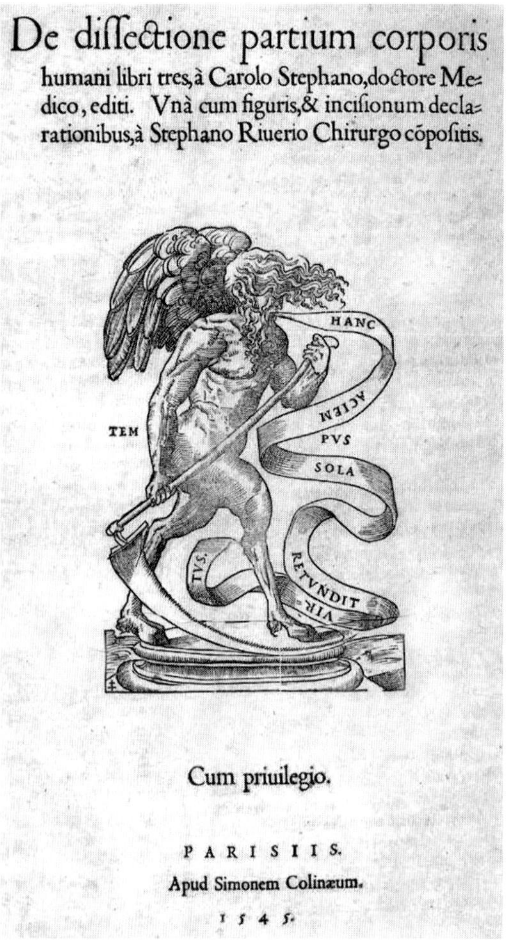

Fig. 1.1 Title page of Stephanus' De dissectione partium corporis humani (1545) (Courtesy History & Special Collections for the Sciences, Louise M. Darling Biomedical Library, University of California, Los Angeles)

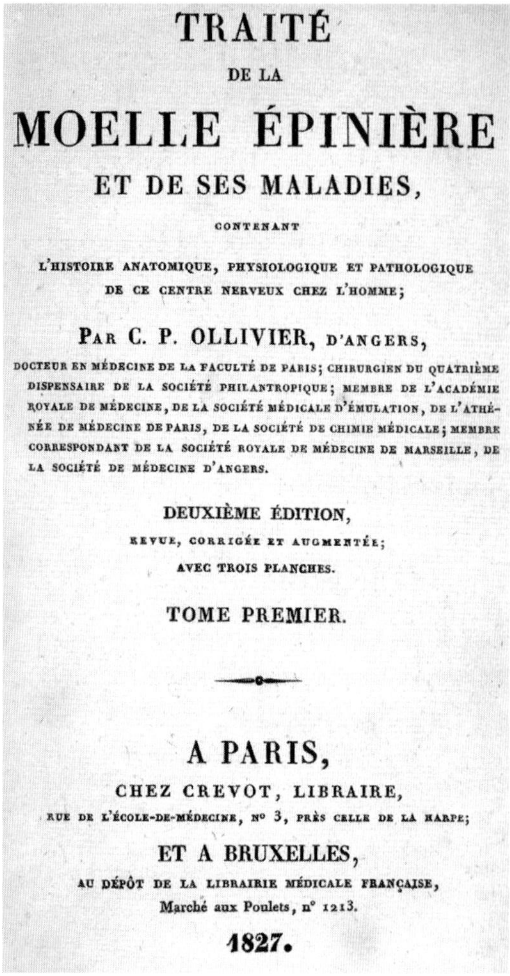
TRAITÉ

DE LA

MOELLE ÉPINIÈRE

ET DE SES MALADIES,

CONTENANT

L'HISTOIRE ANATOMIQUE, PHYSIOLOGIQUE ET PATHOLOGIQUE DE CE CENTRE NERVEUX CHEZ L'HOMME;

PAR C. P. OLLIVIER, D'ANGERS,

DOCTEUR EN MÉDECINE DE LA FACULTÉ DE PARIS; CHIRURGIEN DU QUATRIÈME DISPENSAIRE DE LA SOCIÉTÉ PHILANTROPIQUE; MEMBRE DE L'ACADÉMIE ROYALE DE MÉDECINE, DE LA SOCIÉTÉ MÉDICALE D'ÉMULATION, DE L'ATHÉNÉE DE MÉDECINE DE PARIS, DE LA SOCIÉTÉ DE CHIMIE MÉDICALE; MEMBRE CORRESPONDANT DE LA SOCIÉTÉ ROYALE DE MÉDECINE DE MARSEILLE, DE LA SOCIÉTÉ DE MÉDECINE D'ANGERS.

DEUXIÈME ÉDITION,

REVUE, CORRIGÉE ET AUGMENTÉE;

AVEC TROIS PLANCHES.

TOME PREMIER.

A PARIS,

CHEZ CREVOT, LIBRAIRE,

RUE DE L'ÉCOLE-DE-MÉDECINE, Nº 3, PRÈS CELLE DE LA HARPE;

ET A BRUXELLES,

AU DÉPÔT DE LA LIBRAIRIE MÉDICALE FRANÇAISE,

Marché aux Poulets, nº 1213.

1827.

Fig. 1.2 Title page of Ollivier's Traité de la Moelle Épiniere (1827) (Courtesy History & Special Collections for the Sciences, Louise M. Darling Biomedical Library, University of California, Los Angeles)

1.1.2 Nomenclature and Terminology

The term syringomyelia, describing a tube-like cavity within the spinal cord, was first applied in 1827 by Ollivier d'Angers (Fig. 1.2). He thought that the central canal of the spinal cord was not a normal finding. In 1865, Schüppel described a case of hydromyelia as an upward expansion of the central canal, which then ended in a cavity. By 1890, it was recognised that the central canal is always present (Bruhl 1890). Simon (1875) preferred the term syringomyelia as being more general than hydromyelia, which he defined as hydropic widening of the central canal. For many years the distinction between syringomyelia and hydromyelia became blurred, leading to the invention of terms such as "hydrosyringomyelia" or "syringohydromyelia". Modern imaging techniques have drawn attention to persistence of the central canal as a non-pathological finding, which is best termed hydromyelia. Some have suggested that persistence of the central canal in patients who sustain spinal cord injury or in individuals who have tonsillar ectopia, may explain the development of syringomyelia in these individuals, while others with cord injuries or tonsillar ectopia do not develop syringomyelia (Milhorat et al. 1994).

Schüppel also cited the case of Brunner's in which there was communication with the fourth ventricle. We now appreciate that communication between spinal cord cavities and the fourth ventricle is present in only a small number of cases (West and Williams 1980). The once-presumed communication between a syrinx cavity and the fourth ventricle in patients with cerebellar tonsillar ectopia also led to the now-abandoned distinction between "communicating" and "non-communicating" forms of syringomyelia (Barnett et al. 1973b). On the other hand, isolated spinal cord cavities rarely, but occasionally, do communicate with the subarachnoid space (Milhorat et al. 1995).

1.1.3 First Descriptions of Tonsillar Ectopia

In 1881 Theodor Langhans described tonsillar ectopia and suggested that, by obstructing flow at the foramen magnum, it might result in syringomyelia. In 1883 Cleland described nine infants with spina bifida who had various cerebral anomalies, including hydrocephalus and anencephalus. Elongation of the cerebellar tonsils is evident in his figure 6 (specimen 1). In 1891 Chiari provided his first description of hindbrain abnormalities in association with hydrocephalus. His 1896 publication was more detailed and focused specifically on changes in the cerebellum, pons and medulla. He described four abnormalities, differing in degree of cerebellar abnormality (Table 1.1). In 1894 Arnold added a case of an

Table 1.1 The four varieties of Chiari malformations

Type I: Downward displacement of the cerebellar tonsils and the medial portion of the inferior cerebellar lobes
Type II: Downward displacement of the tonsils, vermis and at least a part of a lengthened fourth ventricle
Type III: Downward displacement of [nearly] the entire cerebellum, out of the cranial cavity, into the cervical area
Type IV: Hypoplasia of the region of the cerebellum without displacement of this structure into the spinal canal

infant with tonsillar descent below the foramen magnum. In 1943 Lichtenstein, a pathologist, also postulated that there was a relationship between tonsillar descent and syringomyelia. We now recognise that there are two general categories of syringomyelia: (a) syringomyelia associated with tonsillar descent (Chiari malformation) and (b) primary spinal syringomyelia, in which the pathology is entirely confined to the spinal cord and its meninges (Williams 1991).

1.1.4 Other Forms of Syringomyelia

Strümpel (1880) may have been the first to identify a case of syringomyelia after trauma. This condition was also recognised by Schlesinger (1895), but the major description was provided by Barnett (Barnett 1973a; Barnett et al. 1973b). Barnett (1973b) also noted that delayed syringomyelia might occur after both severe and less severe spinal injury. Earlier discussions and treatises on syringomyelia also tended to include spinal cord tumour cysts under the broad category of syringomyelia (Barnett and Rewcastle 1973). While spinal cord tumours may be associated with true syringomyelia cavities, notably when the tumour obstructs or narrows the spinal subarachnoid space, syrinx cavities need to be distinguished from tumour cysts, which are often high in protein and represent a different entity, from both physiological and treatment perspectives.

1.2 Elucidation of Clinical Features

Aspects of the motor and sensory deficits caused by syringomyelia had been defined by the end of the nineteenth century, permitting the diagnosis of syringomyelia in a living patient (Kahler and Pick 1879; Schultze 1882). In 1869 Charcot described dissociated anaesthesia with absent upper extremity reflexes and atrophy in one or both upper limbs, particularly the hands. He also described the severe joint deformities, especially the shoulder joints, which characteristically may occur in areas of absent pain sensation also involving the upper trunk (Charcot 1868). Duchenne first called attention to muscular atrophy in association with sensory abnormalities in 1853 and differentiated this condition from the muscular dystrophy that bears his name. Gowers, in his 1886 textbook, provided a more detailed description of the various clinical manifestations of syringomyelia. Milhorat et al. (1999) compiled a comprehensive list of symptoms linked with syringomyelia associated with tonsillar ectopia.

The motor and sensory deficits encountered in patients with primary spinal syringomyelia also relate to the level and degree of spinal cord injury. Foster and Hudgson (1973) described the sometimes-sudden ascent of the sensory level in patients with post-traumatic syringomyelia, not infrequently precipitated by spells of coughing or straining. They also called attention to the fact that it may be difficult to distinguish deficits due to the cord injury from those due to syrinx formation.

1.3   Theories of Pathogenesis

Many theories have surfaced over the course of the years, relating to the origin of syringomyelia cavities. These have implicated inflammation, including specific diseases such as syphilis and arachnoiditis, possibly leading to glial proliferation (Hallopeau 1870), with subsequent degenerative changes resulting in cavity formation (Schultze 1882). A variety of other mechanisms have since been proposed, including congenital abnormalities, neoplasia, ischaemia and processes leading to oedema of the cord (Klekamp and Samii 2002).

The observations of Cleland (1883) and of Chiari (1891, 1896) suggested to them that syrinx cavities fill from the fourth ventricle. Based on this concept, Gardner and Angel (1958) developed the theory of a water hammer effect as the filling mechanism of syrinx cavities. Ellertson and Greitz's (1939) studies tended to strengthen this concept of syrinx communication with the fourth ventricle, but their fluorescein dye experiments also raised the possibility of transparenchymal fluid migration from the

subarachnoid space. Ball and Dayan (1972) suggested that fluid enters the syrinx cavity via the Virchow-Robin spaces during Valsalva manoeuvres, propelled by epidural venous distension. The cerebellar tonsils were postulated to prevent upward propagation of the CSF pulse wave. Brierley (1950) injected a suspension of India ink into the subarachnoid space of rabbits and noted some of this material in the perivascular spaces of the cord. Studies by Rennels et al. (1985) with horseradish peroxidase established fluid flow into the tissues of the neuraxis by a "paravascular" pathway. Stoodley et al. (1996) was able to demonstrate that fluid migrates into the cord along the Virchow-Robin spaces, evidently propelled by the pulsation of arterioles in these spaces. Milhorat et al. (1994) suggested that persistence of the central canal of the spinal cord might play a role in the likelihood of syrinx formation. A currently widely accepted theory proposed by Oldfield is that systolic pressure waves cause the impacted tonsils to act as pistons exerting pressure on the relatively closed spinal subarachnoid space, thereby driving fluid into the spinal cord (Oldfield et al. 1994).

Expansion of the cystic cavity, once formed, also raised questions. Both Barnett et al. (1973a) and Williams (1970, 1991) considered venous expansion in the area below the injury as a significant factor.

Spinal haemorrhage and necrosis were, at one time, believed to be the basis of post-traumatic syringomyelia (Barnett et al. 1973a). Diffusion of fluid from blood vessels was also suggested. Barnett (1973b) also observed that syrinx formation might occur following relatively minor spinal injuries not necessarily associated with immediate neurological impairment, thereby raising doubts about these theories. Partial obstruction of the subarachnoid space is now considered to be the underlying pathophysiology of many forms of primary spinal syringomyelia (Batzdorf 1991). Arachnoid scarring, sometimes referred to as arachnoiditis in the older literature, is believed to act in a manner analogous to how the cerebellar tonsils behave in Chiari-related syringomyelia, preventing unimpaired transmission of the CSF pulse wave along the spinal subarachnoid space. Alterations in the cord parenchyma due to injury may facilitate inflow of CSF into the cord. Focal membranes, such as are seen in arachnoid cysts, are believed to result in syringomyelia by a similar mechanism (Holly and Batzdorf 2006).

It is also known that a small percentage of patients have a family history of syringomyelia. The epidemiology of syringomyelia is discussed in Chap. 2 of this publication, and the genetics of Chiari are covered in Chap. 5. Modern theories of pathogenesis are described in more detail in Chap. 6.

1.4 Development of Imaging Methods

The development of methods of imaging a syrinx cavity, even though it was only visualised indirectly, represented a major advance over localisation by neurological examination alone. Thus, a radiographic finding of bony spinal canal expansion was a useful aid to the diagnosis of suspected syringomyelia in a patient with appropriate clinical signs or symptoms, even before oil contrast myelography allowed one to visualise the expanded spinal cord (Boijsen 1954). Imaging the syringomyelia cord with oxygen was described in 1949 (Marks and Livingston 1949). Variability in cord diameter on air myelography, in relation to patient position, was reported in 1966 (Westberg 1966). Pantopaque myelography, demonstrating a distended cervical spinal cord, followed by air myelography with the patient in upright position, permitted demonstration of collapse of a distended cord in relation to changes in body position (Conway 1967). Real advances were, however, possible only after the introduction of water-soluble contrast material. Experience with computerised tomography (CT) following instillation of such media was reported in 1980 (Aubin et al. 1981). This included the significant observation that contrast could be imaged within the syrinx cavity on delayed CT scans. Magnetic resonance (MR) imaging, in addition to showing the cord cysts in great detail and allowing the demonstration of tumours, had the great advantage of not being invasive. By comparison, myelography required needle puncture of the

theca, potentially changing the fluid dynamics within the spinal CSF channels. A very early MR image was published in 1983 (Batnitzky et al. 1983), and many refinements in technique over the ensuing years have yielded the exquisitely detailed studies currently available. MR technology has also provided insights into the physiology of syringomyelia (Enzmann and Pelc 1989). Constructive interference in steady-state MR images (CISS) is an example of recent refinements, with superior visualisation of subarachnoid webs that may indicate potential benefits from surgery (Korogi et al. 2000; Roser et al. 2010). Future advances in technology will undoubtedly add additional information.

A further account of the history of imaging of syringomyelia is provided in Chap. 21 of this publication.

1.5 Treatment

The earliest attempts at treatment of syringomyelia were directed at relieving the fluid collection within the spinal cord, beginning in 1892, with open cyst aspiration (Abbe and Coley 1892), followed by myelotomy in 1921 (Elsberg 1921) and 1926 (Poussepp 1926) and insertion of a drain into the cystic cavity in 1936 (Frazier and Rowe 1936). Percutaneous cyst aspiration was described in 1966 (Westberg 1966). Tantalum drains and plastic tubing were placed in 1949 (Kirgis and Echols 1949). The use of Pantopaque (Myodil) by injection to obliterate the cyst was proposed in 1981 (Schlesinger et al. 1981). Penfield and Coburn's patient of 1938, although often cited, evidently had a Chiari malformation without syringomyelia.

Noting that in the few cases in which fluid had been surgically evacuated, there was no significant effect on the condition, and also on the basis that syrinx cavities seemed to be caused by glial proliferation, radiation therapy was proposed in 1905 (Raymond 1905). As late as 1955, it was stated in Brain's textbook that radiation therapy was the generally accepted form of treatment of syringomyelia.

Recognising the coexistence of hydrocephalus and syringomyelia, Bernini and Krayenbühl

(1969) suggested ventricular shunting of such patients. Although of interest from a theoretical point of view, the results were disappointing. More local diversion of CSF in the spinal subarachnoid space has shown somewhat better results (Vengsarkar et al. 1991; Lam et al. 2008). Technical improvements in syrinx drainage followed, notably syrinx-to-peritoneal shunting (Edgar 1976), subarachnoid shunting (Tator et al. 1982; Isu et al. 1990; Iwasaki et al. 1999) and syrinx-to-pleural cavity shunting (Williams and Page 1987). Gardner et al.'s (1977) novel concept of syrinx drainage by performing a "terminal ventriculostomy" was unsuccessful in many patients, in large part because it did not address the filling mechanism of syrinx cavities (Williams and Fahy 1983).

Prior to the advent of modern imaging techniques, specifically CT myelography and MR, the belief was still widely held that in most cases a communication existed between the fourth ventricle and the syrinx cavity in patients with Chiari-related syringomyelia. Gardner and Angel (1958) postulated that syrinx cavities fill from the fourth ventricle because of membranous outlet obstruction of the fourth ventricle and recommended plugging of the obex via a posterior fossa approach. Inasmuch as he had to perform a posterior fossa craniotomy to gain access to the obex, it remains difficult to distinguish benefits that might have resulted from the exposure from those due to the obex plugging per se. This received confirmation in the observations of Logue and Edwards (1981). Obex plugging has been abandoned for surgical management of syringomyelia.

Major advances in treatment came about because of a better understanding of the pathophysiology of syringomyelia. For a syrinx cavity to reduce in size, it appears to be necessary to establish free communication between the cranial and spinal subarachnoid spaces. This allows the pulsatile energy within the CSF, transmitted from the cranial cavity to act on the pial surface of the cord (Paré and Batzdorf 1998) which becomes attenuated as it passes down towards the caudal end of the spinal canal. There has therefore been a general trend away from syrinx drainage

procedures whenever possible (Sgouros and Williams 1995; Batzdorf et al. 1998). Nowadays shunting is considered appropriate only when other approaches are not possible (Batzdorf 2000). The currently practised surgical approaches are directed at establishing free communication between the cranial and spinal subarachnoid spaces, best achieved by posterior fossa decompression without, or more commonly with, duraplasty, especially in adults. Reduction of the cerebellar tonsils, first described by Bertrand (1973), is practised by some with modifications. Similar subarachnoid decompression approaches have been employed in primary spinal syringomyelia and have been particularly successful in situations where there is a focal obstruction of the subarachnoid space, such as in syringomyelia associated with arachnoid cysts and in some instances of post-traumatic syrinx (Williams 1991; Batzdorf 2005).

1.6   Previous Monographs

Syringomyelia has remained a challenging problem and has puzzled investigators for many years, particularly with respect to its pathogenesis and optimal management. Reflecting advances in our understanding of the disorder, a number of volumes devoted to this unusual disease entity have appeared over the years, beginning with Schlesinger's book in 1895. Later volumes by Barnett (Barnett 1973a, b; Barnett and Rewcastle 1973; Barnett et al. 1973a, b), Foster and Hudgson (1973), Batzdorf (1991), Tamaki et al. (2001), Anson et al. (1997) and by Klekamp and Samii (2002) each brought a timely update of the understanding current at the time. Excellent reviews were also provided by Schliep (1978) and by Aschoff (1993).

References

Abbe R, Coley WB (1892) Syringomyelia: operation, exploration of the cord; withdrawal of fluid. J Nerv Ment Dis 19:512–520
Anson JA, Benzel EC, Awad IA (1997) Syringomyelia and the Chiari malformations. The American Association of Neurological Surgeons, Park Ridge

Arnold J (1894) Myelocyste, Transposition von Gewebskeimen und Sympodie. Beitr Path Anat 16:1–28

Aschoff A (1993) 100 years syrinx surgery – a review. Acta Neurochir 123:176–177

Aubin ML, Vignaud J, Jardin C et al (1981) Computed tomography in 75 clinical cases of syringomyelia. AJNR Am J Neuroradiol 2:199–204

Ball MJ, Dayan AD (1972) Pathogenesis of syringomyelia. Lancet 2:799–801

Barnett HJM (1973a) Trauma and syringomyelia, chapter 9. In: Barnett HJM, Foster JB, Hudgson P (eds) Syringomyelia. WB Saunders, London

Barnett HJM (1973b) Syringomyelia consequent on minor to moderate trauma, chapter 13. In: Barnett HJM, Foster JB, Hudgson P (eds) Syringomyelia. WB Saunders, London

Barnett HJM, Rewcastle NB (1973) Syringomyelia and tumours of the nervous system, chapter 17. In: Barnett HJM, Foster JB, Hudgson P (eds) Syringomyelia. WB Saunders, London

Barnett HJM, Jousse AT, Ball MJ (1973a) Pathology and pathogenesis of progressive cystic myelopathy as a late sequel to spinal cord injury, chapter 14. In: Barnett HJM, Foster JB, Hudgson P (eds) Syringomyelia. WB Saunders, London

Barnett HJM, Foster JB, Hudgson P (1973b) In: Barnett HJM, Foster JB, Hudgson P (eds) Syringomyelia. WB Saunders, London

Batnitzky S, Price HI, Gaughan MJ et al (1983) The radiology of syringohydromyelia. Radiographics 3:585–611

Batzdorf U (1991) Syringomyelia: current concepts in diagnosis and treatment. Williams and Wilkins, Baltimore

Batzdorf U (2000) Primary spinal syringomyelia. A personal perspective. Neurosurg Focus 8:1–4

Batzdorf U (2005) Primary spinal syringomyelia. J Neurosurg Spine 3:429–435

Batzdorf U, Klekamp J, Johnson JP (1998) A critical appraisal of syrinx cavity shunting procedures. J Neurosurg 89:382–388

Benini A, Krayenbühl H (1969) Ein neuer chirurgischer Weg zur Behandlung der Hydro- und Syringomyelie. Schwciz Mcd Wochenschr 99:1137–1142

Bertrand G (1973) Dynamic factors in the evolution of syringomyelia and syringobulbia. Clin Neurosurg 20:322–333

Boijsen E (1954) Cervical spinal canal in intraspinal expansive processes. Acta Radiol 42:101–115

Brain R (1955) Diseases of the nervous system, 5th edn. Oxford University Press, London, p 683

Brierley JB (1950) The penetration of particulate matter from the cerebrospinal fluid into the spinal ganglia, peripheral nerves, and perivascular spaces of the central nervous system. J Neurol Neurosurg Psychiatry 13:203–215

Bruhl (1890) Contribution à l'étude de la Syringomyélie. Paris [cited in Schlesinger H (1895) Die Syringomyelie. Franz Deuticke, Leipzig/Wien]

Brunner (1688) Bonet's sepulchretum, 2nd edn, book 1. Geneva, p 394 [cited in Schlesinger H (1895) Die Syringomyelie. Franz Deuticke, Leipzig/Wien]

Charcot JM (1868) Sur quelques arthropathies qui paraisent dépendre d'une lésion du cerveau ou de la moelle épinière. Arch Physiol Norm Path (Paris) 1:161–178

Charcot JM, Joffroy A (1869) Deux cas d'atrophie musculaire progressive avec lésions de la substance grise et des faisceaux antérolatéraux de la moelle épinière. Arch Physiol Norm Pathol (Paris) 2:354–367, 629–649, 744–760

Chiari H (1891) Ueber Veränderungen des Kleinhirns infolge von Hydrocephalie des Grosshirns. Dtsch Med Wochenschr 42:1172–1175

Chiari H (1896) Über Veränderungen des Kleinhirns, des Pons und der Medulla Oblongata in Folge von Congenitaler Hydrocephalie des Grosshirns. Denkschr Akad Wissensch (Wien) 63:71–116

Cleland J (1883) Contribution to the study of spina bifida, encephalocele, and anencephalus. J Anat Physiol 17:257–292

Conway LW (1967) Hydrodynamic studies in syringomyelia. J Neurosurg 27:501–514

Duchene (1853). Cited in Schlesinger H (1895) Die Syringomyelie. Franz Deuticke, Pub., Leipzig/Wien

Edgar RE (1976) Surgical management of spinal cord cysts. Paraplegia 14:21–27

Ellertson AB, Greitz T (1939) Myelocystographic and fluorescein studies to demonstrate communication between intramedullary cysts and the cerebrospinal fluid space. Acta Neurol Scand 45:418–430

Elsberg CA (1921) Surgery of intramedullary affections of the spinal cord: anatomic basis and technique with report of cases. JAMA 59:1532–1536

Enzmann DR, Pelc NJ (1989) CSF dynamics in normal and syringomyelia patients using phase contrast cine MR (abstr). In: Society of Magnetic Resonance in Medicine, Berkeley

Foster JB, Hudgson P (1973) The clinical features of communicating syringomyelia, chapter 3. In: Barnett HJM, Foster JB, Hudgson P (eds) Syringomyelia. WB Saunders, London

Frazier CH, Rowe SN (1936) The surgical treatment of syringomyelia. Ann Surg 103:481–497

Gardner WJ, Angel J (1958) The cause of syringomyelia and its surgical treatment. Cleve Clin Q 25:4–8

Gardner WJ, Bell HS, Poolos PN et al (1977) Terminal ventriculostomy for syringomyelia. J Neurosurg 46:609–617

Gowers WR (1886) A manual of diseases of the nervous system, vol 1. Churchill, London, pp 433–443

Hallopeau FH (1870) Note sur un fait de sclérose diffuse de la moelle avec lacune au centre de cet organe, altération de la substance grise et atrophie musculaire. Gaz Mèdicale de Paris 25 [cited by Simon T (1875) Ueber Syringomyelie und Geschwulstbildung im Rückenmarke. Arch Psychiatr Nervenkr 5:144]

Holly LT, Batzdorf U (2006) Syringomyelia associated with intradural arachnoid cysts. J Neurosurg Spine 5:111–116

Isu T, Iwasaki Y, Akino M et al (1990) Syringosubarachnoid shunt for syringomyelia associated with

Chiari malformation (type 1). Acta Neurochir (Wien) 107:152–160

Iwasaki Y, Koyanagi I, Hida K et al (1999) Syringo-subarachnoid shunt for syringomyelia using partial hemilaminectomy. Br J Neurosurg 13:41–45

Kahler O, Pick A (1879) Beitrag zur Lehre von der Syringo- und Hydromyelie. Vierteljahrschr Prakt Heilk 142:20–41 [cited in Schliep G (1978) Syringomyelia and Syringobulbia, chapter 10. In: Vinken PJ and Bruyn GW (eds) Handbook of clinical neurology, vol 32. Elsevier/North-Holland Biomedical Press, Amsterdam]

Kirgis HD, Echols DH (1949) Syringo-encephalomyelia. J Neurosurg 6:368–375

Klekamp J, Samii M (2002) Syringomyelia: diagnosis and treatment. Springer, Berlin/Heidelberg

Korogi HT, Shigematsu Y, Sugahara T et al (2000) Evaluation of syringomyelia with three-dimensional constructive interference in a steady state (CISS) sequence. J Magn Reson Imaging 11:120–126

Lam S, Batzdorf U, Bergsneider M (2008) Thecal shunt placement for treatment of obstructive primary syringomyelia. J Neurosurg Spine 9:581–588

Langhans T (1881) Ueber Höhlenbildung im Rückenmark als Folge von Blutstauung. Arch Path Anat U Physiol U f Klin Med 85:1–25

Lichtenstein BW (1943) Cervical syringomyelia and syringomyelia-like states associated with Arnold-Chiari deformity and platybasia. Arch Neurol Psychiatry 49:881–894

Logue V, Edwards MR (1981) Syringomyelia and its surgical treatment – an analysis of 75 patients. J Neurol Neurosurg Psychiatry 44:273–284

Marks JH, Livingston KE (1949) The cervical subarachnoid space with particular reference to syringomyelia and the Arnold-Chiari deformity. Radiology 52:63–68

Milhorat TH, Kotzen RM, Anzil AA (1994) Stenosis of the central canal of the spinal cord in man: incidence and pathological findings in 232 autopsy cases. J Neurosurg 80:716–722

Milhorat TH, Capocelli AL, Anzil AA et al (1995) Pathological basis of spinal cord cavitation in syringomyelia: analysis of 105 autopsy cases. J Neurosurg 82:802–812

Milhorat TH, Chou MW, Trinidad EM et al (1999) Chiari I malformation redefined: clinical and radiographic findings for 364 symptomatic patients. Neurosurgery 44:1005–1017

Oldfield EH, Muraszko K, Shawker TH et al (1994) Pathophysiology of syringomyelia associated with Chiari I malformation of the cerebellar tonsils. Implications for diagnosis and treatment. J Neurosurg 80:3–15

Ollivier d'Angers CP (1827) Traite de la moelle epiniere et de ses maladies. Crevot, Paris, pp 178–183

Paré LS, Batzdorf U (1998) Syringomyelia persistence after Chiari decompression as a result of pseudo-meningocele formation: implications for syrinx pathogenesis: report of three cases. Neurosurgery 43:945–948

Penfield W, Coburn DF (1938) Arnold-Chiari malformation and its operative treatment. Arch Neurol Psychiatry 40:328–336

Poussepp L (1926) Traitement opératoire dans deux cas de syringomyélie. Rev Neurol 45:1171–1179

Raymond F (1905) La syringomyélie. Rev Gén Clin Thér 19:817–818

Rennels ML, Gregory TF, Blaumanis OR et al (1985) Evidence for a "paravascular" fluid circulation in the mammalian central nervous system, provided by the rapid distribution of tracer protein throughout the brain from the subarachnoid space. Brain Res 326:47–63

Roser F, Ebner FH, Sixt C et al (2010) Defining the line between hydromyelia and syringomyelia. A differentiation is possible based on electro-physiological and magnetic resonance imaging studies. Acta Neurochir (Wien) 152:213–219

Schlesinger H (1895) Die Syringomyelie. Franz Deuticke, Leipzig/Wien

Schlesinger EB, Antunes JL, Michelsen WJ et al (1981) Hydromyelia: clinical presentation and comparison of modalities of treatment. Neurosurgery 9:356–365

Schliep G (1978) Syringomyelia and syringobulbia, chapter 10. In: Vinken PJ, Bruyn GW (eds) Handbook of clinical neurology, vol 32. Elsevier/North-Holland Biomedical Press, Amsterdam

Schultze F (1882) Ueber Spalt-Höhlen- und Gliombildung im Rückenmarke und in der Medulla Oblongata. Virchows Archiv Pathol Anatol 87:510–540

Schüppel O (1865) Über Hydromyelus. Archiv Heilkd 6:289–315

Sgouros S, Williams B (1995) A critical appraisal of drainage in syringomyelia. J Neurosurg 82:1–10

Simon T (1875) Ueber Syringomyelie und Geschwulstbildung im Röckenmarke. Arch Psychiatr Nervenkr 5:120–163

Stephanus C (1545) De dissectione partium corporis humani. Colinaeum, Paris

Stoodley MA, Jones NR, Brown C (1996) Evidence for rapid fluid flow from the subarachnoid space into the spinal cord central canal in the rat. Brain Res 707:155–164

Strümpell A (1880) Beiträge zur Pathologie des Rückenmarks. Spastische Spinalparalysen. Arch Psychiatr Nervenkr 10:676–717

Tamaki N, Batzdorf U, Nagashima T (2001) Syringomyelia: current concepts in pathogenesis and management. Springer, Tokyo

Tator CH, Meguro K, Rowed DW (1982) Favorable results with syringosubarachnoid shunts for treatment of syringomyelia. J Neurosurg 56:517–523

Vengsarkar U, Panchal VG, Tripathi PD et al (1991) Percutaneous thecoperitoneal shunt for syringomyelia. J Neurosurg 74:827–831

West RJ, Williams B (1980) Radiographic studies of the ventricles in syringomyelia. Neuroradiology 20:5–16

Westberg G (1966) Gas myelography and percutaneous puncture in the diagnosis of spinal cord cysts. Acta Radiol Suppl 252:7–67

Williams B (1970) The distending force in the production of communicating syringomyelia. Lancet 2:41–42

Williams B (1991) Pathogenesis of syringomyelia, chapter 4. In: Batzdorf U (ed) Syringomyelia: current concepts in diagnosis and treatment. Williams and Wilkins, Baltimore

Williams B, Fahy G (1983) A critical appraisal of "terminal ventriculostomy" for the treatment of syringomyelia. J Neurosurg 58:188–197

Williams B, Page N (1987) Surgical treatment of syringomyelia with syringopleural shunting. Br J Neurosurg 1:63–80

Epidemiology

2

Enver Bogdanov

Contents

With Aysylu Zabbarova

E. Bogdanov
Neurology and Rehabilitation Department,
Kazan State Medical University and Republican
Clinical Hospital of Republic of Tatarstan,
Kazan, Russia
e-mail: enver_bogdanov@mail.ru

2.1 Introduction

Syringomyelia is a polyaetiological disorder, characterized by abnormal fluid-filled cavities within the spinal cord. It causes typical neurological symptoms and signs as it expands. Many associated disorders and anomalies that can cause syringomyelia have been described (Williams 1995), including Chiari malformation type 1, trauma, intramedullary tumours and inflammation. Despite the ready availability of diagnostic methods and surgical treatments for syringomyelia in developed countries, this pathology continues to present medical and social problems. Syringomyelia accounts for about 5 % of paraplegias (Sedzimir et al. 1974; Williams 1990) and the quality of life for patients with syringomyelia is generally lower than that of the general population, being comparable with that of patients with heart failure or malignant neoplasms (Sixt et al. 2009).

2.2 Geographical and Ethnic Variation

The mean prevalence of MRI-confirmed syringomyelia ranges, in different countries, between 2 and 13 per 100,000 inhabitants (Table 2.1). There are also some small regions where the prevalence is even higher, reaching levels of 80–130 per 100,000 population (Borisova et al. 1989). The ratio of males to females varies between 1:2 and equal (Brickell et al. 2006; Sakushima et al. 2012; Sirotkin 1972).

G. Flint, C. Rusbridge (eds.), *Syringomyelia*,
DOI 10.1007/978-3-642-13706-8_2, © Springer-Verlag Berlin Heidelberg 2014

The recorded incidence and prevalence of syringomyelia have not been constant through time. Between 1949 and 1978, for example, in southwest Germany, recorded cases fell from 25 to less than 1 case per year, per 100,000 inhabitants (Hertel and Ricker 1978; Schergna and Armani 1985). It was suggested that the enormous change in living habits over this period might have accounted for the decrease. In contrast, an epidemiological study in New Zealand found that the incidence of syringomyelia increased between 1961 and 2001, from 0.76 to 4.70 cases per year, per 100,000 population (Brickell et al. 2006). This increasing incidence might have been due to the changing ethnic composition of the population. There are clear ethnic differences in the prevalence of syringomyelia and its associated conditions (Table 2.2), although the extent to which these variations are due to environmental influences, as opposed to genetic factors, remains unknown. Pacific people and Maori have a higher prevalence of syringomyelia than other ethnic groups, and the percentage of Maori and Pacific people in the New Zealand population increased over the study period in the Brickell et al. survey. The population of Pacific people in particular grew 11 times faster than did other ethnic groups. A second possible reason for the increase in recorded incidence in New Zealand is, of course, simply the increased detection of syringomyelia, brought about by improved access to MR imaging.

The Tartar population in the Volga-Ural region of Russia, including Bashkortostan, Tatarstan and other areas, suffers from a particularly high

Table 2.1 Prevalence of syringomyelia

Prevalence (per 100,000 inhabitants)	Geographical region	Reference source
1.94	Japan	Sakushima et al. (2012)
7	USA	Kurtzke (1996)
8.2	New Zealand	Brickell et al. (2006)
12.6	Tatarstan, Russia	Authors' data (2011)

Table 2.2 Ethnic differences in syringomyelia and related disorders

Disorders	Geographical region	Ethnic group	Prevalence (per 100,000 inhabitants)	Reference source
Syringomyelia	New Zealand	Pacific people	18.4	Brickell et al. (2006)
		Maori	15.4	
		Caucasians and other	5.4	
Syringomyelia associated with CM1	New Zealand	Pacific people	16.1	Brickell et al. (2006)
		Maori	8.3	
		Caucasians and other	3.2	
Syringomyelia	Russia, Bashkortostan	Tartars	130	Borisova et al. (1989)
		Russians	0.5–12	
		Bashkirs	0.32–0.6	
Syringomyelia associated with CM1	Russia, Tatarstan	Tartars	14.8	Authors' data (2011)
		Russians (mainly)	9	
Chiari malformations with and without of syringomyelia	Russia, Tatarstan	Tartars	33.4	Authors' data (2011)
		Russians (mainly)	23.8	
Syringomyelia associated with scoliosis	New Zealand	Maori and Pacific people	Children with scoliosis more likely than Caucasians to have syringomyelia	Ratahi et al. (2002)
Syringomyelia	USA	African-Americans and Caucasians	Syringomyelia more prevalent in African-Americans	Tipton and Haerer (1970)

Table 2.3 Geographical distribution of syringomyelia and related disorders

Disorders	Countries and regions with high prevalence (per 100,000 inhabitants)	Countries and regions with low prevalence (per 100,000 inhabitants)	Reference sources
Syringomyelia	*Germany* Southwest	*Germany* Northeast	Hertel and Ricker (1978)
	Italy Piedmont, Valle d'Aosta, Toscana and Marche		Ciaramitaro et al. (2011)
	Russia Central regions in the valleys of the rivers Volga, Kama, Vyatka, Belaya	*Russia* South regions	Borisova et al. (1989)
	Russia Bashkortostan East and Northwest (80–130) Tatarstan North (63–83) Samara region Northeast (43–62)	*Russia* Bashkortostan Southwest (0.3–0.6) Tatarstan Southeast (4.3–5.5) Samara region South (6–20)	Sirotkin (1972) Borisova et al. (1989) Borisova and Mirsaev (2007) Authors' data. (2011)
Chiari malformations with and without of syringomyelia	*Russia* Tatarstan North (100–148)	*Russia* Tatarstan Southeast (9–14)	Authors' data (2011)
Craniovertebral anomalies	*India* Uttar Pradesh, Bihar, Rajasthan, part of Gujarat		Goel (2009)
Basilar impression associated with Chiari malformation	*Brazil* Northeast		Da Silva et al. (2011)
Sagittal synostosis associated with Chiari malformation	*Finland*		Leikola et al. (2010)

prevalence of syringomyelia, at 130 per 100,000 inhabitants. In contrast, the prevalence among other ethnic groups, mainly Bashkirs and Russians, in the same geographic region, was no more than 12 per 100,000 population (Borisova et al. 1989; Borisova and Mirsaev 2007). Our own data, collected since 1998, revealed a less pronounced difference in the prevalence of syringomyelia between the Tartars and other groups, at 15 and 9 per 100,000 inhabitants, respectively. In addition, the prevalence among both Tartars and other ethnic groups varied significantly across different regions of Tatarstan, ranging between 3.7 and 93 per 100,000 adults in Tartars and between 2 and 92 per 100,000 in a population composed mainly of Russians.

Elsewhere in the world, the distribution of syringomyelia and related conditions, by country,

region and even small territories, is extremely non-uniform (Table 2.3, Fig. 2.1). Such differences have been linked to environmental factors, for example, the size of a community, the distance between a patient's place of residence and a diagnostic centre, the degree of physical exertion exercised by the individual as part of his or her profession, the number of siblings in the patient' family, the order of his or her birth and the infant mortality rate in the patient's family (Borisova et al. 1989; Hertel and Ricker 1978; Sirotkin 1972). Most of the patients with syringomyelia tend to come from large families and originate from the second half of the birth order. Infant mortality is especially high among the brothers and sisters of syringomyelia patients. Patients are more likely to live in small towns and are more likely to be employed in occupations involving

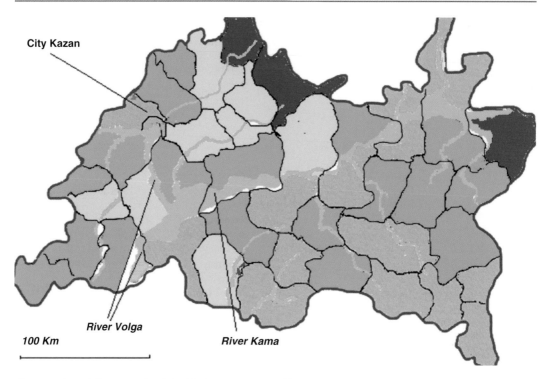

Fig. 2.1 Map of Tatarstan (Russia) with the prevalence of syringomyelia (per 100,000 adult inhabitants). *Red* = very high prevalence (>50); *yellow* = high prevalence (30–50); *green* = moderate prevalence (10–30); *blue* = low prevalence (<10). Regions with very high prevalence of syringomyelia are situated in a compact area in northern Tatarstan (Unpublished authors' data 2011)

hard physical labour. The high prevalence of syringomyelia in the north of Tatarstan may be associated not just with the predominance of the Tartar population in this region but also the employment of these people, mainly in physically demanding jobs in agriculture (author's own data). Interestingly, however, syringomyelia prevalence may also vary with the soil type (Sirotkin 1972).

2.3   Causes of Syringomyelia

A study analysing autopsy results over a 38-year period identified 175 patients with tubular cavitations of the spinal cord. Just over a half of these cases were male and the mean age was just over 40 but with a range from 1 day to 87 years old. Non-neoplastic syringomyelia was found in 60 %, neoplastic cysts in 10 % and syringomyelia ex vacuo (i.e. atrophic syringes occurring with myelomalacia) in 30 % (Milhorat 2000). The reported frequency of the main causes of syringomyelia does, however, vary between clinical and MRI studies (Table 2.4).

The cause of syringomyelia varies between different age groups, with Chiari malformation type 2 being the most common cause in younger patients, whereas in adolescents and adults, Chiari malformation type 1 predominates. In older age groups the cause of the syringomyelia may not always be apparent, and cases are more likely to be given the label of idiopathic (Sakushima et al. 2012).

2.3.1   Chiari Malformations

Most cases of syringomyelia are associated with Chiari malformation type 1, which in turn comprises the commonest abnormality encountered at the craniovertebral junction. It is characterized by underdevelopment of the posterior cranial

Table 2.4 Syringomyelia by cause

Underlying cause	Proportion of all causes of syringomyelia (%)	Geographical region	Reference source
Chiari malformation type 1	26	Germany	Roser et al. (2010)
	32	UK	Williams (1995)
	48	Japan	Sakushima et al. (2012)
	48	Italy	Ciaramitaro et al. (2011)
	50	New Zealand	Brickell et al. (2006)
	77	USA	Speer et al. (2003)
Chiari malformation type 2	4.6	Italy	Ciaramitaro et al. (2011)
	8	Japan	Sakushima et al. (2012)
	2–14	USA	Speer et al. (2003)
Trauma	4	USA	Speer et al. (2003)
	8	Japan	Sakushima et al. (2012)
	10	New Zealand	Brickell et al. (2006)
	19	Germany	Roser et al. (2010)
	24	UK	Williams (1995)
Tumours	0.4	USA	Speer et al. (2003)
	3	UK	Williams (1995)
	5.2	Japan	Sakushima et al. (2012)
	12	Germany	Roser et al. (2010)
	32	Croatia	Orsolic et al. (1998)
Inflammations of the spinal cord and meninges	2	Germany	Roser et al. (2010)
	4	USA	Speer et al. (2003)
	4.4	New Zealand	Brickell et al. (2006)
	5	Japan	Sakushima et al. (2012)
Idiopathic	13–25	Japan	Sakushima et al. (2012)
	16	New Zealand	Brickell et al. (2006)
	28	Germany	Roser et al. (2010)

fossa with overcrowding of an otherwise normally developed hindbrain (Milhorat et al. 1999; Nishikawa et al. 1997). A ubiquitous feature is compression of the retrocerebellar CSF spaces, and about nine out of ten cases have a tonsillar herniation that is at least 5 mm below the level of foramen magnum. Very commonly there are also radiographic signs of cranial base dysplasia, of varying degree (Milhorat et al. 1999). Chiari malformation type 1 has a reported male to female ratio of between 1:0.7 and 1:3.7 (Da Silva et al. 2011; Meadows et al. 2000; Milhorat et al. 1999; Takeuchi et al. 2007). The reported rate of Chiari malformation type 1 as an incidental finding on MRI of the brain ranges from 0.04 to 0.9 % (Meadows et al. 2000; Morris et al. 2009; Vernooij et al. 2007). The reported incidence is higher from studies using high-resolution MRI sequences. One study reported cerebellar tonsillar herniation in as many as 14.4 % of patients presenting with neck pain and/or upper limb symptoms (Takeuchi et al. 2007).

The reported occurrence of syringomyelia in association with Chiari malformation type 1 ranges from 65 to 80 % (Speer et al. 2003). Chiari type 1-related syringomyelia has also been reported as an incidental finding on MRI (Meadows et al. 2000; Nishizawa et al. 2001).

Chiari malformation type 2 is found only in patients with myelomeningocele. It is the leading cause of death in affected individuals under the age of 2, and up to 15 % of patients with early clinical manifestation of Chiari malformation type 2 die by the age of 3 years and nearly a third of survivors have some form of permanent neurological disability (Stevenson 2004). Outcomes in older children, presenting with myelopathy and/or pain, are much better, ranging from 79 to

Table 2.5 Pathologies leading to Chiari type 1 hindbrain hernias

Cranial constriction
Spinal cord tethering
Cranial settling
Intracranial hypertension
Intraspinal hypotension

Table 2.6 Causes of hindbrain hernias

Chiari malformation type 1	57 %
Chiari malformation type 2	1.5 %
Basilar impression/invagination	18–64 %
Hydrocephalus	3–23 %
Tethered cord syndrome	7 %
Craniosynostosis	0.7–17 %

100 % improvement in symptoms following surgery. The prevalence of Chiari malformation type 2 in the general population is 1 in 3,600.

Chiari malformation type 2 is associated with syringomyelia in 35 % of cases (Speer et al. 2003), and it accounts for up to 8 % of the total cases of syringomyelia, with a higher percentage in paediatric practice.

Borderline tonsillar herniation, 2–4 mm below the foramen magnum, has an estimated prevalence of 2.6 per 100,000 population, from all MRI scans of the brain (Takeuchi et al. 2007). Syringomyelia was found in just over half of these patients (Milhorat et al. 1999).

The definition of Chiari malformation type 1 is evolving from that of a simple anatomical description to the concept of it representing the clinical expression of a number of different pathologies. Five broad mechanisms causing cerebellar tonsillar have been described (Table 2.5) (Milhorat et al. 2010; De Souza et al. 2011). These include those which affect the development of the craniocervical structures. For example, the development of Chiari malformation type 1 was seen in 29 % of patients suffering from rickets and in 73 % of all cases of Crouzon's disease. A tight filum terminale has an associated Chiari malformation type 1 in 10 % of cases. Twenty-four percent of pseudotumour cerebri patients had inferiorly displaced cerebellar tonsils. In addition, venous sinus occlusion can be the cause of reversible hindbrain herniation (Novegno et al. 2008). The frequency of these different causes of cerebellar herniation is very variable (Table 2.6) and also has ethno-geographical differences (Da Silva et al. 2011; Milhorat et al. 1999, 2009, 2010; Novegno et al. 2008; Strahle et al. 2011a). Our own observation of 900 adult patients with Chiari malformations, over a 10-year period,

found basilar impression in 17 % and non-syndromic craniosynostosis in 7.4 %. The incidence of hydrocephalus, when defined as an Evans' index greater than 0.30, was present in as many as 54 % of patients. In contrast, the prevalence of basilar impression associated with Chiari malformation in the northeast of Brazil was more than 60 % (Da Silva et al. 2011). It may well be that differences in the frequency of cranial constriction, cranial settling and mild deformations of cranial shape can explain ethno-geographical differences in syringomyelia prevalence.

2.3.2 Post-traumatic Syringomyelia

The causes of spinal cord injury vary from country to country, depending on social and economic factors. Post-traumatic syringomyelia was previously thought to be an infrequent but serious sequel to such injuries, and clinical and CT studies suggested that it occurred with an incidence of between 1 and 5 % (Barnett et al. 1971; Biyani and El Masry 1994; El Masry and Biyani 1996). Since the introduction of MRI, the reported radiological incidence has increased up to 22 % (Burt 2004; Squier and Lehr 1994), which is consistent with the frequency of 17–20 % identified in post-mortem studies (Squier and Lehr 1994; Wozniewicz et al. 1983). Cystic necrosis of the spinal cord, confined to the level of injury, is generally considered to be a myelomalacic cavity and not syringomyelia, but asymptomatic cavitations, extending above and below the levels of injury, are often detected radiologically in victims of spinal cord injury, and these outnumber cases of symptomatic post-traumatic syringomyelia. Which asymptomatic cavities are likely to become symptomatic and over what length of time is, however, unknown. Progression may depend upon the original mechanism of injury or a variety of conditions inherent to the individual or both (Byun et al. 2010; Ohtonari et al. 2009).

Males are more likely to be victims of spinal cord injury than are females, in a ratio of about 6:1 (Burt 2004; El Masry and Biyani 1996). The interval between injury and diagnosis ranges from 2 months to 34 years (Biyani and El Masry 1994; El Masry and Biyani 1996). Full neurological recovery following the original spinal cord injury does not eliminate the possibility of post-traumatic syringomyelia developing later.

2.3.3 Syringomyelia in Patients with Non-traumatic Arachnoiditis

Syringomyelia is a rare sequel (less than 1 %) of infectious and non-infectious central nervous system inflammatory disease (Williams 1995). There are two main mechanisms by which inflammation may lead to the formation of syringomyelia: arachnoiditis and myelitis. Infection may also be a factor precipitating the onset of symptoms in Chiari-associated syringomyelia, in up to 7 % of patients (Milhorat et al. 1999).

Primary spinal syringomyelia is commonly secondary to post-inflammatory scarring, which leads to obstruction to the normal spinal CSF flow. Arachnoiditis might also cause syrinx formation by causing obliteration of the spinal microvasculature, leading to local cord ischaemia. Patterns of arachnoiditis seen range from focal meningeal cicatrix formation to diffuse adhesive spinal arachnoiditis (Caplan et al. 1990).

Foramen magnum arachnoiditis, in the absence of Chiari malformations, is a rare cause of syringomyelia (Klekamp et al. 2002). The mean interval between the presumed causative event (meningitis or trauma) and the development of syringomyelia-related symptoms can be up to 10 years. Compared with patients with Chiari malformation type 1, individuals with syringomyelia due to foramen magnum arachnoiditis have a much poorer long-term outcome.

A stable clinical course was demonstrated in only 14 % of patients in whom surgery was not performed. Following surgery, 57 % of patients will have recurrence of symptoms within 5 years of the procedure.

Non-infectious inflammatory diseases of the nervous system are also sometimes associated with syringomyelia (Ravaglia et al. 2007; Zabbarova et al. 2010) and transient syringomyelia is occasionally encountered and associated with various types of non-infectious myelitis. Syringomyelia also occurs in 4.5 % of patients with multiple sclerosis (Weier et al. 2008) and in 16 % of patients with neuromyelitis optica (Devic's disease) (Kira et al. 1996). Reversible hydromyelia has been reported in patients with transverse myelitis (Wehner et al. 2005).

Syringomyelia arising as a complication of tuberculous meningitis is rare, in the context of the overall incidence and prevalence of this disease (Kaynar et al. 2000). Published literature consists, for the most part, of single case studies or small series, reporting patients who developed syringomyelia as a late complication of tuberculous meningitis. Examples of gross pathology include intradural extramedullary tuberculomas (Gul et al. 2010; Muthukumar and Sureshkumar 2007), tuberculous meningitis with a cranial nerve palsy (Katchanov et al. 2007) and spinal tuberculous arachnoiditis (Paliwal et al. 2011).

Spinal intramedullary haematoma is an uncommon lesion, and spontaneous, non-traumatic, intramedullary haemorrhage, without any obvious underlying pathology, is distinctly rare. Predisposing conditions that have been reported include pregnancy and childbirth, spinal angioma, spinal artery aneurysm, haemophilia and syringomyelia (Leech et al. 1991). The latter condition was originally described by Gowers in 1904 and consequently has been termed Gowers' syringal haemorrhage (Sedzimir et al. 1974). A slowly developing haematomyelia, within an existing syringomyelia cavity, may originate from a torn intraspinal vein, which is deprived of its normal neural and glial support (Ayuzawa et al. 1995). Trauma is not a predisposing cause of such haemorrhages.

2.3.4 Idiopathic Syringomyelia

Idiopathic tubular cavitations of the spinal cord account for between 13 and 28 % of all reported cases of syringomyelia (Brickell et al. 2006; Roser et al. 2010; Sakushima et al. 2012). A study of adult patients presenting to a neurosurgical department, with an MRI diagnosis of syringomyelia, found that 28 % had a central canal with no underlying associated pathology (Roser et al. 2010). A distinguishing feature of these lesions was that there was no accompanying clinical or radiological progression. A study of 794 MRI investigations of the spinal cord, for a variety of indications, found 1.5 % of patients had a filiform intramedullary cavity (Petit-Lacour et al. 2000). These patients did not have any other anatomical factors predisposing to syringomyelia and they, too, were clinically asymptomatic.

Various terms have been used to refer to idiopathic syringomyelia including hydromyelia, idiopathic localized hydromyelia and syringohydromyelia (Roy et al. 2011). Primary or idiopathic hydromyelia is typified by a slitlike expansion of the central canal, without any pathology of CSF dynamics, congenital or acquired (Holly and Batzdorf 2002; Novegno et al. 2008; Roser et al. 2010). Idiopathic, slitlike or "filiform" cavities usually represent a benign condition, and in 50 % of these patients, medical assessment may reveal alternative conditions as being responsible for the presenting symptoms (Holly and Batzdorf 2002).

An explanation for many apparently idiopathic syringomyelia cavities may be simple persistence of the embryonic central canal of the cord (Holly and Batzdorf 2002). This structure is still present at birth but becomes progressively obliterated during childhood and adolescence. Clinical and experimental studies have shown that expansion of the central canal is an early, non-specific and potentially reversible manifestation of disturbed intraspinal fluid circulation, caused by both internal and external factors (Josephson et al. 2001; Milhorat et al. 1993; Petit-Lacour et al. 2000; Weier et al. 2008).

Some cases of syringomyelia that appear to be idiopathic may actually be associated with morphometric abnormalities of the skull, in particular a small posterior fossa, with resultant compression of the subarachnoid cerebrospinal fluid (CSF) pathways (Bogdanov et al. 2004; Chern et al. 2011). This so-called Chiari 0 malformation represents a very small cohort of patients within the spectrum of all individuals with Chiari malformation, and the diagnosis of Chiari 0 malformation can only be made after other aetiologies of syringomyelia have been eliminated conclusively.

2.4 Natural History and Presentation by Age

Clinical manifestations of type 1 Chiari malformation vary according to the age at which they first appear (Klekamp and Samii 2002; Luciano 2011; Vannemreddy et al. 2010). Symptoms are often caused by compression of the brainstem, and in patients under 2 years of age, this often manifests with stridor, crying, apnoea, cyanosis, increased muscle tone and life-threatening respiratory problems. In older children the greatest problem is the development of scoliosis secondary to syringomyelia and an ataxic gait. In both adolescents and adults, chronic brainstem compression may be manifested by occipital headache, nystagmus and hyperaesthesia in the trigeminal nerve territory. In children, onset of clinical features may be associated with the rapidly growing cerebellum, and later resolution of symptoms can be related to increasing skull volume and gradual ascent of the child's cerebellar tonsils (Klekamp and Samii 2002; Novegno et al. 2008).

Of patients diagnosed with Chiari malformation type 1 on MRI, the reported number that is asymptomatic varies between a third and a half (Benglis et al. 2011; Elster and Chen 1992; Meadows et al. 2000; Novegno et al. 2008; Wu et al. 1999). The frequency of asymptomatic syringomyelia has been reported as being 23 % (Sakushima et al. 2012).

Most patients with syringomyelia and Chiari malformation type 1 first become symptomatic during adult life (Table 2.7). Adults diagnosed with Chiari malformation type 1 are more likely to have an associated syringomyelia than are children: 14–58 % of children and 59–76 % of adults (Aitken et al. 2009). The mean age at onset

Table 2.7 Incidence of tonsillar herniation in different age groups

Age group	Takeuchi et al. (2007) (%)	Authors' data (2011)		
		Chiari type 1, without syringomyelia (%)	Chiari type 1, with syringomyelia (%)	Chiari type 1, all cases (%)
<29	5	27	10	19
30–39	20	17	21.7	19
40–49	12	29	38	33
50–59	17	19	20	20
60–69	17	8	10	9
>70	12	–	0.3	0.1

of symptoms in patients with Chiari malformation type 1 is between 11 and 25 years (Aitken et al. 2009; Milhorat et al. 1999). The mean age at onset of symptoms of syringomyelia is between 28 and 40 years (Brickell et al. 2006; Sakushima et al. 2012).

Syringobulbia was found in between 1 and 6 % in patients with syringomyelia (Sakushima et al. 2012; Tubbs et al. 2009).

Syringomyelia is a disorder that can have a varying prognosis (Table 2.8). The course of symptoms after initial diagnosis is not uniform, with deterioration in 20–51 %, 10–80 % remaining unchanged and 11 % improving (Table 2.8). Spontaneous reduction of tonsillar herniation is uncommon, but may occur, in 11–18 % of cases (Novegno et al. 2008). Spontaneous resolution of syringomyelia in adult patients with cerebellar ectopia is rare, although cases have been reported (Perrini 2012). Probable mechanisms include spontaneous drainage between the syrinx and the subarachnoid space or restoration of abnormal CSF dynamics at the craniovertebral junction (Bogdanov et al. 2000, 2006; Kyoshima and Bogdanov 2003; Perrini 2012).

A study of patients with Chiari malformation type 1, who initially elected for nonsurgical management, found no significant change in the mean volume of cerebellar herniation over a 4-year period. There was, however, worsening CSF flow at the foramen magnum in 16 %, but there was also an improvement in flow in 31 %. Development of a spinal cord syrinx was seen in only 5 % and spontaneous resolution of an existing syrinx in 2 % (Strahle et al. 2011b). Ten percent of patients went on to undergo surgical treatment. Other series have reported that, overall, surgical management is required for 29–44 % patients with Chiari malformation type 1 (Benglis

Table 2.8 Clinical course of syringomyelia

Clinical course	%	Reference source
Acute presentation	11	Bogdanov and Mendelevich (2002)
Deterioration	20–51	Bogdanov and Mendelevich (2002)
Slow/moderate progressive	>47	Borisova and Mirsaev (2007)
Rapid progressive	15–20	Nakamura et al. (2009)
Stop after progression	5–6	Sakushima et al. (2012)
Unchanged at 10 years or more	10–80	Bogdanov and Mendelevich (2002), Boman and Livanainen (1967), Borisova and Mirsaev (2007), Nakamura et al. (2009), Sakushima et al. (2012)
Improved	11	Sakushima et al. (2012)
Collapse of cavity	10	Bogdanov and Mendelevich (2002)
Spontaneous remission	3.2	Sakushima et al. (2012)
Dead (or the status was unknown) during 40 years of observation	5.8–20	Boman and Livanainen (1967), Brickell et al. 2006

et al. 2011; Milhorat et al. 1999). Surgical management is performed in 69 % of patients with syringomyelia in Japan (Sakushima et al. 2012). In the paediatric population syringomyelia often (94 %) remains stable in children managed nonsurgically (Singhal et al. 2011).

A retrospective analysis of 103 adult patients with un-operated hindbrain-related syringomyelia looked at the prognostic significance of syrinx size and morphology. Patients with the widest cavities, as measured by their anteroposterior diameter, presented with a short duration of symptoms and a rapidly progressive clinical course. Those with smaller diameter cavities had symptoms of longer duration and a slower rate of progression (Bogdanov and Mendelevich 2002).

Little is known about effect of syringomyelia on life expectancy or what is the most common cause of death of patients with Chiari-associated syringomyelia. Death rates in patients with syringomyelia ranged from 6 to 20 % in studies involving 30 and 40 years of observation (Boman and Livanainen 1967; Borisova et al. 1989; Brickell et al. 2006) and do not exceed the overall rate in the population. Chiari malformation type 1 can very occasionally be associated with respiratory and cardiovascular compromise, which can potentially lead to sudden death (De Souza et al. 2011). The overall risk of such catastrophes must be small and unless a patient reports himself or herself as having suffered blackouts, brought on by Valsalva-like manoeuvres, then surgery still remains an option, rather than an essential treatment. There have been cases reported of people dying in motor vehicle collisions and who have been found, at subsequent post-mortem examination, to harbour a previously asymptomatic Chiari malformation. Forced hyperextension of the neck, to a degree not normally expected to cause serious injury, leads, presumably, to lethal medullary contusion, caused by the herniated cerebellar tonsils. Reported cases are rare and are mostly children, so this sort of tragedy may be related to the increased mobility and poorer musculature of the neck (James 1995; Mäkelä 2006; Rickert et al. 2001; Wolf et al. 1998). It would be wrong, therefore, to advocate surgery for Chiari malformations, solely on the basis that the patient is at marginally increased risk of injury during a road traffic accident.

2.5 Inheritance of Chiari and Syringomyelia

It has been reported that 3–12 % of patients with Chiari malformation type 1 have a family history of Chiari malformation (Milhorat et al. 1999; Schanker et al. 2011). The incidence of a positive family history in our Chiari population was 4.7 %, and the mean prevalence of familial cases was 2 per 100,000 adult inhabitants but ranging from less than 1 to over 100 per 100,000 adult inhabitants, with the highest prevalence found in 2 neighbouring villages in the northern region of Tatarstan. The highest prevalence of familial cases of syringomyelia and Chiari malformation was in the regions with the highest prevalence of all cases of this pathology (Figs. 2.1, 2.2 and 2.3). Genetic studies would help clarify the nature of the prevalence of sporadic and hereditary forms of disease.

Evidence of a genetic contribution to Chiari type 1 malformation and syringomyelia comes from at least three sources: familial aggregation, twin studies and known genetic syndromes associated with Chiari and syringomyelia (Speer et al. 2003). One study identified 31 pedigrees, in which two or more individuals were affected with Chiari malformation type 1 and syringomyelia (Speer et al. 2000). In this study, when MRI of asymptomatic first-degree relatives of affected patients was obtained, 21 % were diagnosed as having Chiari malformation type 1 and syringomyelia. There were no cases of isolated familial syringomyelia without an underlying Chiari malformation, suggesting that familial syringomyelia is more accurately classified as familial Chiari type 1-associated syringomyelia (see Chap. 5).

Chiari malformation with syringomyelia occurs in association with a variety of syndromes of established inheritance patterns (Table 2.9) (Speer et al. 2003). These syndromic cases are likely to account for less than 1 % of the total Chiari population. It has been suggested that the underlying gene or genes involved in Chiari malformation type 1 and syringomyelia will have pleiotropic[1] effects, influencing bone morphology at the skull base, posterior fossa volume and the extent of cerebellar tonsillar herniation (Speer et al. 2000). Such pleiotropic manifestations may or may not be clinically relevant, but one possible condition within such a pleiotropic spectrum may be the Chiari 0 malformation, which is found in individuals with volumetrically small posterior fossa, some of whom have been shown to respond to decompressive surgery.

The genetics of Chiari malformation are discussed in more detail in Chap. 5 of this book.

---

[1] When a single gene influences more than one phenotypic characteristic.

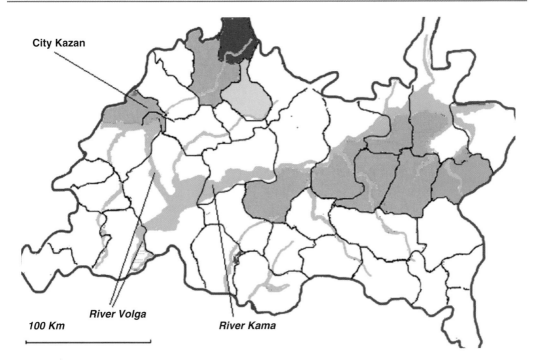

Fig. 2.2 Map of Tatarstan (Russia) with the prevalence of familial cases of Chiari malformation/syringomyelia (per 100,000 adult inhabitants). *Red*=very high prevalence (117.4); *yellow*=high prevalence (34.8); *green*=moderate prevalence (17.6); *grey*=low prevalence (<10). *White* reveals regions without familial cases of Chiari malformation/syringomyelia (Authors' data 2011)

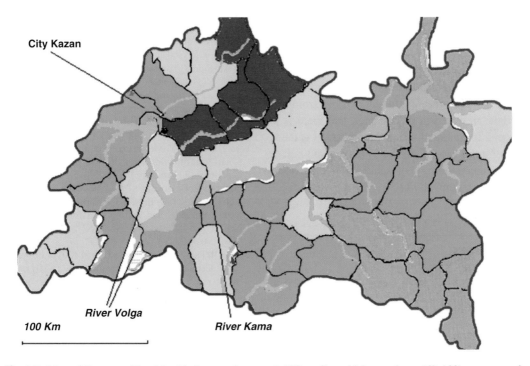

Fig. 2.3 Map of Tatarstan (Russia) with the prevalence of Chiari malformations with or without syringomyelia (per 100,000 adult inhabitants). *Red*=very high prevalence (>100); *yellow*=high prevalence (60–100); *green*=moderate prevalence (20–60); *grey*=low prevalence (<20) (Authors' data 2011)

Table 2.9 Inherited syndromes associated with Chiari and syringomyelia

Achondroplasia
Cleidocranial dysplasia
Crouzon's syndrome
Cystic fibrosis
Familial osteosclerosis
Growth hormone deficiency
Paget's disease of bone
Klippel-Feil sequence/syndrome
Hypophosphataemic rickets

Conclusions

The prevalence of syringomyelia varies widely in different geographic regions and between ethnic groups. These variations can probably be explained by ethno-geographical differences of cranial construction and cranial settling, including mild deformations of cranial shape. Most cases of syringomyelia are associated with Chiari malformation type 1. Among patients with Chiari malformation type 1, with or without syringomyelia, up to 50 % are asymptomatic. Some patients not undergoing surgical treatment may have a favourable disease course with minimal progression of clinical signs and, in a minority, spontaneous reduction of their hindbrain hernia or even resolution of their syringomyelia cavity.

There are clearly limitations as to how far we can draw meaningful conclusions from the data presented in this chapter, and there is a need for international collaboration in gathering more data, if we are to understand better the epidemiology of Chiari malformations and syringomyelia.

References

Aitken L, Lindan C, Sidney S et al (2009) Chiari type I malformation in a paediatric population. Pediatr Neurol 40:449–454

Ayuzawa S, Tsukada A, Enomoto T et al (1995) Intrasyringal hemorrhage of the cervical cord associated with Chiari type I malformation. Neurol Med Chir 35:243–246

Barnett H, Jousse A, Morley T et al (1971) Post-traumatic syringomyelia. Paraplegia 9(1):33–37

Benglis D, Covington D, Bhatia R et al (2011) Outcomes in pediatric patients with Chiari malformation type I followed up without surgery. J Neurosurg Pediatr 7: 375–379

Biyani A, El Masry W (1994) Post-traumatic syringomyelia: a review of the literature. Paraplegia 32: 723–731

Bogdanov E, Mendelevich E (2002) Syrinx size and duration of symptoms predict the pace of progressive myelopathy: retrospective analysis of 103 unoperated cases with craniocervical junction malformations and syringomyelia. Clin Neurol Neurosurg 104:90–97

Bogdanov E, Ibatullin M, Mendelevich E (2000) Spontaneous drainage in syringomyelia: magnetic resonance imaging findings. Neuroradiology 42: 676–678

Bogdanov E, Heiss J, Mendelevich E et al (2004) Clinical and neuroimaging features of "idiopathic" syringomyelia. Neurology 62(5):791–794

Bogdanov E, Heiss J, Mendelevich E (2006) The post-syrinx syndrome: stable central myelopathy and collapsed or absent syrinx. J Neurol 253(6):707–713

Boman K, Livanainen M (1967) Prognosis of syringomyelia. Acta Neurol Scand 43:61–68

Borisova N, Mirsaev T (2007) Syringomyelia in Bashkortostan: epidemiologic and pathogenesis data. Zh Nevrol Psikhiatr Im SS Korsakova 107(3):56–60

Borisova N, Valikova I, Kutchaeva G (1989) Syringomyelia (in Russian). Meditcina, Moscow

Brickell K, Anderson N, Charleston A et al (2006) Ethnic differences in syringomyelia in New Zealand. J Neurol Neurosurg Psychiatry 77:989–991

Burt A (2004) The epidemiology, natural history and prognosis of spinal cord injury. Curr Orthop 18: 26–32

Byun M, Shin J, Hwang Y et al (2010) Decompressive surgery in a patient with posttraumatic syringomyelia. J Korean Neurosurg Soc 47:228–231

Caplan L, Norohna A, Amico L (1990) Syringomyelia and arachnoiditis. J Neurol Neurosurg Psychiatry 53:106–113

Chern J, Gordon A, Mortazavi M et al (2011) Pediatric Chiari malformation type 0: a 12-year institutional experience. J Neurosurg Pediatr 8:1–5

Ciaramitaro P, Baldovino S, Roccatello D et al (2011) Chiari and Syringomyelia Consortium: a model of multidisciplinary and sharing path for rare diseases. Neurol Sci 32(Suppl 3):S271–S273. doi:10.1007/s10072-011-0725-y

Da Silva J, Dos Santos A, Melo L et al (2011) Posterior fossa decompression with tonsillectomy in 104 cases of basilar impression, Chiari malformation and/or syringomyelia. Arq Neuropsiquiatr 69(5):817–823

De Souza R-M, Zador Z, Frim D (2011) Chiari malformation type I: related conditions. Neurol Res 33(3):278–284

El Masry W, Biyani A (1996) Incidence, management, and outcome of posttraumatic syringomyelia. In memory of Mr. Bernard Williams. J Neurol Neurosurg Psychiatry 60:141–146

Elster A, Chen M (1992) Chiari I malformations: clinical and radiologic reappraisal. Radiology 183:347–353

Goel A (2009) Basilar invagination, Chiari malformation, syringomyelia: a review. Neurol India 57(3):235–246

Gul S, Celebi G, Kalayci M et al (2010) Syringomyelia and intradural extramedullary tuberculoma of the spinal cord as a late complication of tuberculous meningitis. Turk Neurosurg 20(4):561–565

Hertel G, Ricker K (1978) A geomedical study on the distribution of syringomyelia in Germany. In: den Hartog JW et al (eds) Neurology. Excerpta Medica, Amsterdam

Holly L, Batzdorf U (2002) Slitlike syrinx cavities: a persistent central canal. J Neurosurg 97(2 Suppl): 161–165

James D (1995) Significance of chronic tonsillar herniation in sudden death. Forensic Sci Int 75(2–3): 217–223

Josephson A, Greitz D, Klason T et al (2001) A spinal thecal sac constriction model supports the theory that induced pressure gradients in the cord cause edema and cyst formation. Neurosurgery 48:636–646

Katchanov J, Bohner G, Schultze J et al (2007) Tuberculous meningitis presenting as mesencephalic infarction and syringomyelia. J Neurol Sci 260(1–2): 286–287

Kaynar M, Kocer N, Belgin E et al (2000) Syringomyelia as a late complication of tuberculous meningitis. Acta Neurochir (Wien) 142:935–939

Kira J, Kanai T, Nishimura Y et al (1996) Western versus Asian types of multiple sclerosis: immunogenetically and clinically distinct disorders. Ann Neurol 40:569–574

Klekamp J, Samii M (2002) Syringomyelia: diagnosis and treatment. Springer, Berlin

Klekamp J, Giorgio I, Batzdorf U et al (2002) Syringomyelia associated with foramen magnum arachnoiditis. J Neurosurg 97(Suppl 3): 317–322

Kurtzke J (1996) Neuroepidemiology. In: Bradley W, Daroff R, Marsden C (eds) Neurology in clinical practice, vol 1. Butterworth, Philadelphia

Kyoshima K, Bogdanov E (2003) Spontaneous resolution of syringomyelia: report of two cases and review of the literature. Neurosurgery 53:762–768

Leech R, Pitha J, Brumback R (1991) Spontaneous haematomyelia: a necropsy study. JNNP 54:172–174

Leikola J, Koljonen V, Valanne L et al (2010) The incidence of Chiari malformation in nonsyndromic, single suture craniosynostosis. Childs Nerv Syst 26(6):771–774

Luciano M (2011) Chiari malformation: are children little adults? Neurol Res 33(3):272–277

Mäkelä J (2006) Arnold-Chiari malformation type I in military conscripts: symptoms and effects on service fitness. Mil Med 171(2):174–176

Meadows J, Kraut M, Guarnieri M et al (2000) Asymptomatic Chiari type I malformations identified on magnetic resonance imaging. J Neurosurg 92: 920–926

Milhorat T (2000) Classification of syringomyelia. Neurosurg Focus 8(3):1

Milhorat T, Nobandegani F, Miller J et al (1993) Noncommunicating syringomyelia following occlusion of central canal in rats. Experimental model and histological findings. J Neurosurg 78(2): 274–279

Milhorat T, Chou M, Trinidad E et al (1999) Chiari I malformation redefined: clinical and radiographic findings for 364 symptomatic patients. Neurosurgery 44:1005–1017

Milhorat T, Bolognese O, Nishikawa M et al (2009) Association of Chiari malformation type I and tethered cord syndrome: preliminary results of sectioning filum terminale. Surg Neurol 72:20–35

Milhorat T, Nishikawa M, Kula R et al (2010) Mechanisms of cerebellar tonsil herniation in patients with Chiari malformations as guide to clinical management. Acta Neurochir (Wien) 152:1117–1127

Morris Z, Whiteley W, Longstreth W et al (2009) Incidental findings on brain magnetic resonance imaging: systematic review and meta-analysis. BMJ 339:b3016. doi:10.1136/bmj.b3016

Muthukumar N, Sureshkumar V (2007) Concurrent syringomyelia and intradural extramedullary tuberculoma as late complications of tuberculous meningitis. J Clin Neurosci 14(12):1225–1230

Nakamura M, Ishii K, Watanabe K et al (2009) Clinical significance and prognosis of idiopathic syringomyelia. J Spinal Disord Tech 22(5):372–375

Nishikawa M, Sokamoto H, Hakuba A et al (1997) Pathogenesis of Chiari malformation: a morphometric study of the posterior cranial fossa. J Neurosurg 86:40–47

Nishizawa S, Yokoyama T, Yokota N et al (2001) Incidentally identified syringomyelia associated with Chiari I malformations: is early interventional surgery necessary? Neurosurgery 49(3):637–640

Novegno F, Caldarelli M, Massa A et al (2008) The natural history of the Chiari type I anomaly. J Neurosurg Pediatr 2:179–187

Ohtonari T, Nishihara N, Ota T et al (2009) Rapid reduction of syrinx associated with traumatic hypotension by direct surgery. Neurol Med Chir 49:66–70

Orsolic K, Bielen I, Vukadin S et al (1998) Incidence of syringomyelia in Croatia. Neurol Croat 47(3–4): 239–243

Paliwal V, Kumar A, Rahi S et al (2011) Charcot foot in post-tubercular spinal arachnoiditis may indicate emerging dorsal cord syringomyelia. Neurol India 59:299–301

Perrini P (2012) Spontaneous resolution of syringomyelia in adult patient with tight cisterna magna. Neurol Sci 33(6):1463–1467

Petit-Lacour M, Lasjaunias P, Iffenecker C et al (2000) Visibility of the central canal on MRI. Neuroradiology 42(10):756–761

Ratahi E, Crawford H, Thompson J et al (2002) Ethnic variance in the epidemiology of scoliosis in New Zealand. J Pediatr Orthop 22:784–787

Ravaglia S, Bogdanov E, Pichiecchio A et al (2007) Pathogenetic role of myelitis for syringomyelia. Clin Neurol Neurosurg 109(6):541–546

Rickert C, Grabellus F, Varchmin-Schultheiss K et al (2001) Sudden unexpected death in young adults with chronic hydrocephalus. Int J Legal Med 114(6): 331–337

Roser F, Ebner F, Sixt C et al (2010) Defining the line between hydromyelia and syringomyelia. A differentiation is possible based on electrophysiological and magnetic resonance imaging studies. Acta Neurochir (Wien) 152(2):213–219

Roy A, Slimack N, Ganju A (2011) Idiopathic syringomyelia: retrospective case series, comprehensive review, and update on management. Neurosurg Focus 31(6):E15

Sakushima K, Tsuboi S, Ichiro Y et al (2012) Nationwide survey on the epidemiology of syringomyelia in Japan. J Neurol Sci 313(1-2):147–152

Schanker B, Walcott B, Nahed B et al (2011) Familial Chiari malformation: case series. Neurosurg Focus 31(3):E1

Schergna E, Armani M (1985) Epidemiological and clinical studies of syringomyelia in the Padova province. Minerva Med 76(37):1699–1704

Sedzimir C, Roberts J, Occleshaw J et al (1974) Gowers' syringal haemorrhage. J Neurol Neurosurg Psychiatry 37:312–315

Singhal A, Bowen-Roberts T, Steinbok P et al (2011) Natural history of untreated syringomyelia in pediatric patients. Neurosurg Focus 31(6):E13

Sirotkin V (1972) Regional peculiarities of syringomyelia as a medical genetic problem. Sov Genet 6(1): 129–134

Sixt C, Riether F, Will B et al (2009) Evaluation of quality of life parameters in patients who have syringomyelia. J Clin Neurosci 16:1599–1603

Speer M, George T, Enterline D et al (2000) A genetic hypothesis for Chiari I malformation with or without syringomyelia. Neurosurg Focus 8(3):12

Speer M, Enterline D, Mehltretter L (2003) Chiari type I malformation with or without syringomyelia: prevalence and genetics. J Genet Couns 12(4): 297–311

Squier M, Lehr R (1994) Post-traumatic syringomyelia. J Neurol Neurosurg Psychiatry 57:1095–1098

Stevenson K (2004) Chiari type II malformation: past, present, and future. Neurosurg Focus 16(2):E5

Strahle J, Muraszko K, Buchman S et al (2011a) Chiari malformation associated with craniosynostosis. Neurosurg Focus 31(3):E2

Strahle J, Muraszko K, Kapurch J et al (2011b) Natural history of Chiari malformation type I following decision for conservative treatment. J Neurosurg Pediatr 8(2):214–221

Takeuchi K, Yokoyama T, Junji I et al (2007) Tonsillar herniation and the cervical spine: a morphometric study of 172 patients. J Orthop Sci 12:55–60

Tipton A, Haerer A (1970) Syringomyelia in Mississippi. J Miss State Med Assoc 11:533–637

Tubbs R, Bailey M, Barrow W et al (2009) Morphometric analysis of the craniocervical juncture in children with Chiari I malformation and concomitant syringobulbia. Childs Nerv Syst 25(6):689–692

Vannemreddy P, Nourbakhsh A, Willis B et al (2010) Congenital Chiari malformations. Neurol India 58: 6–14

Vernooij M, Ikram M, Tanghe H et al (2007) Incidental findings on brain MRI in the general population. N Engl J Med 357:1821–1828

Wehner T, Ross J, Ransohoff R (2005) Fluid in the flute: reversible hydromyelia. J Neurol Sci 236(1–2):85–86

Weier K, Naegelin Y, Thoeni A et al (2008) Non-communicating syringomyelia: a feature of spinal cord involvement in multiple sclerosis. Brain 131(Pt 7):1776–1782

Williams B (1990) Post-traumatic syringomyelia, an update. Paraplegia 28:296–313

Williams B (1995) The cystic spinal cord. J Neurol Neurosurg Psychiatry 58:59–90

Wolf D, Veasey S, Wilson S et al (1998) Death following minor head trauma in two adult individuals with the Chiari I deformity. J Forensic Sci 43(6):1241–1243

Wozniewicz B, Filipowicz K, Swiderska S et al (1983) Pathophysiological mechanism of traumatic cavitation of the spinal cord. Paraplegia 21:312–317

Wu Y, Chin C, Chan K et al (1999) Pediatric Chiari I malformations: do clinical and radiologic features correlate? Neurology 53:1271–1276

Zabbarova A, Davletshina R, Mikhailov A et al (2010) Hydromyelia in demyelinating and disimmune myelitis. Neurol Bull 42(1):115–120

Anatomy and Physiology

3

Roy Weller

Contents

R. Weller
Clinical Neurosciences,
Faculty of Medicine, University of Southampton,
Southampton, England, UK
e-mail: row@soton.uk

3.1   Introduction

Syringomyelia and hydrocephalus, from whatever cause, are characterised by the abnormal accumulation of fluid within cavities in the central nervous system (CNS), suggesting that there is a failure of fluid drainage systems in these conditions.

Extracellular fluid in the CNS consists of cerebrospinal fluid (CSF) and interstitial fluid (ISF). CSF is produced by the choroid plexuses and circulates through the ventricular system and the subarachnoid spaces of the brain and spinal cord. Drainage of CSF is partly into the blood through arachnoid granulations and villi and partly along lymphatic drainage pathways, mostly associated with the cribriform plate of the ethmoid bone (Johnston et al. 2004). Interstitial fluid is larger in volume than CSF: in humans 250 mL compared with 140 mL of CSF (Bergsneider 2001). Derived from the blood, ISF and solutes circulate through the narrow extracellular spaces of the CNS and drain out with soluble brain metabolites, along basement membranes of capillaries

G. Flint, C. Rusbridge (eds.), *Syringomyelia*,
DOI 10.1007/978-3-642-13706-8_3, © Springer-Verlag Berlin Heidelberg 2014

and arteries to lymph nodes (Carare et al. 2008; Weller et al. 2009b). Disturbances of CSF drainage result in hydrocephalus and syringomyelia, whereas failure of ISF drainage appears to play a role in the aetiology of neurodegenerative diseases, particularly Alzheimer's disease (Weller et al. 2009c, 2011).

This chapter reviews the production, circulation and drainage of cerebrospinal fluid and interstitial fluid from the central nervous system and how the balance between the two fluids is disturbed in hydrocephalus and syringomyelia. Some attention is also given to pathologies not directly related to syringomyelia but which serve to illustrate how metabolic consequences of altered CSF and water movement in the CNS might account for some of the hitherto unexplained phenomena relating to syringomyelia.

3.2 Choroid Plexus and the Production of CSF

Cerebrospinal fluid is produced by the choroid plexuses at the rate of approximately 350 µL/min in humans (Davson et al. 1987). The major choroid plexuses are in the lateral and third ventricles and in the fourth ventricle, from which the plexuses protrude through the foramina of Luschka into the subarachnoid space. Microscopic examination of the choroid plexus reveals two major components, namely the stroma and the choroid plexus epithelium (Fig. 3.1) (Wolburg and Paulus 2010). The stroma contains blood vessels, meningeal cells and sheaths of collagen (Alcolado et al. 1986). In contrast with the brain, there is little barrier in the plexus blood vessels to the passage of macromolecules into the stroma itself. This is reflected in the entry of contrast media into the choroid plexus and its resultant visualisation by imaging techniques. Leptomeningeal cells in the choroid plexus generate the collagen bands that constitute the major bulk of the stroma. With advancing age, these leptomeningeal cells produce spheres of collagen that become calcified (Alcolado et al. 1986), to such an extent that they are visible in skull x-rays of older individuals.

The anatomical substrate of the blood-CSF barrier is the choroid plexus epithelium, which is derived from the ependymal lining of the ventricles (Johanson et al. 2008). Choroid plexuses are formed by the invagination of leptomeninges into the ventricular cavities and by modification of the ventricular ependymal lining into choroid plexus epithelium. Histological and ultrastructural techniques have shown that the choroid plexus epithelium is composed of cuboidal cells. These are coated by basement membrane on their basal surface, which abuts onto the stroma, and by microvilli on the ventricular surface (Wolburg and Paulus 2010). Tight junctions bind the apical

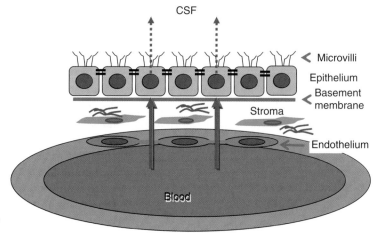

Fig. 3.1 Choroid plexus and the formation of CSF. Fluid and solutes pass freely from the blood through the fenestrated epithelium of choroid plexus capillaries into the stroma (*red arrows*). CSF is produced by filtration through the choroid plexus epithelial cells

Choroid plexus and the formation of CSF

portions of these epithelial cells together. CSF is formed by the net transport of water, sodium chloride, potassium and bicarbonate ions from the choroid plexus stroma, through the epithelial cells, into the ventricles (Fig. 3.1) (Johanson et al. 2008). This process involves the enzymes carbonic anhydrase C, sodium and potassium ATPases, and aquaporin-1 (AQP1), which reside in the choroid plexus epithelial cells (Johanson et al. 2008; Wolburg and Paulus 2010; Yool 2007). Acetazolamide reduces CSF production by inhibiting carbonic anhydrase C and by reducing the amount of AQP1 through an alteration in protein transcription (Ameli et al. 2012). CSF in humans is produced at a rate of 0.3–0.6 mL/min, or 500–600 mL/day. In those smaller mammals that have been studied, CSF is replaced approximately four times per day (Johanson et al. 2008). A small proportion of CSF appears to be derived, additionally, from brain interstitial fluid (Johanson et al. 2008).

3.3 Circulation and Drainage of the CSF

CSF leaves the ventricular system via the foramina of Luschka and Magendie and flows into the basal cisterns and the cisterna magna. It circulates through the ventricles and the basal cisterns and across the foramen magnum in a pulsatile manner (see Sect. 3.5.2), the pulses being derived from the vascular system (Weller 1995).

There are two major routes of drainage of CSF from the subarachnoid channels (Johnston et al. 2004): (a) alongside cranial and spinal nerve roots, particularly the olfactory nerves as they pass through the cribriform plate of the ethmoid bone, and (b) directly into the blood via arachnoid granulations and villi associated with major cranial venous sinuses.

3.3.1 The Ventricular System and Ependyma

The cerebral ventricular system is lined by ependyma, which develops during foetal life. In the postnatal brain and in the adult brain, ependyma

consists of a single layer of ciliated cuboidal epithelial cells (Del Bigio 1995), but in the adult human brain, there are frequently areas of the ventricular walls that are devoid of ependyma, leaving the subependymal glia exposed to ventricular CSF. Ependymal cells are joined by gap junctions and lack the tight barrier function of choroid plexus epithelium so that, even in brains with intact ependyma, tracers injected into the ventricles pass freely into the periventricular tissue, particularly into the white matter (Abbott 2004). The central canal of the spinal cord is well defined in the foetus and is also lined by ependyma. However, in the adult human spinal cord, the central canal is usually very small or obliterated and marked only by a small, closely packed nest of ependyma cells.

3.3.2 Leptomeninges and the Subarachnoid Space

The human brain and spinal cord are encased in layers of meninges. On the outer surface, and abutting the bones of the skull and spine, is the tough collagenous dura mater, the outer layer of which forms the inner periosteum of the skull. Within the dura, the leptomeninges consist of two major layers; the outer is the arachnoid mater and is applied to the inner aspect of the dura mater. Separated from the arachnoid by the subarachnoid space is the pia mater. The arachnoid and pia are connected by many sheetlike trabeculae of arachnoid-coated collagen that traverse the subarachnoid space and suspend the leptomeningeal arteries and veins within the CSF (Fig. 3.2) (Weller 2005). As arteries penetrate the surface of the cortex, the arachnoid coating is reflected onto the surface of the brain as the pia mater and a single layer of pia mater also accompanies the artery into the surface of the brain (Fig. 3.2) (Zhang et al. 1990). Scanning electron microscope studies have also shown that the pia mater on the brain and spinal cord is reflected onto blood vessels in the subarachnoid space and thus separates CSF in the subarachnoid space from the brain and spinal cord (Figs. 3.2 and 3.3) (Hutchings and Weller 1986; Nicholas and Weller 1988; Weller 2005). The pia mater is usually only one cell

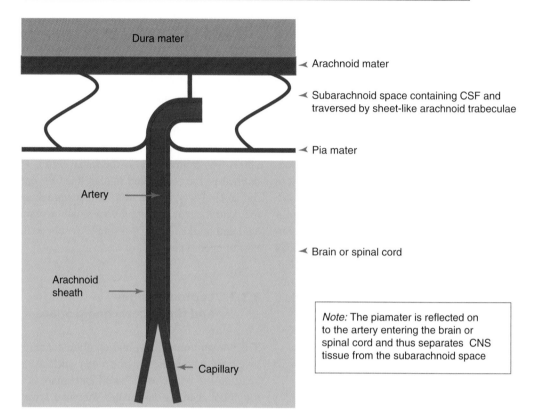

Fig. 3.2 A diagram summarising the arrangement of meninges on the surface of the human brain and spinal cord. Arachnoid mater is closely applied to the dura mater; sheetlike trabeculae cross the subarachnoid space to link arachnoid to the pia mater on the surface of the brain or spinal cord. Pia mater is reflected from the surface of the brain onto the surface of arteries and veins in the subarachnoid space, thus separating CSF in the subarachnoid space from the brain and spinal cord. A thin layer of pia mater extends alongside arteries as they penetrate the brain or spinal cord

thick and contains intercellular junctions, but it is uncertain how impermeable the pia mater is to the passage of water and macromolecules. Larger particles, such as erythrocytes in subarachnoid haemorrhage, do not penetrate the intact pia mater although inflammatory cells can migrate through this thin cell layer (Hutchings and Weller 1986). Underlying the pia mater, there are bundles of collagen that surround arteries and veins in the subpial space (Alcolado et al. 1988).

The layout of leptomeninges coating the spinal cord differs somewhat from the arrangement of the leptomeninges surrounding the cerebral hemispheres and the brain stem. Arachnoid mater coating the spinal cord is composed of several layers (Nicholas and Weller 1988) (Fig. 3.4). The outer arachnoid is firmly applied to the inner surface of the dura mater. A series of intermediate layers of arachnoid mater are attached to this parietal layer, and they either spread out over the dorsal and ventral aspects of the spinal cord or form the dorsal, dorsolateral and anterior ligaments. Dentate ligaments on the lateral aspect of the spinal cord (Fig. 3.4) are formed of collagenous sheets that connect the dura to the substantial layer of subpial collagen that surrounds the

Fig. 3.3 Scanning electron micrograph of the surface of the brain as viewed from the subarachnoid space. A leptomeningeal artery spreads its branches over the surface of the pia mater, and before the branches penetrate the brain, the pia mater is reflected on to the surface of the artery (*arrow*) (Reproduced with permission from Hutchings and Weller (1986)). ×75

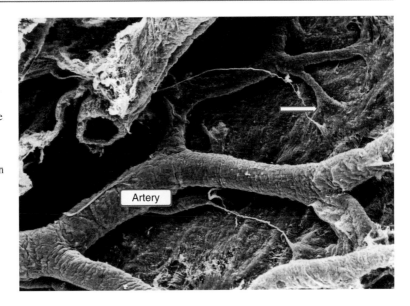

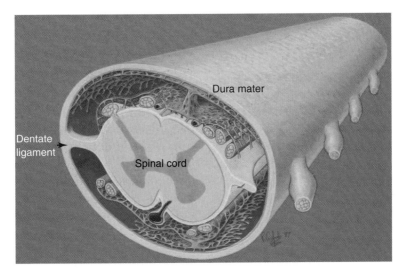

Fig. 3.4 Diagram showing the arrangements of the leptomeninges surrounding the spinal cord. An outer layer of arachnoid mater (*blue*) is applied to the inner aspect of the dura mater. Highly perforated intermediate layers of arachnoid (*green*) arise from the outer arachnoid to coat the dorsal and ventral surfaces of the spinal cord. There is a prominent dorsal ligament and less robust dorsolateral ligaments are also present. The dentate ligaments connect the layer of subpial collagen (*white*) with the collagenous dura (Reproduced with permission from Nicholas and Weller (1988))

spinal cord. The surface of the dentate ligaments is coated by arachnoid mater (Nicholas and Weller 1988). Functionally, the intermediate layers of arachnoid around the spinal cord may act as baffles, modifying the propagation of pressure waves within the CSF passing up and down the spinal subarachnoid channels.

3.3.3 Lymphatic Drainage of the Cerebrospinal Fluid

In smaller mammals such as rats, mice and rabbits and even in larger mammals such as sheep, the major pathways for drainage of CSF appear to be alongside cranial and spinal nerve roots to

Fig. 3.5 Coronal section through the olfactory bulbs, cribriform plate and nasal mucosa of a rat that had received an injection of Indian ink into the CSF. Black Indian ink is seen in the subarachnoid space inferior to the olfactory bulbs. Channels cross the cribriform plate adjacent to branches of the olfactory nerve and allow Indian ink to drain into the lymphatics of the nasal mucosa (*arrow*) (Reproduced with permission from Kida et al. (1993)). Haematoxylin and eosin ×40

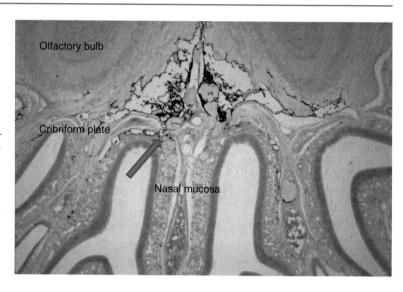

regional lymph nodes. This lymphatic drainage of cranial CSF is via well-defined channels that run alongside branches of the olfactory nerves, as they pass through the cribriform plate of the ethmoid bone to nasal lymphatics (Fig. 3.5) (Johnston et al. 2004; Kida et al. 1993). Channels formed by leptomeningeal cells in the subarachnoid space join nasal lymphatics, and when tracers are injected into the cisterna magna in the rat, they drain to lymph nodes in the neck in less than 1 min (Kida et al. 1993). Although there are arachnoid villi in the rat, they are small and mostly associated with the dorsal aspect of the olfactory bulbs (Kida et al. 1993). It is estimated that at least 50 % of cranial CSF in the rat drains to cervical lymph nodes by the nasal route, and this has implications for immunological reactions in the central nervous system (Cserr and Knopf 1992; Weller et al. 2010).

3.3.4 Drainage of Cerebrospinal Fluid via Arachnoid Villi and Granulations

In humans, the brain is much larger than in other mammals and the volume of CSF is much greater. Similarly, the sizes of arachnoid granulations and villi associated with the superior sagittal sinus and other cerebral and spinal sinuses are also much greater (Upton and Weller 1985). In humans, therefore, CSF drains directly back into

the blood, via arachnoid granulations and villi, as well as through the cribriform plate and nasal lymphatics. However, the balance of amounts of CSF draining via these two routes is still unclear (Johnston et al. 2004).

Structurally, arachnoid granulations and villi are extensions of the leptomeninges, protruding through perforations in the dura mater, into venous sinuses (Fig. 3.6a) (Kida and Weller 1993; Kida et al. 1988). CSF appears to percolate through a mesh of collagenous trabeculae, which is coated by arachnoid cells and located in the centre of the villus or granulation. The CSF finally reaches the venous endothelium via channels in a compacted layer of leptomeningeal cells that caps each granulation or villus (Upton and Weller 1985) (Fig. 3.6b, c). Tracer studies in monkeys suggest that CSF then drains through the venous endothelial cells by a bulk flow mechanism that entails the transport of macrovacuoles across the endothelial cells (Tripathi and Tripathi 1974). Despite the large size of some arachnoid granulations, drainage of CSF appears to be restricted to an apical area some 300 μm in diameter (Upton and Weller 1985).

3.3.5 Other Routes of Drainage of the Cerebrospinal Fluid

In addition to these major drainage pathways for CSF, through venous endothelium and via

Fig. 3.6 Arachnoid granulations in the human brain. (**a**) Diagram showing the relationship between the brain, subarachnoid space (*blue*) and the superior sagittal sinus (*SSS*). Arachnoid granulations extend through the dura from the subarachnoid space into the superior sagittal sinus and its lateral extension. (**b**) Histological section through the length of an arachnoid granulation. CSF from the subarachnoid space (*SAS*) passes into channels in the collagenous core (*red*) of the granulation and then through channels in the arachnoid cap of the granulation (**) to reach the endothelium lining the venous sinus. Haematoxylin van Gieson ×40. (**c**) Diagram showing the main features of an arachnoid granulation with channels leading from the subarachnoid space to the endothelium (*red*) of the superior sagittal sinus (SSS) (Reproduced with permission (a, c) from Dr. Shinya Kida and (b) from Upton and Weller (1985))

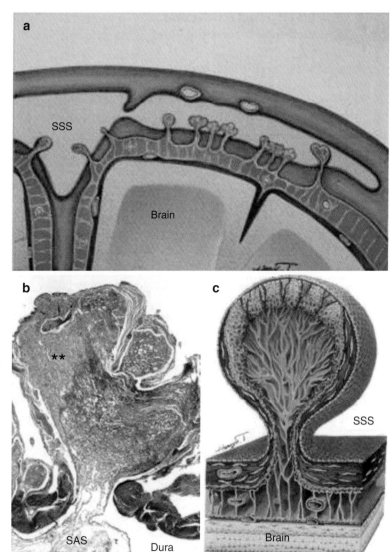

nasal and spinal lymphatics, some may also be absorbed directly into blood vessels in periventricular tissue (Johnston et al. 2004).

3.4 Interstitial Fluid (ISF)

In common with most other tissues of the body, the central nervous system has interstitial fluid within the extracellular spaces. In contrast with most other tissues, there are no conventional lymphatics in the central nervous system to drain interstitial fluid to regional lymph nodes. However, there are well-defined perivascular lymphatic pathways in the CNS by which interstitial fluid and solutes drain from the brain and spinal cord. These run along the basement membranes in the walls of capillaries and arteries, to reach regional lymph nodes (Weller et al. 2009b). Perivascular lymphatic drainage of interstitial fluid appears to be largely separate from the CSF drainage, with only 15 % of ISF leaking into the CSF (Szentistvanyi et al. 1984). This is contrary to some established concepts that the CSF acts as a sink for metabolites from the brain, a concept that needs to be re-examined in the light of more recent work on the drainage of interstitial fluid (Carare et al. 2008; Weller et al. 2009b).

3.4.1 The Blood–brain Barrier and Production of Interstitial Fluid

The blood–brain barrier (BBB) is one of the major systems that regulate homoeostasis and the constancy of the neuronal environment in the CNS. The BBB is located in the capillary endothelial cells of the brain and spinal cord and appears to be induced by the presence of perivascular astrocytic and neuronal processes; it is characterised by the tightness of intercellular junctions and the relative absence of trans-endothelial vesicular transport (Fig. 3.7a) (Abbott et al. 2006; Nag et al. 2011). Although water may pass freely across the blood–brain barrier, other molecules are actively transported from blood to brain; many substances are blocked from entering the CNS by the blood–brain barrier.

The volume of interstitial fluid in the human brain has been estimated at approximately 280 mL (Bergsneider 2001). It is produced partly from the blood and partly from the metabolites produced by the CNS tissue itself. The estimated range of drainage of ISF is 0.11–0.29 μL/min/g of tissue (Abbott 2004); this is comparable with the drainage of ISF from other organs (Szentistvanyi et al. 1984). Although the study of ISF has been largely overshadowed by concentration of research on CSF, the production and drainage of ISF has implications particularly for neurodegenerative disorders, neuroimmunological diseases (Weller et al. 2010), hydrocephalus and syringomyelia.

Fluid in the central nervous system is increased in three main types of oedema. *Cytotoxic oedema* occurs in the very early stages of damage to the CNS, particularly in grey matter, when cells are deprived of oxygen or glucose and die (Marmarou 2007). As ATP production ceases, ion pumps at the cell membrane no longer function and allow the influx of sodium and other electrolytes into the cell, followed by water, with the result that cells swell and burst. *Vasogenic oedema* results from the breakdown of the blood–brain barrier following tissue damage in the CNS and the outpouring of fluid, proteins and other solutes into the brain tissue (Marmarou 2007; Nag et al. 2011). The third type is *interstitial oedema*

(Weller 1998) due to the infusion of CSF into the white matter in hydrocephalus and syringomyelia (see Sects. 3.4.2 and 3.5.2). Accumulation of interstitial oedema fluid reflects the failure of interstitial fluid drainage pathways to accommodate increased ISF in the extracellular spaces of the CNS.

3.4.2 Circulation and Drainage of Interstitial Fluid

Fluid and nutrients cross the blood–brain barrier at the capillary endothelial cells and diffuse through the narrow extracellular spaces of the brain to supply neurons and glial cells (Abbott 2004; Abbott et al. 2006; Marmarou 2007) (Fig. 3.7a, b). Interstitial fluid and soluble metabolites then diffuse through the extracellular spaces (Syková and Nicholson 2008) to drain by bulk flow along the basement membranes in the walls of capillaries and arteries (Fig. 3.7b) within CNS tissue and leptomeninges (Carare et al. 2008; Weller et al. 2009b).

Evidence for perivascular lymphatic drainage pathways is derived from a series of experimental studies, initially using radioactive tracers that showed rapid elimination of interstitial fluid and solutes from the brain to cervical lymph nodes (Szentistvanyi et al. 1984). The detailed anatomy of the drainage pathway was later elucidated using fluorescent tracers and confocal microscopy (Carare et al. 2008). When fluorescent dextran is injected into grey matter of the mouse brain, it initially spreads diffusely through the extracellular spaces and then, within 5 min, is present in the basement membranes in the walls of capillaries and arteries in the brain and leptomeninges (Carare et al. 2008). It appears that interstitial fluid and solutes drain to the lymph nodes at the base of the skull from the walls of the carotid artery (Weller et al. 2009b). The motive force that drives perivascular drainage is thought to be the contrary, or reflection, wave that follows the pulse wave passing along cerebral artery walls; in this model, the contrary wave drives interstitial fluid out of the brain in the reverse direction to the flow of blood (Schley et al. 2006).

Fig. 3.7 Production and drainage of interstitial fluid. (**a**) Transmission electron micrograph of a capillary and surrounding brain tissue in the human cerebral cortex. Endothelial cells, joined by tight junctions (*TJ*), surround the lumen of the capillary and are coated on the abluminal surface by basement membrane (*BM*). Neuronal and glial processes are tightly packed together and separated by a very narrow extracellular space. ×14,000. (**b**) Diagram to show the passage of fluid and soluble nutrients from a capillary, through the narrow extracellular spaces, to neighbouring neurons (*red line*) and the drainage of fluid and soluble metabolites out of the brain along perivascular basement membranes in the walls of capillaries and arteries (*green line*) (Reproduced with permission (a) from Preston et al. (2003))

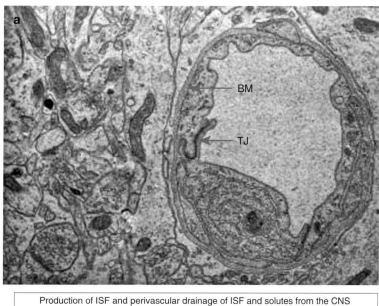

Production of ISF and perivascular drainage of ISF and solutes from the CNS

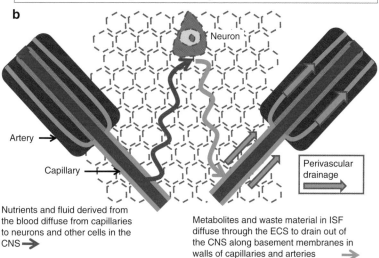

Nutrients and fluid derived from the blood diffuse from capillaries to neurons and other cells in the CNS ➡

Metabolites and waste material in ISF diffuse through the ECS to drain out of the CNS along basement membranes in walls of capillaries and arteries ➡

Although it is not possible to perform tracer studies in humans, there is one natural tracer that strongly indicates the presence of a perivascular lymphatic drainage pathway in the human brain, similar to that in the mouse. Amyloid-β (Aβ) is derived from amyloid precursor protein and is one of the peptides that accumulate within the brain in Alzheimer's disease (Duyckaerts and Dickson 2011). Aβ also accumulates in the walls of capillaries and arteries in the brain and leptomeninges as cerebral amyloid angiopathy (Biffi and Greenberg 2011; Weller et al. 2009c, 2011)

(Fig. 3.8a, b). The pattern of perivascular accumulation of Aβ is exactly the same as the distribution of fluorescent tracers defining interstitial fluid drainage pathways (Carare et al. 2008; Weller et al. 2009b). This strongly suggests that soluble Aβ is draining out of the brain along perivascular interstitial fluid drainage pathways (Biffi and Greenberg 2011; Weller et al. 2011). Furthermore, biochemical studies have shown that the accumulation of Aβ in the walls of the carotid arteries ceases at the base of the skull (Shinkai et al. 1995), suggesting that interstitial

Fig. 3.8 Amyloid-β is deposited in the perivascular interstitial fluid drainage pathways in human brain as cerebral amyloid angiopathy. (**a**) Deposition of amyloid-β (*brown*) in the basement membrane surrounding a cortical capillary. Immunocytochemistry for amyloid-β ×750. (**b**) Leptomeningeal artery (*top*) extends a branch into the cerebral cortex. Amyloid-β (*brown*) is deposited in the basement membranes between the smooth muscle cells of the tunica media (*arrow*) suggesting that soluble amyloid-β drains out of the brain along perivascular pathways. Immunocytochemistry for amyloid-β ×200 (Reproduced with permission (a) from Preston et al. (2003) and (b) from Weller et al. (1998))

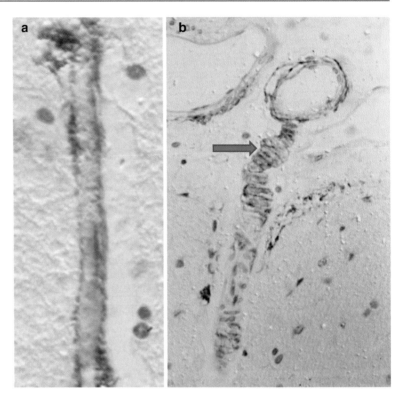

fluid with soluble Aβ drains from the artery wall to adjacent cervical lymph nodes in a similar way to that observed in experimental animals.

Although it is mainly the brain that is affected by amyloid angiopathy in Alzheimer's disease, amyloid also accumulates in artery walls in the spinal cord in the familial British dementia (Revesz et al. 2009). This suggests that interstitial fluid and solutes drain from the spinal cord along perivascular pathways by a system similar to that observed in the brain.

3.5 Pathology of the Cerebrospinal Fluid

Pathology of the CSF falls into two main categories (Weller 1998):

(a) Meningitis and haemorrhage in which inflammatory cells, erythrocytes or tumour cells are released into the CSF following infection, subarachnoid haemorrhage and invasion of the subarachnoid space by primary or metastatic tumours.

(b) Obstruction to the flow of CSF that results in hydrocephalus in the brain and syringomyelia in the spinal cord.

3.5.1 Meningitis and Subarachnoid Haemorrhage

Bacterial and fungal infections of the subarachnoid space result in an outpouring of polymorphonuclear leucocytes and protein from the blood into the CSF (Brown and Gray 2008; Weller 1998). Inflammatory cells remain mostly confined to the subarachnoid space and do not, in general, invade the underlying brain or spinal cord tissue. The pia mater, subpial collagen and the tightly packed astrocyte processes, which form the glia limitans on the surface of the brain and spinal cord, appear to act as a barrier to the entry of infection and inflammatory cells into the CNS. Often the only reaction at the surface of the brain is proliferation of microglia. In tuberculous meningitis, however, caseating granulomata not only involve the leptomeninges but also extend into the surface of the brain or involve cranial nerve roots; there is invasion of the CSF by lymphocytes and high protein levels may be attained in the CSF (Brown and Gray 2008). One of the major complications of both pyogenic and tuberculous meningitis is inflammation in the walls of leptomeningeal arteries, thrombosis of their lumina and infarction of the underlying CNS tissue (Brown and Gray 2008). In the long term, bacterial meningitis may result in fibrosis of the leptomeninges, interfering with drainage of cerebrospinal fluid and resulting in hydrocephalus and syringomyelia.

In viral infections and in autoimmune disease, such as Guillain-Barré syndrome, there is a rise in the level of protein and the presence of lymphocytes in the CSF, indicating a breakdown in the blood-CSF barrier. The major complications of these conditions are not so much in the CSF but result from the involvement of brain tissue (encephalitis) or involvement of cranial and spinal nerve roots (autoimmune neuritis) (Weller 1998).

Subarachnoid haemorrhage results from rupture of a saccular aneurysm or an arteriovenous malformation or may follow an episode of trauma (Ferrer et al. 2008). Fresh arterial blood floods into the subarachnoid space and may spread widely over the surface of the brain and spinal cord and fill the cisterns at the base of the brain. Frequently there is extension of the haemorrhage into the brain itself resulting in a fatal intracerebral haemorrhage. If the patient survives the initial episode, the arteries that are surrounded by blood in the subarachnoid space may go into spasm resulting in cerebral infarction. The long-term effects of the subarachnoid haemorrhage may be fibrosis of the leptomeninges, disturbance of CSF drainage and hydrocephalus (Ferrer et al. 2008).

Both primary and metastatic tumours can invade the cerebrospinal fluid, and the main effect of this invasion is damage to cranial and spinal nerves and extension of tumour cells into the surface of the brain or spinal cord. Tumours in the ventricles, aqueduct or subarachnoid space may also block the drainage of CSF, resulting in hydrocephalus (Weller 1998).

3.5.2 Obstruction of CSF Flow and Drainage

Interference with the flow and drainage of CSF within the ventricular system of the brain or in the subarachnoid spaces overlying the brain and spinal cord may result in hydrocephalus or syringomyelia. There are many causes of hydrocephalus affecting the brain, occurring at any time from infancy to old age (Harding and Copp 2008). Congenital malformations, primary and metastatic tumours in the brain and fibrosis or tumours in the subarachnoid space may all interfere with the flow of CSF from ventricles to the subarachnoid space and its elimination via arachnoid granulations and lymphatic drainage pathways. The resulting dilatation of the ventricular system is associated with a number of pathological changes in periventricular tissue, particularly around the lateral ventricles. In the acute stages of hydrocephalus, the ependyma becomes stretched and flattened and may rupture, allowing CSF to infuse freely into the periventricular white matter and resulting in interstitial oedema (Weller 1998) (Fig. 3.9a–c). This stage may be followed by destruction and gliosis of white matter and severe dilatation of the ventricles (Fig. 3.9d). In human infants that develop hydrocephalus before the sutures of the skull bones have fused, ventricular dilatation, head enlargement and severe attenuation of the cerebral mantle may ensue (Harding and Copp 2008). Damage to nerve fibres in periventricular white matter in hydrocephalus is difficult to detect as it occurs over a protracted time period. It is only in the acute stages of hydrocephalus, when the tissue is oedematous, that axonal degeneration is obvious (Weller and Shulman 1972). As the interstitial oedema of the acute stages of hydrocephalus subsides, the periventricular white matter becomes gliotic.

Compared with white matter, the grey matter of the cerebral cortex and the basal ganglia are relatively well preserved in hydrocephalus (Fig. 3.9b, c). This may be due to a number of factors including the restricted nature of the extracellular space in grey matter, which prevents the entry of fluid (Weller and Wisniewski 1969)

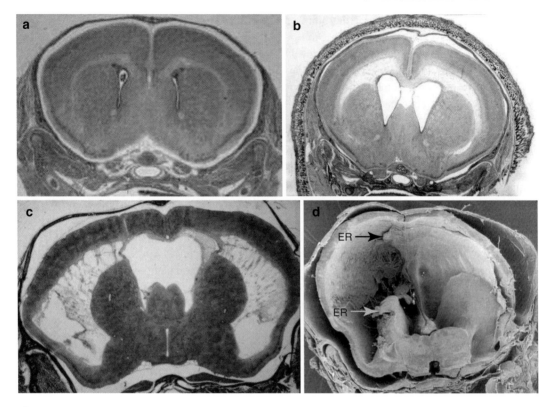

Fig. 3.9 Coronal sections of mouse brains showing progressive hydrocephalus with interstitial oedema and destruction of the white matter. (**a**) Normal mouse brain with small lateral ventricles. Haematoxylin and eosin ×8. (**b**) Early stages of hydrocephalus with dilatation of the lateral ventricles and severe interstitial oedema of the white matter. Haematoxylin and eosin ×8. (**c**) Severe destruction of the oedematous white matter in hydroceph- alus but with relatively good preservation of the central grey matter and cerebral cortex. Phosphotungstic acid haematoxylin (PTAH) ×8. (**d**) Scanning electron micrograph of a severely hydrocephalic mouse brain showing extensive dilatation of the lateral ventricles and rupture of the ependyma (*ER*) ×6 (Reproduced with permission (a–c) from Weller (1998))

and the more efficient perivascular drainage of interstitial fluid from grey matter compared with white matter (see Sect. 3.6.2)

3.6   Syringomyelia

Syringomyelia can be defined as an elongated fluid-filled cavity in the central regions of the spinal cord. Syrinx, a shepherd's (pan) pipe, describes the shape of the syringomyelic cyst, often tapered at the upper and lower ends. The cervical region of the spinal cord is most frequently involved, and four types of syringomyelia have been described (Fernandez et al. 2009):

Type I syringomyelia is associated with obstruc- tion of the foramen magnum with a Chiari type 1 malformation or another obstructive lesion, such as fibrosis or tumour.

Type II syringomyelia is without obstruction of the foramen magnum and is so-called idiopathic.

Type III syringomyelia is associated with other diseases of the spinal cord such as spinal tumours, traumatic lesions of the cord and spinal arachnoiditis.

Type IV is hydromyelia usually associated with hydrocephalus. Hydromyelia is when the central canal is dilated and may be lined by normal ependyma; in the later stages, the ependyma is

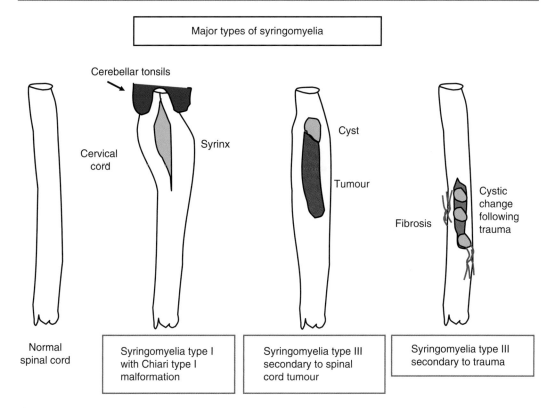

Fig. 3.10 Diagram to illustrate the major types of syringomyelia

replaced by glial tissue. Dilatation may be focal and more pronounced in the lumbar spinal cord. Hydromyelia may be an isolated finding and asymptomatic, or it may be part of a more complex syndrome (Harding and Copp 2008).

3.6.1 Aetiology of Syringomyelia

Figure 3.10 summarises the aetiology of the main types of syringomyelia.

Most cases of syringomyelia and almost 90 % of cases of type 1 syringomyelia are associated with Chiari malformations. Conversely, some 40–75 % of Chiari type 1 malformations have associated syringomyelia (Fernandez et al. 2009). Of the four types of Chiari malformation, type 1 has been defined radiographically as cerebellar tonsillar herniation, or ectopia of 5 mm or greater below the foramen magnum (Sekula et al. 2011; Ellison et al. 2004) (Figs. 3.11 and 3.12).

Maldevelopment of the skull results in reduced length of the occipital portion of the clivus, whereas the sphenoid portion is often normal. Platybasia and abnormalities of the occipital condyles and atlas are also seen. As a result of the malformations, the volume of the posterior fossa is effectively reduced, whereas the volume of the cerebellum is normal.

Cerebellar tonsillar herniation in the Chiari type 1 malformation appears to be the result of a normal cerebellar mass in a small posterior fossa and is thus secondary to the bony abnormality (Goel 2001). Syringomyelia in this case is a tertiary event and is thought to be due to disturbance of CSF flow through the foramen magnum (Heiss et al. 1999; Wetjen et al. 2008) (see Sect. 5.1.2). Other types of Chiari malformation may be associated with further abnormalities of the skull or brain, and in Chiari type 2 malformation, there is an associated myelomeningocoele and hydrocephalus (Harding and Copp 2008).

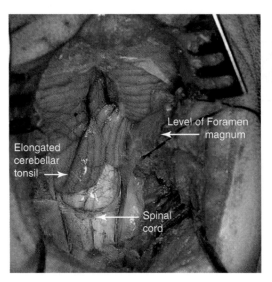

Fig. 3.11 A view of Chiari type 1 malformation at surgery. The posterior aspect of the cerebellum and spinal cord has been exposed by removing the bone of the foramen magnum. Elongated cerebellar tonsils extend through the foramen magnum posterior to the spinal cord (Reproduced with permission from Ellison et al. (2004))

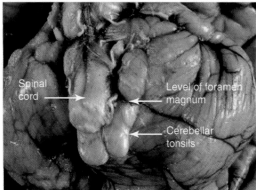

Fig. 3.12 Chiari type 1 malformation in a post-mortem brain. A fixed post-mortem brain at the level of the foramen magnum, viewed from the front. The spinal cord has been cut away to reveal the elongated cerebellar tonsils on its dorsal aspect (Reproduced with permission from Ellison et al. (2004))

Patients with a posterior fossa arachnoid cyst may develop acquired Chiari malformation and syringomyelia due to displacement of the cerebellar tonsils through the foramen magnum (Galarza et al. 2010).

Although the majority of cases of syringomyelia appear to be due to cranio-cervical malformations that are present at birth, the average age of presentation is approximately 35 years (Fernandez et al. 2009).

3.6.2 Pathology of Syringomyelia

Exposure of the syringomyelic spinal cord at surgery or at post-mortem usually results in collapse of the cavity. The full extent of a syrinx is, therefore, more adequately visualised by MRI. At post-mortem examination, the spinal cord in cross-section reveals a cystic space in the centre of the cord that is often asymmetrical and extending laterally towards one or other dorsal root entry zone (Fig. 3.13a). Microscopically, the syrinx may be totally separate from the

central canal or may be partly lined by ependyma. A syrinx of long-standing is often lined by a layer of dense gliotic scar tissue (Fig. 3.13b) (Harding and Copp 2008). Acute syringomyelia induced experimentally (Williams and Weller 1973) shows disruption of the ependyma of the spinal cord, interstitial oedema of the cord tissue surrounding the syrinx and associated nerve fibre damage and reactive astrocytosis (Fig. 3.14). This suggests that fluid may be forced into the tissue around the syrinx as in hydrocephalus (Sect. 3.4.2). Similar tissue oedema may be seen in syringomyelia in humans and other species (Harding and Copp 2008).

At the level of the syrinx, ascending sensory tracts are often damaged, including those in the dorsal columns and the spinothalamic tracts. Locally, anterior horn motor neurons may be damaged. Remotely, above and below the syrinx, long tracts may show changes due to the damage at the level of the syrinx (Harding and Copp 2008).

In type III syringomyelia, there is a cavity in the cord associated with tumour, trauma or arachnoiditis. Oedema fluid derived from a spinal tumour appears to be a precursor of a tumour-associated syringomyelia (Baggenstos et al. 2007) in which the syrinx may be irregular in shape and lined by tumour. Following spinal cord

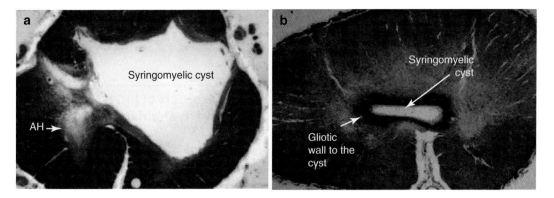

Fig. 3.13 Transverse sections of spinal cords with syringomyelia. (**a**) A large asymmetrical syringomyelic cyst extends towards one dorsal root entry zone. Anterior horn of grey matter (*AH*) on the opposite side of the cord. Weigert-Pal stain ×4. (**b**) Although this long-standing syringomyelic cyst in the spinal cord is small, it is surrounded by a thick layer of purple-stained gliosis (*arrow*). Phosphotungstic acid haematoxylin (PTAH) ×6

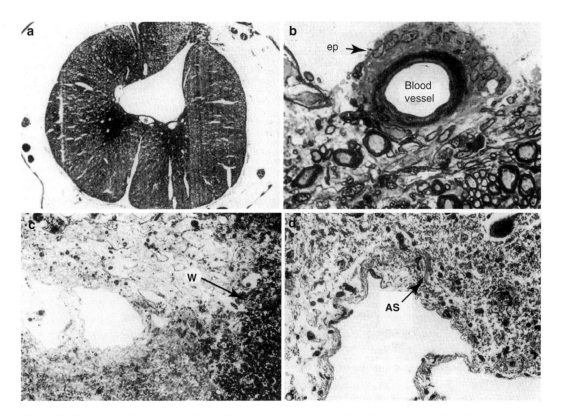

Fig. 3.14 Experimental syringomyelia.(**a**) Transverse section of the spinal cord showing a syringomyelic cyst extending towards one dorsal root entry zone. Haematoxylin and eosin ×8. (**b**) Histology of the wall of the syrinx showing disrupted ependyma (*ep*) partly surrounding a blood vessel. Toluidine blue-stained resin section ×720. (**c**) Interstitial oedema in the acute stage of syringomyelia; a damaged nerve fibre is present at the edge of the oedematous region (*W*). Toluidine blue-stained resin section ×120. (**d**) The oedematous wall of the cyst shows reactive astrocytosis (*AS*). Haematoxylin and eosin ×120 (Reproduced with permission from Williams and Weller (1973))

injury, a syringomyelic cavity may be associated with arachnoiditis and tethering of the spinal cord or may be due to myelomalacia resulting from direct damage or ischemia of the cord linked to the trauma (Falci et al. 2009).

3.6.3 Dynamics of CSF Movement at the Foramen Magnum

Recent data on the dynamics of CSF flow at the foramen magnum are mainly derived from phase-contrast MRI (Ambarki et al. 2007; Battal et al. 2011). The model presented is that of a rigid skull containing three incompressible elements, namely brain, CSF and blood (Ambarki et al. 2007). CSF has a viscosity close to that of water and is distributed in three spaces that communicate with each other, the cerebral ventricles and the cranial and spinal subarachnoid spaces. Both the brain and spinal cord float in the CSF, and the surface of the CNS is crossed by a vascular network of arteries and veins. The overall intracranial volume remains constant, and the Monro-Kellie doctrine describes the blood, brain and CSF as incompressible. If the volume of one of the intracranial components increases, static mechanisms force one or both of the other components out of the cranial cavity, to maintain a constant intracranial volume. Pulsations of intracranial arteries result in a cyclical expansion of cerebral blood volume, which is transferred as pulsations in the CSF (Ambarki et al. 2007). Maintenance of intracranial volume is by expulsion of CSF from the cranial to the spinal subarachnoid space, which itself is expandable due to distensibility of the spinal dural sac, which acts as a mediator of compliance. CSF oscillates through the foramen magnum in response to pulsatile cerebral blood flow. This results in a coupling between changes in blood volume and CSF volume (Ambarki et al. 2007). Disturbance of the normal free flow of CSF through the foramen magnum appears to be a major factor responsible for the formation of a syrinx in the cervical spinal cord (Heiss et al. 1999; Wetjen et al. 2008). However, failure of absorption or drainage of extracellular fluid may also play a role, either in the pathogenesis of a syringomyelic cavity or in maintaining the volume of fluid within it (Koyanagi and Houkin 2010).

3.7 Disorders of Interstitial Fluid and Its Drainage

Maintaining a constant external environment for neurons within the central nervous system depends upon homoeostasis of the interstitial fluid, itself achieved through the control of nutrients, metabolites and other soluble materials in the extracellular compartment of the CNS. Entry of fluid and solutes into the interstitial fluid is controlled by the blood–brain barrier (Abbott 2004), and their elimination is along perivascular pathways in the narrow basement membranes in the walls of capillaries and arteries (see Sect. 3.3.2). Drainage of antigens by this route from the brain and spinal cord may play a role in immunological protection of the central nervous system and in neuroimmunological disease (Weller et al. 2009b, 2010). Equally important are the neurodegenerative diseases, such as Alzheimer's disease, in the category of *protein-elimination failure arteriopathies* (*PEFA*) that are associated with failure of drainage of interstitial fluid and solutes from the CNS (Weller et al. 2008, 2009b; Carare 2013).

3.7.1 Cerebral Amyloid Angiopathy and Alzheimer's Disease

Alzheimer's disease is characterised, pathologically, by the accumulation of neurofibrillary tangles within neurons and deposition of insoluble amyloid-β (Aβ) in brain parenchyma and in artery walls, as cerebral amyloid angiopathy. Some 5 % of cases of Alzheimer's disease are familial disorders of Aβ production, caused by defects in the amyloid precursor protein and presenilin genes (Bertram and Tanzi 2011). In the majority of cases of Alzheimer's disease, however, age is the major risk factor and failure of elimination of Aβ from the brain with age appears to be a major causative factor in the disease. Several mechanisms for the elimination of Aβ from the brain have been identified; they include the enzyme neprilysin in brain parenchyma and vessel walls, absorption of Aβ into the blood and drainage of soluble Aβ out of the brain along perivascular pathways (Weller et al. 2009c, 2011). As cerebral arteries age, elasticity in the walls is reduced and elimination of Aβ along perivascular pathways appears to be less efficient (Schley et al. 2006; Weller et al. 2009a). Failure of elimination of Aβ results in the deposition of Aβ as insoluble plaques (Duyckaerts and Dickson 2011), a rise in soluble Aβ in brain tissue (Lue et al. 1999; McLean et al. 1999) and loss of homoeostasis of the neuronal environment, leading to the cognitive decline we see in Alzheimer's disease. Although it is not the only factor in the aetiology of Alzheimer's disease, failure of perivascular drainage of soluble Aβ appears to play an important role.

Deposition of amyloid is mainly in the cortex and to a lesser extent in the basal ganglia, but the white matter is also affected in Alzheimer's disease. Leukoaraiosis is the accumulation of fluid in the subcortical white matter that is detectable by CT and MRI in a proportion of patients with Alzheimer's disease. The blood supply for subcortical white matter is from leptomeningeal arteries on the surface of the brain; long thin arteries penetrate the cortex to supply the underlying white matter. Accumulation of fluid in the subcortical white matter in leukoaraiosis is associated with severe cerebral amyloid angiopathy of leptomeningeal arteries (Roher et al. 2003); it appears that deposition of Aβ in artery walls interferes with the drainage of fluid from the subcortical white matter.

3.7.2 Interrelationships Between Cerebrospinal Fluid and Interstitial Fluid

CSF fills the ventricles and cerebral and spinal subarachnoid spaces, functioning as a buoyancy fluid for the brain and spinal cord. Interstitial fluid plays a role in maintenance of homoeostasis within the parenchyma of the brain and spinal cord. Although largely separate in their functions

and drainage systems, there are areas of interface between CSF and interstitial fluid. On the one hand, a small proportion of interstitial fluid leaks into the CSF during drainage along the artery walls (Szentistvanyi et al. 1984), and on the other hand, tracers, such as horseradish peroxidase, injected into the subarachnoid space, diffuse along perivascular spaces into the CNS (Rennels et al. 1985). Despite the connections between the two fluids, failure of drainage of one is not compensated by increased drainage of the other. In acute hydrocephalus, for example, CSF enters periventricular white matter resulting in interstitial oedema. As outlined in Sect. 3.4.2 and Fig. 3.9, interstitial oedema affects the white matter, but grey matter areas such as the basal ganglia and cortex are largely spared in hydrocephalus. This suggests that drainage of interstitial fluid along artery walls from grey matter is maintained in hydrocephalus, whereas such a drainage system in the white matter is overloaded and cannot cope with the infusion of CSF. It is still unclear why CSF, accumulating within the ventricles of the brain in hydrocephalus and in the spinal cord in syringomyelia, does not drain along perivascular pathways in the surrounding brain or spinal cord tissue. It is possible that perivascular drainage of interstitial fluid is limited and is unable to cope with the excess volume of CSF when drainage of the latter is impaired. Similarly, the failure of elimination of Aβ by perivascular drainage from grey matter is not compensated by elimination of fluid and Aβ into the CSF. In fact, the level of Aβ is reduced in the CSF in Alzheimer's disease (Mawuenyega et al. 2010).

Conclusions

Balanced production and elimination of CSF plays a significant role in maintaining physical stability of the brain and spinal cord. Similarly, the balance between production and elimination of interstitial fluid ensures the stable tissue environment for neurological activity. Disturbances in the elimination of CSF and interstitial fluid result in retention of fluid and solutes in the CNS. CSF and interstitial fluid are largely separate in their production and elimination, and although there is an interface between the two fluids systems, neither system appears to compensate fully for deficiencies in the other. Facilitating drainage of CSF would have major effects in the treatment of hydrocephalus and syringomyelia, whereas facilitating the elimination of interstitial fluid and the soluble metabolites that it contains would have a major effect on the treatment of neurodegenerative diseases. On the other hand, increasing the capacity to drain extracellular fluid along perivascular pathways may reduce the fluid in hydrocephalic ventricles and syringomyelic cysts, and increasing the drainage of interstitial fluid into CSF would facilitate the elimination of soluble metabolites from the brain in cerebral amyloid angiopathy and Alzheimer's disease.

References

Abbott NJ (2004) Evidence for bulk flow of brain interstitial fluid: significance for physiology and pathology. Neurochem Int 45:545–552

Abbott NJ, Rönnbäck L, Hansson E (2006) Astrocyte-endothelial interactions at the blood–brain barrier. Nat Rev Neurosci 7:41–53

Alcolado JC, Moore IE, Weller RO (1986) Calcification in the human choroid plexus, meningiomas and pineal gland. Neuropathol Appl Neurobiol 12:235–250

Alcolado R, Weller RO, Parrish EP et al (1988) The cranial arachnoid and pia mater in man: anatomical and ultrastructural observations. Neuropathol Appl Neurobiol 14:1–17

Ambarki K, Baledent O, Kongolo G et al (2007) A new lumped-parameter model of cerebrospinal hydrodynamics during the cardiac cycle in healthy volunteers. IEEE Trans Biomed Eng 54:483–491

Ameli PA, Madan M, Chigurupati S et al (2012) Effect of acetazolamide on aquaporin-1 and fluid flow in cultured choroid plexus. Acta Neurochir Suppl 113:59–64

Baggenstos MA, Butman JA, Oldfield EH et al (2007) Role of edema in peritumoral cyst formation. Neurosurg Focus 22:E9

Battal B, Kocaoglu M, Bulakbasi N et al (2011) Cerebrospinal fluid flow imaging by using phase-contrast MR technique. Br J Radiol 84:758–765

Bergsneider M (2001) Evolving concepts of cerebrospinal fluid. Neurosurg Clin N Am 36:631–638

Bertram L, Tanzi RE (2011) Genetics of Alzheimer's disease. In: Dickson DW, Weller RO (eds) Neurodegeneration: the molecular pathology of dementia and movement disorders. Wiley-Blackwell, Chichester, pp 51–61

Biffi A, Greenberg SM (2011) Cerebral amyloid angiopathy: a systematic review. J Clin Neurol 7:1–9

Brown E, Gray F (2008) Bacterial infections. In: Love S, Louis DN, Ellison DW (eds) Greenfield's neuropathology. Hodder Arnold, London, pp 1391–1445

Carare RO, Bernardes-Silva M, Newman TA et al (2008) Solutes, but not cells, drain from the brain parenchyma along basement membranes of capillaries and arteries. Significance for cerebral amyloid angiopathy and neuroimmunology. Neuropathol Appl Neurobiol 34:131–144

Carare RO, Hawkes CA, Jeffrey M, Kalaria RN, Weller RO (2013) Cerebral amyloid angiopathy, prion angiopathy, CADASIL and the spectrum of protein elimination failure angiopathies (PEFA) in neurodegenerative disease with a focus on therapy. Neuropathology and applied neurobiology 39(6): 593–611. doi:10.1111/nan.12042

Cserr HF, Knopf PM (1992) Cervical lymphatics, the blood–brain barrier and the immunoreactivity of the brain: a new view. Immunol Today 13:507–512

Davson H, Welch K, Segal MB (1987) Physiology and pathophysiology of the cerebrospinal fluid. Churchill Livingstone, Edinburgh

Del Bigio MR (1995) The ependyma: a protective barrier between brain and cerebrospinal fluid. Glia 14:1–13

Duyckaerts C, Dickson DW (2011) Neuropathology of Alzheimer's disease and its variants. In: Dickson DW, Weller RO (eds) Neurodegeneration: the molecular pathology of dementia and movement disorders. Wiley-Blackwell, Chichester, pp 62–91

Ellison D, Love S, Chimelli L et al (2004) Neuropathology: a reference text of CNS pathology, 2nd edn. Mosby, Edinburgh

Falci SP, Indeck C, Lammertse DP (2009) Posttraumatic spinal cord tethering and syringomyelia: surgical treatment and long-term outcome. J Neurosurg Spine 11:445–460

Fernandez AA, Guerrero AI, Martinez MI et al (2009) Malformations of the craniocervical junction (Chiari type I and syringomyelia: classification, diagnosis and treatment). BMC Musculoskelet Disord 10(Suppl 1):S1

Ferrer I, Kaste M, Kalimo H (2008) Vascular diseases. In: Love S, Louis DN, Ellison DW (eds) Greenfield's neuropathology. Hodder Arnold, London, pp 121–240

Galarza M, López-Guerrero AL, Martínez-Lage JF (2010) Posterior fossa arachnoid cysts and cerebellar tonsillar descent: short review. Neurosurg Rev 33:305–314

Goel A (2001) Is syringomyelia pathology or a natural protective phenomenon? J Postgrad Med 47:87–88

Harding BN, Copp AJ (2008) Malformations. In: Love S, Louis DN, Ellison DW (eds) Greenfield's neuropathology. Hodder Arnold, London, pp 335–479

Heiss JD, Patronas N, DeVroom HL et al (1999) Elucidating the pathophysiology of syringomyelia. J Neurosurg Pediatr 91:553–562

Hutchings M, Weller RO (1986) Anatomical relationships of the pia mater to cerebral blood vessels in man. J Neurosurg 65:316–325

Johanson CE, Duncan JA 3rd, Klinge PM et al (2008) Multiplicity of cerebrospinal fluid functions: new challenges in health and disease. Cerebrospinal Fluid Res 5:10

Johnston M, Zakharov A, Papaiconomou C et al (2004) Evidence of connections between cerebrospinal fluid and nasal lymphatic vessels in humans, non-human primates and other mammalian species. Cerebrospinal Fluid Res 1:2–15

Kida S, Weller RO (1993) Morphological basis for fluid transport through an around ependymal, arachnoidal and glial cells. In: Raimondi AJ (ed) Intracranial cyst lesions. Springer, New York, pp 37–52

Kida S, Yamashima T, Kubota T et al (1988) A light and electron microscopic and immunohistochemical study of human arachnoid villi. J Neurosurg 69:429–435

Kida S, Pantazis A, Weller RO (1993) CSF drains directly from the subarachnoid space into nasal lymphatics in the rat. Anatomy, histology and immunological significance. Neuropathol Appl Neurobiol 19:480–488

Koyanagi I, Houkin K (2010) Pathogenesis of syringomyelia associated with Chiari type 1 malformation: review of evidences and proposal of a new hypothesis. Neurosurg Rev 33:271–284

Lue LF, Kuo YM, Roher AE et al (1999) Soluble amyloid beta peptide concentration as a predictor of synaptic change in Alzheimer's disease. Am J Pathol 155:853–862

Marmarou A (2007) A review of progress in understanding the pathophysiology and treatment of brain edema. Neurosurg Focus 22:E1

Mawuenyega KG, Sigurdson W, Ovod V et al (2010) Decreased clearance of CNS beta-amyloid in Alzheimer's disease. Science 330:1774

McLean CA, Cherny RA, Fraser FW et al (1999) Soluble pool of Abeta amyloid as a determinant of severity of neurodegeneration in Alzheimer's disease. Ann Neurol 46:860–866

Nag S, Kapadia A, Stewart DJ (2011) Review: molecular pathogenesis of blood–brain barrier breakdown in acute brain injury. Neuropathol Appl Neurobiol 37:3–23

Nicholas DS, Weller RO (1988) The fine anatomy of the human spinal meninges. A light and scanning electron microscopy study. J Neurosurg 69:276–282

Preston SD, Steart PV, Wilkinson A et al (2003) Capillary and arterial amyloid angiopathy in Alzheimer's disease: defining the perivascular route for the elimination of amyloid beta from the human brain. Neuropathol Appl Neurobiol 29:106–117

Rennels ML, Gregory TF, Blaumanis OR et al (1985) Evidence for a 'paravascular' fluid circulation in the mammalian central nervous system, provided by the rapid distribution of tracer protein throughout the brain from the subarachnoid space. Brain Res 326: 47–63

Revesz T, Holton JL, Lashley T et al (2009) Genetics and molecular pathogenesis of sporadic and hereditary cerebral amyloid angiopathies. Acta Neuropathol 118:115–130

Roher AE, Kuo Y-M, Esh C et al (2003) Cortical and leptomeningeal cerebrovascular amyloid and white matter pathology in Alzheimer's disease. Mol Med 9:112–122

Schley D, Carare-Nnadi R, Please CP et al (2006) Mechanisms to explain the reverse perivascular transport of solutes out of the brain. J Theor Biol 238: 962–974

Sekula RFJ, Arnone GD, Crocker C et al (2011) The pathogenesis of Chiari I malformation and syringomyelia. Neurol Res 33:232–239

Shinkai Y, Yoshimura M, Ito Y et al (1995) Amyloid beta-proteins 1–40 and 1-42(43) in the soluble fraction of extra- and intracranial blood vessels. Ann Neurol 38: 421–428

Syková E, Nicholson C (2008) Diffusion in brain extracellular space. Physiol Rev 88:1277–1340

Szentistvanyi I, Patlak CS, Ellis RA et al (1984) Drainage of interstitial fluid from different regions of rat brain. Am J Physiol 246:F835–F844

Tripathi BJ, Tripathi RC (1974) Vacuolar transcellular channels as a drainage pathway for cerebrospinal fluid. J Physiol 239:195–206

Upton ML, Weller RO (1985) The morphology of cerebrospinal fluid drainage pathways in human arachnoid granulations. J Neurosurg 63:867–875

Weller RO (1995) Fluid compartments and fluid balance in the central nervous system. In: Williams PL (ed) Gray's anatomy. Churchill Livingstone, Edinburgh, pp 1202–1224

Weller RO (1998) Pathology of cerebrospinal fluid and interstitial fluid of the CNS: significance for Alzheimer disease, prion disorders and multiple sclerosis. J Neuropathol Exp Neurol 57:885–894

Weller RO (2005) Microscopic morphology and histology of the human meninges. Morphologie 89:22–34

Weller RO, Shulman K (1972) Infantile hydrocephalus: clinical, histological, and ultrastructural study of brain damage. J Neurosurg 36:255–265

Weller RO, Wisniewski H (1969) Histological and ultrastructural changes with experimental hydrocephalus in adult rabbits. Brain 92:819–828

Weller RO, Massey A, Newman TA et al (1998) Cerebral amyloid angiopathy: amyloid beta accumulates in putative interstitial fluid drainage pathways in Alzheimer's disease. Am J Pathol 153:725–733

Weller RO, Subash M, Preston SD et al (2008) Perivascular drainage of amyloid-beta peptides from the brain and its failure in cerebral amyloid angiopathy and Alzheimer's disease. Brain Pathol 18:253–266

Weller RO, Boche D, Nicoll JA (2009a) Microvasculature changes and cerebral amyloid angiopathy in Alzheimer's disease and their potential impact on therapy. Acta Neuropathol 118:87–102

Weller RO, Djuanda E, Yow HY et al (2009b) Lymphatic drainage of the brain and the pathophysiology of neurological disease. Acta Neuropathol 117:1–14

Weller RO, Preston SD, Subash M et al (2009c) Cerebral amyloid angiopathy in the aetiology and immunotherapy of Alzheimer disease. Alzheimers Res Ther 1(2):6

Weller RO, Galea I, Carare RO et al (2010) Pathophysiology of the lymphatic drainage of the central nervous system: implications for pathogenesis and therapy of multiple sclerosis. Pathophysiology 17:295–306

Weller RO, Love S, Nicoll JAR (2011) Elimination of Aβ from the brain, its failure in Alzheimer's disease and implications for therapy. In: Dickson DW, Weller RO (eds) Neurodegeneration: the molecular pathology of dementia and movement disorders. Wiley-Blackwell, Chichester, pp 97–101

Wetjen NM, Heiss JD, Oldfield EH (2008) Time course of syringomyelia resolution following decompression of Chiari malformation type I. J Neurosurg Pediatr 1: 118–123

Williams B, Weller RO (1973) Syringomyelia produced by intramedullary fluid injection in dogs. J Neurol Neurosurg Psychiatry 36:467–477

Wolburg H, Paulus W (2010) Choroid plexus: biology and pathology. Acta Neuropathol 119:75–88

Yool AJ (2007) Aquaporins: multiple roles in the central nervous system. Neuroscientist 13:470–485

Zhang ET, Inman CB, Weller RO (1990) Interrelationships of the pia mater and the perivascular (Virchow-Robin) spaces in the human cerebrum. J Anat 170:111–123

Developmental Anatomy

4

Guirish A. Solanki

Contents

G.A. Solanki
Department of Paediatric Neurosurgery,
Birmingham Children's Hospital,
Birmingham, B4 6NH England, UK
e-mail: guirish.solanki@bch.nhs.uk

4.1 Early Development of the Nervous System

Formation of the central nervous system (CNS) during embryonic life takes place in distinct stages. The three most important are gastrulation, primary neurulation and secondary neurulation. Gastrulation includes the ability of the ectodermal layer to develop the neuroectoderm, by a process known as neural induction. Primary neurulation forms the whole of the CNS, down to and including the conus, by closure of the developing neural tube. Secondary neurulation is the stage during which the cauda equina and the sacral elements are formed by a process of cavitation of a caudal cell mass. Secondary neurulation is not important for the development of Chiari or syringomyelia, which are both effects of primary neurulation.

4.1.1 Gastrulation

Early in the 2nd week of development, prior to implantation of the blastocyst, its inner cell mass (the embryoblast) develops into a two-layered structure, made up of a primitive ectoderm (the epiblast) and a primitive endoderm (the hypoblast). By the beginning of the third week, a 'primitive streak' has appeared on the dorsal surface of the ectodermal layer. This structure develops at what will become the caudal end of the embryo, but at the cranial end of the streak itself, a distinct elevation forms, as a result of proliferation of cells. This structure is known as

G. Flint, C. Rusbridge (eds.), *Syringomyelia*,
DOI 10.1007/978-3-642-13706-8_4, © Springer-Verlag Berlin Heidelberg 2014

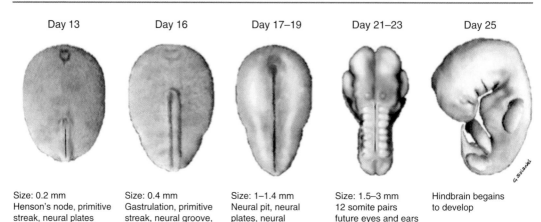

Day 13	Day 16	Day 17–19	Day 21–23	Day 25
Size: 0.2 mm Henson's node, primitive streak, neural plates (caudal end)	Size: 0.4 mm Gastrulation, primitive streak, neural groove, trilaminar embryo	Size: 1–1.4 mm Neural pit, neural plates, neural groove visible	Size: 1.5–3 mm 12 somite pairs future eyes and ears are obvious	Hindbrain begains to develop

Fig. 4.1 Gastrulation and primary neurulation Embryo stages from development of Hensen's node on day 13 to closure of anterior neuropore on day 25

Hensen's node, and cells arising here begin to migrate into the interface between the ectoderm and endoderm, to form the mesodermal layer. This stage is known as gastrulation as it results in the formation of the primitive gut cavity, but it also defines the period in which the three basic germ cell layers form. Those mesodermal cells that migrate along the midline give rise to the notochord. The immediately overlying ectodermal cells then begin to develop into the neural plate, by a process referred to as neural induction. This neural plate becomes the source of the majority of neurons and glial cells in the mature mammal (Fig. 4.1).

4.1.2 Primary Neurulation

Further development of the neural plate begins the process of primary neurulation. This sees the plate begins to invaginate, between neural folds on each side of the midline. Cells at the top of the neural folds are referred to as neural crest cells. The neural folds then begin to fuse at several points, concomitant with the appearance of the budding somites.[1]

The main driving force for the shaping of the neural plate seems to be a medially directed movement of cells, with intercalation in the midline, leading to a narrowing and lengthening of the plate, a process known as convergent extension[2] (Keller et al. 2000; Copp et al. 2003), illustrated in Fig. 4.2. The result of this process is the formation of a tubular structure, below the surface of the ectoderm, by week 4 of development (Table 4.1). The cranial end of this neural tube (the anterior neuropore) seals by the 25th day, and its location, in the mature central nervous system, is represented by the lamina terminalis. The caudal end of the neural tube (the posterior neuropore) closes between 26 and 28 days (Norman et al. 1995) (Fig. 4.3).

This infolding of the neural plate is usually described as starting at the craniocervical junction and proceeding both rostrally and caudally, in a 'zipper'-like fashion. Recent evidence suggests, however, that the closure actually occurs simul-

---

[1] A somite, or primitive segment, is a division of the body of an animal. Somites form the vertebral column, dermis and skeletal muscle. They are derived from the paraxial mesoderm.

[2] Convergent extension is a mechanism of cellular morphogenesis, whereby cells within a structure converge and extend possibly by the action of actin-myosin contractions at cellular boundaries. The process is under the control of myosin regulatory chains found at these boundaries, which direct contraction of cell boundaries perpendicular to the axis of elongation and elongation along this axis. Structures that undergo convergent extension become elongated and thinned out without any net increase in cell volume or number. It is an important mechanism in the formation, extension and shaping of the neural tube.

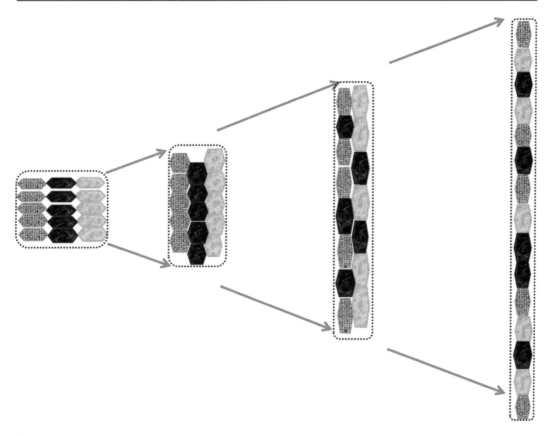

Fig. 4.2 Illustration depicting the mechanism of convergent extension. This results in gene-regulated convergence (narrowing) along one axis and extension (lengthening or elongation) in a perpendicular axis. The three cell layers first converge and intercalate causing constriction. Further morphogenesis occurs with contraction of exact cell boundaries perpendicular to growth direction and redistribution of cells into two layers along the growth axis with elongation in a sequential fashion. Finally reducing the cellular layer numbers on one axis (convergence) and adding these cells along the perpendicular elongation axis causes extension. Both gastrulation and primary neurulation cellular morphogenesis depend on effective convergent extension

Table 4.1 Stages in cranial neural tube closure

Shape of neural tube	Stage	Process
Biconvex	Inner biconvex morphology of neural folds	Expansion of the cranial mesoderm
Transitional	Dorsolateral neural plate bending	Under sonic hedgehog homologue signalling the apices of the neural folds begin to come into apposition in the dorsal midline
Biconcave	Midline approximation of neural folds	Contraction of subapical actin microfilaments is thought to be the process that pulls the folds together towards the midline
	Dorsal neural crest cell migration	Emigration of the neural crest occurs as the midline approximates and thins down. Timing differs between cranial and spinal ends
	Ventral plate neuroepithelial cell deposition	Maintenance of a proliferative neuroepithelium
Tubular	Midline neural plate	Believed to be an apoptotic process
	Neural tube separation from dorsal epithelium	Apical apoptotic cell death is involved in epithelial remodelling following closure

Fig. 4.3 Primary neurulation.
The ectoderm germ layer by a
process of columnarisation
forms a thickening, the flat
neural plate. The neural plate
then grooves and develops a
medial hinge point, folds in
upon itself, developing
bilateral dorsolateral hinge
points and neural crests. As
the neural folds are pushed
upwards and towards the
midline by the expanding
paraxial mesoderm, the neural
crest cells separate from the
neuroectoderm which begins
to separate from the ectoderm
by a process of apoptosis.
This process is achieved by
neural plate switching from
expressing E-cadherin to
N-cadherin and N-CAM
expression. This allows the
approximating neural tube in
the midline to recognise as the
same tissue and close the
neural tube

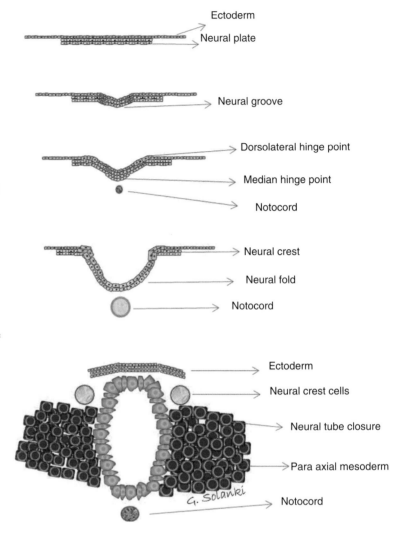

taneously at multiple sites. In the mouse embryo, for example, neural tube closure initiates at three distinct locations, with an intermittent pattern of subsequent closure (Golden and Chernoff 1993). A study of neural tube defects in human embryos indicated that five closure sites exist (Van Allen et al. 1993), and other investigators have confirmed these views (Ahmad and Mahapatra 2009; Nakatsu et al. 2000), suggesting that the mode of closure in humans is different from that in other animal species. Sites identified as points of initiation include the future cervical region, the mesencephalic-rhombencephalic boundary, the anterior neuropore and the posterior neuropore. The existence of multiple simultaneous closure points help to explain why neural tube defects

occur preferentially at certain sites. Examples include the lumbosacral myelomeningocoele and frontal and occipital meningo-encephalocoeles.

It is also becoming clear that neural tube closure is dependent on an apoptotic process, rather than just a proliferative growth of cells that meet in the midline. In an experimental study in chicken embryos, the apoptosis inhibitor Zvad-fmk[3] was shown to prevent cell death in the neural plate and to inhibit neural tube closure.

---

[3] Zvad-fmk   (carbobenzoxy-valyl-alanyl-aspartyl-[O-methyl]-fluoromethylketone) is a cell-permeant pan caspase inhibitor that irreversibly binds to the catalytic site of caspase proteases. In this way it inhibits the induction of apoptosis.

Furthermore, the way in which brain and spinal cord components of the neural tube close differs. In the spinal region, the neural tube closes first, and outward migration of neural crest cells only begins several hours after this process is complete (Franz 1992). This contrasts with the cranial closure, where outward migration of the neural crest cells occurs before closure. Indeed, it is likely that neural crest migration is required to trigger the neural tube closure at this level.

Primary neurulation subserves the future development of the whole of the central nervous system. As a result, the vast majority of CNS anomalies, ranging from fatal deformities such as anencephaly to open neural tube defects, occur during this stage. The causes of most of these brain anomalies are still unknown (Norman et al. 1995), although advances in genetics and developmental embryology, as well as various clinical studies, looking at congenital conditions and their causes, genetic or otherwise, have found new mutations. Their effects on children and adults with brain anomalies or malfunctions are identifying an increasing number of responsible chromosomal aberrations, single gene mutations and extrinsic teratogens.

The period of time for which a deformed embryo survives is determined by the type and location of the neural tube defects. Almost all embryos with total dysraphism die by 5 weeks of gestation, and those with an opening over the rhombencephalon die by 6.5 weeks. In contrast, those with a defect at the frontal and parietal regions may survive beyond 7 weeks (Nakatsu et al. 2000). For example, even when there is severe failure of neural tube closure anteriorly, such as leading to anencephaly, the foetus may survive even to birth, although the condition is always fatal thereafter. This suggests that, in terms of survival of an embryo, normal development of the hindbrain is more important than development of the forebrain or the distal spine.

Spina bifida occurs from failure of posterior tube closure. Two varieties may arise, referred to as spina bifida aperta and spina bifida occulta. In the former, the neural elements are openly exposed with sometimes leaking CSF through thin dysplastic skin. Its most severe form leads to an open neural tube placode with cauda equina

nerves lying outside of the spinal canal in a myelomeningocoele pouch. Less severe forms include dermal sinuses and meningocoele sacs. In spinal bifida occulta the anomaly includes open laminae and perhaps a neural tube lesion but covered by intact muscle and skin.

4.1.3   Molecular Control of Primary Neurulation

Differentiation of ectodermal cells into skin cells is regulated by the action of a protein, known as bone morphogenetic protein (BMP). Normally BMP4 causes ectodermal cells to differentiate into epidermis. During neural induction, however, two proteins, known as Noggin and Chordin, are produced by the notochord and its enveloping mesoderm. They diffuse locally into the overlying ectoderm and inhibit the activity of BMP4, allowing these cells to differentiate into neural cells. Thereafter closure of the dorsal neural tube is patterned in two stages, midline neural plate closure and neural tube separation from the dorsal epithelium. It is believed that these processes are brought about by a combination of programmed cell death, on the one hand, and epithelial remodelling, on the other hand, probably modulated once again by BMP4.

Development of the dorsal neural plate (the alar plate) is controlled by its flanking ectodermal plate. Initial growth of the ventral part (the basal plate) is organised by the notochord, which regulates much of the development of the nervous system (Jessell et al. 2000). The ventral neural tube is subsequently patterned by the protein sonic hedgehog homologue (SHH).[4] Sonic hedgehog plays a key role in regulating vertebrate organ formation, including organisation of the brain and growth of digits on limbs. It also controls cell division of adult stem cells and has been implicated in the development of some cancers, such as medulloblastomas, which mostly

---

[4] Sonic hedgehog homologue (SHH) is one of three proteins in the mammalian signalling pathway family called hedgehog; desert hedgehog (DHH) and Indian hedgehog (IHH) are the other two. Sonic hedgehog was named after Sega's video game character Sonic the Hedgehog.

occur in the region of the hindbrain. Sonic hedgehog can function in different ways, according to the cellular substrate upon which it acts. It also has different effects on the cells of the developing embryo, depending on its concentration. Basal (floor) plate-derived SHH subsequently signals to other cells in the neural tube and is essential for proper specification of ventral neuron progenitor domains.

SHH binds to a protein, named protein-patched homologue 1 (PTCH1). This then results in uncoupling of PTCH from a receptor named smoothened. This in turn results in activation of the Gli family of transcription factors (Gli1, Gli2 and Gli3), which are the ultimate effectors of this SHH signalling. In this context SHH acts as a morphogen, inducing cell differentiation dependent on its concentration. At low concentrations it promotes formation of ventral interneurons; at higher concentrations it induces motor neuron development, and at highest concentrations it induces floor plate differentiation. Failure of SHH-modulated differentiation results in holoprosencephaly, a condition where there is failure of midline clefting of the forebrain, with cortex crossing the midline, often associated with agenesis of the corpus callosum and a single midline thalamic mass.

4.2 Development of the Spinal Cord

As the spinal part of the neural tube develops, neuroblasts proliferate in two zones, creating the characteristic butterfly-shaped mantle of grey matter seen in cross section. The lateral walls of the tube thicken but leave a shallow, internal, longitudinal groove called the sulcus limitans, which separates the developing grey matter into a dorsal (alar) plate and a ventral (basal) plate. The sulcus limitans extends the length of the spinal cord and beyond to the mesencephalon. Cell bodies in the alar plate form the nuclei, which make up the uninterrupted dorsal column of grey matter (Fig. 4.4). These nuclei receive and relay input from somatic and visceral afferent neurons, whose fibres run in the dorsal roots of spinal nerves. In the basal plate, cells likewise form an uninterrupted column of ventral grey matter that extends the length of the cord. Axons of these efferent neurons project motor fibres to skeletal muscle and make up the ventral roots of the spinal nerves. Further proliferation and bulging of alar and basal plates results in the formation of the external longitudinally running dorsal median septum and ventral median sulcus.

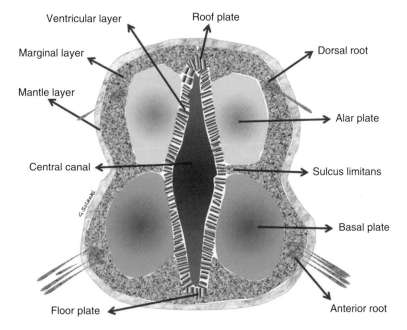

Fig. 4.4 The spinal cord
Three layers (ventricular, mantle and marginal) develop from the neural tube.
The ventricular layer contains undifferentiated neurons.
The grey matter of the spinal cord will develop from differentiating neurons in the mantle layer and the white matter from the nerve fibres in the marginal layer

Concurrently the lumen of the neural tube becomes reduced to a small central canal. Addition of longitudinally running intersegmental axons, long ascending and descending axons and incoming dorsal root sensory fibres, on the outside of this grey matter, creates a marginal layer. Beginning in the 4th month, these fibres acquire myelin sheaths and form the white matter of the cord.

4.3 Formation of the Brain

Progressive dilatation and folding into flexures of the cranial end of the neural tube creates three distinct, primitive brain vesicles, the prosencephalon, the mesencephalon and the rhombencephalon. The mesencephalon remains undivided, to form the future cerebral peduncles and quadrigeminal plate. The alar and basal plates of the prosencephalon, on the other hand, will divide to form the telencephalon and diencephalon, respectively. The optic vesicles, which will develop into the optic nerves, retinas and irises, expand out from lateral extensions of the diencephalon. The cerebral hemispheres develop from the dorsal alar plate of the telencephalon. The basal and alar rhombencephalic plates will form the metencephalon (future pons and cerebellum) and myelencephalon (future medulla oblongata). Different parts of the future basal ganglia (nuclei basales) arise separately, the caudate nucleus and the putamen from the alar plate telencephalon and the globus pallidus, from basal plate diencephalon. The thalamus and hypothalamus also arise from basal plate diencephalon.

4.3.1 The Brainstem

Neuroblasts of the brainstem develop in a manner similar to those in the spinal cord. Alar and basal plates form sensory and motor columns of cells that supply cranial nerves, but the topographical layout of these nuclei differs in the brainstem, as compared with the cord. The mesencephalon remains undivided and consists of the basal midbrain and alar quadrigeminal plate. The pons consists of two parts, the basis pontis and the pontine tegmentum. The former is ventrally located and is phylogenetically newer. The latter is the older portion, is dorsal in position and is continuous with the medulla. The pontine tegmentum and the medulla together form the floor of the fourth ventricle. Here, the alar and basal plates are separated by a sulcus limitans, but unlike in the spinal cord, they are disposed laterally and medially, instead of dorsal and ventral. With continued development, alar and basal plates shift laterally but retain their respective functions, with the alar plates containing afferent nuclei and the basal plates forming efferent nuclei. Portions of the alar plate migrate ventrally and form the inferior olivary nucleus. Nuclei of the basis pontis migrate there from the alar plate. They receive synapses of cortically originating fibres. Medullary pyramids consist of fibres from the cerebral cortex and develop on the ventral surface near the midline

4.3.2 The Cerebellum

Caudal to the mesencephalon lies the metencephalon, which is the rostral portion of the hindbrain. It differentiates into two major structures, the cerebellum and the pons. At the rostral edge of the roof of the fourth ventricle lie the rhombic lips, which arise from the dorsolateral alar plates of the rhombencephalon. At about the fifth or sixth week, these lips start forming the cerebellar primordia. Their growth and infolding into each other causes them to fuse in the midline, creating the cerebellar plate, which covers the fourth ventricle caudal to the mesencephalon. Although the cerebellum accounts for approximately 10 % of the human brain's volume, it contains over 50 % of the total number of neurons in the brain. The cerebellum, like the frontal lobe, is the last of the structures to develop. Chiari tonsillar descent, for example, has not been identified earlier than 10 weeks on antenatal ultrasound scans (Blaas et al. 2000). Another example of the effect of disordered

Table 4.2 Components of the basal and alar plates

Basal plate components	Alar plate components
Nucleus of cranial nerve VI	Vestibulocochlear components of cranial nerve VIII
Motor components to muscle of branchiomeric origin of cranial nerves V and VII	Trigeminal sensory for pain and temperature, cranial nerve V
Superior salivary nucleus of cranial nerve VII	Solitary nucleus for taste and visceral sensation of cranial nerves VII, IX and X
	Pontine nuclei in the basis pontis upon which corticofugal fibres terminate

development and growth on this late maturation is seen in severe prematurity,[5] where cerebellar function and volume may be affected. Recent evidence shows that individuals born very preterm have significantly smaller cerebella than their term-born peers, and that this difference remains statistically significant after controlling for whole brain volume and other potentially confounding variables (Allin et al. 2001).

4.3.3   The Cranial Nerves

By the 5th week of gestation, all cranial nerves are recognisable except for the olfactory and optic nerves. The pure motor cranial nerves (III, IV, VI and XII) have no external ganglia and arise from the basal (motor) plate. Sensory nerves have conspicuous ganglia near the brain and most have motor components, except for the eighth. Apart from the third and fourth cranial nerves, which arise from the midbrain, the 5th to the 12th cranial nerves arise from the rhombencephalon (Table 4.2). *Hox* genes play an important role in temporospatial development of motor neurons of the trigeminal and facial nerves, as we will see later.

---

[5] Severe prematurity or extremely premature or extremely low GA (gestational age) refers to the youngest of premature newborns, usually born at 27 weeks' gestational age or younger. These infants also have an extremely low birth weight defined as a birth weight of less than 1,000 g (2 lb, 3 oz).

4.3.4   The Ventricular System

The cranial part of the neural canal (lumen of neural tube) forms the ventricular system of the brain. The shape of the ventricles is determined by the brain folding around the two primary flexures (cephalic and cervical), forming three primitive vesicles, during week 4 of gestation. These bends arise as a result of tremendous cell proliferation, occurring within the confined space of the cranial vault, causing the neural tube to buckle as the brain develops. Towards the end of week 4 and early into week 5, the primitive 3-vesicle brain divides further to become a 5-vesicle structure. Each vesicle contains its own ventricle (Table 4.3). The prosencephalon gives rise to paired lateral telencephalic vesicles, which become the cerebral hemispheres. It also forms the diencephalon, from which the optic vesicles also extend. During week 6, in the 5-vesicle stage, the pontine flexure develops. This divides the rhombencephalon into a rostral metencephalon, which will form the pons and cerebellum, and a caudal myelencephalon, which becomes the medulla. Later, the disproportionate expansion of the cerebral hemispheres alters the configuration of the lateral ventricles, which become 'C'-shaped. These flexures also create specific narrowings within the ventricles. The foramina of Monro are located at the level of the telencephalon/diencephalon division. The cerebral aqueduct remains as a relatively simple tubular channel within the unflexed mesencephalon. During the fifth and sixth weeks, the roof of the fourth ventricle thins out in the midline to form the foramen of Magendie and, laterally, the foramen of Luschka (Melsen 1974; Koseki et al. 1993). By approximately the 7th week, a connection between the fourth ventricle and the subarachnoid space is established. The foramina of Luschka and Magendie lie at the division of the rostral metencephalon and caudal myelencephalon. More caudally, below the cervical flexure, the central canal lies within and along the spinal cord.

The development of the three primary vesicles (5th week) and subsequently, at 7 weeks, the five secondary vesicles (telencephalon, diencephalon,

Table 4.3 Development of the flexures, ventricular system and foramina

Timing	Event	Flexures	Primitive vesicles	Secondary vesicles	Future ventricles
Early 4th week Day 22	Neural tube closure and primary neurulation start	Cephalic and Cervical	Prosencephalon Mesencephalon Rhombencephalon		
5th week	Primary vesicles subdivide. Future foramina of Monro will form between forebrain and midbrain	Cephalic	Prosencephalon	Telencephalic Diencephalic	Paired lateral ventricles Third ventricle
	Does not divide		Mesencephalon	Mesencephalic	Cerebral aqueduct
	Pontine flexure develops. Separates pons and cerebellum from medulla at level of future foramina of Luschka and Magendie	Pontine	Rhombencephalon	Metencephalic Myelencephalic	Fourth ventricle
	Cervical or cervicomedullary flexure separates medulla from the spinal cord (future foramen magnum)	Cervical			Vestigial central canal of the spinal cord

mesencephalon, metencephalon and myelencephalon) is accomplished by the development of flexures. These flexures may also help maintain the CSF between them in a state of tension, so as to expand the ventricular system in an asymmetric way. Our ventricular system was moulded by flexural kinks into different shapes and sizes, aided by the moulding weight of the developing brain around it (Fig. 4.5). The hydrostatic tension within the ventricles acts as a vital scaffold upon which the parenchyma develops and grows. Premature unfolding of a particular flexure will impact on the CSF tension within the corresponding vesicle and almost certainly cause a degree of collapse of the dorsal structures upon it. Hypothetically, if the distal pontine flexure – which develops around the seventh week, between the pons, cerebellum and medulla oblongata – and/or the cervical flexure were to 'unkink', then this could result in lesser tension in the metencephalic vesicle and a smaller posterior fossa, as seen in occipital somite (skull base) development anomalies. On the other hand, if there was a continuous caudal CSF leak, as we see with leaking myelomeningocoeles, then the normal tension within the ventricular system would be reduced. The effect would be a sequential collapse of dorsal structures upon the floppy metencephalic and myelencephalic vesicle centres, causing a small posterior fossa and its caudal dislocation. An inward suction/decompression effect on the most rostral part of the ventricle could also occur, leading to flattening of the forehead. This may hypothetically explain why foetuses develop the typical lemon appearance of the forehead and the banana sign[6] on ultrasounds of myelomeningocoele and Chiari II malformation. It may also help explain the tectal

---

[6] An early cranial ultrasound may give indirect signs of myelomeningocoele-derived loss of CSF and hindbrain hernia, even before the actual spinal lesion can be observed. At the level of the cerebellum and cistern magna, unwinding of the nearest (pontine) flexure, due to CSF leakage in the lumbosacral spine, likely releases the hydrostatic CSF pressure maintaining the posterior fossa 'scaffold' and causes descent and herniation of the cerebellar vermis through the foramen magnum, giving the cerebellum the appearance of a banana. Frontally, on both sides of the metopic suture (in between the two frontal bones), a depression or buckling occurs, giving the anterior calvarium the pointed shape of a lemon (the 'lemon sign'). Both signs are associated with and the consequence of spina bifida aperta and associated with Chiari II malformation. Once the CSF tension drops through the pontine flexure, the whole ventricular axis may be affected. It is interesting to note that, if the spinal leak is sealed antenatally by the second trimester, the Chiari II malformation is less severe or does not occur.

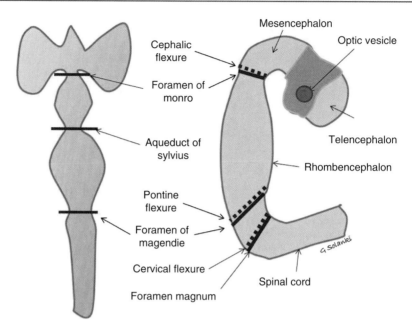

Fig. 4.5 Development of the ventricular system Neural canal develops two flexures and three vesicles. Remodelling and mantle laying of grey matter deforms the canal further into three flexures and five vesicles. The two original flexures are at the level of the foramen of Monro and foramen magnum. Above the future foramina of Monro, the prosencephalon divides into two vesicles, the mesencephalon and diencephalon. A further flexure, known as the pontine flexure, develops in the rhomben-cephalon, splitting it into a rostral metencephalon (the future pons and cerebellum) and a caudal myelencephalon (the future medulla oblongata). This occurs at the level of the future lateral foramina of Luschka and medial fora-men of Magendie. Flexures help maintain tension within the ventricles, which may act as an internal scaffold for the mantle layer cellular proliferation

beaking and neuronal migration disorders seen in association with Chiari II malformations and myelomeningocoele.

4.4 Development of Mesodermal Elements

The neural tube and its future coverings develop hand in hand. As the folding of the neural tube progresses, it becomes surrounded ventrally by the mesoderm-derived notochord, dorsolater-ally by the paraxial mesoderm and neural crest cells and in the midline dorsally, by the ectoderm.

4.4.1 Somite Development

Somites are masses of mesoderm, distributed along the two sides of the neural tube, that will eventually become dermis (dermatome), skeletal muscle (myotome) and vertebrae (sclerotome). During the 4th week of gestation, 42 somites are formed. These are made up of 4 occipital somites, 8 cervical, 12 thoracic and 5 lumbar; the remain-der are sacrococcygeal (Muller and O'Rahilly 1980; Gasser 1976; Arcy 1965) . Each somite then differentiates into an outer dermatome, an inner myotome and a medial sclerotome (Fig. 4.6). Because the sclerotome differentiates before the other two components, the term 'der-momyotome' is sometimes used to describe the combined dermatome and myotome. Each sclero-tome has three parts, a hypocentrum, a centrum and a neural arch. The first four sclerotomes go on to form the skull base and the foramen mag-num. The hypocentrum forms different structures at each level (see Table 4.4). The sclerotomes are ventromedial to the neural tube and will surround the notochord and go on to form the vertebral bodies. This topography means that the skull base develops ventral to the rostral notochord (Melsen 1974).

Fig. 4.6 Budding somite derived from paraxial mesoderm The sclerotome lies ventro-medially, adjacent to the neural tube. After its detachment the remaining somite is known as dermomyotome. The dermo-myotome splits to form the dermatome and the myotome and then the myotome splits into epimeres, which form the deep muscles of the back, and hypomeres, which form the musculature of the lateral and anterior body wall

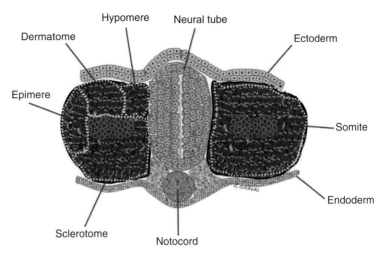

Table 4.4 Structures developed from occipital and first two spinal sclerotomes

Origin	Process/division	Anatomical part
Neural crest cell derived	Membranous ossification	Skull vortex and calvarium
All four occipital sclerotomes, derived from the paraxial mesoderm	Enchondrosis	Skull base
1st and 2nd occipital sclerotomes		Clivus – basiocciput
3rd occipital sclerotome	Exoccipital bone	Jugular tubercles
4th occipital sclerotome (proatlas)	Hypocentrum	Anterior tubercle of clivus
	Centrum	Dens apex
		Apical ligament
	Ventral neural arch	Basion - anterior margin of foramen magnum
		Occipital condyles
		Midline third occipital condyle
	Lateral neural arch	Cruciate ligament
		Alar ligaments
	Caudal neural arch	C2 lateral mass
		Superior portion of posterior arch of C1
	Dorsal fusion of first 4 sclerotomes	Posterior margin of FM
		Occipital bone
1st spinal sclerotome	Hypocentrum	Anterior arch of C1
	Centrum	Dens
	Neural arch	Inferior portion of posterior arch of C1
	Hypocentrum	Disappears
2nd spinal sclerotome	Centrum	Body of axis
	Neural arch	Facets
		Posterior arch of atlas

The clivus and the occipital bone and, hence, the foramen magnum are derived from the four occipital somites. The first two occipital sclerotomes give rise to the basiocciput (Fig. 4.7). The tip of clivus, the anterior tubercle of the C1, the dens apex and the apical ligament are derived from the fourth occipital sclerotome, otherwise referred to as the proatlas (Menezes 1996; Gladstone and Wakeley 1925; Gasser 1976). The anterior margin of the foramen magnum, as well as the occipital condyles and the midline third occipital condyle (Fig. 4.8), arises from the ventral portion of the proatlas (Prescher et al. 1996). The cruciate ligament and the alar ligaments arise from the lateral part of proatlas. The C2 lateral mass and the superior portion of the posterior arch of the atlas develop from the caudal proatlas. The

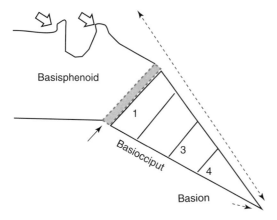

Fig. 4.7 The clivus The clivus is made up from the basisphenoid, the basiocciput and the sphenooccipital synchondrosis (*closed arrow*), as well as the anterior and posterior clinoids – otherwise referred to as the basiendosphenoid (*open arrows*). It also includes the basion, which forms the anterior lip of foramen magnum. The basiocciput is formed by the occipital sclerotomes. The basion is formed by the 4th occipital sclerotome, or proatlas. Anomalies of the 4th occipital sclerotome are associated with Chiari malformations

posterior rim of the foramen magnum and the occiput develop from the dorsal fusion of the first four (occipital) sclerotomes. The odontoid process and the atlas vertebra are formed from the first spinal sclerotome. The atlas shows several ossification centres in development (Keynes and Stern 1988). While the lateral masses of C2 are present at birth, complete ossification may not occur until about 3 years of age when a complete ring may then be seen. The dens is the central portion of the first sclerotome, which fuses with the axis body. The neural arch of this first spinal sclerotome proceeds to form the posterior and inferior portion of the C1 arch (Menezes 1995; Koseki et al. 1993). With further development, the hypocentrum of the second spinal sclerotome disappears, but the centrum goes on to form the body of the axis body. Division of the neural arch forms the facets and the posterior arch of the axis vertebra (Keynes and Stern 1988). In summary, most of the dens develops from the first spinal sclerotome, but the terminal portion of the odontoid process arises from the proatlas, and the most inferior portion of the axis body is formed by the second spinal sclerotome (Table 4.4).

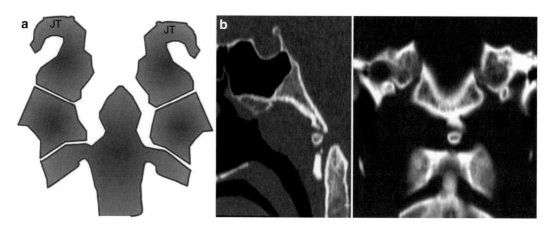

Fig. 4.8 (**a**) Bony structures related to the lateral boundaries of the foramen magnum. In higher vertebrates, the foramen magnum is surrounded by a ring of four bones. They arise from the third occipital sclerotome. The basioccipital bone lies in front of the opening, the two exoccipitals lie to either side, and the larger supraoccipital lies posteriorly. The jugular tubercles (*JT*) arise from the two exoccipital bones, which lie lateral to the foramen

magnum. (**b**) Third occipital condyle. (*a*) CT sagittal. (*b*) Coronal multiplanar reconstruction. The third occipital condyle (condylus tertius or median occipital condyle) was first described by J.F. Meckel in 1815. It is a bony process in the anterior midline of the foramen magnum, forming a rudimentary articulation above the C1 arch. It sometimes persists into adult life

4.4.2 Development of the Skull

The skull develops by two different processes. The calvarium and facial bones develop by membranous ossification (Kessel and Gruss 1991; Christ and Wilting 1992; Dietrich and Kessel 1997) as does the occipital skull above the nuchal line, although this component is thought to arise, originally, from neural crest cells, rather than from the paraxial mesoderm. The skull base and the remainder of the occipital bone develop from a cartilaginous framework, in which deposition of bone occurs. This process is driven mainly by distorting forces generated by the developing brain. Just as remodelling of the anterior cranial fossa occurs as the prosencephalon folds down, posterior fossa expansion occurs following the growth of its neural contents. In response to the pontine and medullary enlargement, the clivus elongates at the basiocciput and lowers the front margin of the foramen magnum. Downward cerebellar displacement pushes the opisthion downward and backward. These processes result from a combination of endochondral resorption and sutural growth.

Some parts of the skull base also continue to develop later in life, in response to the growth of surrounding structures. For example, growth of the sphenooccipital and sphenopetrosal synchondrosis, along with adjacent endochondral and intramembranous ossification, results in an elongation of the clivus and the posterior skull base (Menezes 1998). This process can continue until late adolescence and will ultimately model the final shape and size of the posterior fossa.

4.4.3 Genetic Control of Mesodermal Growth

The process of segmentation at the craniocervical junction and along the spine is tightly regulated by control genes. Proteins promoted by these genes modulate the transcription of specific downstream genes, thereby controlling morphogenesis and providing specific identify for each vertebra (Lufkin et al. 1992). The main genetic groups involved in mesodermal and neuroectodermal development of the craniocervical junction are the *SHH* genes, for basal development, the *Hox* genes[7] for dorsal neural folding and tube closure and the *PAX* genes[8] for segmentation. Subsequent re-segmentation of the sclerotomes then occurs, to establish vertebral boundaries. This process seems to be independently controlled by two regulatory genes of the *PAX* family (Koseki et al. 1993).

Following segmentation, the *Hox* genes play a critical role. They are part of the developmental-genetic toolkit[9] and contain the phylogenetically highly conserved homeobox[10] domain. *Hox* genes regulate the establishment of the body plan in a temporospatial manner. They achieve this by the phenomenon of colinearity.[11] *Hox* genes are ordered in a linear fashion, precisely correlated with the order of both the segments and regions they affect and with the timing in which they are affected. Any mutation leading to a loss or gain in the gene cluster causes precise and specific similar changes in the affected segments and regions. The precise identity of each

---

[7] *HOX* genes organise dorsal neural folding and tube closure. This happens in the craniocaudal plane. At the same time sonic hedgehog and *PAX* genes are working on the basal plane and segmentation at each somite, respectively.

[8] *PAX* genes encode for a family of closely related transcription factors (TGF). In their absence segmental development fails. For example, PAX1/PAX9 double-mutant mice completely lack the medial derivatives of the sclerotomes, the vertebral bodies, intervertebral discs and the proximal parts of the ribs.

[9] The developmental-genetic toolkit consists of a small fraction of the genes in an organism's genome whose products control its overall development.

[10] A homeobox is a 180-base pairs long DNA sequence found within genes that are involved in the regulation of patterns of anatomical development (morphogenesis). These homeobox genes switch on cascades of other genes by using transcription factors. The homeobox encodes a protein domain (the homeodomain) which when expressed binds to DNA in a sequence-specific manner.

[11] Colinear property of Hox genes – the sequence of *Hox* genes matches the sequence in which they act along the body axes. *Hox* colinearity is pivotal in embryogenesis and is described in three ways: functional colinearity describes the order in which *Hox* genes act along a body axis, spatial colinearity refers to the spatial order in which the *Hox* genes are expressed and temporal colinearity is the time sequence in which they are expressed.

Table 4.5 Human CNS malformations

Days of gestation	Event	Resultant malformation
0–18	Formation of 3 germ layers and neural plate	Death or unclear effect
18	Formation of neural plate and groove	Anterior midline defects
22–23	Appearance of optic vessels	Hydrocephalus (18–60 days)
24–26	Closure of anterior neuropore	Anencephaly
26–28	Closure of posterior neuropore	Cranium bifidum, spina bifida cystica, spina bifida occulta
32	Vascular circulation	Microcephaly (30–130 days)
		Migration anomalies
33–35	Splitting of prosencephalon to make paired telencephalon	Holoprosencephaly
70–100	Formation of corpus callosum	Agenesis of the corpus callosum

hindbrain and prevertebral segment (and for every segment along the embryo) is controlled by *Hox* genes.

It is likely that a number of malformations have a basis in anomalies of regulatory gene function or of their signalling molecules, starting early in the gastrulation phase and continuing into primary neurulation (Table 4.5). The dorsally placed hindbrain and the craniocervical junction are particularly sensitive to *Hox* gene anomalies and/or disruption. In the hindbrain, cells in each rhombomere[12] do not cross established boundaries and are programmed to form only one precise part of the hindbrain (Fraser et al. 1990; Lumsden 1990). In this way, rhombomeres 2 and 3 induce formation of the motor neurons of the trigeminal nerve, rhombomeres 4 and 5 are responsible for the motor nerves of the facial nerve and rhombomeres 6 and 7 for the glossopharyngeal and vagus nerves. Retinoic acid treatment has been shown to alter the expression boundaries of homeobox genes and to cause homeotic transformations in the hindbrain (Marshall et al. 1992; Kessel 1993; Alexander et al. 2009) and within the vertebrae (Kessel and Gruss 1991). Marshall and colleagues reported in 1992 that retinoic acid alters

hindbrain *HOX* code[13] and induces transformation of rhombomeres r2/r3 into an r4/r5 identity.[14] A main feature of this rhombomeric phenotype is that the trigeminal motor nerve is transformed to a facial identity. Neural crest cells derived from rhombomeres r2/r3 also express posterior *HOX* markers, suggesting that the retinoic acid-induced transformation extends to multiple components of the first branchial arch (Marshall et al. 1992). Such anomalies also extend to the craniovertebral junction, where a

---

[12] Rhombomeres (r) are eight distinct segments of the neural tube located distal to the cephalic flexure. They determine the pattern of maturation of the rhombencephalon (developing hindbrain) into its final parts – pons, cerebellum and medulla. Each rhombomere develops its own set of ganglia and nerves. Transcription factors (T-box) have been linked to the proper development of migrating cells in the region extending from one rhombomere to another.

[13] The *HOX* code is an ordered molecular system of positional values provided by the *HOX* genes. The *HOX* code is responsible for the patterning of hindbrain, craniofacial structures, vertebrae and limbs.

[14] While rhombomeres were discovered and histologically characterised in the early nineteenth century, only recently has their role in development become known. In all vertebrates, rhombomeres and branchial nerves (cranial nerves V, VII, IX for branchial arches I, II and III) are organised in a pair-wise fashion, such that the motor neurons of trigeminal nerve arise from r2 and r3, the facial and auditory neurons arise from r4 and r5 and the glossopharyngeal and vagus neurons extend caudal to r6. This specificity is controlled by the *HOX* genes. The segmental specification for each rhombomere within the hindbrain neuroectoderm remains, despite surgical transplantation into the next even-/odd-numbered rhombomere. In contrast, spinal nerve segmentation depends entirely on the pattern of somites. This implies that cranial nerve patterning is brought about by factors intrinsic to rhombomeres and to the attached neural crest cell populations. The patterns of the neuroectoderm and of the peripheral nervous system (PNS) are specified early in hindbrain development and cannot be influenced by tissue transplantation. In rhombomeres without neural crest cells (odd-numbered r3 and r5), transplantation leads to neurons migrating back to their appropriate (original) rhombomere nerve root exit site rather than the closest exit site in the transplanted rhombomeres for that root.

Fig. 4.9 Anterior homeotic transformation. Mutation of the *Hox* gene (loss of function) results in C1 arch fusion to the occiput. This artist's rendering of a cervical spine, in a coronal view, shows fusion of the occipital condyle to the C1 lateral mass on the right side

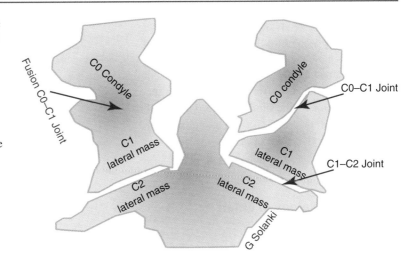

variety of homeotic transformations[15] can occur. When there is loss of a *Hox* gene, the corresponding region fails to segment from its cranial neighbour. This anomaly produces an anterior homeotic transformation, where the C1 arch will remain fused to the occiput and clivus. When there is a gain of function in the Hox gene, a posterior homeotic transformation occurs, where the distal clivus is assimilated into C1 or C1 into the tip of the dens (Fig. 4.9). Teratogen-induced disturbance of Hox gene expression, or mutation in the Hox genes themselves, can cause alterations in the morphology or number of cervical vertebra that are formed. Inactivation of the HOX-d3 gene in mice, for example, produces mutations with assimilation of the atlas into the basiocciput and failure of occipital somite development, resulting in a small or contracted occiput and leading to a small posterior fossa (Condie and Capecchi 1993).

4.5 Developmental Anomalies of the Craniocervical Junction

The endochondral skull base of foetuses with Chiari malformations is shorter than normal and elevated in relation to the spinal axis (Marin-Padilla and Marin-Padilla 1981). This underdevelopment of the occipital bone results in a short and small posterior fossa of inadequate volume for the normal hindbrain. A secondary effect is elongation of the odontoid process, the so-called dolicho-odontoid process, or dolichoid dens. This is often associated with a short basiocciput, and these two features result in basilar invagination, an appearance seen not uncommonly with Chiari malformations.

Anomalies of development of the proatlas and the spinal sclerotomes may lead to segmentation failures of the proatlas and development of occipital vertebrae (Tominaga et al. 2002; Rao 2002; Koseki et al. 1993; Gasser 1976). Hindbrain herniation is seen in 33 % of affected children. Another anomaly is the Klippel-Feil deformity, where there is failure of segmentation between the fourth occipital and the first spinal sclerotome (VonTorklus and Gehle 1972; Menezes 1995; Gehweiler et al. 1983). Basilar invagination is a secondary phenomenon, with associated hindbrain herniation, in about 40 % of cases.

A number of anomalies of the craniofacial skeleton are associated with the Chiari malformations and syringomyelia (Thompson and Rudd 1976). Craniofacial syndromes, which include lambdoid synostosis, severe brachyturricephaly[16] or pansynostosis, are quite likely to have an associated Chiari I malformation (Koseki et al. 1993).

---

[15] Homeotic transformation means that a normal body part is replaced by a body part which is regularly found in other regions. This can be anterior or posterior.

[16] Brachyturricephaly is an abnormal head shape where there are sagittal narrowing, coronal widening and increase in skull height, generally seen in syndromic craniosynostosis and bicoronal synostosis.

This may not be regarded as an essential component of the syndromic phenotypes but can be seen as a secondary effect of the cranioce-phalic mismatch, be this supratentorial or infratentorial. Indeed, calvarial augmentation surgery often resolves the hindbrain hernia in such cases, without the need for foramen magnum decompression (Iskandar et al. 2004; Frias et al. 1988; Nakai et al. 1995; Solanki et al. 2009).

4.5.1 Embryology of Chiari Malformations

Several different theories have been considered in explaining the embryogenesis or origins of Chiari malformations (Thompson and Rudd 1976), but a unifying theory has yet to emerge. Based on our current understanding of gastrulation and neurulation, the onset for the Chiari malformations lies in the embryonic period, somewhere between the 3rd and the 5th week and is likely to happen prior to, during and following closure of the neural tube. The association of Chiari I malformation with other spine, skull, somatic and craniofacial abnormalities, which are the result of mesodermal maldevelopment, would suggest a paraxial mesoderm origin of Chiari malformations and point towards a common pathway for these insults (Lee et al. 2003; Tubbs et al. 2003; Tubbs and Oakes 2005) (Table 4.6). The association of craniosynostosis and Chiari I malformation is well documented and is strongest in cases of syndromic, multi-suture and lambdoid synostosis. Nearly a 100 % association is noted with Kleeblatschadel.[17] The incidence of Chiari I malformation in Crouzon syndrome is about 70 % but is much lower in syndromes such as Apert (2 %) (Cinalli et al. 2005). It is most likely that the Chiari malformations arise from anomalies of the mesoderm, resulting in axial skeletal defects but with a range of associated neurological anomalies, proportionate

---

[17] The Kleeblattschadel deformity is a form of craniosynostosis where there are prominent temporal bones, leading to a clover leaf-type appearance of the skull.

Table 4.6 Associations reported with Chiari malformations

Group	Syndrome or anomaly
Craniosynostosis	Antley-Bixler syndrome
	Apert syndrome
	Crouzon syndrome
	Jackson-Weiss syndrome
	Kleeblattschädel syndrome
	Lambdoid synostosis
	Loeys-Dietz syndrome type I
	Metopic synostosis
	Pansynostosis
	Pfeiffer syndrome
	Seckel syndrome
	Shprintzen-Goldberg syndrome
Hydrocephalus	Obstructive hydrocephalus
Endocrine	Very rare in achondroplasia
	Acromegaly
	Growth hormone deficiency
	Hyperostosis
	Craniometaphyseal dysplasia
	Erythroid hyperplasia
	Osteopetrosis
	Paget disease
	Bone mineral deficiency
	Familial vitamin D-resistant rickets
	Familial hypophosphataemic rickets
Haematology	Sickle-cell disease with hypertrophy of diploic layer
Cutaneous/ neurocutaneous disorders	Acanthosis nigricans
	Blue rubber bleb nevus syndrome
	Giant congenital melanocytic nevi
	LEOPARD syndrome
	Macrocephaly-cutis marmorata telangiectatica
	Neurofibromatosis type I
	Phacomatosis pigmentovascularis type II
	Waardenburg syndrome
Spinal neurulation defects	
Primary neurulation	Lipomeningomyelocoele
Secondary neurulation	Caudal regression syndrome
Spinal somitic defects	Atlantoaxial assimilation
	Basilar impression
	Odontoid retroflexion
	Klippel-Feil syndrome
	Spondyloepiphyseal dysplasia

Table 4.6 (continued)

Group	Syndrome or anomaly
Space-occupying lesions	Posterior fossa
	Supratentorial
	Spinal cord
	Congenital space-occupying lesions
Other	Beckwith-Wiedemann syndrome
	CHERI syndrome
	*Ch*iari 1 malformation with or without cleft palate, deviant *E*EG or *e*pilepsy and *r*etarded *i*ntelligence with delayed language development (Haapanen 2007)
	Cloacal exstrophy
	Costello syndrome
	Cystic fibrosis
	Ehlers-Danlos syndrome
	Fabry disease
	Kabuki syndrome
	Situs inversus
	Williams-Beuren syndrome
	Pierre-Robin syndrome

Modified from Loukas et al. (2011)

Table 4.7 Theories of pathogenesis of Chiari malformations

Caudal traction
Hindbrain dysgenesis and developmental arrest
Lack of embryological ventricular distension
Hydrocephalus and hydrodynamic theory of Gardner
Small posterior fossa/hindbrain overgrowth theory

to the extent of the mesodermal disturbance. Many features of Chiari malformations, including neuronal migration anomalies,[18] are now believed to be secondary, rather than primary (Gardner et al. 1975) (Table 4.7). What was previously considered as a primary neuronal migration anomaly, as part of the Chiari II presentation, may in fact occur secondary to physical changes resulting from an open spina bifida. The loss of tension within the ventricular system distorts the brain parenchyma with a dorso-caudal movement. This elongation of parenchyma may lead to loss of cortical rugosity, sulcation anomalies, beaking of the tectum and so on.

Both genetic and environmental factors, including teratogens, might also play a role in the development of Chiari malformations. For example, administration of a single dose of vitamin A to pregnant hamsters, early during the morning of their 8th day of gestation, induces the formation of type 1 and type 2 Chiari malformations (Marin-Padilla and Marin-Padilla 1981). The critical defect arises from inhibition of a diffusible retinoid inducing factor, during gastrulation, causing a primary paraxial mesodermal insufficiency. The consequent underdevelopment of occipital somite, leading to a short clivus and a small occipital bone, results in a shallow posterior fossa (Tominaga et al. 2002). This, coupled with the later, rapid development, leads to a range of hindbrain abnormalities consistent with Chiari I and II malformations, as well as other mesenchymal anomalies. Interference with induction by the prechordal plate[19] at or before stage 8 (18 days) would also be expected to affect future development, particularly of the mediobasal part of the neural plate. Such anomalies occur by the 4th week post-ovulation (Muller and O'Rahilly 1980). Failure of the pontine flexure to form normally during primary neurulation from the 28th to 29th day of gestation may lead to formation of elongated brainstem and Chiari I and II malformations. Signs of Chiari malformations have certainly been noted on antenatal ultrasound as early as 10 weeks (Blaas et al. 2000), and there is evidence for accelerated growth of the cerebellum in the 20th week; this,

---

[18] Neuronal migration anomalies are a wide spectrum of developmental malformations of the cortex caused by disruption to its normal process of formation, which includes proliferation, migration and organisation (lamination, gyration and sulcation). The most well known are, for example, megalencephaly (proliferation), lissencephaly (migration) and heterotopias (organisation).

[19] 'Prechordal plate' and 'prochordal plate' are essentially synonymous terms referring to the horseshoe-shaped band of thickened endoderm rostral to the notochord. The prechordal plate starts as a thickening of the endoderm at the cranial end of the primitive streak. It is located at the anterior end of the notochord, which appears in early embryos as an integral part of the roof of the foregut. It contributes mesodermal type cells to the surrounding tissue. Cells derived from the prechordal plate become incorporated into the cephalic mesenchyme, which is thought to contribute, later, to the meninges. Failure of induction leads to cyclopia, holoprosencephaly and other mediobasal defects.

in the presence of arrested occipital somite development, may cause the typical hindbrain herniation seen in the commoner Chiari types I and II.

4.5.2   Chiari II Malformation

Chiari II malformation is virtually always present in neonates with open spinal dysraphism. The anatomical severity and resultant physiological effects of the malformation vary from one child to another. We encounter a range, from a near-normal-sized posterior fossa with no real descent of the vermis or brainstem to other children that may be affected by permanent nocturnal central hypoventilation, requiring noninvasive ventilation (Bhangoo et al. 2006).

The open neural tube defect arises during primary neurulation. Failure of developmental closure of the caudal neural tube results in an unfolded neural tube, known as neural placode, exposed to the dorsal surface in the midline. CSF leaks through the defect into the amniotic sac, resulting in chronic CSF hypovolemia and hypotension within the developing neural tube. This creates a small ventricular system and inadequate dilatation of the future fourth ventricle. It also fails to induce the posterior cranial fossa perineural mesenchyme (McLone and Knepper 1989). The dominant features of Chiari II malformation, up to 20 weeks of gestation, are the result of these developmental failures. After 20 weeks the accelerated and disproportionate growth of the cerebellum dominates (Beuls et al. 2003; Paek et al. 2000; Bouchard et al. 2003; Sutton et al. 1999). Both cerebellum and brainstem are eventually forced to develop within a smaller than normal posterior fossa and consequently herniate through both the tentorial hiatus and the foramen magnum.

In lambs, adding a myelotomy to experimentally induced dysraphic lesions leads to formation of a hindbrain hernia that is similar to that observed in the human Chiari II malformation. Further, repair of myelomeningocoele in a human foetus reverses the hindbrain herniation and restores gross anatomy of the vermis (Bouchard et al. 2003; Sutton et al. 1999). The posterior fossa will expand in time to allow fur-

ther normal growth of both the cerebellum and brainstem.

CSF hypotension in the supratentorial brain may also impair neuronal migration, producing various associated malformations of the nervous tissue. Although histologically normal, the cerebral cortex in patients with Chiari II malformation is abnormal in gross appearance. The gyri are abnormally numerous and small, although the term polymicrogyria is best avoided because of its association with an abnormal four-layered cortex that is not present in Chiari II malformation; the term polygyria is to be preferred (McLendon et al. 1985). Partial-to-total agenesis of the corpus callosum is seen in a third of patients with Chiari II malformation; nearly two thirds of those have below average intelligence (Venes et al. 1986).

Multiple ventricular anomalies are found commonly in the patient with Chiari II malformation. The fourth ventricle, which is typically small and poorly visualised, is frequently displaced into the cervical canal, along with its choroid plexus. The aqueduct is similarly small and rarely seen on routine imaging, although this probably does not contribute significantly to the hydrocephalus (Peach 1965). The third ventricle is rarely enlarged but may take on a narrow-angled appearance, giving rise to the term 'shark tooth deformity'. The lateral ventricular appearance varies from nearly normal to severely deformed and hydrocephalic. Colpocephaly[20] is common, with the occipital horns disproportionately enlarged compared with the frontal horns. This finding is often present, even in patients with myelomeningocoele who do not have hydrocephalus. It frequently persists in patients in whom a shunt has been placed. 'Beaking' of the frontal horns is occasionally seen, when the frontal horns point

---

[20] Colpocephaly refers to an abnormal appearance of the ventricular system of the brain in which there is asymmetric dilatation of the occipital horns but with normal-sized frontal horns. It is common in Chiari malformation II. It is thought to be related to an intrauterine disturbance that occurs between the second and sixth months of pregnancy. The finding may be indirectly suggested on ultrasound by the so-called lemon sign, which occurs due to depression of the calvarium at the bilateral frontal suture lines, giving the calvarium the appearance of a lemon.

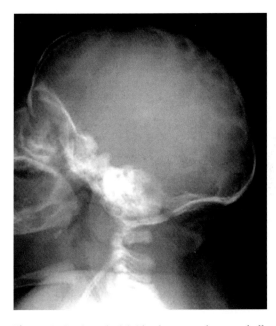

Fig. 4.10 Luckenschadel Also known as lacunar skull, this condition is a dysplasia of the membranous skull vault. Two variants are described. Craniolacunia is the name given when the grooves in the skull are limited to the inner table. In craniofenestrae there are palpable defects involving both the inner and outer tables. It is associated with Chari malformations, particularly Chiari II malformation (up to 80 %). It is believed that the defect is not so much due to pressure from within but rather an abnormality of collagen development and ossification

inferiorly. This finding is attributed to interdigitations of the cerebral hemispheres in the affected region (Rauzzino and Oakes 1995).

In addition to the anomalies of the brain, typical skull malformations are frequently found in association with Chiari II malformation. The foramen magnum is often enlarged, a finding which obviates the need for suboccipital craniectomy in many patients undergoing surgery for symptomatic Chiari II malformation. Luckenschadel scalloping of the petrous pyramid (Fig. 4.10) and shortening of the clivus are common findings on computerised tomography scanning (Naidich et al. 1980).

A description of the pathological and radiological types of Chiari variants is given in Table 4.8. MRI findings are described in Table 4.9.

The widened foramen magnum provides one of the key components of any herniation, which is an incompetent orifice between two compartments. This raises questions regarding the perceived merits of expanding an already widened or incompetent hernia orifice to treat the hindbrain 'hernia'. Indeed the most reasonable treatment of any hernia is to tighten the orifice; release of a constricted orifice is reserved for those cases

Table 4.8 Chiari pathological classification and new radiological variants

Chiari	Description	Association
I	Herniation of the cerebellar tonsils 5 mm below the foramen magnum	Association with craniosynostosis, skull base anomalies and craniocephalic mismatch
II	Herniation of the cerebellar vermis and 4th ventricle	Associated with myelomeningocele, defect, hydrocephalus syringomyelia and neurological deficits
	Low-lying tentorium with low torcula	
	Occipital lobe often posterior to cerebellum	
III	Cerebellum, brainstem, 4th ventricular herniation with occipital or occipito-cervical meningoencephalocoele	Most serious form of Chiari malformation. Hydrocephalus may be present. Severe neurological deficits, incompatible with survival
IV	Cerebellar hypoplasia, 4th ventricle communicates with cisterna magna, no hindbrain hernia	Dandy-Walker-type malformation
Proposed new variants		
0	Patients with headaches and other symptoms of Chiari malformation or syringomyelia and no tonsillar hernia or tonsillar hernia less than 3 mm	Abnormal CSF flow the posterior fossa or foramen magnum as the suspected cause for syringomyelia (Tubbs et al. 2001)
1.5	A Chiari is seen in combination with brainstem herniation through the foramen magnum	Obex below the foramen magnum. Flat medulla oblongata. Mean backward angulation of the odontoid process in relation to the C2 body was 84°. Fifty percent have syringomyelia. Patients may not respond well to posterior fossa decompressive surgery especially if syringomyelia is present

Table 4.9 MRI findings in Chiari II malformation

Location	Abnormality	Cause
Infratentorial	Metencephalon/posterior fossa mismatch	Variably reduced space for the cerebellum and brainstem into a smaller than normal posterior fossa
Inferior vermis	Peg-like cerebellar tonsillar descent	The inferior vermis herniates into the foramen magnum and wraps around the posterior surface of the cord
Medulla	Cervicomedullary kink	The medulla is stretched downwards into the foramen magnum, while the cervical cord is anchored by the dentate ligaments, resulting in the cervicomedullary kink
Cerebellar hemispheres	Cerebellar hemispheres expand around the brainstem, occupying the cerebellopontine angles. Upward cerebellar herniation through the tentorial hiatus	The posterior fossa volume mismatch causes the cerebellum to move forward and be upright creating a distinctive appearance, the 'standing-up' cerebellum
Tentorium cerebelli	Steep angle of the tentorium	
Torcula	Displaced inferiorly	Pushed down nearly into level of foramen magnum along with steep tentorium
Vascular	Venous hypertension	Anomalies of the skull base, tight posterior fossa
Height of posterior fossa	Height from level of foramen magnum to apex of tentorium is increased	
Occipital lobes	Lie posterior to the cerebellum instead of above	
Occipital lobes	Stenogyria[a]	Crowding of the cerebral lobe gyri with loss of sulcal CSF and increased density
4th ventricle	The fourth ventricle is usually small or even completely effaced	
Tectal beaking	The inferior colliculi may be hypertrophied or fused, and point posteriorly to form the tectal beak	
Suprapineal recess of the 3rd ventricle	The suprapineal recess of the third ventricle and the interthalamic mass are especially prominent	
Corpus callosum	Commissural anomalies are commonly associated	
Membranous skull	Lacunar skull or luckenschädel	Disorganisation of the collagenous outer meninges (from which the membranous calvarium forms) produces irregularity of the surfaces of the inner and outer table of the skull
Hydrocephalus	Consistent finding within 48–72 h of repair of the spinal dysraphism	Once the caudal leakage is repaired, the amount of CSF increases in the ventricular system

[a]This is a radiological term describing compaction of otherwise normal gyri, such that they become small, with loss of intervening CSF. This feature is seen commonly in association with Chiari II malformation malformations

of strangulated hernia. It is therefore interesting to learn that performing a posterior, supratentorial calvarial augmentation, in children with craniosynostosis, can lead to regression of an associated Chiari malformation, without recourse to augmentation of the posterior fossa or decompression of the foramen magnum (Solanki et al. 2009, 2011; Farooq et al. 2011; White et al. 2009).

4.6   Morphometric Studies

From the foregoing discussions it may reasonably be suggested that idiopathic Chiari I malformation is the result of mesodermal defects that create a congenitally small posterior fossa (Atkinson et al. 1998; Badie et al. 1995; Nishikawa et al. 1997). A mismatch between the size of the posterior fossa and its contents leads to neural element compression and herniation through the foramen magnum (Tubbs et al. 2002). In children with Chiari I malformation, the anteroposterior dimension, the width and the volume of the posterior fossa are significantly lower than in controls (Furtado et al. 2009; Milhorat et al. 1999; Rodrigues and Solanki 2008; Rodrigues et al. 2009). So too is the ratio of posterior fossa volume to the overall intracranial volumes. Indeed, posterior fossa volumes may be some 23 % smaller in Chiari I patients compared to controls (Vemaraju et al. 2009; Milhorat et al. 1999). In contrast, a small body of evidence suggests that there is no difference in the size of the posterior fossa in patients with tonsillar ectopia, as compared with controls (Vega et al. 1990). The weight of evidence, however, points to a comparatively smaller size of the posterior fossa, in relation to the supratentorial compartment, in Chiari-affected patients (Badie et al. 1995; Solanki et al. 2009; Frias et al. 1988; Nakai et al. 1995; Vemaraju et al. 2009; Rodrigues et al. 2009; Milhorat et al. 1999).

Morphometric studies also reveal a larger sagittal diameter and a greater area of the foramen magnum compared to controls in both Chiari and Chiari II patients. The shape of the foramen magnum is also altered and expanded, from a normal ovoid to a more rounded opening, particularly in Chiari II malformations (Vemaraju et al. 2009). Contrast this with achondroplasia, a condition where accelerated fusion of the basiocciput and supraocciput occurs. Here the foramen magnum is narrow with a reduced area and sagittal stenosis.[21] Achondroplasia is also associated with macrocephaly, venous hypertension and ventriculomegaly, and yet there is no herniation of the hindbrain. Interestingly, in achondroplasia, the abnormalities often result in upward displacement of the brainstem, sometimes in conjunction with angulation of the pons and medulla oblongata (Nakai et al. 1995; Frias et al. 1988). This may explain the fact that Chiari type I malformation is somewhat rare in the achondroplastic population.

Conclusions

The SHH, HOX and PAX genes are crucial in the normal development of the brain and spinal cord, and many of their influences are mediated through the notochord organiser. It is very probable that both Chiari I and Chiari II malformations have a paraxial mesodermal origin, with a variable expression of their anomaly. It is now seen as less likely that Chiari II malformations are a disorder of neuronal migration, despite the presence of heterotopias[22] in some cases. Indeed, one could argue that Chiari II malformation malformations represent an exaggerated form of Chiari I malformation, resulting from an open neural tube defect that leaks CSF, causing caudal slump of the cerebrum and cerebellum.

The Chiari II malformation first becomes visible by the 10th to 12th weeks on ultrasound imaging. There is now good evidence to suggest that foetal surgery for Chiari II malformation improves motor outcomes, reverses the hindbrain hernia and reduces need for shunting after birth. This does mean, however, that a decision to reverse it must be taken urgently in such cases (Gehweiler et al. 1983).

References

Ahmad FU, Mahapatra AK (2009) Neural tube defects at separate sites: further evidence in support of multi-site closure of the neural tube in humans. Surg Neurol 71(3):353–356

Alexander T, Nolte C, Krumlauf R (2009) Hox genes and segmentation of the hindbrain and axial skeleton. Annu Rev Cell Dev Biol 25:431–456

Allin M, Matsumoto H, Santhouse AM et al (2001) Cognitive and motor function and the size of the cerebellum in adolescents born very pre-term. Brain 124(1):60–66

Arcy LB (1965) Developmental anatomy: a textbook and laboratory manual of embryology. WB Saunders Co., Philadelphia

Atkinson JLD, Kokmen E, Miller GM (1998) Evidence of posterior fossa hypoplasia in the familial variant of adult Chiari I malformation: case report. Neurosurgery 42(2):401

---

[21] Sagittal stenosis: narrow in the anterior-posterior diameter.

[22] Heterotopia refers to normal tissue present at an abnormal site. Heterotopia within the brain is often divided into three groups: subependymal heterotopia, focal cortical heterotopia and band heterotopia.

Badie B, Mendoza D, Batzdorf U (1995) Posterior fossa volume and response to suboccipital decompression in patients with Chiari I malformation. Neurosurgery 37(2):214

Beuls E, Vanormelingen L, Van Aalst J et al (2003) The Arnold-Chiari type II malformation at midgestation. Pediatr Neurosurg 39(3):149–158

Bhangoo R, Sgouros S, Walsh AR et al (2006) Hindbrain-hernia-related syringomyelia without syringobulbia, complicated by permanent nocturnal central hypoventilation requiring non-invasive ventilation. Childs Nerv Syst 22(2):113–116

Blaas HG, Eik-Nes SH, Isaksen C (2000) The early diagnosis of neural tube defects. J Med Screen 7:169–174

Bouchard S, Davey MG, Rintoul NE et al (2003) Correction of hindbrain herniation and anatomy of the vermis after in utero repair of myelomeningocele in sheep. J Pediatr Surg 38(3):451–458

Christ B, Wilting J (1992) From somites to vertebral column. Ann Anat 174(1):23–32

Cinalli G, Spennato P, Sainte-Rose C et al (2005) Chiari malformation in craniosynostosis. Childs Nerv Syst 21(10):889–901

Condie BG, Capecchi MR (1993) Mice homozygous for a targeted disruption of Hoxd-3 (Hox-4.1) exhibit anterior transformations of the first and second cervical vertebrae, the atlas and the axis. Development 119(3):579–595

Copp AJ, Greene NDE, Murdoch JN (2003) The genetic basis of mammalian neurulation. Nat Rev Genet 4(10):784–793

Dietrich S, Kessel M (1997) The vertebral column. In: Thorogood P (ed) Embryos, genes and birth defects. Wiley, Chichester, pp 281–302

Farooq U, Solanki GA, Lo W et al (2011) Regression of chronic hindbrain hernia following posterior calvarial augmentation in children: new insights into pathology of hindbrain hernia. Paper presented at the 2011 autumn meeting of the Society of British Neurological Surgeons, October 2011. Br J Neurosurg 25(5):554–579, Abstracts

Franz T (1992) Neural tube defects without neural crest defects in splotch mice. Teratology 46(6):599–604

Fraser SE, Keynes RJ, Lumsden A (1990) Segmentation in the chick embryo hindbrain is defined by cell lineage restriction. Nature 344:431–435

Frias JL, Williams JL, Friedman WA (1988) Magnetic resonance imaging in the assessment of medullary compression in achondroplasia. Arch Pediatr Adolesc Med 142(9):989

Furtado SV, Reddy K, Hegde AS (2009) Posterior fossa morphometry in symptomatic pediatric and adult Chiari I malformation. J Clin Neurosci 16(11):1449–1454

Gardner E, O'Rahilly R, Prolo D (1975) The Dandy-Walker and Arnold-Chiari malformations: clinical, developmental, and teratological considerations. Arch Neurol 32(6):393

Gasser RF (1976) Early formation of the basicranium in man. In: Bosma JF (ed) Symposium on development of the basicranium. Department of Health Education and Science Publication (NIH), Bethesda, pp 29–43

Gehweiler JA, Daffner RH, Roberts L (1983) Malformations of the atlas vertebra simulating the Jefferson fracture. Am J Roentgenol 140(6):1083–1086

Gladstone RJ, Wakeley CPG (1925) Variations of the occipito-atlantal joint in relation to the metameric structure of the cranio-vertebral region. J Anat 59(Pt 2):195

Golden JA, Chernoff GF (1993) Intermittent pattern of neural tube closure in two strains of mice. Teratology 47(1):73–80

Haapanen ML (2007) CHERI: time to identify the syndrome? J Craniofac Surg 18(2):369–373

Iskandar BJ, Quigley M, Haughton VM (2004) Foramen magnum cerebrospinal fluid flow characteristics in children with Chiari I malformation before and after craniocervical decompression. J Neurosurg Pediatr 101(2):169–178

Jessell TM, Kandel ER, Schwartz HJ (2000) Induction and Patterning of the Nervous System Ch 52 1019–1041, In Kandel ER, Schwartz JH, Jessell TM (eds). Principles of Neural Science, 4th ed. McGraw-Hill, New York

Keller R, Davidson L, Edlund A et al (2000) Mechanisms of convergence and extension by cell intercalation. Philos Trans R Soc Lond B Biol Sci 355(1399):897–922

Kessel M (1993) Reversal of axonal pathways from rhombomere 3 correlates with extra Hox expression domains. Neuron 10:379–393

Kessel M, Gruss P (1991) Homeotic transformations of murine vertebrae and concomitant alteration of Hox codes induced by retinoic acid. Cell 67(1):89–104

Keynes RJ, Stern CD (1988) Mechanisms of vertebrate segmentation. Development 103(3):413–429

Koseki H, Wallin J, Wilting J et al (1993) A role for Pax-1 as a mediator of notochordal signals during the dorso-ventral specification of vertebrae. Development 119(3):649–660

Lee J, Hida K, Seki T et al (2003) Pierre-Robin syndrome associated with Chiari type I malformation. Childs Nerv Syst 19(5):380–383

Loukas M et al (2011) Associated disorders of Chiari type I malformations. Neurosurg Focus 31(3):E3

Lufkin T, Mark M, Hart CP et al (1992) Homeotic transformation of the occipital bones of the skull by ectopic expression of a homeobox gene. Nature 359(6398):835–841

Lumsden A (1990) The cellular basis of segmentation in the developing hindbrain. Trends Neurosci 13:329–335

Marin-Padilla M, Marin-Padilla TM (1981) Morphogenesis of experimentally induced Arnold-Chiari malformation. J Neurol Sci 50(1):29–55

Marshall H, Nonchev S, Sham MH et al (1992) Retinoic acid alters hindbrain Hox code and induces transformation of rhombomeres 2/3 into a 4/5 identity. Nature 360(6406):737–741

McLendon RE, Crain BJ, Oakes WJ et al (1985) Cerebral polygyria in the Chiari type II (Arnold-Chiari) malformation. Clin Neuropathol 4(5):200

McLone DG, Knepper PA (1989) The cause of Chiari II malformation: a unified theory. Pediatr Neurosurg 15(1):1–12

Melsen B (1974) The cranial base; the postnatal development of the cranial base studied histologically on human autopsy material. Acta Odontol. Scand. 1974;32(Supp 62): American Journal of Orthodontics 66(6):689–691

Menezes AH (1995) Primary craniovertebral anomalies and the hindbrain herniation syndrome (Chiari I): data base analysis. Pediatr Neurosurg 23(5):260–269

Menezes AH (1996) Congenital and acquired abnormalities of the craniovertebral junction. In: Youmans J (ed) Neurological surgery. WB Saunders, Philadelphia, pp 1035–1089

Menezes AH (1998) Embryology, development and classification of disorders of the craniovertebral junction. In: Dickman CA, Sonntag VKH, Spetzler RF (eds) Surgery of the craniovertebral junction. Thieme Medical Publishers, New York, pp 3–12

Milhorat TH, Chou MW, Trinidad EM et al (1999) Chiari I malformation redefined: clinical and radiographic findings for 364 symptomatic patients. Neurosurgery 44(5):1005

Muller F, O'Rahilly R (1980) The human chondrocranium at the end of the embryonic period, proper, with particular reference to the nervous system. Am J Anat 159(1):33–58

Naidich TP, Pudlowski RM, Naidich JB et al (1980) Computed tomographic signs of the Chiari II malformation. Part I: skull and dural partitions. Radiology 134(1):65–71

Nakai T, Asato R, Miki Y et al (1995) A case of achondroplasia with downward displacement of the brain stem. Neuroradiology 37(4):293–294

Nakatsu T, Uwabe C, Shiota K (2000) Neural tube closure in humans initiates at multiple sites: evidence from human embryos and implications for the pathogenesis of neural tube defects. Anat Embryol 201(6):455–466

Nishikawa M, Sakamoto H, Hakuba A et al (1997) Pathogenesis of Chiari malformation: a morphometric study of the posterior cranial fossa. J Neurosurg 86(1):40–47

Norman MG, McGillivray BC, Kalousek DK (1995) Congenital malformations of the brain. Pathological, embryological, clinical, radiological and genetic aspects. Oxford University Press, New York

Paek BW, Farmer DL, Wilkinson CC et al (2000) Hindbrain herniation develops in surgically created myelomeningocele but is absent after repair in fetal lambs. Am J Obstet Gynecol 183(5):1119–1123

Peach B (1965) Arnold-Chiari malformation: anatomic features of 20 cases. Arch Neurol 12(6):613

Prescher A, Brors D, Adam G (1996) Anatomic and radiologic appearance of several variants of the craniocervical junction. Skull Base Surg 6(2):83

Rao PVV (2002) Median (third) occipital condyle. Clin Anat 15(2):148–151

Rauzzino M, Oakes WJ (1995) Chiari II malformation and syringomyelia. Neurosurg Clin N Am 6(2):293

Rodrigues D, Solanki GA (2008) Morphological features of the posterior fossa in Chiari malformation. Paper presented at the 36th annual meeting of the International Society for Paediatric Neurosurgery, Cape Town, South Africa, October 2008. Childs Nerv Syst 24:1225–1280, Abstracts

Rodrigues D, Vemaraju R, Furtado N, et al (2009): Paediatric Foramen Magnum dimensions in the Chiari malformations and syringomyelia: A comparative review. Proceedings of the 153rd Meeting of the Society of British Neurological Surgeons: Oral Abstracts of the Platform Presentations, British Journal of Neurosurgery, 23(2):111–135

Rodrigues D, Vemaraju R, Roy D et al (2009) Factors associated with syringomyelia in children with chronic hindbrain herniation. Br J Neurosurg 23(2):111–135

Solanki GA, Pettorini BL, Rodrigues D et al (2009) Effect of fixed calvarial augmentation on hindbrain hernia. Paper presented at the 37th annual meeting of the International Society for Pediatric Neurosurgery, Los Angeles, CA, USA, October 2009. Childs Nerv Syst 251:1345–1380

Solanki GA, Rodrigues D, Evans M et al (2011) Development of a radiographic criteria for surgical assessment of outcome following posterior calvarial augmentation. Paper presented at the 39th annual meeting of the International Society for Pediatric Neurosurgery, Goa, India, October, 2011. Childs Nerv Syst 27:1751–1850, Abstracts

Sutton LN, Adzick NS, Bilaniuk LT et al (1999) Improvement in hindbrain herniation demonstrated by serial fetal magnetic resonance imaging following fetal surgery for myelomeningocele. JAMA 282(19): 1826–1831

Thompson MW, Rudd N (1976) The genetics of spinal dysraphism. In: Morley TP (ed) Current controversies in neurosurgery. WB Saunders, Philadelphia, pp 126–146

Tominaga T, Takahashi T, Shimizu H et al (2002) Rotational vertebral artery occlusion from occipital bone anomaly: a rare cause of embolic stroke. J Neurosurg 97(6):1456–1459

Tubbs RS, Elton S, Grabb P, et al. Analysis of the posterior fossa in children with the Chiari 0 malformation. Neurosurgery. 2001; 48:1050–1055

Tubbs RS, Oakes WJ (2005) Beckwith-Wiedemann syndrome in a child with Chiari I malformation. J Neurosurg Pediatr 103(2):172–174

Tubbs RS, Dockery SE, Salter G et al (2002) Absence of the falx cerebelli in a Chiari II malformation. Clin Anat 15(3):193–195

Tubbs RS, Smyth MD, Wellons JC 3rd et al (2003) Hemihypertrophy and the Chiari I malformation. Pediatr Neurosurg 38(5):258–261

Van Allen MI, Kalousek DK, Chernoff GF et al (1993) Evidence for multi-site closure of the neural tube in humans. Am J Med Genet 47(5):723–743

Vega A, Quintana F, Berciano J (1990) Basichondrocranium anomalies in adult Chiari type I malformation: a morphometric study. J Neurol Sci 99(2–3):137–145

Venes JL, Black KL, Latack JT (1986) Preoperative evaluation and surgical management of the Arnold-Chiari II malformation. J Neurosurg 64(3):363–370

VonTorklus D, Gehle W (1972) The upper cervical spine. Regional anatomy, pathology and traumatology. In: ThiemeVerlag G (ed) A Systemic radiological atlas and textbook. Grune & Stratton, New York, pp 1–99

White N, Evans M, Dover MS et al (2009) Posterior calvarial vault expansion using distraction osteogenesis. Childs Nerv Syst 25(2):231–236

Genetics of Chiari Malformation and Syringomyelia

5

Guy Rouleau

Contents

With Zoha Kibar

G. Rouleau
Department of Medicine, CHU Sainte-Justine
Research Center, University of Montreal,
Montreal, QC, Canada
e-mail: guy.rouleau@umontreal.ca

5.1   Introduction

Chiari malformations are among the most common congenital abnormalities of the craniovertebral junction (Tubbs et al. 2008b). They encompass various degrees of herniation of inferior cerebellar structures, resulting in an overcrowding at the foramen magnum and altered cerebrospinal flow across the craniovertebral junction. Classification is based on the location and degree of herniation of the cerebellar tonsils and adjacent structures. Type I is the most common form of Chiari malformation and consists of a caudal descent of the cerebellar tonsils through the foramen magnum into the vertebral canal. It is a leading cause of syringomyelia and occurs in association with bony abnormalities at the craniovertebral junction. The most common of these is a small and shallow posterior fossa, with flattening of the squamous occipital bone (Tubbs et al. 2008b). Other associated abnormalities include kinking and inferior displacement of the medulla, angulation of the cervicomedullary junction and ventriculomegaly. Chiari malformation type II typically occurs in conjunction with myelomeningocoele and hydrocephalus. In addition to herniation of the cerebellar tonsils, the cerebellar vermis, fourth ventricle and medulla also protrude through the foramen magnum. Chiari malformations types III and IV are very rare conditions. Type III is structurally similar to type II malformation but with a coexistent low occipital or high cervical encephalocoele. Type IV is characterised by cerebellar

G. Flint, C. Rusbridge (eds.), *Syringomyelia*,
DOI 10.1007/978-3-642-13706-8_5, © Springer-Verlag Berlin Heidelberg 2014

hypoplasia with no hindbrain herniation (Hurlbert and Fehlings 1998).

Chiari types II, III and IV are very different from Chiari I embryologically, and little is known, at present, about the genetics of these forms of hindbrain hernia. The following discussions, therefore, relate in the main to the Chiari type I malformation.

5.2 Epidemiology and Clinical Presentation

If we accept that the diagnosis of Chiari type I malformation can only be confirmed by magnetic resonance imaging, then our best estimates of the prevalence of the condition, or at least the underlying anatomical abnormality, are likely to be given by reviews of MRI scans (Hurlbert and Fehlings 1998). Not surprisingly, estimated numbers have increased significantly with advances in MRI technology, and a review of all brain images in one hospital, over a 43-month period (22,591 individuals in total), produced a figure of 0.77 % (Meadows et al. 2000). This figure could be an overestimate since the study was conducted in a hospital population that is biased towards symptomatic patients with an increased incidence of anatomical abnormalities. Alternatively, this figure still could be an underestimate because of the under-diagnosed asymptomatic individuals in the normal population (Speer et al. 2003). Chiari type I malformation has a higher incidence in females than males (3:2) (Hurlbert and Fehlings 1998).

Nearly a third of patients with Chiari type I malformation become symptomatic (Hurlbert and Fehlings 1998). Initial presentation can occur in the paediatric population but is usually delayed until the third, fourth or fifth decade (Tubbs et al. 2007). Patients with Chiari type I may present with a variety of symptoms and signs, ranging from slight headache to severe neurological deficits and permanent nervous system damage, depending upon whether or not there is an associated syringomyelia. The most common symptom of Chiari is pain (60–70 %), usually occipital and upper cervical in location and often induced or exacerbated by Valsalva manoeuvres such as laughing, sneezing and coughing. Other common features are visual disturbances (78 %) and otoneurological symptoms (74 %), as well as those arising from an associated syringomyelia (Speer et al. 2003).

5.3 Aetiology and Pathogenesis

Whilst tonsillar herniation can be produced by pathologies causing increased intracranial pressure, including trauma, hydrocephalus, intracranial masses and benign intracranial hypertension, most cases of Chiari malformation are congenital in nature. The aetiology of congenital hindbrain hernias is probably multifactorial and almost certainly involves some genetic determinants. The majority of cases of Chiari that we regard as being congenital in origin is sporadic with no family history. Only about 1 % of the total number of Chiari type I malformations occur as part of a genetic syndrome (Speer et al. 2003; Tubbs et al. 2008b).

Several theories have been put forward to explain the embryological basis of Chiari type I malformation but with no single hypothesis being able to account for all aspects of the condition (Tubbs et al. 2008b; Sarnat 2007). Clearly, molecular studies are required and will be important, if we are to gain a better understanding of the underlying pathogenic mechanisms. The most widely accepted explanation, currently, is the 'crowding theory'. This proposes that a small posterior fossa volume, relative to the total cranial volume, results in herniation of the cerebellar tonsils into the vertebral canal. Essentially, we have a volume discrepancy between the posterior fossa of the cranium and the neural tissue residing within it. This explanation implies that the primary developmental defect is mesodermal, involving the cranial base, rather than being a primary disorder of the neuroectodermal tissue (Sarnat 2007). Morphometric studies in human patients certainly indicate that the posterior fossa is small and shallow in Chiari type I patients, compared to the normal population, while the total cranial volume is not reduced. These studies also suggest that the fundamental defect may involve underdevelopment of the occipital somites, originating from the paraxial mesoderm (Nishikawa et al. 1997; Karagöz et al. 2002; Aydin et al. 2005; Sekula et al. 2005; Trigylidas et al. 2008). In hamsters,

Chiari type I malformation can be induced experimentally by administration of a single dose of vitamin A, a substance known to affect mesodermal development, on day 8 of embryonic life. These laboratory studies suggest that the defect of Chiari type I malformation involves the somitic mesoderm at the basicranium and craniovertebral junction. An insufficiency of the paraxial mesoderm after the closure of the neural folds could lead to underdevelopment of the basichondrocranium, resulting in a posterior fossa that is too small and shallow (Marin-Padilla and Marin-Padilla 1980). Another study demonstrated that the structures affected in both Chiari type I and type II malformations are neural crest derived, and hence the defect could be neuroectodermal in origin (Matsuoka et al. 2005).

Syringomyelia is encountered in anywhere between 30 and 85 % of patients with Chiari type I malformation (Speer et al. 2003). It is possible that some or all of these cases are simply another consequence of a single developmental defect involving posterior fossa size. If so, they would share the same underlying genetic lesions. Alternatively, the development of syringomyelia could be determined by a different set of genetic modifiers that modulate the Chiari type I genetic background.

5.4   Genetic Influences

A genetic basis for Chiari type I malformation is supported by three major lines of evidence: (1) familial aggregation, (2) twin studies and (3) association with other genetic conditions.

5.4.1   Familial Aggregation and Clustering

A number of case studies have reported familial aggregation and clustering of Chiari type I malformation, suggesting a genetic basis to the pathogenesis of this condition in at least a proportion of patients (Table 5.1). A large study of 364 patients with Chiari type I malformation found that 12 % had a close relative with Chiari (Milhorat et al. 1999). Another large retrospective institutional study, looking at 500 surgically treated paediatric

Chiari type I malformations, reported a positive family history of approximately 3 % (Tubbs et al. 2011). Familial Chiari malformation is probably under-diagnosed because many affected relatives may be asymptomatic. Indeed, about one in five asymptomatic first-degree relatives of Chiari type I patients were also found to have Chiari malformations on MRI (Speer et al. 2000).

Families with Chiari type I malformation showed both vertical (mother-to-child) and male-to-male (father-to-son) transmission[1] consistent with an autosomal dominant mode of inheritance. Since the disease frequency in these affected families is less than what would be expected from pure Mendelian inheritance, Chiari type I malformation is thought to be incompletely penetrant.[2] Other pedigree studies, however, have implicated autosomal recessive mode of inheritance for Chiari type I malformation (Table 5.1). Most likely, the pattern of inheritance is oligogenic, i.e. determined by the cumulative effect of variants in several genes, albeit with variable penetrance.

A few cases have been reported of familial syringomyelia without an associated Chiari type I malformation (Robenek et al. 2006; Koç et al. 2007), although another study found no cases of familial syringomyelia in the absence of Chiari type I malformation, in a cohort of over 150 families (Speer et al. 2003). It may be that cases of 'isolated' familial syringomyelia have a volumetrically small posterior fossa without overt tonsillar herniation (Mavinkurve et al. 2005).

5.4.2   Twin Studies

Classical twin studies compare the occurrence of the same trait or disease in monozygotic and dizygotic twins. Monozygotic twins develop from a single fertilised egg and therefore have identical genetic material. Dizygotic twins derive

---

[1] Father-to-son transmission of a trait usually indicates that this trait is transmitted in a dominant fashion on an autosomal chromosome and not on the X chromosome.

[2] Penetrance is the proportion of individuals carrying a particular variant of a gene that also express an associated trait (phenotype). Penetrance is said to be incomplete or reduced when some individuals fail to express the trait, even though they carry the disease-causing mutation.

Table 5.1 Studies of families affected with Chiari type I malformation, with or without syringomyelia

Proposed inheritance	Number of families	Affected members	Reference study
Autosomal dominant with reduced penetrance	21 families	Parent–child, siblings, avuncular pairs[a], cousins	Milhorat et al. (1999)
	23 families	Parent–child, siblings, avuncular pairs, cousins	Boyles et al. (2006)
	1 family	Two brothers	Robenek et al. (2006)
	31 families	Parent–child, siblings, avuncular pairs, cousins	Speer et al. (2000)
	1 family	2 monozygotic twins and first-degree relatives	Stovner et al. (1992)
	1 family	3 generations	Coria et al. (1983)
	1 family	3 affected members	Giménez-Roldán et al. (1978)
Autosomal recessive	21 families	Siblings, avuncular pairs, cousins	Milhorat et al. (1999)
Multifactorial	3 families	Parent–child, monozygotic twins, avuncular pairs and cousins	Szewka et al. (2006)
Undetermined	3 families	2 mother–daughter pairs and 1 father–daughter pair	Schanker et al. (2011)
	15 families	15 surgically treated cases with positive family history including 3 pairs of affected siblings	Tubbs et al. (2011)
	1 family	4 generations	Tubbs et al. (2004a)
	1 family	3 sisters	Weisfeld-Adams et al. (2007)
	31 families	Parent–child, siblings, avuncular pairs, cousins	Speer et al. (2000)
	1 family	2 sisters	Mavinkurve et al. (2005)
	1 family	Monozygotic twin sisters and the daughter of one sister	Atkinson et al. (1998)
	1 family	2 siblings	Stovner and Sjaastad (1995)
	1 family	2 siblings	Herman et al. (1990)

[a]An avuncular relationship describes that between uncles and their nieces and nephews

from two eggs that were fertilised independently from two different sperm cells at the same time. These twins, like any other siblings, share 50 % of their genes.

Comparing the concordance[3] of monozygotic twins for a trait or disease with that of dizygotic twins provides an estimate of the extent to which genetic variation contributes to that trait or disease. A higher concordance in monozygotic as opposed to dizygotic twins indicates a genetic contribution to the trait under study (Boomsma et al. 2002). Several twin studies of Chiari type I malformation have reported an almost 100 % concordance in monozygotic twins (Stovner et al. 1992; Iwasaki et al. 2000; Szewka et al. 2006; Miller

et al. 2008; Tubbs et al. 2008a; Solth et al. 2010). Only five studies were examined for an associated syringomyelia, and three sets of twins were found to be discordant for this phenotype (Stovner et al. 1992; Iwasaki et al. 2000; Tubbs et al. 2008a), whilst two other sets were concordant for the absence of syringomyelia (Miller et al. 2008; Solth et al. 2010). Another report described syringomyelia in monozygotic twin brothers who were discordant for Chiari type I malformation (Tubbs et al. 2004b). A unique report of a monozygotic triplets described differing degrees of tonsillar descent; one triplet was affected by Chiari type I malformation and syringomyelia, whilst the other two asymptomatic siblings had tonsillar descent of 4 and 2.5 mm, respectively (Cavender and Schmidt 1995). A study of three pairs of dizygotic twins revealed that one pair of sisters was

---

[3]Concordance refers to the occurrence of the same trait in both members of a pair of twins.

concordant for Chiari type I malformation with syringomyelia. A second pair of sisters had Chiari type I malformation but only one of them had syringomyelia. In a third pair, one sister had Chiari type I malformation with syringomyelia while the female co-twin had neither (Speer et al. 2003). Collectively, these studies indicate a higher concordance of Chiari type I malformation between monozygotic than dizygotic twins, further supporting a genetic basis for Chiari type I malformation. Clearly, additional, larger twin studies are needed to confirm these findings and to investigate further twin concordance for syringomyelia associated with Chiari type I malformation.

5.4.3 Association with Known Genetic Syndromes

Co-segregation[4] of one condition, with one or more other known genetic conditions, suggests a genetic basis for the first condition. The assumption is that a common genetic defect is responsible for the various abnormal phenotypes within the complete syndrome. Chiari type I has been associated with several known genetic disorders or syndromes (Table 5.2). The majority of these disorders affect bone structures, for example, achondroplasia and Crouzon syndrome, or pathways involved in axial mesodermal growth and differentiation, for example, Williams syndrome and Shprintzen–Goldberg syndrome. The causative genes have been identified for some of these conditions and are mainly regulators of signalling pathways or transcription factors.[5] A few are implicated in essential cellular functions, such as chromatin methylation and proteolysis. DNA methylation plays an important role in regulation of gene expression during development and differentiation (Qureshi and Mehler 2011). Proteolysis is the process by which proteins are hydrolysed into small peptides and removed or cleaved for cell signalling (Maupin-Furlow 2011). The genes

are hypothesised to have pleiotropic effects[6] on the manifestation of cerebellar tonsil herniation, occipital hypoplasia, syringomyelia and other phenotypes.

Alternatively, Chiari type I malformation could be acquired secondarily in some of these diseases, for example, in cystic fibrosis, consequent upon constant Valsalva, from recurrent coughing or wheezing or as a result of metabolic and electrolyte imbalances (Patel et al. 2011).

Genomic deletions or duplications, on chromosome 7q and chromosome 16p, have been associated with Chiari type I malformation (Pober and Filiano 1995; Mercuri et al. 1997; Ferrero et al. 2007; Schaaf et al. 2011). These rearranged chromosomal regions contain a large number of biologically plausible candidate genes for Chiari type I, including *TBX6*, on chromosome 16p, that encodes a transcription factor important in establishing mesodermal identity and which can have a role in the aetiology of congenital spinal anomalies (Schaaf et al. 2011). A more comprehensive and systematic research of these regions is needed to identify the underlying genetic lesions and to understand their pathogenic role in the development of Chiari type I malformation.

5.5 Molecular Studies of Chiari in Humans

While Chiari type I malformation has a tendency to aggregate in families, it is rarely segregating in a classical Mendelian fashion. It is believed to be a complex trait that could be either oligogenic or polygenic, i.e. resulting from a large number of genetic variants, each contributing small effects. One cannot exclude the possibility of unknown environmental or nongenetic influences that may interact with these predisposing genetic factors to modulate the incidence of the Chiari type I with or without syringomyelia phenotype.

Studies of alleles[7] that influence other complex diseases could provide some indication of

---

[4] Co-segregation is the tendency for closely linked genes or traits to segregate or be inherited together.

[5] A transcription factor is a protein that binds to specific DNA sequences and controls the transcription or flow of genetic information from DNA to mRNA.

[6] Pleiotropy is a phenomenon in which one gene can influence two or more phenotypic traits.

[7] Different alleles of a gene refer to alternative forms of the gene; usually they are only very minor sequence differences between different alleles of any gene.

Table 5.2 Summary of genetic diseases and syndromes that can be associated with Chiari type I malformation

Syndrome (phenotype MIM#[a])	Locus	Gene	Gene function	References
Signalling transducers				
Achondroplasia (MIM# 100800)	4p16.3	*FGFR3* (fibroblast growth factor receptor 3)	Transmembrane growth factor receptor that mediates FGF signalling during development	Nakai et al. (1995), Bauer et al. (2005), Caldarelli et al. (2007), Richette et al. (2008)
Costello syndrome (MIM# 218040)	11p15.5	*HRAS* (v-Ha-ras Harvey rat sarcoma viral oncogene homologue)	Member of the Ras oncogene family that functions in signal transduction pathways	Gripp et al. (2010), White et al. (2005)
Crouzon syndrome (MIM# 123500) Apert's syndrome (MIM#101200)	10q26.13	*FGFR2* (fibroblast growth factor receptor-2)	Transmembrane growth factor receptor that mediates FGF signalling during development	Cinalli et al. (1995), Park et al. (1995), Reardon et al. (1994)
Hajdu–Cheney syndrome (MIM# 102500)	1p12-p11	*NOTCH2* (Notch gene homologue 2)	Notch type 1 transmembrane protein that plays a role in bone metabolism	Di Rocco and Oi (2005), Simpson et al. (2011)
Klippel–Feil syndrome (MIM# 118100)	8q22.1	*GDF6* (growth/differentiation factor 6)	Bone morphogenetic protein that regulates the formation of skeletal joints in the limbs, skull and axial skeleton	Tubbs et al. (2003), Tassabehji et al. (2008)
Loeys–Dietz syndrome type 1 (MIM# 609192)	9q22.33	*TGFBR1* (transforming growth factor, beta receptor 1)	Serine/threonine protein kinase that functions in TGF-beta signalling	Loeys et al. (2005)
Neurofibromatosis type I (MIM# 162200)	17q11.2	*NF1* (neurofibromin)	Negative regulator of the Ras signal transduction pathway	Tubbs et al. (2003), (2004a), Yohay (2006)
Noonan syndrome-1 (MIM# 163950)	12q24.13,	*PTPN11* (protein tyrosine phosphatase, non-receptor type 11)	Protein tyrosine kinase that plays a role in signalling via the RAS-mitogen activated protein kinase (MAPK) pathway	Croonen et al. (2008), Holder-Espinasse and Winter (2003)
Paget's disease of bone (MIM# 602080)	Genetically heterogeneous	*PDB4* (Paget's disease of bone 4)	*PDB4*: undetermined function	Otsuka et al. (2004), Richards et al. (2001)
	5q31	*SQSTM1* (sequestosome 1)	SQSTM1: binds ubiquitin and regulates activation of the nuclear factor kappa-B (NF-κB) signalling pathway	
	5q35.3	*TNFRSF11A* (tumour necrosis factor receptor super family, member 11a)	*TNFRSF11A*: member of the TNF-receptor super family, an essential mediator for osteoclast and lymph node development	
	18q21.33			
Transcription factors				
Chromosome 1p32-p31 deletion syndrome (MIM# 613735)	1p32-p31	*NF1A* (nuclear factor 1)	CAAT box transcription factor, plays a major role in development	Lu et al. (2007)

Syndrome (phenotype MIM#)	Locus	Gene	Gene function	References
Cleidocranial dysplasia (MIM#600211)	6p21.1	RNX2 (runt-related transcription factor 2)	Transcription factor, a key modulator of osteoblast differentiation	Vari et al. (1996), Ziros et al. (2008)
Combined pituitary hormone deficiency-4 (MIM#262700)	1q25.2	LHX4 (LIM-homeobox 4)	Transcription factor, functions during the development of the mammalian pituitary gland and the nervous system	Machinis et al. (2001), Tajima et al. (2007)
Type II blepharophimosis–ptosis–epicanthus inversus syndrome (BPES) (MIM# #110100)	3q22.3	FOXL2 (Forkhead box L2)	Forkhead transcription factor important in ovarian development	Paquis et al. (1998), Crisponi et al. (2001)
Velocardiofacial syndrome (MIM#192430)	1.5–3.0-Mb hemizygous deletion of 22q11.2	Some cases are caused by mutations in TBX1 (T-box 1)	TBX1: transcription factor with a conserved DNA-binding domain, the T-box	Hultman et al. (2000), Yagi et al. (2003)
Miscellaneous functions				
Cystic fibrosis (MIM# 219700)	7q31.2	CFTR (cystic fibrosis transmembrane conductance regulator)	Member of the ATP-binding cassette (ABC) transporter super family, functions as a chloride channel	Bobadilla et al. (2002), Patel et al. (2011)
Hypophosphatemic rickets (MIM# 307800)	Xp22.11	PHEX (phosphate-regulating endopeptidase homologue, X-linked)	Zinc-dependent metalloprotease, found in the cell-surface membrane of osteoblasts, osteocytes and odontoblasts	Caldemeyer et al. (1995) The HYP Consortium (1995)
Idiopathic growth hormone deficiency (MIM# 173100)	17q23.3	GH1 (growth hormone)	Growth hormone	Tubbs et al. (2003), Alatzoglou and Dattani (2010)
Kabuki syndrome (MIM# 147920)	12q12-q14	MLL2 (myeloid/lymphoid or mixed-lineage leukaemia 2)	Trithorax–group histone methyltransferase, important in the epigenetic control of active chromatin states	Ciprero et al. (2005), Ng et al. (2010)
Miller–Dieker lissencephaly syndrome (MIM#247200)	17p13.3	PAFAH1B1 (platelet-activating factor acetylhydrolase, isoform Ib)	Inactivating enzyme for platelet-activating factor, important for neuronal migration	Nagamani et al. (2009)
Shprintzen–Goldberg syndrome (MIM# 182212)	15q21.1	FBN1 (fibrillin 1) in some cases	Extracellular matrix glycoprotein that serves as a structural component of 10–12 nm calcium-binding microfibrils	Sood et al. (1996), Greally (2006)
Associated genes unknown				
Macrocephaly–capillary malformation (MIM# 602501)	Unknown		Unknown	Garavelli et al. (2005),Conway et al. (2007)

(continued)

Table 5.2 (continued)

Syndrome (phenotype MIM#[a])	Locus	Gene	Gene function	References
Primary basilar impression (MIM#109500)	Unknown		Unknown	Bentley et al. (1975)
Chromosome 16p11.2 rearrangements	Unknown		Unknown	Schaaf et al. (2011)
William's syndrome or chromosome 7q11.23 deletion syndrome (MIM#194050)	Hemizygous deletion of 1.5–1.8 Mb on chromosome 7q11.23		Unknown	Ferrero et al. (2007), Mercuri et al. (1997), Pober and Filiano (1995)

[a]MIM: Mendelian Inheritance in Man is a catalogue of human genes and genetic disorders (http://www.ncbi.nlm.nih.gov/omim/)

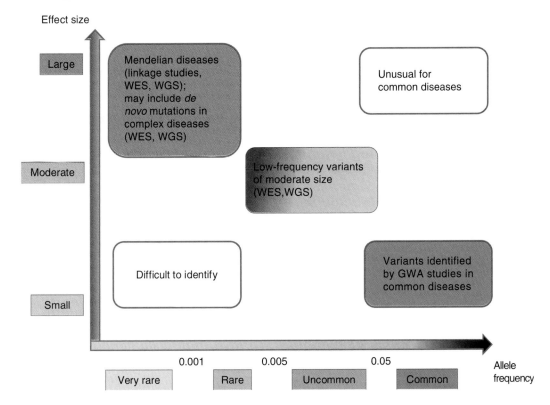

Fig. 5.1 Feasibility of gene identification studies by allele frequency and effect size in Mendelian and complex human diseases. Rare variants that have a large effect on the phenotype in Mendelian diseases can be identified in linkage studies where one investigates the segregation of a genetic marker with the disease phenotype in large multiple families affected with the disease. Very rare Mendelian diseases that are present in few small families are not amenable to this kind of linkage analysis and can only be identified if one sequences the whole exome (WES) or the whole genome (WGS) of the few affected individuals in order to identify the mutation specific to the phenotype. Recent genomics studies have implicated the presence of de novo (new) mutations in complex diseases that can only be identified by WES and/or WGS to identify the new mutation present in the affected individual and absent in parents. On the other end of the spectrum, common variants that have a small effect on the phenotype in complex diseases are identified by genome-wide association studies where one determines the association of a marker allele with the phenotype in a large cohort of cases and controls. *Abbreviations*: *WES* whole exome sequencing, *WGS* whole genome sequencing, *GWA* genome wide association

what might be taking place with Chiari type I malformation and syringomyelia. There is considerable heterogeneity both as regards the frequency and as regards the strength of effect of the alleles described to date (Fig. 5.1). At one end of the spectrum are high risk alleles, segregating in large families affected with Mendelian diseases. These can be identified easily by family-based linkage studies that aim at identifying a polymorphic genetic marker allele[8] that seg- regates strongly with the disease phenotype in a family.[9] At the other extreme, gene identification in complex traits remains a challenge. A number of common alleles have been found to be associated with common phenotypes, as predicted from the common disease/common variant hypothesis.

---

[8] A genetic marker refers to a short sequence of DNA with a known location on a chromosome. This marker is polymorphic when there are two or more allelic forms in the same population and the most common allele has a frequency of 0.99 or less.

[9] The principle of a linkage study is the following: if a disease runs in a family, one could look for genetic markers that run exactly the same way as the disease in the family. A marker allele that segregates with the disease is said to be linked to the disease. In this case, we assume that the gene that causes the disease and the marker allele are in the same area of the genome. Since we know the location of the genetic marker in the genome, we can deduce the location of the disease gene.

These common variants are usually identified by genetic association studies that investigate the association between common genetic variation and disease in a large numbers of study subjects. This type of analysis requires a dense set of polymorphic markers that capture a substantial proportion of common variation across the genome (for genome-wide association studies or GWAS[10]) or across a set of biologically plausible candidate genes (for candidate gene association studies) (Frazer et al. 2009). Common variants seem to have modest effect sizes.[11] Even when combined, their impact on overall population variance and predictive power[12] is limited. For many traits, associated variants have explained only a small proportion of estimated heritability.[13] A significant proportion of this undetermined heritability, known as 'missing heritability', may be attributable to variants that are of low frequency (<0.01 in frequency) with intermediate penetrance effects, which cannot be detected by conventional gene-discovery approaches mentioned above (Manolio et al. 2009). Recently, a role for rare de novo mutations is emerging in the genetic architecture of some of the complex traits, particularly those that decrease the reproductive fitness and incur a large degree of selection against the phenotype (Gillis and Rouleau 2011).

Gene identification studies of Chiari type I malformation and syringomyelia have been hindered by their complex aetiologies and inheritance patterns. Two approaches have been adopted or suggested in an attempt to identify the responsible genes and the underlying molecular pathogenic mechanisms. These are candidate gene studies and genome-wide linkage studies.

5.5.1 Candidate Genes Studies

A number of biologically plausible candidate genes, derived from mouse models, have been proposed for Chiari type I malformation, including the *Hox* genes, *Pax* genes, *FGFR2* and *Noggin*. The *Hox* gene family controls the development of the occipital bone and ectopic expression[14] of *Hox-2.3* results in dysplasia or deficiency of occipital, basisphenoid and atlas bones in transgenic[15] mice (McLain et al. 1992). The *Pax* group of genes codes for transcription factors with a conserved DNA-binding domain that have important roles in mesodermal segmentation and vertebral development. In particular, *Pax1* plays an important role in somitic segmentation and proper sclerotomal differentiation in the cervico-occipital transitional zone (Chi and Epstein 2002). *FGFR2* is transmembrane protein conserved across evolution and known to be critical for the normal development of multiple organ systems, including the craniofacial skeleton. The most common cause of Crouzon syndrome, a well-known craniosynostosis, is a mutation in *FGFR2, and* Chiari type I malformation is a common feature of Crouzon syndrome (Park et al. 1995). *Noggin* is required for growth and differentiation of the somites of the paraxial mesoderm (see Chap. 4). Noggin knockout mice show various defects, affecting neural and axial skeletal defects (McMahon et al. 1998). *Noggin* was analysed in 33 cases of Chiari type I malformation but no variant was identified, which suggests that this gene is not a common genetic factor involved in Chiari type I malformation (Speer et al. 2003).

---

[10] GWAS (genome-wide association studies) involve scanning hundreds to thousands of samples, either as case–control cohorts or in family trios, utilising hundreds of thousands of genetic markers located throughout the genome. This analysis identifies regions with statistically significant differences in allele frequencies between cases and controls, pointing to their role in disease.

[11] Effect size measures the strength of the relationship between the variant and the phenotype in a study population.

[12] Variants identified through association studies as significantly associated with disease susceptibility may be used in a *genetic predictive test* to classify disease risk in individual.

[13] Heritability is a measure of how much variation of a trait within a population is due to genes compared to variation due to environment.

[14] Ectopic expression is the expression of a gene in an abnormal place in an organism.

[15] A transgenic mouse contains additional, artificially introduced genetic material in every cell. This can confer a gain of function if the mouse produces a new protein or a loss of function if the integrated DNA interrupts another gene.

5.5.2 Linkage Studies

To date, only one linkage study[16] of human Chiari type I malformation has been conducted in a collection of 23 families with 71 affected individuals. This detected significant linkage of Chiari type I malformation to two genomic regions, on chromosomes 9q21.33–33.1 (31.3 Mb) and 15q21.1–22.3 (12.3 Mb) (Boyles et al. 2006). These two regions were too large for positional candidate gene cloning efforts whereby disease genes are identified using only knowledge of their approximate chromosomal location. A large candidate region identified by a linkage or an association study will most likely contain a large number of genes to be analysed, hence making this cloning procedure long and tedious. Interestingly, the region on chromosome 15 harbours a biologically plausible gene for Chiari type I malformation, fibrillin 1. This has been linked to a human syndrome called Shprintzen–Goldberg syndrome, which has Chiari type I malformation as a distinguishing characteristic (Boyles et al. 2006). These studies also demonstrated significant heritability of posterior fossa volume, supporting the presence of a genetic basis for this condition. Results from both studies should be interpreted cautiously as they are complicated by probable genetic heterogeneity[17] and the multifactorial aetiology of Chiari type I malformation.

5.6 Canine Models for Chiari and Syringomyelia

Chiari type I malformation in humans is similar to a condition called Chiari-like malformation that is common in several toy breed dogs including two genetically related dog breeds, the Cavalier King Charles Spaniels and Griffon Bruxellois (Rusbridge and Knowler 2003;

Rusbridge et al. 2009). Chiari-like malformation is present in almost 100 % of Cavalier King Charles Spaniels (Cerda-Gonzalez et al. 2009), and in a recent study of 56 Griffon Bruxellois dogs, the condition was found at a frequency of 6 in 10 (Rusbridge et al. 2009). Canine Chiari-like malformation therefore provides a spontaneously occurring, natural model of Chiari type I malformation in humans. In affected dogs, the caudal fossa is small relative to the entire cranial cavity (Cerda-Gonzalez and Dewey 2010), and the cerebellum is disproportionally large especially with dogs with early-onset syringomyelia (Shaw et al. 2012). As with humans, Chiari-like malformation in the dog is thought to involve an insufficiency of the occipital bones, producing a small caudal fossa (Rusbridge et al. 2009). The bony changes consist of a shortening of the basicranium, a shorter and vertical supraoccipital bone and a compensatory lengthening of the parietal bone. The latter characteristic does allow for accommodation of the forebrain, but there is insufficient room for the hindbrain, resulting in displacement of the neural structures into and through the foramen magnum (Rusbridge et al. 2009).

There is also a strong association between Chiari-like malformation and syringomyelia in dogs, which is thought to be related to obstruction of cerebrospinal fluid (CSF) movement across the craniovertebral junction (Rusbridge and Knowler 2003).

The high incidence of Chiari-like malformation in the Cavalier King Charles Spaniel and Griffon Bruxellois, as compared to other breeds, suggests the involvement of genetic factors in the aetiology of this disease (Rusbridge and Knowler 2003, 2004). Canine Chiari-like malformation does not segregate in Mendelian fashion in affected families, suggesting that this condition is oligogenic, polygenic or complex in origin, which could implicate environmental factors as well. The heritability of syringomyelia was estimated to be 0.37 (±0.15 standard error), indicating a moderate genetic effect on susceptibility to development of syringomyelia (Lewis et al. 2010). This heritability estimate implies that ~37 % of the trait is due to genetic factors.

---

[16] A genome-wide linkage scan refers to a screen of the whole genome for segregation of a marker allele with the phenotype.

[17] Genetic heterogeneity is a phenomenon in which many alleles of the same gene or of different genes cause the same phenotype.

Purebred dogs represent an invaluable tool for mapping and cloning genes affecting human health (Karlsson and Lindblad-Toh 2008). More than 450 diseases have been identified in dogs, and of these around 360 are homologues of common human disorders. These conditions can be studied and traced more easily when large dog pedigrees are available in established registries. The dog population has a unique history that is characterised by founder effects[18] and periodic population bottlenecks.[19] This, along with stringent breeding programmes, led to a closed genetic pool among dogs of each breed (Ostrander et al. 2000; Sutter and Ostrander 2004). There are some 350 breeds of dogs, and the high prevalence of specific diseases in many of these genetically homogeneous breeds suggests that a limited number of genes underlie each disease (Shearin and Ostrander 2010). These circumstances are mirrored, in part, in isolated human populations, such as the Finns and Icelanders. This situation can be used advantageously in genetic mapping studies, as such populations have limited variation in their gene pools, which reduces the chances of disease heterogeneity (Varilo and Peltonen 2004).

Most dog breeds are less than 200 years old and thus have long linkage disequilibrium[20] blocks, making them particularly amenable to linkage disequilibrium mapping with fewer markers and fewer dogs as compared to humans (Hyun et al. 2003; Sutter et al. 2004). This approach has been successful in mapping and identifying many genes predisposing to Mendelian as well as complex traits in the dog (Karlsson et al. 2007; Karlsson and

Lindblad-Toh 2008; Patterson et al. 2008; Wilbe et al. 2010). Notably, a genome-wide association study in 81 affected dogs and 57 controls, from the Nova Scotia Duck Tolling Retriever breed, identified five loci associated with a systemic lupus erythematosus-related disease. This demonstrated the power of linkage disequilibrium mapping in the dog, even in a small cohort of less than 100 cases and 100 controls, to identify pathways involved in human complex diseases (Wilbe et al. 2010).

The dog model is the only known naturally occurring animal model for Chiari type I malformation and syringomyelia. The high prevalence of Chiari-like malformation in the Cavalier King Charles Spaniel and Griffon Bruxellois breeds, along with the genetic homogeneity within these breeds, should help identify the defective gene(s) in the dog and then provide an entry point for a parallel search for mutations in the human orthologue(s)[21] in Chiari type I and syringomyelia. We can hope to identify key genes, proteins and molecular pathways involved in normal and abnormal development of structures of the human craniovertebral junction.

5.7   Future Studies

To date, no genetic factor predisposing to Chiari type I malformation and syringomyelia has been identified in humans. Identification of such genes by classical linkage analysis, association studies and positional cloning strategies is hindered by the complex nature of the inheritance of the disease along with its multifactorial aetiology. The candidate gene approach where one investigates genes that are biologically plausible (e.g. genes that are important for development of the craniovertebral junction) has not been successful so far because little is known about the molecular mechanisms underlying the pathogenesis of Chiari type I and syringomyelia. Identification of the Chiari gene(s), as for all other complex diseases, faces other major difficulties. These include epistasis, which is the effect that genetic variants have on each other,

---

[18] Founder effect occurs when a small group of individuals from a genetically diverse population migrates away and forms a new colony. Because the new colony will be composed only of genes from those few individuals, its genetic diversity will be reduced compared to the parent population.

[19] Population bottleneck is an evolutionary event characterised by a marked reduction in population size followed by the survival and expansion of a small random sample of the original population.

[20] Linkage disequilibrium is the nonrandom association of alleles at two or more loci. The strength of LD depends on many factors including the number of founders and the number of generations over which recombination has driven the decay of LD.

[21] Orthologues are genes in different species that originated from a single gene of the last common ancestor.

genetic alterations that occur during gametogenesis or after fertilisation and imprinting, which is the phenomenon in which only one of the two alleles of a gene may be expressed (Dean 2003). Finally, we always have to take into account the influence of various unknown environmental factors.

Powerful advances in genomics technologies have the potential, in the future, to revolutionise the exploration of the molecular genetics of Chiari I and syringomyelia. We are entering an exciting era, when we can sequence the 'whole genome' of an individual, in a cost-effective manner and in a short period. The next generation sequencing technologies will allow whole genome mutation analysis, with no prior assumptions regarding gene function and identification of low-frequency variants that increase disease susceptibility in affected individuals. A similar approach can focus on sequencing only protein-coding exons,[22] which comprise about 1 % of the human genome sequence. Exon-containing genomic fragments are isolated using oligonucleotide capture libraries,[23] followed by next generation sequencing.[24] A major challenge remains, however, with such innovative technologies, as regards the management and analysis of the massive data sets that will be generated (Majewski et al. 2011).

Genetic defects other than point mutations[25] could be involved in the pathogenesis of Chiari type I and syringomyelia. Data have emerged on the role of DNA copy number variants[26] as an important cause of neurodevelopmental conditions and birth defects. The novel technology of array comparative genomic hybridisation can survey the whole genome and detect large segments of genomic imbalance that are usually detectable by karyotyping,[27] as well as smaller copy number variants (Vissers et al. 2005). Using whole genome array comparative genomic hybridisation, several groups have shown that pathogenic copy number variants are a frequent cause of structural malformations in foetuses and newborns (Choy et al. 2010).

Epigenetic modifications[28] including DNA methylation could play an important role in the development of Chiari malformation. Assays that interrogate the whole genome for epigenetic regulatory modifications, for example, chromatin immunoprecipitation combined with DNA microarrays,[29] will enable us to explore the epigenomic influences on Chiari malformations (Schones and Zhao 2008). Another key regulator of gene expression is the recently discovered class of small RNA molecules, known as microRNAs. These play important regulatory roles in developmental timing and patterning, cellular differentiation, organogenesis and apoptosis (Chang et al. 2008). Several methodologies, including cloning, northern blotting, real-time RT-PCR and in situ hybridisation, have been developed and applied successfully in microRNA profiling (Li and Ruan 2009).

Conclusions

Chiari type I malformation, with or without syringomyelia, is a complex trait, with predisposing genetic influences. We are still in the early stages of identifying these genetic factors, and progress is hampered by the complexity of this trait. We are, however, witnessing a rapid expansion of high resolution technologies which, when coupled with the canine Chiari-like malformation model, will help us define these genetic factors and

---

[22] An exon is a sequence of DNA that codes information for protein synthesis that is transcribed to messenger RNA.

[23] Oligonucleotide capture libraries are pooled libraries of thousands of probes that will hybridise against and capture the coding exons.

[24] Next generation sequencing is the most recently developed high-throughput sequencing method that produces thousands or millions of sequences at once.

[25] A point mutation is when a single base pair is altered.

[26] A copy number variant is a segment of DNA ranging from 1 kb to several megabases in size that is caused by deletions, duplications, triplications, insertions or translocations.

[27] Karyotyping is a laboratory test that provides a picture of all the chromosomes from an individual's cells.

[28] Epigenetics is the study of heritable changes in gene expression or cellular phenotype caused by mechanisms other than changes in the DNA sequence.

[29] A DNA microarray or a DNA chip is a collection of microscopic DNA spots attached to a solid surface.

better understand the pathophysiology of human Chiari malformations. We may then be in a better position to advise affected patients about any likely inheritance of their condition.

References

Alatzoglou KS, Dattani MT (2010) Genetic causes and treatment of isolated growth hormone deficiency-an update. Nat Rev Endocrinol 6:562–576

Atkinson JL, Kokmen E, Miller GM (1998) Evidence of posterior fossa hypoplasia in the familial variant of adult Chiari I malformation: case report. Neurosurgery 42:401–403

Aydin S, Hanimoglu H, Tanriverdi T et al (2005) Chiari type I malformations in adults: a morphometric analysis of the posterior cranial fossa. Surg Neurol 64: 237–241

Bauer AM, Mueller DM, Oró JJ (2005) Arachnoid cyst resulting in tonsillar herniation and syringomyelia in a patient with achondroplasia. Case report. Neurosurg Focus 19:E14

Bentley SJ, Campbell MJ, Kaufmann P (1975) Familial syringomyelia. J Neurol Neurosurg Psychiatry 38: 346–349

Bobadilla JL, Macek M Jr, Fine JP et al (2002) Cystic fibrosis: a worldwide analysis of CFTR mutations–correlation with incidence data and application to screening. Hum Mutat 19:575–606

Boomsma D, Busjahn A, Peltonen L (2002) Classical twin studies and beyond. Nat Rev Genet 3:872–882

Boyles AL, Enterline DS, Hammock PH et al (2006) Phenotypic definition of Chiari type I malformation coupled with high-density SNP genome screen shows significant evidence for linkage to regions on chromosomes 9 and 15. Am J Med Genet A 140: 2776–2785

Caldarelli M, Novegno F, Vassimi L et al (2007) The role of limited posterior fossa craniectomy in the surgical treatment of Chiari malformation type I: experience with a pediatric series. J Neurosurg 106:187–195

Caldemeyer KS, Boaz JC, Wappner RS et al (1995) Chiari I malformation: association with hypophosphatemic rickets and MR imaging appearance. Radiology 195:733–738

Cavender RK, Schmidt JH 3rd (1995) Tonsillar ectopia and Chiari malformations: monozygotic triplets. Case report. J Neurosurg 82:497–500

Cerda-Gonzalez S, Dewey CW (2010) Congenital diseases of the craniocervical junction in the dog. Vet Clin North Am Small Anim Pract 40:121–141

Cerda-Gonzalez S, Olby NJ, McCullough S et al (2009) Morphology of the caudal fossa in Cavalier King Charles Spaniels. Vet Radiol Ultrasound 50:37–46

Chang S, Wen S, Chen D et al (2008) Small regulatory RNAs in neurodevelopmental disorders. Hum Mol Genet 18:R18–R26

Chi N, Epstein JA (2002) Getting your Pax straight: Pax proteins in development and disease. Trends Genet 18:41–47

Choy KW, Setlur SR, Lee C et al (2010) The impact of human copy number variation on a new era of genetic testing. BJOG 117:391–398

Cinalli G, Renier D, Sebag G et al (1995) Chronic tonsillar herniation in Crouzon's and Apert's syndromes: the role of premature synostosis of the lambdoid suture. J Neurosurg 83:575–582

Ciprero KL, Clayton-Smith J, Donnai D et al (2005) Symptomatic Chiari I malformation in Kabuki syndrome. Am J Med Genet A 132A:273–275

Conway RL, Pressman BD, Dobyns WB et al (2007) Neuroimaging findings in macrocephaly-capillary malformation: a longitudinal study of 17 patients. Am J Med Genet 143A:2981–3008

Coria F, Quintana F, Rebollo M et al (1983) Occipital dysplasia and Chiari type I deformity in a family. Clinical and radiological study of three generations. J Neurol Sci 62:147–158

Crisponi L, Deiana M, Loi A et al (2001) The putative forkhead transcription factor FOXL2 is mutated in blepharophimosis/ptosis/epicanthus inversus syndrome. Nat Genet 27:159–166

Croonen EA, van der Burgt I, Kapusta L et al (2008) Electrocardiography in Noonan syndrome PTPN11 gene mutation–phenotype characterization. Am J Med Genet 146A:350–353

Dean M (2003) Approaches to identify genes for complex human diseases: lessons from Mendelian disorders. Hum Mutat 22:261–274

Di Rocco F, Oi S (2005) Spontaneous regression of syringomyelia in Hajdu-Cheney syndrome with severe platybasia. Case report. J Neurosurg 103(2 Suppl): 194–197

Ferrero GB, Biamino E, Sorasio L et al (2007) Presenting phenotype and clinical evaluation in a cohort of 22 Williams-Beuren syndrome patients. Eur J Med Genet 50:327–337

Frazer KA, Murray SS, Schork NJ et al (2009) Human genetic variation and its contribution to complex traits. Nat Rev Genet 10:241–251

Garavelli L, Leask K, Zanacca C et al (2005) MRI and neurological findings in macrocephaly-cutis marmorata telangiectatica congenita syndrome: report of ten cases and review of the literature. Genet Couns 16: 117–128

Gillis RF, Rouleau GA (2011) The ongoing dissection of the genetic architecture of autistic spectrum disorder. Mol Autism 2:12

Giménez-Roldán S, Benito C, Mateo D (1978) Familial communicating syringomyelia. J Neurol Sci 36: 135–146

Greally MT (2006) Shprintzen-Goldberg syndrome. In: Pagon RA, Bird TD, Dolan CR, Stephens K (eds) GeneReviews [Internet]. University of Washington, Seattle

Gripp KW, Hopkins E, Doyle D et al (2010) High incidence of progressive postnatal cerebellar enlargement in Costello syndrome: brain overgrowth associated with HRAS mutations as the likely cause of structural brain and spinal cord abnormalities. Am J Med Genet 152A:1161–1168

Herman MD, Cheek WR, Storrs BB (1990) Two siblings with the Chiari I malformation. Pediatr Neurosurg 16:183–184

Holder-Espinasse M, Winter RM (2003) Type 1 Arnold-Chiari malformation and Noonan syndrome: a new diagnostic feature? Clin Dysmorphol 12:275

Hultman CS, Riski JE, Cohen SR et al (2000) Chiari malformation, cervical spine anomalies, and neurologic deficits in velocardiofacial syndrome. Plast Reconstr Surg 106:16–24

Hurlbert RJ, Fehlings MG (1998) The Chiari malformations. In: Engler GL, Cole J, Merton WL (eds) Spinal cord diseases diagnosis and treatment. Marcel Dekker, New York

Hyun C, Filippich LJ, Lea RA et al (2003) Prospects for whole genome linkage disequilibrium mapping in domestic dog breeds. Mamm Genome 14:640–649

Iwasaki Y, Hida K, Onishi K et al (2000) Chiari malformation and syringomyelia in monozygotic twins: birth injury as a possible cause of syringomyelia – case report. Neurol Med Chir (Tokyo) 40:176–178

Karagöz F, Izgi N, Kapíjcíjoğlu Sencer S (2002) Morphometric measurements of the cranium in patients with Chiari type I malformation and comparison with the normal population. Acta Neurochir (Wien) 144:165–171

Karlsson EK, Lindblad-Toh K (2008) Leader of the pack: gene mapping in dogs and other model organisms. Nat Rev Genet 9:713–725

Karlsson EK, Baranowska I, Wade CM et al (2007) Efficient mapping of mendelian traits in dogs through genome-wide association. Nat Genet 39:1321–1328

Koç K, Anik I, Anik Y et al (2007) Familial syringomyelia in two siblings: case report. Turk Neurosurg 17:251–254

Lewis T, Rusbridge C, Knowler P et al (2010) Heritability of syringomyelia in Cavalier King Charles spaniels. Vet J 183:345–347

Li W, Ruan K (2009) MicroRNA detection by microarray. Anal Bioanal Chem 394:1117–1124

Loeys BL, Chen J, Neptune ER et al (2005) A syndrome of altered cardiovascular, craniofacial, neurocognitive and skeletal development caused by mutations in TGFBR1 or TGFBR2. Nat Genet 37:275–281

Lu W, Quintero-Rivera F, Fan Y et al (2007) NFIA haploinsufficiency is associated with a CNS malformation syndrome and urinary tract defects. PLoS Genet 3:e80

Machinis K, Pantel J, Netchine I et al (2001) Syndromic short stature in patients with a germline mutation in the LIM homeobox LHX4. Am J Hum Genet 69:961–968

Majewski J, Schwartzentruber J, Lalonde E et al (2011) What can exome sequencing do for you? J Med Genet 48:580–589

Manolio TA, Collins FS, Cox NJ et al (2009) Finding the missing heritability of complex diseases. Nature 2009(461):747–753

Marin-Padilla M, Marin-Padilla TM (1980) Morphogenesis of experimentally induced Arnold–Chiari malformation. J Neurol Sci 50:29–55

Matsuoka T, Ahlberg PE, Kessaris N et al (2005) Neural crest origins of the neck and shoulder. Nature 436:347–355

Maupin-Furlow J (2011) Proteasomes and protein conjugation across domains of life. Nat Rev Microbiol 10:100–111

Mavinkurve GG, Sciubba D, Amundson E et al (2005) Familial Chiari type I malformation with syringomyelia in two siblings: case report and review of the literature. Childs Nerv Syst 21:955–959

McLain K, Schreiner C, Yager KL et al (1992) Ectopic expression of Hox-2.3 induces craniofacial and skeletal malformations in transgenic mice. Mech Dev 39:3–16

McMahon JA, Takada S, Zimmerman LB et al (1998) Noggin-mediated antagonism of BMP signaling is required for growth and patterning of the neural tube and somite. Genes Dev 12:1438–1452

Meadows J, Kraut M, Guarnieri M et al (2000) Asymptomatic Chiari type I malformations identified on magnetic resonance imaging. J Neurosurg 92:920–926

Mercuri E, Atkinson J, Braddick O et al (1997) Chiari I malformation in asymptomatic young children with Williams syndrome: clinical and MRI study. Eur J Paediatr Neurol 1:177–181

Milhorat TH, Chou MW, Trinidad EM et al (1999) Chiari I malformation redefined: clinical and radiographic findings for 364 symptomatic patients. Neurosurgery 44:1005–1017

Miller JH, Limbrick DD, Callen M et al (2008) Spontaneous resolution of Chiari malformation Type I in monozygotic twins. J Neurosurg Pediatr 2:317–319

Nagamani SCS, Zhang F, Shchelochkov OA et al (2009) Microdeletions including YWHAE in the Miller-Dieker syndrome region on chromosome 17p13.3 result in facial dysmorphisms, growth restriction, and cognitive impairment. J Med Genet 46:825–833

Nakai T, Asato R, Miki Y et al (1995) A case of achondroplasia with downward displacement of the brain stem. Neuroradiology 37:293–294

Ng SB, Bigham AW, Buckingham KJ et al (2010) Exome sequencing identifies MLL2 mutations as a cause of Kabuki syndrome. Nat Genet 42:790–793

Nishikawa M, Sakamoto H, Hakuba A et al (1997) Pathogenesis of Chiari malformation: a morphometric study of the posterior cranial fossa. J Neurosurg 86:40–47

Ostrander EA, Galibert F, Patterson DF (2000) Canine genetics comes of age. Trends Genet 16:117–124

Otsuka F, Inagaki K, Suzuki J et al (2004) Skull Paget's disease developing into Chiari malformation. Endocr J 51:391–392

Paquis P, Lonjon M, Brunet M et al (1998) Chiari Type I malformation and syringomyelia in unrelated patients with blepharophimosis. Report of two cases. J Neurosurg 89:835–838

Park WJ, Theda C, Maestri NE et al (1995) Analysis of phenotypic features and FGFR2 mutations in Apert syndrome. Am J Hum Genet 57:321–328

Patel AJ, Raol VH, Jea A (2011) Rare association between cystic fibrosis, Chiari I malformation, and hydrocephalus in a baby: a case report and review of the literature. J Med Case Reports 5:366

Patterson EE, Minor KM, Tchernatynskaia AV et al (2008) A canine DNM1 mutation is highly associated with the syndrome of exercise-induced collapse. Nat Genet 40:1235–1239

Pober BR, Filiano JJ (1995) Association of Chiari I malformation and Williams syndrome. Pediatr Neurol 12:84–88

Qureshi IA, Mehler MF (2011) Advances in epigenetics and epigenomics for neurodegenerative diseases. Curr Neurol Neurosci Rep 11:464–473

Reardon W, Winter RM, Rutland P et al (1994) Mutations in the fibroblast growth factor receptor 2 gene cause Crouzon syndrome. Nat Genet 8:98–103

Richards PS, Bargiota A, Corrall RJ (2001) Paget's disease causing an Arnold-Chiari type 1 malformation: radiographic findings. AJR Am J Roentgenol 176: 816–817

Richette P, Bardin T, Stheneur C (2008) Achondroplasia: from genotype to phenotype. Joint Bone Spine 75: 125–130

Robenek M, Kloska SP, Husstedt IW (2006) Evidence of familial syringomyelia in discordant association with Chiari type I malformation. Eur J Neurol 13:783–785

Rusbridge C, Knowler SP (2003) Hereditary aspects of occipital bone hypoplasia and syringomyelia (Chiari type I malformation) in cavalier King Charles spaniels. Vet Rec 15:107–112

Rusbridge C, Knowler SP (2004) Inheritance of occipital bone hypoplasia (Chiari type I malformation) in Cavalier King Charles Spaniels. J Vet Intern Med 18: 673–678

Rusbridge C, Knowler S, Pieterse L et al (2009) Chiari-like malformation in the Griffon Bruxellois. J Small Anim Pract 50:386–393

Sarnat HB (2007) Disorders of segmentation of the neural tube: Chiari malformations. Handb Clin Neurol 87: 89–103

Schaaf CP, Goin-Kochel RP, Nowell KP et al (2011) Expanding the clinical spectrum of the 16p11.2 chromosomal rearrangements: three patients with syringomyelia. Eur J Hum Genet 19:152–156

Schanker BD, Walcott BP, Nahed BV et al (2011) Familial Chiari malformation: case series. Neurosurg Focus 31: E1

Schones DE, Zhao K (2008) Genome-wide approaches to studying chromatin modifications. Nat Rev Genet 9:179–191

Sekula RF Jr, Jannetta PJ, Casey KF et al (2005) Dimensions of the posterior fossa in patients symptomatic for Chiari I malformation but without cerebellar tonsillar descent. Cerebrospinal Fluid Res 2:11

Shaw TA, McGonnell IM, Driver CJ et al (2012) Increase in cerebellar volume in cavalier king Charles spaniels with Chiari-like malformation and its role in the development of syringomyelia. PLoS One 7:e33660

Shearin AL, Ostrander EA (2010) Leading the way: canine models of genomics and disease. Dis Model Mech 3:27–34

Simpson MA, Irving MD, Asilmaz E et al (2011) Mutations in NOTCH2 cause Hajdu-Cheney syndrome, a disorder of severe and progressive bone loss. Nat Genet 43:303–305

Solth A, Barrett C, Holliman D et al (2010) Chiari malformation in female monozygotic twins. Br J Neurosurg 24:607–608

Sood S, Eldadah ZA, Krause WL et al (1996) Mutation in fibrillin-1 and the Marfanoid-craniosynostosis (Shprintzen-Goldberg) syndrome. Nat Genet 12: 209–211

Speer MC, George TM, Enterline DS et al (2000) A genetic hypothesis for Chiari I malformation with or without syringomyelia. Neurosurg Focus 8:E12

Speer MC, Enterline DS, Mehltretter L et al (2003) Chiari type I malformation with or without syringomyelia: prevalence and genetics. J Genet Couns 12:297–311

Stovner LJ, Sjaastad O (1995) Segmental hyperhidrosis in two siblings with Chiari type I malformation. Eur Neurol 35:149–155

Stovner LJ, Cappelen J, Nilsen G et al (1992) The Chiari type I malformation in two monozygotic twins and first-degree relatives. Ann Neurol 31:220–222

Sutter NB, Ostrander EA (2004) Dog star rising: the canine genetic system. Nat Rev Genet 5: 900–910

Sutter NB, Eberle MA, Parker HG et al (2004) Extensive and breed-specific linkage disequilibrium in Canis familiaris. Genome Res 14:2388–2396

Szewka AJ, Walsh LE, Boaz JC et al (2006) Chiari in the family: inheritance of the Chiari I malformation. Pediatr Neurol 34:481–485

Tajima T, Hattori T, Nakajima T et al (2007) A novel missense mutation (P366T) of the LHX4 gene causes severe combined pituitary hormone deficiency with pituitary hypoplasia, ectopic posterior lobe and a poorly developed sella turcica. Endocr J 54:637–641

Tassabehji M, Fang ZM, Hilton EN et al (2008) Mutations in GDF6 are associated with vertebral segmentation defects in Klippel-Feil syndrome. Hum Mutat 29: 1017–1027

The HYP Consortium (1995) A gene (PEX) with homologies to endopeptidases is mutated in patients with X-linked hypophosphatemic rickets. Nat Genet 11: 130–136

Trigylidas T, Baronia B, Vassilyadi M et al (2008) Posterior fossa dimension and volume estimates in pediatric patients with Chiari I malformations. Childs Nerv Syst 24:329–336

Tubbs RS, McGirt MJ, Oakes WJ (2003) Surgical experience in 130 pediatric patients with Chiari I malformations. J Neurosurg 99:291–296

Tubbs RS, Rutledge SL, Kosentka A et al (2004a) Chiari I malformation and neurofibromatosis type 1. Pediatr Neurol 30:278–280

Tubbs RS, Wellons JC 3rd, Blount JP et al (2004b) Syringomyelia in twin brothers discordant for Chiari I malformation: case report. J Child Neurol 19:459–462

Tubbs RS, Lyerly MJ, Loukas M et al (2007) The pediatric Chiari I malformation: a review. Childs Nerv Syst 23:1239–1250

Tubbs RS, Hill M, Loukas M et al (2008a) Volumetric analysis of the posterior cranial fossa in a family with four generations of the Chiari malformation Type I. J Neurosurg Pediatr 1:21–24

Tubbs RS, Shoja MM, Ardalan MR et al (2008b) Hindbrain herniation: a review of embryological theories. Ital J Anat Embryol 113:37–46

Tubbs RS, Beckman J, Naftel RP et al (2011) Institutional experience with 500 cases of surgically treated pediatric Chiari malformation Type I. J Neurosurg Pediatr 7: 248–256

Vari R, Puca A, Meglio M (1996) Cleidocranial dysplasia and syringomyelia. Case report. J Neurosurg Sci 40: 125–128

Varilo T, Peltonen L (2004) Isolates and their potential use in complex gene mapping efforts. Curr Opin Genet Dev 14:316–323

Vissers LE, Veltman JA, van Kessel AG et al (2005) Identification of disease genes by whole genome CGH arrays. Hum Mol Genet 14:R215–R223

Weisfeld-Adams JD, Carter MR, Likeman MJ et al (2007) Three sisters with Chiari I malformation with and without associated syringomyelia. Pediatr Neurosurg 43:533–538

White SM, Graham JM Jr, Kerr B et al (2005) The adult phenotype in Costello syndrome. Am J Med Genet A 136(2):128–135

Wilbe M, Jokinen P, Truvé K et al (2010) Genome-wide association mapping identifies multiple loci for a canine SLE-related disease complex. Nat Genet 42:250–254

Yagi H, Furutani Y, Hamada H et al (2003) Role of TBX1 in human del22q11.2 syndrome. Lancet 362: 1366–1373

Yohay KH (2006) The genetic and molecular pathogenesis of NF1 and NF2. Semin Pediatr Neurol 13: 21–26

Ziros PG, Basdra EK, Papavassiliou AG (2008) Runx2: of bone and stretch. Int J Biochem Cell Biol 40: 1659–1663

The Filling Mechanism

6

Marcus Stoodley

Contents

With Lynne Bilston, Andrew Brodbelt, Sarah Hemley
and Johnny Wong

M. Stoodley
Neurosurgery Unit, Australian School of Advanced
Medicine, Macquarie University, Sydney,
NSW, Australia
e-mail: marcus.stoodley@mq.edu.au

6.1 Introduction

Syringomyelia is one of the most enigmatic conditions affecting the central nervous system. The seemingly simple nature of these intramedullary cysts belies the complexity that meets any serious investigation of the filling mechanisms. The pathophysiology may at first appear tantalizingly simple, yet closer inspection reveals complexity, and a satisfactory explanation remains elusive.

A myriad of theories have been proposed. Hydrodynamic theories generally assume that syrinx fluid is cerebrospinal fluid (CSF) that has entered the cord as a result of perturbations of pulsations in the subarachnoid space, caused by an associated Chiari malformation, arachnoiditis, or other abnormalities obstructing the subarachnoid space. Other theories propose that the fluid is not CSF, being formed predominantly from interstitial fluid. Suggested mechanisms include cord tethering, stretching the cord apart, and the Venturi effect in the subarachnoid space, expanding the cord by suction. Recent theories have proposed that disruptions of the blood-spinal cord barrier or alterations of aquaporin expression or function may result in excess fluid accumulation in the cord. Despite the plethora of theories, the pathophysiology of syringomyelia remains perplexing.

At a fundamental level, the volume of fluid and pressure in a syrinx are determined by the flow of fluid into and out of the cavity. A syrinx can only enlarge if net inflow exceeds net

G. Flint, C. Rusbridge (eds.), *Syringomyelia*,
DOI 10.1007/978-3-642-13706-8_6, © Springer-Verlag Berlin Heidelberg 2014

outflow; enlargement may therefore occur due to either increased inflow or decreased outflow. In addition to such factors, there may be local tissue characteristics that limit or permit syrinx expansion and influence internal pressure and the effect that it has on cord neurological function.

Syringomyelia is associated with many conditions, and the filling mechanism may, of course, be different in each case. Whether a syrinx is an expansion of the central canal (canalicular) or is outside the central canal (extracanalicular) and whether the subarachnoid space is affected by the associated condition may be important factors determining the underlying pathophysiology. Furthermore, there may be different mechanisms for initial cyst formation and subsequent cyst enlargement (Brodbelt and Stoodley 2003).

Essential, but still unresolved aspects of the condition include the composition of syrinx fluid and the pressure within syrinx cavities relative to the subarachnoid space. Each of these will be discussed, following a general outline of the history of theories regarding syringomyelia pathogenesis.

6.2   History of Filling Mechanism Theories

Original descriptions of syringomyelia were garnered from autopsy studies. The pathological appearances were therefore of a collapsed cavity, rather than the tense cyst, exerting pressure on the surrounding cord tissue, that is now familiar to neurosurgeons. Initial theories regarding pathogenesis were accordingly not focused on fluid dynamics. Chiari and Ollivier D'Angers both suggested that syrinx cavities were developmental defects of the central canal or spinal cord (Newton 1969; Ollivier 1827). A subsequent theory was that the cavities were formed secondary to tissue loss, and attention turned to ischaemia as a possible cause (Joffroy and Achard 1887). Early experimental studies continued to focus on tissue loss and vascular effects of arachnoid inflammation and scarring (Hall et al. 1975; McLaurin et al. 1954; Woodard and Freeman 1956). Ischemic tissue loss was considered by

Caplan and colleagues to be an important component of syringomyelia associated with arachnoiditis, although the authors suggested that alterations of CSF dynamics could contribute to cavity formation (Caplan et al. 1990).

Traumatic birth then received attention as a possible causative factor. It was suggested that the high pressure applied to the foetal head during a difficult labour and the use of forceps may increase venous pressure, displace the cerebellar tonsils, cause the central canal to rupture, or cause haemorrhage that results in arachnoiditis (Newman et al. 1981; Williams 1977; Hida et al. 1994).

A hydrodynamic aetiology was first proposed by Cleland, who suggested that brainstem abnormalities led to hydrocephalus and dilation of the central canal (Cleland 1883). Gardner refined this theory, proposing that obstruction of the outlets of the fourth ventricle led to both hydrocephalus and an enlarged central canal which, in extreme cases, would rupture and manifest as myelomeningocele (Gardner 1959; Gardner and Angel 1958). Williams proposed an alternative explanation by which fluid could be forced from the fourth ventricle into the central canal, implicating mobile cerebellar tonsils as a variable plug that would lead to pressure differentials between the head and the spine (Williams 1969, 1972).

A hydrodynamic mechanism, forcing CSF from the spinal subarachnoid space across the cord parenchyma, was first proposed by Ball and Dayan, who suggested that increases in CSF pressure caused by coughing and sneezing would force fluid into the cord (Ball and Dayan 1972). Different pathways and dynamics of transmedullary CSF flow have subsequently been proposed by Oldfield and colleagues (Heiss et al. 1999; Oldfield et al. 1994), Stoodley and colleagues (Bilston et al. 2003, 2006, 2010; Brodbelt et al. 2003a, b; Stoodley et al. 1997, 1999, 2000), Carpenter and colleagues (2003), Klekamp and colleagues (2001), and Elliott and colleagues (2009).

Rather than increased flow into syrinx cavities, some authors have argued that the problem is a blockage of fluid outflow. This was first proposed by Aboulker, who postulated that blockage at the foramen magnum prevented CSF from draining from the central canal into the fourth ventricle (Aboulker 1979). Similarly, Koyanagi and Houkin suggested that fluid accumulates because of an impairment in extracellular fluid absorption (Koyanagi and Houkin 2010), and Klekamp has suggested that blockage of perivascular spaces or cord tethering could affect outflow (Klekamp 2002).

Over the last two decades, some authors have suggested sources of fluid other than CSF. Greitz argued that an increase in intramedullary pulse pressure results in expansion of the cord and that the expanded space fills with extracellular fluid (Greitz 2006). Chang and Nakagawa proposed that syrinx fluid comes from the central canal when there is a lowering of the adjacent subarachnoid pressure (Chang and Nakagawa 2004). Levine has suggested that pressure exerted by a Chiari malformation causes an increase in the spinal cord venous pressure, with vascular damage allowing plasma filtrate to pass across the vessel walls (Levine 2004).

Investigating detailed fluid physiology is often impossible in patients and difficult in experimental animals. Over recent years, computational and physical modelling techniques have been used to investigate numerous theories regarding CSF physiology in the subarachnoid and perivascular spaces (Bertram et al. 2008; Bilston et al. 2003, 2006, 2010; Berkouk et al. 2003; Carpenter et al. 2003; Martin et al. 2005; Loth et al. 2001; Elliott et al. 2009). Refinements of these techniques may prove extremely useful in adding to our understanding of syrinx pathophysiology.

Recent attention has turned to molecular and cellular contributions to syrinx pathophysiology. Disruption of the blood-spinal cord barrier as a source of fluid has been proposed by several investigators (Ravaglia et al. 2007; Hemley et al. 2009; Levine 2004). Alterations in aquaporin expression have recently been proposed to either increase fluid load or impair fluid outflow (Nesic et al. 2006).

With improved diagnostic imaging, a greater understanding of the pathological anatomy of syringomyelia has developed. It is now known that syrinx cavities associated with Chiari malformation are expansions of the central canal, whereas those associated with spinal cord injury usually start outside the central canal (Milhorat et al. 1995a, b). It has been demonstrated that syrinx cavities are usually not in communication with the fourth ventricle. New dynamic imaging techniques may prove extremely helpful in understanding syrinx pathophysiology (Gottschalk et al. 2010).

6.3 Syrinx Fluid Composition and Pressure

Two crucial factors that could be indicators of syrinx fluid origins and physiology are its composition and pressure. For example, a biochemical composition similar to that of CSF would provide evidence for an origin from CSF, although extracellular fluid would also remain a possibility. It is generally assumed that the composition of syrinx fluid is identical to that of CSF and that this implies that the origin of the fluid is CSF from the subarachnoid space. In fact, there is little direct evidence to support this concept, with only a number of case reports comparing the composition of syrinx fluid with CSF. Most studies have examined the protein content, and there are minimal data on other biochemical parameters. In a study of nine post-traumatic syrinx patients, Rossier and colleagues reported a higher syrinx protein content of 0.35–3.9 g/L (mean 1.15) when compared with cisternal CSF protein of 0.1–0.44 g/L (mean 0.24) (Rossier et al. 1985). Other authors have reported syrinx protein levels ranging from 0.28 to 2.24 g/L (mean 0.88) and a cisternal CSF protein ranging from 0.14 to 0.28 g/L (mean 0.18) (Barnett 1973; Laha et al. 1975; Nurick et al. 1970; Werner et al. 1969; Freeman 1959). Similarly, the fluid in tumour cases has been reported to have a higher protein content than CSF (Lohle et al. 1994). In contrast, Shannon and colleagues reported identical levels of protein in syrinx fluid and CSF in 10 of 13 post-traumatic syrinx patients treated with a syringotomy (Shannon et al. 1981). In 17 of 48 patients, Schlesinger and co-workers obtained percutaneous aspirates of spinal fluid from the central canal and subarachnoid space (Schlesinger et al. 1981). The syrinx protein content was below 0.5 g/L, which was the same or less than the simultaneous sample obtained from the subarachnoid space.

For a syrinx cavity to enlarge, the pressure within it must exceed the subarachnoid space pressure. The degree of enlargement depends on the pressure difference and the stiffness of the spinal cord tissue. Any proposed mechanism for syrinx expansion must therefore provide an explanation for a higher pressure within the cyst than in the subarachnoid space: simply invoking increases in subarachnoid space pressure is not a sufficient explanation. Of course, spinal pressures are pulsatile, and it may be that the pulsations are more important than mean pressures or that the timing of relationships among syrinx, arterial, and CSF pulsations is important. A vital step in investigating these issues would be to perform simultaneous syrinx and subarachnoid space pressure measurements in awake, ambulatory patients. Pressures within syrinx cavities are obviously difficult to measure directly under these conditions. Pressure measurements taken with patients anaesthetized, under positive pressure ventilation and positioned prone, may have no relationship to the pressure in awake, ambulatory patients. Studies using MRI and computational modelling techniques (Battal et al. 2011; Shaffer et al. 2011) may provide some assessment of CSF flow dynamics, but cannot directly measure pressure, and cannot be used to compare syrinx and subarachnoid space pressures.

In a pioneering study of pressures, Ellertsson and Greitz performed percutaneous measurements of syrinx and subarachnoid space pressures in ten patients (Ellertsson and Greitz 1970). They reported a higher pressure in the syrinx in most patients, but the difference was not significant. Perhaps the most detailed study of pressures in awake patients is that of Heiss and colleagues, who studied cervical and lumbar subarachnoid pressures in patients with Chiari malformation and syringomyelia, both while they were awake and during surgery (Heiss et al. 1999). Compared to controls, they found that cervical subarachnoid mean pressure and pulse pressure were increased and that compliance was reduced. After posterior

fossa decompression, the spinal subarachnoid pressure and pulse pressure returned to normal. They also measured syrinx pressure and subarachnoid pressure during surgery and found the two pressures to be identical (Heiss et al. 1999). Application of a Valsalva manoeuvre during surgery produced no significant difference between cranial and spinal subarachnoid pressures. This is in contrast to a report by Williams, who found that Valsalva manoeuvres created transient differences between spinal and cranial pressures (Williams 1981).

It is apparent that only sparse information exists regarding the crucial elements of syrinx fluid composition and pressure. In our opinion, it is unlikely that a complete understanding of syrinx pathophysiology will unfold without more detailed studies of these aspects in patients.

6.4 Hydrodynamic Mechanisms

Contemporary theories of syringomyelia pathogenesis have largely focused on alterations of CSF pressure, pulsations, and flow that drive fluid into the spinal cord. These are referred to here as 'hydrodynamic mechanisms' and are divided into those that implicate a flow from the fourth ventricle into the central canal and those that involve fluid flowing across the cord parenchyma from the subarachnoid space, mechanisms limiting outflow, and pressure effects on the cord causing dissection of cord tissue by an existing syrinx.

6.4.1 Flow from the Fourth Ventricle

Gardner refined the original hypothesis of Cleland, suggesting that obstruction of the fourth ventricle outlets resulted in expansion of the central canal as part of the same process leading to hydrocephalus (Gardner and Angel 1958). In this model, a 'water-hammer' effect is created, with each arterial pulsation causing an increase in intracranial pressure that is transmitted directly into the central canal, expanding it to form a syrinx (Fig. 6.1). Gardner argued that the

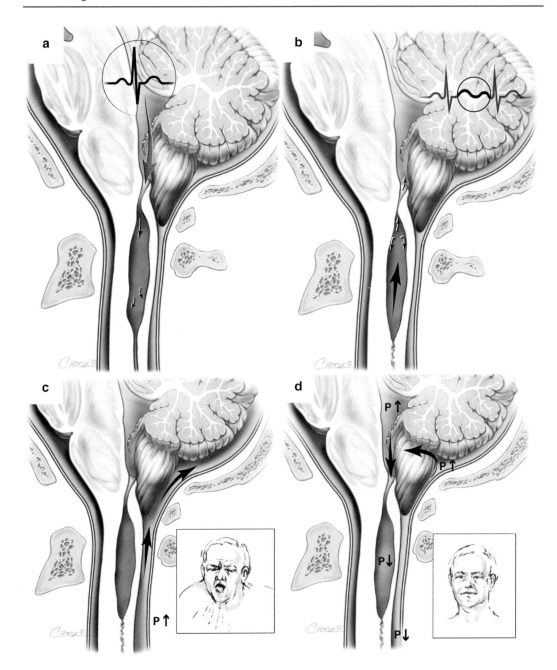

Fig. 6.1 Proposed syrinx filling mechanisms involving fluid flow from the fourth ventricle. Theory proposed by Gardner et al. (1957). (**a**) During systole, CSF is forced into the central canal. (**b**) During diastole the canal is closed and fluid cannot return to the fourth ventricle. Theory proposed by Williams (1970). (**c**) During Valsalva manoeuvres, CSF is forced from the spine into the cisterna magna. (**d**) After relaxing, the cerebellar tonsils act as a valve, preventing fluid returning to the spinal subarachnoid space. Fluid is therefore forced into the fourth ventricle and then into the syrinx. There is now abundant evidence that these theories do not explain the vast majority of syrinxes

subarachnoid space normally forms when the CSF pressure in the fourth ventricle ruptures through the foramina of Magendie and Luschka.

He considered there to be a spectrum of resulting abnormalities, with hydrocephalus, Chiari malformation, and syringomyelia at the less severe end and open myelomeningocele at the more severe end (Gardner and Angel 1958). He also suggested that syringomyelia in association with other conditions such as spinal cord injury was coincidental and that such cases also had an underlying Chiari malformation.

Much of Gardner's hypothesis appears to hold for syringomyelia in association with Chiari II malformation. In these cases, there is continuity between the expanded central canal and the fourth ventricle, and there is hydrocephalus (Milhorat et al. 1995a, b). The hydrocephalus and syringomyelia both resolve with ventricular shunting.

For other types of syringomyelia, which form the majority, there has been an accumulation of strong evidence against Gardner's hypothesis: the subarachnoid space forms prior to the opening of the fourth ventricle outlets during development; there is usually no continuity between the fourth ventricle and the syrinx; the outlets of the fourth ventricle are not always obstructed in cases of Chiari I malformation; and Chiari malformation is not the only condition associated with syringomyelia.

Williams developed an alternative explanation for a force driving fluid from the fourth ventricle into the central canal (Williams 1970, 1972). He proposed that the outlets of the fourth ventricle are not obstructed and that fluid enters the cranial subarachnoid space when the spinal subarachnoid pressure increases with coughing and sneezing (Fig. 6.1). The cerebellar tonsils would then act like a valve to prevent fluid flowing back into the spinal subarachnoid space, resulting in a pressure differential between the cranial and spinal cavities. The only available pathway for fluid in the cranial subarachnoid space to reach the spine to restore pressure equilibrium would then be for it to flow into the fourth ventricle and then to the central canal, causing it to expand.

Evidence against this proposed mechanism includes the fact that syrinx cavities are not usually in continuity with the fourth ventricle and that syringomyelia occurs in association with other posterior fossa abnormalities and tumours that would not be expected to have the same valve mechanism as was proposed for the cerebellar tonsils in Chiari malformation.

The evidence against a direct flow of fluid from the fourth ventricle into the central canal or syrinx is compelling. Although posterior fossa decompression remains the mainstay of treatment for syringomyelia associated with Chiari malformation, this does not appear to be due to correction of the abnormalities proposed by Gardner or Williams. Plugging of the opening of the central canal is no longer recommended as part of this procedure (Vanaclocha et al. 1997; Ball and Dayan 1972).

6.4.2 Trans-parenchymal Flow

If the fluid in syrinx cavities is CSF and it has not reached the cavity directly from the fourth ventricle, it must flow across the cord tissue from the subarachnoid space. There has been much speculation about the possible route of such a fluid flow and the forces driving it.

In contrast to the proposal by Williams, Ball and Dayan suggested that a Chiari malformation would act to prevent spinal CSF from entering the cranial compartment during Valsalva manoeuvres (Fig. 6.2). They then speculated that the resulting increase in spinal CSF pressure could force CSF into perivascular spaces in the cord and that this fluid could coalesce to form a syrinx (Ball and Dayan 1972). Subarachnoid space obstruction from other causes such as post-traumatic arachnoiditis was said to produce a similar mechanism for fluid entry into the cord (Ball and Dayan 1972). The authors pointed to the pathological finding of enlarged perivascular spaces in syrinx cases as evidence for this theory.

Oldfield and colleagues proposed a similar mechanism, whereby the Chiari malformation imparts a piston-like effect on the spinal subarachnoid space, forcing fluid through either the perivascular spaces or interstitial spaces (Fig. 6.2) (Oldfield et al. 1994; Heiss et al. 1999). These authors provided cine-MRI and intra-operative ultrasound evidence of cerebellar tonsil movement in support of their theory, but had no direct evidence for fluid flow into the cord.

Support for a perivascular flow of fluid has arisen from the experimental work of Stoodley

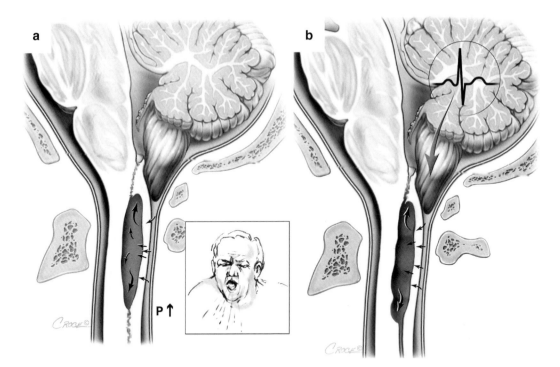

Fig. 6.2 Proposed trans-medullary filling mechanisms. Theory proposed by Ball and Dayan (1972). (**a**) The Chiari malformation acts to isolate the spinal subarachnoid space and that Valsalva manoeuvres increase the subarachnoid space pressure, forcing fluid into the cord. Theory proposed by Oldfield et al. (1994). (**b**) The cerebellar tonsils act as a 'piston' with each systole to increase spinal subarachnoid pressure and force fluid into the cord. These theories cannot explain expansion of a syrinx cavity, because the pressure in the cavity must exceed subarachnoid pressure for it to do so

and colleagues, who used tracers of CSF bulk flow to demonstrate perivascular flow from the subarachnoid space to the central canal in normal animals (Stoodley et al. 1996, 1997), and from Klekamp et al., who showed oedema and enlarged perivascular spaces in a model of arachnoiditis (Klekamp et al. 2001). Further work showed that perivascular flow of CSF from the subarachnoid space occurs in models of canalicular and extracanalicular syringomyelia (Fig. 6.3) (Stoodley et al. 1999; Brodbelt et al. 2003b) and that flow is dependent on arterial pulsations (Stoodley et al. 1997).

A major problem with any proposed explanation for syrinx formation from a transparenchymal flow of CSF from the subarachnoid space is the simple physical fact that increasing pressure on the outside of the cord cannot create an expanding cyst within the cord. For a cavity to enlarge, the pressure within it must exceed the surrounding pressure, and this cannot occur with flow that is driven by an increase in pressure in the subarachnoid space. Several investigators have attempted to address this. Bilston and colleagues have examined the pulsatile properties of fluid flow in perivascular spaces and the subarachnoid space (Bilston et al. 2003, 2010). Using computational modelling, they demonstrated that the anatomical characteristics of the perivascular space could act as a 'leaky' one-way valve for pulsatile CSF flow. In addition, a timing mismatch between the arterial wave and CSF pressure wave arriving at the interface between the subarachnoid space and the perivascular space could act to increase flow (Fig. 6.4). They indicate this occurs when the CSF peak pressure occurs at a different time to the arterial pulse peak pressure, resulting in lower resistance to CSF inflow than outflow (Bilston et al. 2010). It was suggested that Chiari malformation and other obstructions in the subarachnoid space could act to create the timing mismatch.

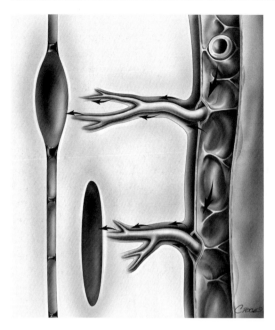

Fig. 6.3 Perivascular spaces as a proposed pathway for CSF flow in both canalicular and extracanalicular syringomyelia. Flow from the subarachnoid space enters the perivascular spaces, which narrow as they penetrate deeper into the cord. Possible mechanisms for such a flow to create a higher mean syrinx pressure than mean subarachnoid pressure include a partial valve effect of the perivascular space and a mismatch in the timing of the arterial and CSF pulse waves (Bilston et al. 2003, 2010)

An alternative explanation is that stenosis of the subarachnoid space could lead to a focal increase in pressure in the spinal cord with Valsalva manoeuvres, the so-called 'elastic jump' (Carpenter et al. 2003). Although computational modelling has shown this to be a theoretical possibility, the magnitude of the effect appears to be too small to be significant (Elliott et al. 2009).

6.4.3 Obstruction of Outflow

It appears likely that there is a continual flow of fluid into the spinal cord and also into syrinx cavities. Unless a syrinx is enlarging, the outflow must equal the inflow. The physiology of fluid outflow is not known, but one possible explanation for syrinx formation and enlargement is the obstruction of outflow. This concept was initiated by Ellertsson and Greitz, who measured syrinx and subarachnoid space pressures in patients, showing higher pressure in syrinx cavities, although this was not significant. They suggested an impairment of outflow, although did not speculate as to the mechanism of this (Ellertsson and Greitz 1970).

Fig. 6.4 A phase difference in pulsations may explain a valvelike effect of perivascular flow. Obstructions of the subarachnoid space could be responsible for slowing the pulse transmission to create a phase mismatch. If the CSF systolic wave arrives at the cord surface during arterial diastole, the perivascular space will be open, and flow will be greater than if the CSF pulse arrives during arterial systole, when the perivascular space will be smaller (Bilston et al. 2010)

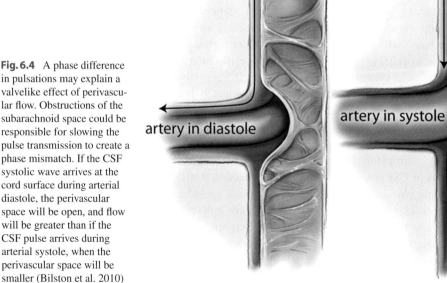

Aboulker suggested that the pressure on the spinal cord at the cervicomedullary junction prevents CSF draining rostrally along the central canal to the fourth ventricle (Aboulker 1979). Although such a rostral flow has been demonstrated in experimental animals, it is not known whether this occurs in humans (Milhorat et al. 1991). Theoretically, fluid could also drain through spinal cord parenchyma, and cord compression might compress the extracellular space or reduce permeability, thus restricting outflow.

Recently, Koyanagi and Houkin have suggested that an increase in spinal venous pressure might impair absorption of extracellular fluid, resulting in accumulation of fluid in the cord and syrinx formation (Koyanagi and Houkin 2010).

There is little clinical or experimental evidence to support or refute these theories. The physiology of fluid outflow from the spinal cord and syrinx cavities is a largely unexplored area that may be important in syringomyelia physiology and is deserving of more research attention.

6.4.4 Transmitted Pressure Effects on Existing Cavities

Rather than fluid being forced into the cord by pressure changes in the subarachnoid space or physiological changes in perivascular flow, an alternative view is that pressure exerted on the cord surface causes rostral-caudal dissection of an existing cavity, leading to enlargement of the cavity. This concept began with the description by Williams of a 'suck and slosh' mechanism for expansion of post-traumatic syrinx cavities. He suggested that increases in pressure in the subarachnoid space cause pressure on a cavity, which then dissects into the surrounding cord tissue, enlarging the potential space for the cavity, which then fills with extracellular fluid (Williams 1992). This mechanism has also been supported by the work of Oldfield and colleagues (Oldfield et al. 1994), who used intra-operative ultrasound to show that the cord and syrinx became compressed with each arterial pulsation and in synchrony with the descent of the cerebellar tonsils of a Chiari malformation. They suggested that this compression would cause extension of the

syrinx cavity and that the fluid filling the cavity came from the subarachnoid space.

These theories rely on the presence of an initial cavity that can subsequently be enlarged by the putative dissection process. It is possible that this may apply to post-traumatic syringomyelia, where initial cavities form from haemorrhage and ischaemia. However, there is no evidence for a similar process in those cases associated with Chiari malformation. In addition, this process could at best explain the enlargement of a syrinx but not an increase in pressure relative to the subarachnoid space.

6.4.5 Summary of Hydrodynamic Theories

The available evidence does not support a fourth ventricular origin for syrinx fluid. There is good evidence that at least some syrinx fluid originates from the subarachnoid space and that the route of this fluid flow is via the perivascular spaces. However, theories that invoke increases in subarachnoid space pressure as the driving force are not sufficient to explain syrinx formation and enlargement. It is possible that complex relationships between CSF and arterial pulsations or the anatomical characteristics of the perivascular spaces explain the accumulation of fluid inside the cord. Pulsations exerted on the surface of the cord may contribute to cord tissue damage but seem insufficient to explain the development of high-pressure cavities. The possible role of perturbations in fluid outflow remains largely unexplored.

6.5 Other Sources of Fluid

None of the hydrodynamic theories have adequately explained syrinx formation and enlargement. Alternative theories have been put forward to suggest that syrinx fluid is not of CSF origin and that hydrodynamic factors driving CSF flow are not responsible. These proposed mechanisms have been used to explain the development of cavities in association with intramedullary tumours, or have suggested that syrinx fluid is derived from interstitial fluid, or originates through abnormalities of the blood-spinal cord barrier or even cellular fluid transport mechanisms.

6.5.1 Tumours

Syringomyelia occurs in association with posterior fossa tumours and with spinal extramedullary and intramedullary tumours. In general, it is reasonable to propose that the filling mechanism in posterior fossa tumour cases may be similar to the process that occurs with Chiari malformation and may be hydrodynamic in origin. Spinal extramedullary tumours may act by causing partial blockage of the subarachnoid space and could be thought of as having a similar underlying aetiology to cases associated with spinal arachnoiditis.

The particular tumour type that is likely to have a unique pathophysiology is the intramedullary tumour. Although expansion of the cord could theoretically result in obstruction of the subarachnoid space, it is our experience that many tumours are small and the subarachnoid space does not appear to be affected in the majority of cases. Intramedullary tumours with particularly high rates of syrinx development include haemangioblastomas and ependymomas (Samii and Klekamp 1994).

A possible explanation for syrinx development in association with intramedullary tumours is that the cystic cavity is part of the tumour itself (Barnett 1973), but for some tumour types at least, the syrinx wall is gliotic tissue (Lohle et al. 1994). There is limited information regarding the composition of tumour-associated syrinx fluid, but there is some evidence that it is high in protein (Lohle et al. 1994), suggesting that the fluid comes directly from the tumour or its vasculature.

It has been suggested that, in haemangioblastomas, the vasculature is leaky and the interstitial pressure is high, leading to extravasation of plasma (Lonser et al. 2006). In support of this hypothesis, Lonser et al. have reported a case demonstrating progressive leakage of contrast medium from a haemangioblastoma into the surrounding cord tissue (Lonser et al. 2006).

Samii and Klekamp argue that the pathophysiology is likely to include some abnormality of CSF flow in addition to secretion of fluid and protein by the tumour. They cite the predominant rostral location of syrinx cavities relative to the tumour and the higher rates of syrinx formation in tumours in the cervical cord to support this view (Samii and Klekamp 1994).

We are not aware of any experimental models of tumour-associated syringomyelia, and the clinical evidence is limited. However, it does seem likely that specific tumour-related factors are more important than CSF dynamics in this type of syrinx.

6.5.2 Interstitial Fluid

Interstitial fluid has been proposed by numerous authors as a source of syrinx fluid. One line of reasoning is that tethering of the cord by arachnoiditis results in tensile radial stress, which lowers the pressure in the cord and leads to inflow of extracellular fluid (Bertram et al. 2008).

Josephson and colleagues provided experimental evidence for a theory that pulse transmission through the cord, past a region of subarachnoid block, would cause expansion of the cord below the block (Josephson et al. 2001). The proposal is that, with each arterial pulsation, the pulse wave in the subarachnoid space is blocked, but the wave in the cord continues, creating a higher pressure in the cord than in the surrounding subarachnoid space, thus expanding the cord. The expanded cord would then fill with extracellular fluid. A similar explanation was proposed and tested using an electrical circuit model of CSF dynamics (Chang and Nakagawa 2003, 2004). In this model, the pressure was transmitted down the central canal, forcing fluid out of this channel, below the level of the subarachnoid block where the surrounding subarachnoid pressure was lower.

Greitz subsequently proposed a somewhat different explanation (Greitz 2006). He suggested that narrowing of the subarachnoid space causes an increase in CSF velocity at the region of narrowing. The increased fluid velocity has a

Venturi effect, lowering the pressure in the subarachnoid space and causing a suction effect on the cord, expanding it during each systole. According to Greitz, extracellular fluid would accumulate in the expanded cord, forming a syrinx (Greitz 2006).

Klekamp suggested that interstitial fluid could be important in canalicular and extracanalicular cavities, by exceeding the normal fluid capacity of the extracellular space. This might occur due to blockage of perivascular spaces, cord tethering, changes in vascular flow, or obstruction of CSF flow (Klekamp et al. 2002).

In common with the hydrodynamic theories, many of the theories proposing an interstitial fluid origin cannot explain a higher pressure in the syrinx than the spinal cord tissue and subarachnoid space. Instead, they imply passive filling of syrinx cavities, which does not fit with our clinical observation that the pressure in many syrinx cavities appears much higher than the surrounding subarachnoid space.

6.5.3 Blood-Spinal Cord Barrier Disruption

Several authors have suggested that fluid crossing a deficient blood-spinal cord barrier may contribute to syrinx fluid (Fig. 6.5). Clinical case reports have supported a role for barrier disruption, by demonstrating contrast enhancement around syrinx cavities on MR scans (Lonser et al. 2006; Ravaglia et al. 2007).

Levine suggested that the changes in pressure above and below a subarachnoid blockage would be transmitted into the veins, with collapse of vessels rostral to a block and dilation of vessels caudal to the block, causing cord parenchymal stress. This stress would lead to tissue destruction and resultant damage to capillaries, and venules would allow plasma filtrate to pass into the cord (Levine 2004).

A particular case could be made for a role of the blood-spinal cord barrier in post-traumatic syringomyelia. It has been demonstrated that the

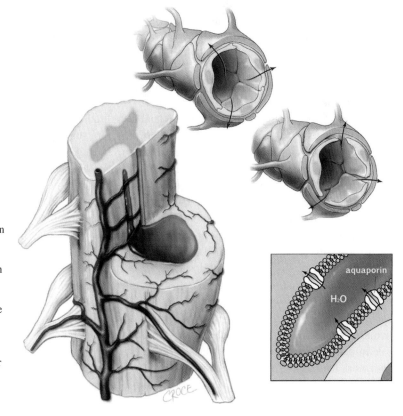

Fig. 6.5 Vascular and tissue sources of fluid or impaired absorption may result in a syrinx pressure higher than the subarachnoid space. *Left*: the syrinx cavity is often in the highly vascular grey matter and surrounded by vessels. *Top* and *top-right*: an impaired blood-spinal cord barrier allows fluid to cross the vessel wall and add to the syrinx volume. *Bottom right*: abnormalities of aquaporin expression may also allow fluid to leak across vessels or may impair absorption of syrinx fluid into the vasculature

barrier is disrupted following spinal cord injury (Mautes et al. 2000), which contributes to spinal cord oedema. In most spinal cord injuries, it is assumed that the barrier is subsequently reconstituted and the oedema subsides. It is possible that a prolonged disruption of the barrier could allow continued fluid leakage and enlargement of an initial haemorrhagic or necrotic cavity. Experimental evidence in a rat model of post-traumatic syringomyelia supports this hypothesis (Hemley et al. 2009).

6.5.4 Aquaporins

The recent discovery of a role of aquaporins in fluid transport in the central nervous system may have implications for syringomyelia pathogenesis. Aquaporin-4 is the most abundant type in the brain and spinal cord and is expressed on astrocyte and ependymal membranes around the blood-brain barrier and brain-CSF interfaces. Studies of aquaporin-4 in spinal cord injury have reported conflicting results, with some authors finding an early downregulation and later upregulation (Nesic et al. 2006) and other investigators finding an early upregulation (Saadoun et al. 2008). It is possible that changes in aquaporin expression could either enhance the movement of water into the central canal or alternatively prevent water from moving from the central canal into the parenchyma. These mechanisms may contribute to the enlargement of the central canal in Chiari-associated syringomyelia. A case of syringomyelia in a patient with anti-aquaporin antibodies has recently been reported, with the authors suggesting that a reduction in aquaporin expression may have resulted in permeability of the blood-spinal cord barrier (Sakabe et al. 2010).

There are very few experimental studies of aquaporins in syringomyelia. Sun and colleagues found a downregulation of aquaporin-4 in the early stages of syrinx formation in a rabbit canalicular model and suggested that this played a role in oedema formation (Sun et al. 2007). Our own work has demonstrated an increase in aquaporin expression around cavities in post-traumatic syringomyelia (Hemley et al. 2013) but not

around cavities in canalicular syringomyelia (Hemley et al. 2012). Regardless of whether aquaporin disturbances play a role in syrinx initiation, our view is that they are likely to have an important function in fluid transport in or out of syrinx cavities.

6.6 Outstanding Questions

At the beginning of this chapter, we suggested that close inspection of the pathophysiology underlying syringomyelia reveals complexity. Unfortunately, rather than elucidating the syrinx filling mechanism, the plethora of theories described above has added to this complexity. Many of the theories provide divergent opinions on basic concepts such as whether syrinx fluid is CSF, interstitial fluid, or plasma; whether the cerebellar tonsils in Chiari malformation allow fluid to pass from the head to the spine or vice versa; whether the subarachnoid space pressure is elevated or reduced; and whether syrinx cavities expand by fluid being forced in or by sucking fluid in. We do not think that major advances will be made in the understanding of syrinx filling mechanisms until the following fundamental questions are answered by careful clinical and experimental studies:

- What is the chemical composition of syrinx fluid in the various types? Is the fluid CSF, interstitial fluid, plasma, or a mixture of these?
- What is the relationship between syrinx pressure and subarachnoid space pressure?
- What is the relationship between syrinx and subarachnoid space pulse pressures?

In addition to these fundamental questions, much greater detail is required regarding fluid inflow and outflow pathways, the role of the blood-spinal cord barrier and aquaporins, and the precise mechanism at play with each associated condition.

Conclusions

Despite the myriad theories proposed regarding syrinx pathogenesis, an objective appraisal would suggest that very little is certain regarding even the fundamental principles. The goal of a single unifying theory remains unlikely to be fulfilled until these are elucidated. It remains likely that different syrinx subtypes have different filling mechanisms and much work remains to be done to clarify these.

References

Aboulker J (1979) Syringomyelia and intra-rachidian fluids. X. Rachidian fluid stasis. Neurochirurgie 25(Suppl 1):98–107

Ball MJ, Dayan AD (1972) Pathogenesis of syringomyelia. Lancet 2(7781):799–801

Barnett HJM (1973) Syringomyelia and tumours of the nervous system. In: Barnett HJM, Foster JB, Hudgson P (eds) Syringomyelia. Saunders, London, pp 245–301

Battal B, Kocaoglu M, Bulakbasi N et al (2011) Cerebrospinal fluid flow imaging by using phase-contrast MR technique. Br J Radiol 84:758–765

Berkouk K, Carpenter PW, Lucey AD (2003) Pressure wave propagation in fluid-filled co-axial elastic tubes. Part 1: basic theory. J Biomech Eng 125(6):852–856

Bertram CD, Bilston LE, Stoodley MA (2008) Tensile radial stress in the spinal cord related to arachnoiditis or tethering: a numerical model. Med Biol Eng Comput 46(7):701–707

Bilston LE, Fletcher DF, Brodbelt AR et al (2003) Arterial pulsation-driven cerebrospinal fluid flow in the perivascular space: a computational model. Comput Methods Biomech Biomed Engin 6(4):235–241

Bilston LE, Fletcher DF, Stoodley MA (2006) Focal spinal arachnoiditis increases subarachnoid space pressure: a modeling study. Clin Biomech (Bristol, Avon) 21:579–584

Bilston L, Stoodley MA, Fletcher DF (2010) The influence of the relative timing of arterial and subarachnoid space pressures pulse waves on spinal perivascular cerebrospinal fluid flow as a possible factor in syrinx development. J Neurosurg 112:808–813

Brodbelt AR, Stoodley MA (2003) Post-traumatic syringomyelia: a review. J Clin Neurosci 10(4):401–408

Brodbelt AR, Stoodley MA, Watling AM et al (2003a) Altered subarachnoid space compliance and fluid flow in an animal model of posttraumatic syringomyelia. Spine 28(20):E413–E419

Brodbelt AR, Stoodley MA, Watling AM et al (2003b) Fluid flow in an animal model of post-traumatic syringomyelia. Eur Spine J 12(3):300–306

Caplan LR, Norohna AB, Amico LL (1990) Syringomyelia and arachnoiditis. J Neurol Neurosurg Psychiatry 53(2):106–113

Carpenter PW, Berkouk K, Lucey AD (2003) Pressure wave propagation in fluid-filled co-axial elastic tubes. Part 2: mechanisms for the pathogenesis of syringomyelia. J Biomech Eng 125(6):857–863

Chang HS, Nakagawa H (2003) Hypothesis on the pathophysiology of syringomyelia based on simulation of cerebrospinal fluid dynamics. J Neurol Neurosurg Psychiatry 74(3):344–347

Chang HS, Nakagawa H (2004) Theoretical analysis of the pathophysiology of syringomyelia associated with adhesive arachnoiditis. J Neurol Neurosurg Psychiatry 75(5):754–757

Cleland J (1883) Contribution to the study of spina bifida, encephalocele, and anencephalus. J Anat Physiol 17:257–291

Ellertsson AB, Greitz T (1970) The distending force in the production of communicating syringomyelia. Lancet 1(7658):1234

Elliott NS, Lockerby DA, Brodbelt AR (2009) The pathogenesis of syringomyelia: a re-evaluation of the elastic-jump hypothesis. J Biomech Eng 131: 044503

Freeman G (1959) Ascending spinal paralysis. J Neurosurg 16:120–122

Gardner WJ (1959) Anatomic anomalies common to myelomeningocele of infancy and syringomyelia of adulthood suggest a common origin. Cleve Clin Q 26:118–133

Gardner WJ, Angel J (1958) The mechanism of syringomyelia and its surgical correction. Clin Neurosurg 6:131–140

Gardner WJ, Abdullah AF, McCormack LJ (1957) The varying expressions of embryonal atresia of the fourth ventricle in adults: Arnold-Chiari malformation, Dandy-Walker syndrome, arachnoid cyst of the cerebellum, and syringomyelia. J Neurosurg 14(6): 591–605

Gottschalk A, Schmitz B, Mauer U et al (2010) Dynamic visualization of arachnoid adhesions in a patient with idiopathic syringomyelia using high-resolution cine magnetic resonance imaging at 3T. J Magn Reson Imaging 32:218–222

Greitz D (2006) Unraveling the riddle of syringomyelia. Neurosurg Rev 29(4):251–263

Hall PV, Muller J, Campbell RL (1975) Experimental hydrosyringomyelia, ischemic myelopathy, and syringomyelia. J Neurosurg 43(4):464–470

Heiss JD, Patronas N, DeVroom HL et al (1999) Elucidating the pathophysiology of syringomyelia. J Neurosurg 91(4):553–562

Hemley S, Tu J, Stoodley M (2009) Role of the blood-spinal cord barrier in post-traumatic syringomyelia. J Neurosurg Spine 11:696–704

Hemley SJ, Bilston LE, Cheng S et al (2012) Aquaporin-4 expression and blood–spinal cord barrier permeability in canalicular syringomyelia. J Neurosurg Spine 17(6):602–612. doi:10.3171/2012.9.SPINE1265

Hemley SJ, Bilston LE, Cheng S et al (2013) Aquaporin-4 expression in posttraumatic syringomyelia. J Neurotrauma 30:1457–1467

Hida K, Iwasaki Y, Imamura H et al (1994) Birth injury as a causative factor of syringomyelia with Chiari type I deformity. J Neurol Neurosurg Psychiatry 57(3): 373–374

Joffroy A, Achard C (1887) De la myelite cavitaire (observations; reflexions; pathogenic des cavites). Arch Physiol Norm Pathol 10:435–472

Josephson A, Greitz D, Klason T et al (2001) A spinal thecal sac constriction model supports the theory that induced pressure gradients in the cord cause edema and cyst formation. Neurosurg Clin N Am 48: 636–645

Klekamp J (2002) The pathophysiology of syringomyelia – historical overview and current concept. Acta Neurochir (Wien) 144:649–664

Klekamp J, Volkel K, Bartels CJ et al (2001) Disturbances of cerebrospinal fluid flow attributable to arachnoid scarring cause interstitial edema of the cat spinal cord. Neurosurgery 48(1):174–185; discussion 185–186

Klekamp J, Iaconetta G, Batzdorf U et al (2002) Syringomyelia associated with foramen magnum arachnoiditis. J Neurosurg 97(3 Suppl):317–322

Koyanagi I, Houkin K (2010) Pathogenesis of syringomyelia associated with Chiari type 1 malformation: review of evidences and proposal of a new hypothesis. Neurosurg Rev 33:271–284

Laha RK, Malik HG, Langille RA (1975) Post-traumatic syringomyelia. Surg Neurol 4(6):519–522

Levine DN (2004) The pathogenesis of syringomyelia associated with lesions at the foramen magnum: a critical review of existing theories and proposal of a new hypothesis. J Neurol Sci 220(1–2):3–21

Lohle PN, Wurzer HA, Hoogland PH et al (1994) The pathogenesis of syringomyelia in spinal cord ependymoma. Clin Neurol Neurosurg 96(4):323–326

Lonser RR, Butman JA, Oldfield EH (2006) Pathogenesis of tumor-associated syringomyelia demonstrated by peritumoral contrast material leakage. Case illustration. J Neurosurg Spine 4(5):426

Loth F, Yardimci MA, Alperin N (2001) Hydrodynamic modeling of cerebrospinal fluid motion within the spinal cavity. J Biomech Eng 123(1):71–79

Martin BA, Kalata W, Loth F et al (2005) Syringomyelia hydrodynamics: an in vitro study based on in vivo measurements. J Biomech Eng 127(7):1110–1120

Mautes A, Weinzierl M, Donovan F et al (2000) Vascular events after spinal cord injury: contribution to secondary pathogenesis. Phys Ther 80:673–687

McLaurin RL, Bailey OT, Schurr PH et al (1954) Myomalacia and multiple cavitations of spinal cord secondary to adhesive arachnoiditis: an experimental study. Arch Pathol 57(2):138–146

Milhorat T, Johnson R, Johnson W (1991) Evidence of CSF flow in rostral direction through central canal of spinal cord in rats. In: Matsumoto S, Tamaki N (eds) Hydrocephalus. Pathogenesis and treatment. Springer, Tokyo, pp 207–217

Milhorat TH, Capocelli AL Jr, Anzil AP et al (1995a) Pathological basis of spinal cord cavitation in syringomyelia: analysis of 105 autopsy cases. J Neurosurg 82(5):802–812

Milhorat TH, Johnson RW, Milhorat RH et al (1995b) Clinicopathological correlations in syringomyelia using axial magnetic resonance imaging. Neurosurgery 37(2):206–213

Nesic O, Lee J, Ye Z et al (2006) Acute and chronic changes in aquaporin 4 expression after spinal cord injury. Neuroscience 143(3):779–792

Newman PK, Terenty TR, Foster JB (1981) Some observations on the pathogenesis of syringomyelia. J Neurol Neurosurg Psychiatry 44(11): 964–969

Newton EJ (1969) Syringomyelia as a manifestation of defective fourth ventricular drainage. Ann R Coll Surg Engl 44(4):194–213

Nurick S, Russell JA, Deck MD (1970) Cystic degeneration of the spinal cord following spinal cord injury. Brain 93(1):211–222

Oldfield EH, Muraszko K, Shawker TH et al (1994) Pathophysiology of syringomyelia associated with Chiari I malformation of the cerebellar tonsils. Implications for diagnosis and treatment. J Neurosurg 80(1):3–15

Ollivier CP (1827) Traité des maladies de la Moelle Épiniè, contenant l'histoire anatomique, physiologique et pathologique de ce centre nerveux chez l'homme. Méquignon-Marvis père et fils, Paris

Ravaglia S, Bogdanov EI, Pichiecchio A et al (2007) Pathogenetic role of myelitis for syringomyelia. Clin Neurol Neurosurg 109:541–546

Rossier AB, Foo D, Shillito J et al (1985) Posttraumatic cervical syringomyelia. Incidence, clinical presentation, electrophysiological studies, syrinx protein and results of conservative and operative treatment. Brain 108(Pt 2):439–461

Saadoun S, Bell B, Verkman A et al (2008) Greatly improved neurological outcome after spinal cord compression injury in AQP4-deficient mice. Brain 131:1087–1098

Sakabe E, Takizawa S, Ohnuki Y et al (2010) Syringomyelia in neuromyelitis optica seropositive for aquaporin-4 antibody. Intern Med 49:353–354

Samii M, Klekamp J (1994) Surgical results of 100 intramedullary tumors in relation to accompanying syringomyelia. Neurosurgery 35(5):865–873; discussion 873

Schlesinger EB, Antunes JL, Michelsen WJ et al (1981) Hydromyelia: clinical presentation and comparison of modalities of treatment. Neurosurgery 9(4):356–365

Shaffer N, Martin B, Loth F (2011) Cerebrospinal fluid hydrodynamics in type I Chiari malformation. [Review]. Neurol Res 33:247–260

Shannon N, Symon L, Logue V et al (1981) Clinical features, investigation and treatment of post-traumatic syringomyelia. J Neurol Neurosurg Psychiatry 44(1): 35–42

Stoodley MA, Jones NR, Brown CJ (1996) Evidence for rapid fluid flow from the subarachnoid space into the spinal cord central canal in the rat. Brain Res 707(2):155–164

Stoodley MA, Brown SA, Brown CJ et al (1997) Arterial pulsation-dependent perivascular cerebrospinal fluid flow into the central canal in the sheep spinal cord. J Neurosurg 86(4):686–693

Stoodley MA, Gutschmidt B, Jones NR (1999) Cerebrospinal fluid flow in an animal model of noncommunicating syringomyelia. Neurosurgery 44(5): 1065–1075; discussion 1075–1076

Stoodley MA, Jones NR, Yang L et al (2000) Mechanisms underlying the formation and enlargement of noncommunicating syringomyelia: experimental studies. Neurosurg Focus 8(3):E2

Sun G, Zhang Q, Wang H (2007) Expression of aquaporin 4 during development of experimental presyrinx state in rabbits. Beijing Da Xue Xue Bao 39:177–181

Vanaclocha V, Saiz-Sapena N, Garcia-Casasola MC (1997) Surgical technique for cranio-cervical decompression in syringomyelia associated with Chiari type I malformation. Acta Neurochir (Wien) 139(6):529–539; discussion 539–540

Werner A, Rossier A, Berney J et al (1969) Apropos of 4 observations on late cervical syringomyelia following medullar injury. Schweiz Arch Neurol Neurochir Psychiatr 104(1):77–86

Williams B (1969) The distending force in the production of communicating syringomyelia. Lancet 2(7622):696

Williams B (1970) The distending force in the production of communicating syringomyelia. Lancet 2(7662):41–42

Williams B (1972) Pathogenesis of syringomyelia. Lancet 2(7784):969–970

Williams B (1977) Difficult labour as a cause of communicating syringomyelia. Lancet 2(8028):51–53

Williams B (1981) Simultaneous cerebral and spinal fluid pressure recordings. 2. Cerebrospinal dissociation with lesions at the foramen magnum. Acta Neurochir (Wien) 59(1–2):123–142

Williams B (1992) Pathogenesis of post-traumatic syringomyelia. Br J Neurosurg 6(6):517–520

Woodard JS, Freeman LW (1956) Ischemia of the spinal cord; an experimental study. J Neurosurg 13:63–72

Mathematical Modelling

7

Novak S.J. Elliott

Contents

With Paul Harris

N.S.J. Elliott
Department of Mechanical Engineering,
Curtin University, Perth, WA, Australia
e-mail: n.s.j.elliott@curtin.edu.au

7.1   Introduction

A model is a representation of objects and processes that, when analysed, may reveal their properties and behaviour (Dym and Ivey 1980). A familiar example in medical research is the animal model. For an animal of sufficient likeness to human anatomy (objects), physiology and pathological response (processes), the outcomes of experiment may be extrapolated to human medicine. The model may refer to the animal itself, especially if purpose bred, or its combination with the treatment protocol to reproduce the desired pathology. For example, animal models of human posttraumatic syringomyelia have been developed using injections of kaolin and quisqualic acid in rats (Stoodley et al. 1999; Brodbelt et al. 2003a). Likewise, physiological or pathophysiological processes acting on normal or abnormal anatomy may be expressed in terms of force and mass balances, according to the laws of mechanics, which are most naturally formulated as mathematical equations. By careful manipulation of these equations, using well-established rules, one may construct a mathematical model—a theoretical representation of a physical system.

Neurosurgeons regularly make judgments involving the mechanical properties of the spinal cord and brain, as part of routine diagnosis and treatment. For example, when examining computed tomography (CT) and static magnetic resonance (MR) images of a Chiari malformation, clinicians will make some estimate of the pressure acting upon and the deformation of the

G. Flint, C. Rusbridge (eds.), *Syringomyelia*,
DOI 10.1007/978-3-642-13706-8_7, © Springer-Verlag Berlin Heidelberg 2014

hindbrain. The opening pressure of the cerebro-spinal fluid (CSF) is taken during lumbar puncture using a column manometer. The protein concentration of the CSF subsequently collected gives an indication of viscosity. During a spinal procedure, the surgeon may gently palpate the exposed spinal cord, in order to determine the degree of scar tissue build-up or the size and location of syrinxes or tumours and may thereby be making an estimate of compliance. Dynamic MR imaging is used to identify CSF flow obstructions, which are areas of high resistance, and the pulse-wave speed of the cerebrospinal fluid can also be appreciated from this imaging modality.

The uncertain surgical prognosis for syringomyelia and the difficulties of carrying out experimental work make mathematical modelling of the mechanics of this condition very attractive for research. Such models do, however, rely upon accurate measurement of mechanical properties of the cerebrospinal system, but these are difficult to obtain due to both the delicate nature of neurological tissues and their inaccessibility in situ. The risks to the patient of making such measurements may also outweigh any benefit gained. Further, the more realistically one attempts to represent the cerebrospinal fluid system, the more complex the mathematics become. For all these reasons, mathematical models of syringomyelia have been slow to evolve. Nonetheless, useful insights are now being made, with models that are consistent with the pathology and adhere to the laws of mechanics (Elliott et al. 2013).

7.2   Background

7.2.1   The Laws of Mechanics

In our everyday lives, we observe and experience certain physical phenomena that occur in a *predictable* way. For example, if a car breaks down and needs to be pushed, it requires a lot of effort to get going, but this becomes easier once the car is moving. While driving, applying the brakes in an emergency will cause the passengers to be thrown forwards against their seatbelts. The harder a golf ball is struck, the more rapidly it

will gain speed. When standing on solid ground, we feel our own weight through the soles of our feet. These events all involve force, motion and strength of materials—'mechanics' as termed by Galileo (Fung 1993)—and may be described by the *laws of mechanics*, a subset of the so-called physical laws of nature. In 1687, Sir Isaac Newton, the English mathematician, physicist and astronomer,[1] published his monograph *Philosophiæ Naturalis Principia Mathematica*, in which he stated three laws of motion:

1. In the absence of any external forces, an object that is still will remain still, and an object that is in motion will continue with constant speed in a fixed direction. An object is thus said to possess *inertia* (Latin 'iners': idle), a tendency to resist any change in its state of rest or motion. A measure of an object's inertia is its mass, i.e. how much 'stuff' the object is made of, which is equal to its density times its volume. The above example of a car braking can be explained by the inertia of the car and its occupants, respectively.

2. Force is equal to mass multiplied by acceleration, where the resulting acceleration is in the same direction as the applied force. So, a golf ball correctly driven down the fairway will reach great speed, whereas it will move much slower when gently putted on the green, even ignoring the friction of the air and grass.

3. For every action, there is an equal and opposite reaction. A person's weight is the force produced by their mass being subjected to the acceleration of gravity towards the centre of earth. Opposing this is a force exerted by the earth of equal size but directed back into the person's feet.

When objects change shape as a result of applied forces—a good example being flowing liquids—we also need to consider the *law of conservation of mass*. This states that the total amount of matter in an isolated system will remain constant over time. Similarly, when temperature changes become appreciable, the *law of conservation of energy*[2] is called into play; e.g.

---

[1] Also natural philosopher, alchemist and theologian.

[2] A generalisation of the laws of thermodynamics.

freshly poured coffee warms the cup (and cools the coffee) due to the transfer of thermal energy.

Conservation appears to be a principle that all laws of nature follow. Newton's laws of motion may be reformulated in terms of *momentum*, i.e. mass multiplied by velocity, which, it turns out, is also conserved. When working with conservation laws, one is essentially keeping a running tally of the various quantities to make sure the budgets balance.

When considering the everyday functioning of the human body, the above laws generally suffice. When working on the very large scales of the cosmos or the very small scales of atoms, additional phenomena become important. These are described by laws of gravitation (Newton, Einstein) and quantum electrodynamics (Feynman), respectively. Laws, however, are simply generalisations of physical behaviour, based on empirical observations. What is so special about them, to earn the title 'law', is their simplicity, universal nature and lasting truth, despite being falsifiable[3] through the possibility of contradictory observations. Newton once said "I have told you how it moves, not why" (Feynman 1965). Laws describe what happens, but theories seek an explanation.

7.2.2 Fundamentals of Biomechanics

Living creatures populate the physical world and are thus subject to the same mechanical laws as inanimate objects. Biomechanics is a relatively modern term applied to a long-established practice, the application of mechanics to biology.[4] In fact, medicine and mechanics evolved symbiotically out of the joint efforts of physical and biological scientists, and it was once not uncommon to be educated and active in both disciplines (Fung 1993; Ethier and Simmons 2007). We consider two notable examples:

1. Thomas Young (1773–1829) was a London physician with a doctorate in physics (Fung 1993). Amongst his numerous contributions was his characterisation of the elastic nature of solid materials, which followed his studies of the human voice. When a force pushes on an object, it will exert a pressure on its surface (pressure equals force divided by area) that will be transmitted as *stress* (σ) and cause the object to become compressed. Likewise, if the force pulls on the surface, the stress causes the object to stretch, producing a state of tension. The ratio of the stress to the fractional change in length, or strain (ε), is termed Young's modulus of elasticity (E) and is a fundamental property of the material, i.e.

$$E = \sigma / \varepsilon. \qquad (7.1)$$

Hard vertebrae have a much larger Young's modulus than the soft dura mater, as a greater stress (about 100 times) is required to produce the same strain. The concept of elasticity is at the foundation of solid mechanics.

2. The Frenchman Jean Louis Marie Poiseuille (1797–1869) was an experimental physiologist with formal training in mathematics and physics (Sutera and Skalak 1993). He was first interested in 'the force of the aortic heart' and so invented the U-tube mercury manometer to measure arterial blood pressure in horses and dogs. Continuing his study of haemodynamics, Poiseuille next turned his attention to the microcirculation. On observing frog mesenteric blood vessels, he noted that red cells would stream in the centre of the vessels, whereas white blood cells tended to stick to the vessel walls. To understand the nature of these flow patterns, he subsequently conducted an extensive series of experiments in small-diameter glass tubes. Fluid flows from high to low pressure, and Poiseuille established the relationship between the fall in driving pressure along the tube (Δp), the length (L) and diameter (D) of the tube and the

---

[3] For its relevance as a demarcation criterion between science and pseudoscience, a hotly debated topic, see, for example, Popper (1998).

[4] At the cellular level is the emerging subdiscipline of mechanobiology, which is attempting to uncover the molecular mechanism by which cells sense and respond to mechanical signals. For a recent overview of this topic, specific to the nervous system, see Bilston and Stucky (2011).

subsequent volumetric flow rate (Q). The fluid property connecting these four quantities is the viscosity (μ), and their relation is known as Poiseuille's law:

$$Q = \left(\pi D^4 / 128\mu L \right) \Delta p. \qquad (7.2)$$

Thus, for a given pressure drop, there will be a greater volumetric flow rate through vessels having a larger diameter or a lower viscosity. Such differences come into play when we compare the calibres of subarachnoid and perivascular spaces and the viscosities of CSF and blood. Mathematics also gives us the converse relation, in that a greater drop in pressure will result from a larger flow rate.

7.2.3 Constructing a Mathematical Model

What mathematics is and its utility are widely misunderstood (Stewart 2011). Mathematics (Greek 'máthēma', to learn) is a branch of science that deals with concepts of quantity, space, structure and change. It is often referred to as the 'language of nature' for its ability to communicate the ideas of physical phenomena. Mathematics has symbols and a grammar for arranging them, but over and above a traditional language, it also includes a system of *reasoning*. We can explain equations in words but seldom the connection between them; herein lies the power of mathematics (Feynman 1965).

The first step in constructing a mathematical model is to decide upon the level of detail. It is not feasible to include every physical feature that influences the phenomenon being studied. Nor, in fact, is this desirable as doing so would only reproduce the complexity inside the 'black box' that we did not understand in the first place. The aim, therefore, is to retain the features with the greatest influence and omit the rest. Every mathematical model is thus a deliberate idealisation of the phenomenon being studied. Choosing what to include is a process of trial and error, guided by the intuition of experience and the comparison of predictions with empirical data (Barenblatt

2003). There is no one 'correct' model of a given system and what to include depends on the question being asked. A useful starting point is to eliminate quantities that are relatively 'small'. For example, the vertebrae are very hard and stiff compared to the meninges and spinal cord, so their shape is much less affected by typical subarachnoid fluid pressures; in mathematical notation, $\varepsilon_{\text{bone}}$ will have a much smaller value than $\varepsilon_{\text{soft tissue}}$. Thus, it may be reasonable to omit the elasticity of the vertebrae when, say, studying the effects of cough-based pressure pulses in the spinal canal. In contrast, if one were interested in spinal trauma, then the much higher forces involved would demand the bone be treated as an elastic material. By convention, mathematicians and engineers would tend to say "we assume the vertebrae are rigid", rather than "we omit the elasticity of the vertebrae"; these statements mean the same thing, and what is being assumed is that omitting these features from the model so will not significantly change the outcome of subsequent calculations and predictions.

Once all of the simplifying assumptions have been made, one can write down a set of equations that govern the system. This is the essence of the mathematical model. The next task is to solve the equations, for which there are two choices: (1) solve them by hand using pen and paper or (2) solve them on a computer. The former is called an *analytical solution* and yields great insight into the underlying phenomenon by obtaining a relation describing it explicitly, e.g. Eq. (7.2). While this approach is preferable, it is usually only possible for the very simplest equations, so instead one often employs computer programs to obtain a *numerical solution*. Computers are digital so they can only store information as a set of discrete samples. As a result, solving an equation on a computer may introduce error due to the continuums of time and space being approximated as a finite number of values. The finer the partitioning, the smaller the error will be but also the more demanding it becomes to compute. Thus, compromise must be made.

To demonstrate that a mathematical model makes reliable predictions, it should be *validated* against empirical data. For example, Eq. (7.2) was derived mathematically from the laws of mechanics by Eduard Hagenbach (1860), and it matched the relationship that Poiseuille obtained from his glass-tube experiments (Sutera and Skalak 1993). Unfortunately, it is often the case with problems in biomechanics that a controlled experiment, equivalent to that of Poiseuille, is not possible. Instead, in these situations, one deconstructs the model into sufficiently general components, such as water flow through a pipe that can be validated separately. Solutions that are obtained via computer also need to be *verified* to ensure that no mistakes were made in the software; simpler versions of the equations can be computed and compared to well-known analytical solutions, such as the speed of pressure waves in a fluid-filled elastic tube (e.g. Cirovic and Kim 2012). Thus, *validation* ensures that the correct equations are being solved, while *verification* ensures that the equations are being solved correctly.

7.2.4 Modelling Predictions

The real usefulness of a mathematical model lies in its predictive capabilities. Once validated, a mathematical model can be used to determine what happens in hypothetical situations and, most prominently, situations that are not amenable to physical observation and measurement. For example, in a model of posttraumatic syringomyelia, the efficacy of various shunt treatments have been evaluated (Elliott et al. 2011). Crucially though, one must ensure that predictions are consistent with the assumptions upon which the model is based (Dym and Ivey 1980). For biological materials, the elasticity as defined in Eq. (7.1) is only applicable for small strains. This means that in a spinal canal model, one would likely have to choose small enough input pressures to ensure that this condition were not violated.

In clinical and animal studies, a sufficiently large cohort is required to make representative predictions. The empirical findings are analysed in terms of their statistical distribution (mean, standard deviation, confidence intervals, etc.) but may not be predicted precisely. In contrast, mathematical models based on Newton's laws of

mechanics are *isolated* from external influences, so there is no random variation, making them *deterministic*, rather than stochastic (Murthy et al. 1990). It is this ability to remove confounding factors that permits analysis with absolute certainty. However, it is a certainty limited to the model itself. The relevance of mathematical predictions to the biological system depends on the degree to which the model is representative of the biological system.

7.3 Mechanics of the Healthy Cerebrospinal System

7.3.1 Solid and Fluid Components

The spinal cord and brain constitute a soft, elastic solid that is housed within the rigid confines of the vertebral canal and cranial cavity. The intervening subarachnoid spaces, which also extend as cavities (ventricles) into the brain, are filled with cerebrospinal fluid (CSF), not unlike sea water. As the cord and brain themselves are also largely water by mass, they float within their bony container but are hitched in place, loosely by the arachnoid trabeculae and, in the case of the cord, more substantially by the denticulate ligaments and filum terminale (see Chap. 3). These elastic connections span the subarachnoid space which is lined by the pia mater along the cord and brain surface and by the arachnoid layer that is adherent to the dura mater that lines the vertebrae and skull (England and Wakeley 2006).

7.3.2 Elastic Properties of the Soft Tissues

The elasticity of any material is determined by its microstructure, and in the case of soft biological tissues, this largely means the quantity and arrangement of collagen and elastin fibres. The collagen protein molecule has a triple-helix structure, and when grouped into fibrils, and subsequently into fibres, it becomes a much stiffer structure than elastin fibres, which are rubbery, convoluted, thin strands (Fung 1993). The spinal dura mostly consists of collagen fibres, densely arranged in longitudinal bundles but with a network of fine elastin fibres threading in all directions (Tunturi 1977; Maikos et al. 2008). In contrast, the spinal pia consists of small bundles of collagenous fibres together with individual collagen and elastin fibres that are all loosely woven into a reticular pattern (Tunturi 1978). The spinal cord parenchyma itself has a negligible amount of collagen and elastin so its elasticity instead depends on the axonal fibres and their myelin sheaths.

Estimates of the Young's moduli for dura, pia and the spinal cord vary widely in the literature, but broadly speaking, the dura is about 100 times stiffer than the pia (i.e. greater E), which in turn is about 100 times stiffer than the soft cord tissue (Elliott et al. 2013). These tissues, like all materials, can only withstand a certain amount of strain before they become permanently damaged; i.e. they no longer recover their original shape when the forces are removed and may, in fact, rupture. The stress corresponding to this 'mechanical failure' is referred to as the *yield strength*. Collagen, for example, has a Young's modulus of 1–1.5 GPa,[5] but as it can only withstand a strain of 10–20 %, its yield strength is much lower, 70–150 MPa (Meyers et al. 2008).[6] The pia's greater stiffness than the spinal cord to which it is attached limits the strain that the cord endures, thereby performing a mechanically protective role (Bertram 2010; Ozawa et al. 2004).

7.3.3 Fluid Pathways

CSF is secreted from the choroid plexus and commences a slow bulk flow from the ventricles, continuing through the subarachnoid space before the fluid is reabsorbed back into the superior sagittal sinus and venous system via the arachnoid villi. The total volume of CSF (about 150 ml) is

replaced about three times daily (Bradbury 1993). Ill-defined amounts of CSF are also filtered from blood plasma and absorbed into the lymphatic system (Brodbelt and Stoodley 2007). In the human cranial subarachnoid space, the arteries and veins reside within pia-like tubular sheaths. The arterial sheaths continue into the brain parenchyma, while the veins lose their sheaths at the pia mater interface (Zhang et al. 1990). Although not proven, it seems likely that the situation is the same in the spinal canal. As the interstitial and cerebrospinal fluids may pass through pores and leaky gap junctions in the pia, the extracellular, perivascular and subarachnoid spaces thus form a single continuous fluid compartment (Rennels et al. 1985; Stoodley et al. 1996; Johanson 2008; Saadoun and Papadopoulos 2010). Superimposed on the bulk CSF flow is a reciprocating flow of more substantial magnitude—measurable with MRI—that is due to the periodic *volume changes* of the blood vessels with the cardiac and respiratory cycles.

7.3.4 Volume Compliance

The volume change of a distensible vessel is related to pressure change through compliance. However, there are two measures of compliance: *static* and *dynamic* (Bertram 2010).

Static compliance is defined as the change in vessel volume resulting from a given change in the pressure acting across the vessel walls:

$$C = \Delta V / \Delta P. \qquad (7.3)$$

i.e. the slope of the volume versus pressure curve, with which most clinicians are familiar. In the main fluid compartment of the cerebrospinal system, the CSF reservoir, it is well established that static compliance is not constant but decreases as the compartment becomes distended. The cranial pressure-volume index (PVI)[7] attempts to describe this filling-volume-dependent quantity with a single value (Marmarou et al. 1975).

---

[5] Pascals (Pa) is the S.I. unit of measure with the prefixes k, M and G denoting quantities of 10^3, 10^6 and 10^9, respectively; pounds per square inch (psi) is the less-commonly used imperial unit of measure.

[6] For $E = 1.5$ GPa and a maximum strain of $\varepsilon = 0.1$ (10 %) Eq. (7.2) can be expressed as $\sigma = E\,\varepsilon$, predicting a yield stress of 150 MPa.

[7] PVI is the notional volume (ml) which, when added to the craniospinal volume, causes a tenfold rise in intracranial pressure (mmH$_2$O).

Heiss et al. (1999) measured the static compliance of the human craniospinal system as ranging between 3 and 15 ml/mmHg. Marmarou et al.'s (1975) measurements on cats suggest that the spinal canal contributes about a third of the total. Conceptualising the cerebrospinal system as collection of compartments (CSF, blood, brain, spinal cord) allows it to be expressed mathematically as a hydraulic *lumped-parameter* model. The compliance and flow resistance between adjacent compartments are 'lumped at' (assigned to) their interface; i.e. these properties are spatially averaged over each compartment and so do not vary within compartments. The solution consists of the discrete compartment pressures as they vary in time. This modelling technique has long been popular in studying disorders of the intracranial CSF system, such as hydrocephalus (e.g. Agarwal et al. 1969; Ambarki et al. 2007), but including intraspinal compartments to investigate syringomyelia has only been attempted in three studies (Chang and Nakagawa 2003, 2004; Elliott et al. 2011). The reason for this disparity is that it is easier to measure the inter-compartmental compliances and resistances of the head than the spinal canal. The cranial volume may be considered constant due to the rigidity of the skull, the so-called Monro-Kellie doctrine, which makes any internal volume (hence pressure) changes well defined. In the spinal canal, the dura mater is surrounded by fluid (distensible veins) and fatty tissue that are necessary for the mobility of the spine so the total compartment volume is variable.

Dynamic compliance is a measure of how *time-varying* changes in pressure and volume are related, as in pulsation. It governs the speed of pressure waves which feature prominently in the spinal canal. A cough elevates the pressure in the thorax that squeezes blood from the thoracic veins into the adjacent epidural veins. Distension of these veins transmits pressure to the spinal subarachnoid space, leading to a travelling pressure wave (Lockey et al. 1975). Williams (1976) was the first to measure the speed of these waves using pressure transducers connected to lumbar puncture needles. A non-invasive technique, using MRI, has recently been developed (Kalata et al. 2009). Wave speeds are typically around 4 m/s.

The propagation of pressure waves in elastic, fluid-filled tubes is a well-studied problem of classical mechanics (Lamb 1898; Womersley 1955). The spinal cord may be thought of as an annular, elastic, solid cylinder, containing an inner cylindrical central canal and sheathed in a tube of pia mater, which in turn is surrounded by an annular cylinder of fluid, the spinal subarachnoid space that is contained by the outer tube of dura mater. A number of mathematical models of the spinal canal have been developed from variants of this system of coaxial tubes (Lockey et al. 1975; Loth et al. 2001; Berkouk et al. 2003; Carpenter et al. 2003; Bertram et al. 2005, 2008; Cirovic 2009; Elliott et al. 2009; Bertram 2009, 2010; Martin et al. 2012; Cirovic and Kim 2012; Elliott 2012; Cheng et al. 2012), elucidating the mechanics of a number of wave modalities.

The wave recorded by Williams (1976), normally described as the 'CSF pulse wave' or the 'subarachnoid pressure wave', is made up of a moving section of cord constriction and an adjacent segment of dura distension. Of the known wave types, this one involves the largest cord motion and so is most easily observed with MRI. Another wave exists in which the cord distends, rather than constricts, but this vanishes as the central canal is obliterated by adulthood (Milhorat et al. 1994). The healthy spinal canal supports at least two further waves, one similar to the previous but also involving lengthwise cord compression and a final wave, almost exclusively involving stretching of the dura (Cirovic 2009; Bertram 2009; Cirovic and Kim 2012). A cough will initiate a pressure pulse in the thoracolumbar region which will set up each of the above wave types in pairs, one wave travelling in the rostral direction and the other in the caudal direction (analogous to the way surface waves radiate from a stone dropped into a pond). These waves will successively reflect at the craniocervical junction and the lumbar cistern, respectively, and vice versa. This may amplify the fluid pressure, and tissue stresses in regions where opposite-moving wave components superimpose. Individual waves will not persist indefinitely though. The motion of fluid and solid spinal components involves kinetic energy (Greek kinētikos, 'to move') that will be lost to internal friction. This friction is termed *viscosity*[8] in fluids and *viscoelasticity* in solids and is responsible for attenuating waves as they travel. Getting the speed of the CSF pulse wave in a mathematical model to match that measured in the human body has become a useful way of validating the model as it ensures that the dynamic compliance is anatomically realistic.

Although pressure waves are induced by abrupt percussive events, they do not induce a significant amount of CSF motion in the spinal subarachnoid space. The alterations in the shape of the cord and dura occur too quickly for the fluid to keep up so the tissue only has a 'massaging' effect, gently stirring the fluid into motion (Bertram 2009). The reciprocating motion of CSF, well known to the clinician, is due to the lower-frequency pulsations of the cardiac cycle (Bertram 2010). The interdependence of pressure drop and flow rate means that the pressure drop along the spinal subarachnoid space changes from positive to negative, and vice versa, twice per cardiac cycle.

7.4 Mechanics of Syringomyelia

7.4.1 Syrinxes

Mechanically, syrinxes provide the cord with additional localised compliance through displacement of the contained fluid when the syrinx is squeezed into a different shape. Williams (1980) hypothesised that a CSF pulse wave would compress the syrinx at one end, causing the fluid to 'slosh' to the other end, akin to squeezing a water balloon, with the syrinx subsequently extending by tissue dissection. In a computer-based mathematical model, Bertram (2009) demonstrated that a CSF pulse wave travelling rostrocaudally induces axial motion of the syrinx fluid relative to the syrinx walls, leading to fluid pressure at the caudal end of the syrinx exceeding spinal subarachnoid space pressure at the same level, and a

distending (tensile) stress at the caudal tip of the syrinx wall. The pulse wave slowed down as it passed the syrinx, agreeing with Cirovic's (2009) analytical prediction, but not enough to induce the substantial sloshing motions of syrinx fluid proposed by Williams. Consequently, the incurred stress had relatively little potential for tearing the cord tissue and concomitant lengthening of the syrinx. It was acknowledged, though, that a higher-resolution model of the spinal cord is needed to better capture the large stress gradients at the ends of the syrinx.

An additional complication arises with the presence of a syrinx—partial wave reflection and refraction. When a pressure wave reaches a syrinx border, some of the wave continues ahead, and the remainder doubles back due to the change in cross-sectional constitution. Given that there are many types of wave, all moving at different speeds, and that overlapping waves sum together (either reinforcing or cancelling each other), the resulting state of fluid pressure/velocity and tissue stress/displacement easily becomes complicated (e.g. see figure 10 in Bertram 2009). This, unfortunately, does not lend the wave mechanics to intuitive theorising, and some wave-based theories, while being admirable attempts to explain the pathophysiology of syrinx filling, are conceptually unphysical (e.g. Greitz 2006).

7.4.2 Syrinxes with Associated CSF Obstruction

Stenosis occurs at the craniocervical junction in the presence of a herniated hindbrain. It also occurs elsewhere along the spinal subarachnoid space due to, most commonly, scar tissue build-up following spinal trauma. These pathologies obstruct the CSF circulation and act as amplification sites for pressure and stress through the wave reflections that they produce. Their frequent juxtaposition with syrinxes has motivated several groups to pursue a mathematical line of enquiry (Berkouk et al. 2003; Carpenter et al. 2003; Bertram et al. 2005; Elliott et al. 2009; Bertram 2010; Cirovic and Kim 2012; Elliott 2012).

---

[8] For example, honey has more viscosity, or is said to be more viscous ('thicker'), than water, and so loses kinetic energy more rapidly as it flows.

Carpenter and colleagues developed a pathogenesis hypothesis based on the theory of shockwaves (Berkouk et al. 2003; Carpenter et al. 2003). They demonstrated in a mathematical model of coaxial tubes that a pulse wave will become steeper as it propagates, much like a beach wave does on reaching shallow water. If the concomitant elevation in pressure difference between the spinal subarachnoid space and the cord/syrinx reaches the maximal value, then a so-called shock-like elastic jump occurs, which is mathematically similar to the beach wave breaking. When this pressure wave reaches a complete stenosis, the incident and reflected components superimpose, creating an abnormally large tissue stress/syrinx pressure that could potentially damage the cord/expand a syrinx. Although the predictions make a fundamental contribution to the mathematical modelling community, subsequent analysis reveals that the proposed mechanism is unlikely to play a role in the human body; the gross dimensions of the spinal canal and its contents only confer marginal shock-like stress/pressure changes (Elliott et al. 2009). When additional features are included in the coaxial tube representation of the spinal system, such as fluid viscosity and the ability to capture a spectrum of frequencies, shock-like phenomena become even less likely. The pressure waves tend to spread out and attenuate rather than steepen and amplify (Bertram et al. 2005).

Numerous medical (Williams 1980, 1986; Oldfield et al. 1994; Fischbein et al. 1999; Brodbelt et al. 2003b) and engineering (Carpenter et al. 2003; Martin et al. 2005; Bertram 2010) investigators have hypothesised various scenarios in which wave-induced fluid exchange across the pia mater could play a role in syrinx formation. In an analytical model with a permeable pia mater, Elliott (2012) showed that pressure waves will attenuate as they travel due to fluid crossing the pia mater, thereby alleviating the tissue stress therein. Furthermore, dilated perivascular spaces, spinal subarachnoid obstructions, and a stiffer and thicker pia mater—all associated with syringomyelia—will increase transpial flux and retard wave travel. An associated mechanism for syrinx formation remains to be investigated.

A rather different situation arises during the cardiac cycle, unaided by pressure waves, when a partial CSF obstruction occurs at the same level as a syrinx. The obstruction itself acts as a flow resistor causing a localised drop in pressure. This was demonstrated in both simplified (Bilston et al. 2006) and anatomically accurate (Cheng et al. 2012) computer models of a rigid-walled spinal subarachnoid space with simulated subarachnoid scar tissue. When one adds in tissue compliance, the partial obstruction is able to move in response to the reciprocating flow through the spinal subarachnoid space, driven by the cardiac cycle. The net effect is a resonant oscillation[9] in pressure gradient about the obstruction, which lowers in frequency and attenuates more rapidly as the obstruction increases in severity. This has been demonstrated in both mathematical modelling (Bertram 2010) and engineering experiments (Martin and Loth 2009; Martin et al. 2010). The mechanical features of the trans-stenosis pressure gradient (including its time-varying nature and non-negligible viscous forces) meant that a Venturi effect,[10] postulated elsewhere as being important (Greitz 2006), was in fact small (Bertram 2010) if not nonexistent (Martin and Loth 2009; Martin et al. 2010). More dramatically, the addition of a syrinx at the same level as the stenosis created a one-way valve. The pressure drop across the stenosis caused the syrinx to be compressed at one end and distended at the other, thereby narrowing the already obstructed spinal subarachnoid pathway. As the flow resistance past the obstruction was higher during (simulated) diastole than systole the result was a one-way valve, *dissociating* the CSF

---

[9] A natural frequency of the cerebrospinal system, coinciding with the cardiac excitation frequency. One familiar example is a playground swing. Pushing a person in a swing at its resonant frequency will make the swing go higher, while pushing the swing at a faster or slower tempo will result in smaller arcs.

[10] The reduction in pressure and increase in velocity that occurs, due to mass conservation alone, when a fluid flows through a narrowed section of pipe (and vice versa). Named after Giovanni Battista Venturi (1746–1822), an Italian physicist, this is an application of Bernoulli's equation; for details see (Tritton 1988; Houghton and Carpenter 2003).

pressure caudal to the stenosis from that rostral to it (Bertram 2010). This longitudinal pressure dissociation had two important ramifications. Firstly, the pressure in the spinal subarachnoid space caudal to the stenosis was higher than that in the underlying syrinx when averaged over the cardiac cycle (also predicted by Chang and Nakagawa 2004). This presents a pressure gradient favouring CSF flow into the syrinx, potentially through the perivascular spaces of penetrating arteries; i.e. a filling mechanism. Secondly, the distending stress at the caudal end of the syrinx was much higher with the one-way valve in operation, in fact high enough (relative to the input pressure amplitude) to raise the possibility of cord tissue rupture and syrinx expansion (Bertram 2010).

While the existing models can predict stresses and strains near a fissure, it is the spinal cord's microstructure that determines the critical conditions for rupture and this has not yet been modelled. The study of *fracture mechanics* provides the relevant mathematical techniques, a discipline born out of the demand for reliable ships and aeroplanes in World War II (Anderson 2005). The empirical data needed to complete such a model (e.g. the material property 'fracture toughness') have not, however, been obtained. A rat model of posttraumatic syringomyelia showed that there is a proliferation of cells following syrinx formation that are involved in glial scar formation (Tu et al. 2010, 2011; Fehlings and Austin 2011). This suggested a mechanism to limit syrinx enlargement, which is consistent with the principles of fracture mechanics.

7.4.3   Cord Tethering

In addition to obstructing CSF flow, subarachnoid scar tissue may tether the cord, constraining its movement. Bertram et al. (2008) mathematically predicted that CSF pulse wave transmission past a tethered section of cord could lead to a distending stress in the underlying tissue. The computed stress values were not large enough to conclude a damaging effect but the simulated tethering did not include flow obstruction and their simultaneous effect remains to be investigated.

7.4.4   Perivascular Pumping

It is a commonly held view that syrinx fluid originates from CSF. This is based on their having a similar chemical composition (Table 17.1) and physical properties (Kiernan 1998; Bloomfield et al. 1998) and is reinforced by the histological studies that establish the perivascular spaces around penetrating arteries as forming a hydraulic connection between the syrinx cavity and the spinal subarachnoid space (Brodbelt and Stoodley 2007). On this premise, a computer model of fluid flow through a perivascular space has been developed (Bilston et al. 2010). The inner surface was cyclically distended to simulate the cardiac pulsation of the enclosed artery and the superficial end of the perivascular space was given a pressure signal, computed from flow-rate measurements in the human spinal subarachnoid space (Bilston et al. 2006). The relative timing of these two cardiac-based pulsations was varied. Provided the two pulses were not in synchrony, a net amount of fluid would be pumped into or out of the cord, with maximal inflow occurring when the pulses were out of phase. It was postulated that interruptions to the local blood supply, such as might be created by scar tissue, could lead to these phase differences (Bilston et al. 2010). Martin et al. (2012) demonstrated that, in fact, there may be a *natural* variation between the timing of the vascular and CSF pulses in the spinal canal. In a computer model that included the entire cardiovascular tree represented as a collection of elastic tubes interacting with a like representation of the spinal subarachnoid space, the vascular-to-CSF pulse delay was found to vary a great deal along the length of the spinal canal depending on craniospinal compliance and vascular anatomy.

Elliott et al. (2011) examined how effective the phasic-pumping mechanism would be when perivascular spaces are incorporated into a lumped-parameter model of the whole cerebrospinal system. The model had compartments representing (1) the spinal cord, (2) the spinal subarachnoid space, (3) the venous bed of the spinal cord, (4) the venous bed of the spinal subarachnoid space and epidural space and (5) a vascular pressure source. Fluid was permitted to exchange between the spinal subarachnoid space and the spinal cord (interstitium). Their pia mater interface was compliant, and similar compliances allowed for collapse of the cord's venous bed and displacement of fluid in the epidural space. The phasic pumping of CSF into the cord was predicted. However, the pressure gradient driving fluid into the cord also constricts the cord, so the two effects are in competition. Thus, for the phasic-pumping mechanism to operate, the spinal cord must have volume compliance due to displacement of blood from the cord venous bed, which is unlikely to be substantial.

7.5 Pathophysiology Yet to Be Modelled

Some aspects of spinal pathophysiology are less amenable to mathematical modelling than others, leaving their mechanics relatively uncharted. We highlight two notable examples.

Greitz proposed a syringogenesis mechanism in which the syrinx fluid is derived from blood plasma, rather than CSF, and that it involves a disruption to the blood-spinal cord barrier (e.g. Greitz 2006). While some mechanical features of the proposed event cascade may require further thought, the spinal arteries certainly provide a favourable pressure gradient for flow into a syrinx. In a recent paper on normal pressure hydrocephalus, Tully and Ventikos (2011) adapted a method from geomechanics for modelling the effects of porosity: the brain parenchyma was treated as an elastic solid matrix, permeated by low-porosity pores (interstitial spaces) and high-porosity fissures (blood vessels) with fluid transport permitted between them (the blood–brain barrier). Such an approach may also prove useful for the spinal cord and would permit investigation of the proposal of oedema as a 'pre-syrinx state' (Fischbein et al. 2000). Before attempting this, however, a better understanding is required of the mechanical interaction between the elastic cord tissue and fluid-filled interstitial pores. Harris and Hardwidge's (2010) computer model

of a porous spinal cord and Elliott's (2012) analytical model of wave-induced fluid transport across the pia mater provide a mathematical starting point.

The herniated hindbrain features prominently in Chiari-based syringomyelia. Williams (1974) built a physical model of the cerebrospinal system that simulated the hindbrain-plugging of the craniocervical junction following a cough. This has not yet been attempted mathematically but others have modelled the simpler problem, when the hindbrain is 'frozen' in position (Roldan et al. 2009). The dynamic range of CSF velocities at the craniocervical junction makes obtaining accurate validation data an additional challenge (Santini et al. 2009; Odéen et al. 2011; Battal et al. 2011).

Conclusions

In our everyday lives, we observe and experience certain physical phenomena that occur in a predictable way. These events may be described by the laws of mechanics which can be used to construct a mathematical model—a theoretical representation of a physical system.

The cerebrospinal system consists of solid and fluid components that interact through their volume compliance. From this single concept, we can gain an appreciation of how:

1. Abrupt pressure impulses, such as from a cough, lead to wave propagation in the spinal canal.
2. Slower pulsation, due to the cardiac cycle, accelerates the fluid in the spinal subarachnoid space back and forth.

An isolated syrinx increases the cord's compliance but does not appear to lead to adverse pressures or stresses. When coupled with an overlying stenosis, however, a one-way valve may be set up in the spinal subarachnoid space that presents favourable circumstances for CSF flow into the syrinx and syrinx elongation by stress-induced tissue rupture. Another one-way valve, in the perivascular spaces, also promotes CSF influx but is limited by the collapsibility of the cord's venous reservoir.

It is hoped that this chapter gives the clinician greater accessibility to mathematical modelling concepts which will facilitate closer collaborations with mathematicians and engineers.

Acknowledgements In addition to the Editors' review, the author would like to thank the following people for useful feedback on the manuscript: Mr. Andrew Brodbelt (The Walton Centre NHS Foundation Trust, UK), Dr. Duncan Lockerby (School of Engineering, University of Warwick, UK), Dr. Richard Howell (Department of Mechanical Engineering, Curtin University, Australia), and Prof. John Heiss (Department of Neurological Surgery, The George Washington University, USA). The author acknowledges the support of the Australian Research Council through project DP0559408, the WA State Centre of Excellence in e-Medicine, and would also like to thank the School of Mathematics, University of Manchester, UK, for hosting him as an honorary visitor during the preparation of the manuscript.

References

Agarwal GC, Berman BM, Stark L (1969) A lumped parameter model of the cerebrospinal fluid system. IEEE Trans Biomed Eng BME-16:45–53

Ambarki K, Baledent O, Kongolo G et al (2007) A new lumped-parameter model of cerebrospinal hydrodynamics during the cardiac cycle in healthy volunteers. IEEE Trans Biomed Eng 54(3):483–491

Anderson TL (2005) Fracture mechanics: fundamentals and applications. CRC Press/Taylor & Francis, Boca Raton

Barenblatt GI (2003) Scaling. Cambridge texts in applied mathematics. Cambridge University Press, Cambridge

Battal B, Kocaoglu M, Bulakbasi N et al (2011) Cerebrospinal fluid flow imaging by using phase-contrast MR technique. Br J Radiol 84:758–765

Berkouk K, Carpenter PW, Lucey AD (2003) Pressure wave propagation in fluid-filled co-axial elastic tubes, part 1: basic theory. ASME J Biomech Eng 125(6): 852–856

Bertram CD (2009) A numerical investigation of waves propagating in the spinal cord and subarachnoid space in the presence of a syrinx. J Fluids Struct 25(7): 1189–1205

Bertram CD (2010) Evaluation by fluid/structure-interaction spinal-cord simulation of the effects of subarachnoid-space stenosis on an adjacent syrinx. ASME J Biomech Eng 132(6):061009

Bertram CD, Brodbelt AR, Stoodley MA (2005) The origins of syringomyelia: numerical models of fluid/structure interactions in the spinal cord. ASME J Biomech Eng 127(7):1099–1109

Bertram CD, Bilston LE, Stoodley MA (2008) Tensile radial stress in the spinal cord related to arachnoiditis

or tethering: a numerical model. Med Biol Eng Comput 46(7):701–707. doi:10.1007/s11517-008-0332-0

Bilston LE, Stucky CL (2011) Mechanotransduction in the nervous system. In: Bilston LE (ed) Neural tissue biomechanics. Studies in mechanobiology, tissue engineering and biomaterials. Springer, Berlin, pp 231–245

Bilston LE, Fletcher DF, Stoodley MA (2006) Focal spinal arachnoiditis increases subarachnoid space pressure: a computational study. Clin Biomech 21(6):579–584

Bilston LE, Stoodley MA, Fletcher DF (2010) The influence of the relative timing of arterial and subarachnoid space pulse waves on spinal perivascular cerebrospinal fluid flow as a possible factor in syrinx developments. J Neurosurg 112(4):808–813

Bloomfield IG, Johnson IH, Bilston LE (1998) Effects of proteins, blood cells and glucose on the viscosity of cerebrospinal fluid. Pediatr Neurosurg 28(5):246–251

Bradbury M (1993) Anatomy and physiology of CSF. In: Schurr PH, Polkey CE (eds) Hydrocephalus. Oxford University Press, Oxford, New York, pp 19–47

Brodbelt A, Stoodley M (2007) CSF pathways: a review. Br J Neurosurg 21(5):510–520

Brodbelt A, Stoodley M, Watling A et al (2003a) Fluid flow in an animal model of post-traumatic syringomyelia. Eur Spine J 12:300–306

Brodbelt AR, Stoodley MA, Watling AM et al (2003b) Altered subarachnoid space compliance and fluid flow in an animal model of posttraumatic syringomyelia. Spine 28(20):E413–E419

Carpenter PW, Berkouk K, Lucey AD (2003) Pressure wave propagation in fluid-filled co-axial elastic tubes, part 2: mechanisms for the pathogenesis of syringomyelia. ASME J Biomech Eng 125(6):857–863

Chang HS, Nakagawa H (2003) Hypothesis on the pathophysiology of syringomyelia based on simulation of cerebrospinal fluid dynamics. J Neurol Neurosurg Psychiatry 74(3):344–347

Chang HS, Nakagawa H (2004) Theoretical analysis of the pathophysiology of syringomyelia associated with adhesive arachnoiditis. J Neurol Neurosurg Psychiatry 75(5):754–757. doi:10.1136/jnnp.2003.018671

Cheng S, Stoodley MA, Wong J et al (2012) The presence of arachnoiditis affects the characteristics of CSF flow in the spinal subarachnoid space: a modelling study. J Biomech 45(7):1186–1191

Cirovic S (2009) A coaxial tube model of the cerebrospinal fluid pulse propagation in the spinal column. ASME J Biomech Eng 131(2):021008

Cirovic S, Kim M (2012) A one-dimensional model of the spinal cerebrospinal-fluid compartment. ASME J Biomech Eng 134(2):021005

Dym CL, Ivey ES (1980) Principles of mathematical modelling. Academic Press Inc, New York

Elliott NSJ (2012) Syrinx fluid transport: modeling pressure-wave-induced flux across the spinal pial membrane. ASME J Biomech Eng 134(3):031006. doi:10.1115/1.4005849

Elliott NSJ, Lockerby DA, Brodbelt AR (2009) The pathogenesis of syringomyelia: a re-evaluation of the elastic-jump hypothesis. ASME J Biomech Eng 131(4):044503

Elliott NSJ, Lockerby DA, Brodbelt AR (2011) A lumped-parameter model of the cerebrospinal system for investigating arterial-driven flow in posttraumatic syringomyelia. Med Eng Phys 33:874–882

Elliott NSJ, Bertram CD, Martin BA et al (2013) Syringomyelia: a review of the biomechanics. J Fluids Struct 40:1–24. doi:10.1016/j.jfluidstructs.2013.01.010

England MA, Wakeley JW (2006) Color atlas of the brain and spinal cord: an introduction to normal neuroanatomy. Mosby, Philadelphia

Ethier CR, Simmons CA (2007) Introductory biomechanics: from cells to organisms. Cambridge University Press, Cambridge

Fehlings MG, Austin JW (2011) Editorial: posttraumatic syringomyelia. J Neurosurg Spine 14(5):570–572

Feynman RP (1965) The character of physical law. M.I.T Press, Cambridge

Fischbein NJ, Dillon WP, Cobbs C et al (1999) The "pre-syrinx" state: a reversible myelopathic condition that may precede syringomyelia. AJNR Am J Neuroradiol 20(1):7–20

Fischbein NJ, Dillon WP, Cobbs C et al (2000) The "pre-syrinx" state: is there a reversible myelopathic condition that may precede syringomyelia? Neurosurg Focus 8(3):1–13

Fung YC (1993) Biomechanics: mechanical properties of living tissues, 2nd edn. Springer, New York

Greitz D (2006) Unravelling the riddle of syringomyelia. Neurosurg Rev 29(4):251–264

Hagenbach E (1860) Ueber die Bestimmung der Zähigkeit einer Flüssigkeit durch den Ausfluss aus Röhren [On the determination of the viscosity of a fluid by flow experiments through tubes]. Annalen der Physik 185(3):385–426. doi:10.1002/andp.18601850302

Harris PJ, Hardwidge C (2010) A porous finite element model of the motion of the spinal cord. In: Constanda C, Pérez ME (eds) Integral methods in science and engineering, vol 2, Computational methods. Birkhäuser, Boston, pp 193–201

Heiss JD, Patronas N, DeVroom HL et al (1999) Elucidating the pathophysiology of syringomyelia. J Neurosurg 91:553–562

Houghton EL, Carpenter PW (2003) Aerodynamics for engineering students, 5th edn. Butterworth-Heinemann, Amsterdam

Johanson CE (2008) Choroid plexus—cerebrospinal fluid circulatory dynamics: impact on brain, growth, metabolism, and repair. In: Conn PE (ed) Neuroscience in medicine, 3rd edn. Human Press, Totown

Kalata W, Martin BA, Oshinski JN et al (2009) MR measurement of cerebrospinal fluid velocity wave speed in the spinal canal. IEEE Trans Biomed Eng 56(6): 1765–1768

Kiernan JA (1998) Barr's the human nervous system, an anatomical viewpoint, 7th edn. Lippincott-Raven, Philadelphia

Lamb H (1898) On the velocity of sound in a tube, as affected by the elasticity of the walls. Manch Literary Philos Soc Memoirs Proc 42:1–16

Lockey P, Poots G, Williams B (1975) Theoretical aspects of the attenuation of pressure pulses within cerebrospinal-fluid pathways. Med Biol Eng 13(6): 861–869

Loth F, Yardimci MA, Alperin N (2001) Hydrodynamic modelling of cerebrospinal fluid motion within the spinal cavity. ASME J Biomech Eng 123:71–79

Maikos JT, Elias RAI, Shreiber DI (2008) Mechanical properties of dura mater from the rat brain and spinal cord. J Neurotrauma 25(1):38–51

Marmarou A, Shulman K, LaMorgese J (1975) Compartmental analysis of compliance and outflow resistance of the cerebrospinal fluid system. J Neurosurg 43:523–534

Martin BA, Loth F (2009) The influence of coughing on cerebrospinal fluid pressure in an in vitro syringomyelia model with spinal subarachnoid space stenosis. Cerebrospinal Fluid Res 6(17):18. doi:10.1186/1743-8454-6-17

Martin BA, Kalata W, Loth F et al (2005) Syringomyelia hydrodynamics: an in vitro study based on in vivo measurements. ASME J Biomech Eng 127(7): 1110–1120

Martin BA, Labuda R, Royston TJ et al (2010) Spinal subarachnoid space pressure measurements in an in vitro spinal stenosis model: implications on syringomyelia theories. ASME J Biomech Eng 132(11): 111007

Martin BA, Reymond P, Novy P et al (2012) A coupled hydrodynamic model of the cardiovascular and cerebrospinal fluid system. Am J Physiol Heart Circ Physiol 302(7):H1492–H1509

Meyers MA, Chen P-Y, Lin AY-M et al (2008) Biological materials: structure and mechanical properties. Prog Mater Sci 53:1–206

Milhorat TH, Kotzen RM, Anzil AP (1994) Stenosis of central canal of spinal cord in man: incidence and pathological findings in 232 autopsy cases. J Neurosurg 80:716–722

Murthy DNP, Page NW, Rodin EY (1990) Mathematical modelling: a tool for problem solving in engineering, physical biological and social sciences. Permagon Press, Oxford

Odéen H, Uppman M, Markl M et al (2011) Assessing cerebrospinal fluid flow connectivity using 3D gradient echo phase contrast velocity encoded MRI. Physiol Meas 32(4):407–421

Oldfield EH, Muraszko K, Shawker TH et al (1994) Pathophysiology of syringomyelia associated with Chiari I malformation of the cerebellar tonsils. Implications for diagnosis and treatment. J Neurosurg 80:3–15

Ozawa H, Matsumoto T, Ohashi T et al (2004) Mechanical properties and function of the spinal pia mater. J Neurosurg Spine 1:122–127

Popper K (1998) Science: conjectures and refutations. In: Cover JA, Curd M (eds) Philosophy of science: the central issues. WW Norton & Co, New York, pp 3–10

Rennels ML, Gregory TF, Blaumanis OR et al (1985) Evidence for a 'paravascular' fluid circulation in the mammalian central nervous system, provided by the rapid distribution of tracer protein throughout the brain from the subarachnoid space. Brain Res 326(1):47–63

Roldan A, Weiben O, Haughton V et al (2009) Characterization of CSF hydrodynamics in the presence and absence of tonsillar ectopia by means of computational flow analysis. AJNR Am J Neuroradiol 30:941–946

Saadoun S, Papadopoulos MC (2010) Aquaporin-4 in brain and spinal cord oedema. Neuroscience 168: 1036–1046

Santini F, Wetzel SG, Bock J et al (2009) Time-resolved three-dimensional (3D) phase-contrast (PC) balanced steady-state free precession (bSSFP). Magn Reson Med 62:966–974

Stewart I (2011) Mathematics of life. Basic Books, New York

Stoodley MA, Jones NR, Brown CJ (1996) Evidence for rapid fluid flow from the subarachnoid space into the spinal cord central canal in the rat. Brain Res 707(2): 155–164

Stoodley MA, Gutschmidt B, Jones NR (1999) Cerebrospinal fluid flow in an animal model of non-communicating syringomyelia. Neurosurgery 44(5): 1065–1077

Sutera SP, Skalak R (1993) The history of Poiseuille's law. Annu Rev Fluid Mech 25:1–19

Tritton DJ (1988) Physical fluid dynamics, 2nd edn. Clarendon, Oxford

Tu J, Liao J, Stoodley MA, Cunningham AM (2010) Differentiation of endogenous progenitors in an animal model of post-traumatic syringomyelia. Spine 35(11):1116–1121

Tu J, Liao J, Stoodley MA et al (2011) Reaction of endogenous progenitor cells in a rat model of post-traumatic syringomyelia. J Neurosurg Spine 14(5): 573–582

Tully B, Ventikos Y (2011) Cerebral water transport using multiple-network poroelastic theory: application to normal pressure hydrocephalus. J Fluid Mech 667: 188–215

Tunturi AR (1977) Elasticity of the spinal cord dura in the dog. J Neurosurg 47(3):391–396

Tunturi AR (1978) Elasticity of the spinal cord, pia, and denticulate ligament in the dog. J Neurosurg 48(6): 975–979

Williams B (1974) A demonstration analogue for ventricular and intraspinal dynamics (DAVID). J Neurol Sci 23:445–461

Williams B (1976) Cerebrospinal fluid pressure changes in response to coughing. Brain 99:331–346

Williams B (1980) On the pathogenesis of syringomyelia: a review. J R Soc Med 73(11):798–806

Williams B (1986) Progress in syringomyelia. Neurol Res 8:130–145

Womersley JR (1955) Method for the calculation of velocity, rate of flow and viscous drag in arteries when the pressure gradient is known. J Physiol 127: 553–563

Zhang ET, Inman CBE, Weller RO (1990) Interrelationships of the pia mater and the perivascular (Virchow-Robin) spaces in the human cerebrum. J Anat 170:111–123

Clinical Presentation

8

Ulrich Batzdorf

Contents

U. Batzdorf
Department of Neurosurgery,
University of California, Los Angeles (UCLA),
Los Angeles, CA, USA
e-mail: ubatzdorf@mednet.ucla.edu

8.1   Underlying Pathologies

Syringomyelia, defined as a tubular or cystic expansion within the spinal cord, containing fluid indistinguishable from cerebrospinal fluid, is generally thought to occur in situations of partial obstruction of the subarachnoid cerebrospinal fluid (CSF) pathways. The most common form of syringomyelia occurs in the presence of cerebellar tonsillar ectopia, generally referred to as a Chiari malformation. The genetic and developmental origins of hindbrain hernias are discussed in Chaps. 4 and 5. Chiari malformation may also be seen in association with other conditions, including achondroplasia (Ryken and Menezes 1994), hypophosphataemic rickets (Caldemeyer et al. 1995) and Paget's disease (Elisevich et al. 1987; Schmidek 1977).

The other major category of syringomyelia is primary spinal syringomyelia, which includes a group of conditions in which the underlying partial obstruction of the subarachnoid channels is entirely confined to the spinal canal. The most common aetiologies of primary spinal syringomyelia are trauma, inflammatory scarring of the leptomeninges and mass effect, such as may be produced by certain tumours or even by intervertebral discs. Syringomyelia caused by a mass compressing the subarachnoid space may be seen with both extradural and intradural tumours. It is important, however, to distinguish between true tumour cysts, which generally contain proteinaceous fluid, and syringomyelic cavities caused by narrowing of the subarachnoid channels by

G. Flint, C. Rusbridge (eds.), *Syringomyelia*,
DOI 10.1007/978-3-642-13706-8_8, © Springer-Verlag Berlin Heidelberg 2014

tumour. Some tumours, typically haemangioblastomas, may have both a true tumour cyst and an associated syringomyelia cavity. Inflammation of the meninges may result from bacterial or fungal infection or from subarachnoid haemorrhage, such as may occur after aneurysmal rupture. It may also be caused by chemical substances, formerly introduced into the CSF pathways for diagnostic purposes (Tabor and Batzdorf 1996). Post-inflammatory scarring of the leptomeninges is usually far more extensive and covers a much wider area of the spinal cord than does the cicatrix caused by spinal cord injury, a fact which has broad implications for treatment of this type of syringomyelia. Trauma tends to produce a more localised or focal obstruction of the subarachnoid channels, which may be more amenable to surgical treatment (Holly et al. 2000). Arachnoid webs and cysts, believed to be developmental in origin, can act in similar fashion, and the resulting obstruction to spinal CSF flow may also be associated with syringomyelia (Holly and Batzdorf 2006).

Distinctions between various forms of primary spinal syringomyelia may overlap to some degree. For instance, it is in the nature of spinal trauma that it may cause displacement fractures of the vertebral bones, angulation of the spine or disc protrusions (Holly et al. 2000), as well as haemorrhage into the meninges. All of these, individually or in combination, may lead to the development of syringomyelia as a result of narrowing of the subarachnoid CSF pathways. With both post-traumatic syringomyelia and post-inflammatory syringomyelia, it may sometimes be difficult to distinguish between the effects of the underlying pathology, i.e. cord injury and meningitis, and the effects of the syrinx itself.

Persistence of the central canal, be this focal or more extensive, is usually not considered to be clinically significant. Some of these patients present when imaging studies have been performed for other reasons, most frequently after motor vehicle accidents but also in patients who have pain of unknown origin. The central canal undergoes involution most rapidly during the first 10 years of life (Yasui et al. 1999), but modern imaging techniques have allowed us to recognise persistence of the central canal in

adults. The shape of the persistent central canal is characteristic, tapering into a thin "line" both caudally and rostrally. Axial images show the residual canal to be perfectly round and located centrally within the cord (Holly and Batzdorf 2002). Persistence of the central canal, focal or even more extensive, is often not considered to be clinically significant, even though some of these patients present with various symptoms of uncertain origin. The term idiopathic syringomyelia is still used by many, but in general, modern imaging techniques have allowed us to recognise a potential pathogenic mechanism in most of these cases.

The mechanism of syrinx formation as a consequence of these various pathologies has been studied by Heiss et al. (2012) and is dealt with in Chap. 6.

8.2 Clinical Features of Chiari Malformations

Headaches brought on by coughing or straining, the classical "tussive headache", is recognised in many patients with Chiari malformation (Milhorat et al. 1999; Mueller and Oró 2004). It is believed to result from the sudden increase in intracranial CSF volume, caused by intracranial and spinal epidural venous engorgement, in a situation where herniated cerebellar tonsils prevent the normal displacement of CSF out of the cranial cavity. Williams (1991) observed that headaches develop a split second after the cough, rather than at the instant of the Valsalva manoeuvre, presumably because of impeded CSF flow at the level of the foramen magnum.

Other manifestations of Chiari malformation may also be helpful in establishing the diagnosis (Milhorat et al. 1999). Involvement of the brainstem by compression, as well as downward traction of the lower cranial nerves, may sometimes give rise to symptoms suggestive of a pharyngeal or throat disorder. Thus, patients may complain of hoarseness, dysphagia or coughing with swallowing and even difficulty moving food about their mouth due to unilateral tongue atrophy. Such patients are often first seen and treated by ear, nose and throat specialists. Tinnitus is also recognised quite frequently in patients with Chiari malformation and, when associated with balance problems such as may also be seen with Chiari malformation, may lead to a quest for an otological source of the patient's symptoms (Kumar et al. 2002; Sperling et al. 2001). Visual disturbances encountered in Chiari malformation relate to impaired ocular movements, due to involvement of brainstem vestibuloocular connections. Patients may complain of oscillopsia, and horizontal, rotatory or downbeat nystagmus may be evident on examination. Cerebellar ataxia and associated gait disturbances may sometimes mimic extrapyramidal disorders. Of various other symptoms that have been associated with Chiari malformation, syncope is one of the more serious (Weig et al. 1991).

8.3 Differential Diagnosis of Chiari Headaches

The key features of Chiari-related headaches are, then, their relationship to any Valsalva-like manoeuvre, their brief duration – often lasting only seconds – and their posterior, suboccipital location. Thus, headaches that are diffuse or primarily temporal, periorbital or located at the vertex, as well as headaches described as lasting all day, are all unlikely to be related to a Chiari malformation. Headaches that originate in the neck muscles may extend into the suboccipital area, by virtue of muscle and ligamentous insertions. They are longer in duration than hindbrain-related headaches and are often relieved by neck support or by optimization of the individual's office or other work station. Testing the range of neck motion or identifying an area of tenderness by palpation may be helpful. These features also help to distinguish headaches reported by patients with fibromyalgia, a condition sometimes presenting with symptoms that mimic those of Chiari malformation (Watson et al. 2011). The distinction is important so that fibromyalgia patients do not undergo inappropriate posterior fossa surgery.

Classical migraine headaches are often preceded by a visual aura of scintillating lights in a portion of the visual field of each eye. They may be accompanied by nausea. There may be a family history of migraine, and certain food items such as chocolate or wine may precipitate episodes.

Neoplasms or other mass lesions in the posterior fossa may generate headaches very similar to those associated with Chiari malformation and may also produce descent of one or both cerebellar tonsils. Such tumours may also cause upper cervical nerve root irritation (Kerr 1961). Posterior fossa mass lesions generally, however, produce headaches of more prolonged duration, sometimes associated with vomiting. Funduscopic examination may demonstrate swollen optic nerve discs or true papilloedema.

The diagnosis of pressure dissociation headaches is sometimes less obvious, particularly when other forms of headache coexist. Headaches of longer duration or more diffuse in character may sometimes be seen in Chiari patients and may be related to the mechanism of upper cervical nerve root irritation suggested by Kerr (1961).

Idiopathic intracranial hypertension (IIH), also referred to as benign intracranial hypertension or pseudotumour cerebri, is sometimes particularly difficult to distinguish from Chiari headaches. The mechanism of increased intracranial volume and pressure in this condition may be due to chronic engorgement of the intracranial veins, as suggested by Rekate (2010), and the increased mass effect may sometimes result in descent of the cerebellar tonsils below the foramen magnum. Headaches due to occult CSF leaks in the spinal canal may also result in downward displacement of the cerebellar tonsils, mimicking Chiari malformation. This situation may also be encountered in some patients with lumboperitoneal shunts (Hoffman and Tucker 1976; Welch et al. 1981).

8.4 Features Caused by the Syrinx Itself

It is recognised that syringomyelia does not develop in every patient with Chiari malformation. The figure varies between different reported series, but perhaps up to 60 % of patients with Chiari malformation also have syringomyelia. While many of these patients present with symptoms related to the hindbrain hernia, the manifestations of syringomyelia may be the dominant presenting complaint. Fortunately, the availability of magnetic resonance imaging has led to much earlier diagnosis of syringomyelia, so that advanced stages of disease are now rarely seen.

The classical description of the neurological presentation of syringomyelia was provided by Gowers (1886), the so-called dissociated sensory pattern, with loss of pain and temperature sensation while vibratory and proprioceptive sensation is preserved. When the sensory loss is predominantly in the shoulder area, it has been referred to as being "cape-like" in distribution. Due to lack of pain perception, patients may develop injuries of the hands or other involved areas, including chronic skin ulcerations. Hand involvement is often asymmetrical, particularly when the syrinx cavity itself is eccentric, as are many cavities. Typically, damage due to the expanded syrinx cavity also results in anterior horn cell destruction at the affected cord levels. This is also often associated with compression and sometimes destruction of long tracts, including the corticospinal tract. Spasticity of the lower extremities may also result from involvement of the corticospinal tracts. Bladder and bowel control could also be affected. Anterior horn cell destruction will affect not only the motor cells innervating the limb muscles, resulting in muscle atrophy, but also cells innervating the axial musculature (Batzdorf et al. 2007). Anterior horn cell destruction in the cervical region may result in hand muscle atrophy. The simultaneous involvement of flexor and extensor muscles results in a typically deformed hand, often referred to as a "claw hand" deformity. Horner's syndrome may also be encountered with cervical or upper thoracic cavities. Involvement of axial musculature may cause weakness of spine support. The anatomical level or levels of cord involvement will, of course, determine the level of neurological deficit. Syringomyelia should also be considered in the differential diagnosis in any young person with scoliosis, since appropriate treatment of the underlying syringomyelia often results in reversal of the deformity (Muhonen et al. 1992).

In post-traumatic syringomyelia, it is often difficult to distinguish deficits resulting from the syrinx cavity from those due to the cord injury itself. It must be noted, however, that there generally is a time interval between the spinal injury and development of post-traumatic syringomyelia and, in the pre-MR era, it was not uncommon for the diagnosis of post-traumatic syringomyelia to be made years after the original spinal injury (Barnett and Jousse 1973; LaHaye and Batzdorf 1988). It should also be recognised that post-traumatic syringomyelia may develop even when the spine injury did not cause major injury to the spinal cord (Barnett 1973). Presumably local bleeding may lead to leptomeningeal scar formation and, in time, to the development of syringomyelia.

In patients with Chiari-related syringomyelia, particularly when associated with syringobulbia (Jonesco-Sisesti 1986), it may be difficult to distinguish the effects of tonsillar and brainstem descent from those of the intramedullary cavitation. Post-inflammatory syringomyelia may pose similar problems when the inflammatory process, i.e. meningitis, has produced injury to the underlying cord parenchyma.

Pain, sometimes poorly localised, is commonly encountered in patients with syringomyelia. Pain may be due to dural distension but is more likely to be neuropathic, originating in the cord itself, with release of substance P and other cytokines (Milhorat et al. 1996) (see Chap. 16). Upper extremity involvement is more frequent due to the location of the syrinx cavity.

Figure 8.1 summarises how symptoms arising from a syrinx or a hindbrain hernia may produce, alone or in combination, a variety of clinical profiles.

8.5   Differential Diagnosis of Syringomyelia Myelopathy

There are, of course, many different causes of myelopathy, several of which are more common than syringomyelia, but syringomyelia should always be considered in the differential diagnosis of any case of spinal cord disease (Honan and

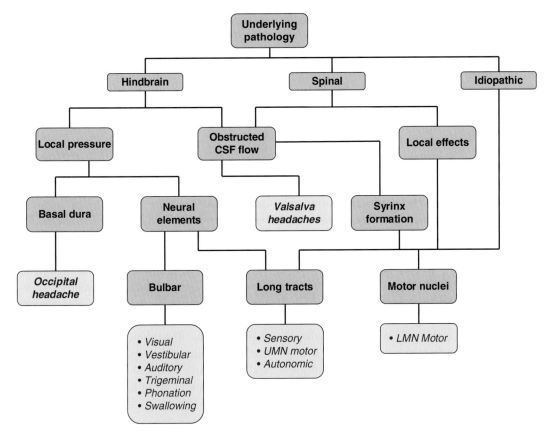

Fig. 8.1 Origin of symptoms. This flowchart illustrates how both the syrinx and its underlying pathology combine to produce a variety of neurological symptoms (Courtesy of Graham Flint)

Williams 1993). The hallmarks of myelopathy associated with syringomyelia include muscle weakness and atrophy at the level of maximal syrinx formation, very often localised to the hands and forearms, in association with long tract signs involving mostly the lower extremities. Pain seen with syringomyelia tends to be diffuse and neuropathic in character. Cervical spondylotic myelopathy is by far the more common cause of myelopathy and is often associated with pain and motor findings in nerve root distribution. Long tract signs may be more prominent than with syringomyelia, and upper extremity reflexes, often absent in syringomyelia, are often preserved and sometimes hyperactive in cervical spondylotic myelopathy. The latter condition results from acquired narrowing of the cervical spinal canal, due to osteophyte formation, and is therefore more likely to be seen in an older patient group than is syringomyelia. Radicular pain is more acute, may be positionally related and may respond to cervical traction.

Other forms of myelopathy, including those due to so-called neurodegenerative disorders, including motor neuron disease and various viral disorders (e.g. HIV and tropical spastic paraparesis), also must be considered. Magnetic resonance imaging is, of course, now fundamental to establishing a correct diagnosis.

8.6   Incidental Findings

The increasing use of magnetic resonance imaging (MRI) studies, in people who have suffered relatively minor injuries and accidents, has led to an increase in the number of patients who have been diagnosed with "small syringomyelia cavities", which are actually moderately distended or simply persisting central canals, of the type commonly referred to as hydromyelic cavities (Holly and Batzdorf 2002). Sometimes one encounters patients with more sizeable, relatively distended cavities which may not be in any way symptomatic and which may not generate any physical signs. It has been suggested that such cavities may represent a form of "compensated hydromyelia", in a manner analogous to the so-called compensated hydrocephalus. On occasion, however, a traumatic origin of such a cavity may be missed, when a history of an injury many years previously is overlooked.

8.7   Natural History and Progression

Symptoms of Chiari malformation and syringomyelia often first develop in adult patients in their 20s or 30s, yet we are dealing with bony and other anatomical features which were, presumably, fully developed at puberty. One possible explanation is that the exertional manoeuvres, which are part of daily living, cause very gradual incremental descent of the tonsils. It is also recognised that trauma, such as a sudden jarring of the head, or prolonged bout of severe coughing may bring about a sudden onset of symptoms in a previously asymptomatic patient. Presumably this is also the result of an increase in tonsillar descent. With syringomyelia similarly, symptoms normally tend to progress gradually, but there are descriptions of sudden symptom development, such as in spinal injury patients following prolonged severe coughing spells (Barnett and Jousse 1973; Foster 1991). Sudden death is extremely rare in patients with Chiari malformation (Friede and Roessmann 1976; Williams 1981), and in most patients the disease progresses either slowly or intermittently. Emergency surgical intervention is rarely, if ever, indicated in these disorders.

When syringomyelia or a Chiari malformation is diagnosed as an incidental finding, there is a potential opportunity for the natural history of the condition to be followed, to determine the rate of progression of the disease in such cases.

Unfortunately few such studies have been carried out. The natural history of syringomyelia is discussed further in Chap. 2.

8.8   Non-specific Symptoms

Reviews of cohorts of patients with Chiari malformation, with or without syringomyelia, have provided extensive lists of presenting symptoms, some of which are non-specific (Mueller and Oró 2004). Wide availability of such lists on the Internet, for patients to view, has made it increasingly difficult for clinicians to obtain an uncontaminated history from many patients. As with many other chronic disorders, symptoms of anxiety, memory impairment, depression and sleep problems are encountered not uncommonly in patients with syringomyelia and Chiari malformation. The clinician must weigh all such symptoms with respect to their specificity and particularly as regards the likelihood of the specific symptom being helped by any surgical intervention.

References

Barnett HJM (1973) Syringomyelia consequent on minor to moderate trauma, chapter 13. In: Barnett HJM, Foster JB, Hudgson P (eds) Syringomyelia. WB Saunders, London

Barnett HJM, Jousse AT (1973) Syringomyelia as a late sequel to traumatic paraplegia and quadriplegia – clinical features, chapter 10. In: Barnett HJM, Foster JB, Hudgson P (eds) Syringomyelia. WB Saunders, London

Batzdorf U, Khoo LT, McArthur DL (2007) Observations on spine deformity and syringomyelia. Neurosurgery 61:370–378

Caldemeyer KS, Boaz JC, Wappner RS et al (1995) Chiari I malformation: association with hypophosphatemic rickets and MR imaging appearance. Radiology 195:733–738

Elisevich K, Fontaine S, Bertrand G (1987) Syringomyelia as a complication of Paget's disease. J Neurosurg 66:611–613

Foster JB (1991) Neurology of syringomyelia, chapter 5. In: Batzdorf U (ed) Syringomyelia, current concepts in diagnosis and treatment. Williams and Wilkins, Baltimore

Friede RL, Roessmann U (1976) Chronic tonsillar herniation. Acta Neuropathol 34:219–235

Gowers WR (1886) A manual of diseases of the nervous system, vol 1. Churchill, London, pp 433–443

Heiss JD, Snyder K, Peterson MM et al (2012) Pathophysiology of primary spinal syringomyelia. J Neurosurg Spine 17:367–380

Hoffman HJ, Tucker WS (1976) Cephalocranial disproportion. A complication of the treatment of hydrocephalus in children. Childs Brain 2:167–176

Holly LT, Batzdorf U (2002) Slitlike syrinx cavities: a persistent central canal. J Neurosurg (Spine 1) 97:161–165

Holly LT, Batzdorf U (2006) Syringomyelia associated with intradural arachnoid cysts. J Neurosurg Spine 5:111–116

Holly LT, Johnson JP, Masciopinto JE et al (2000) Treatment of posttraumatic syringomyelia with extradural decompressive surgery. Neurosurg Focus 8(3):1–6

Honan WP, Williams B (1993) Sensory loss in syringomyelia: not necessarily dissociated. J R Soc Med 86:519–520

Jonesco-Sisesti N (1986) Syringobulbia. In: Ross RT (ed) A contribution to the pathophysiology of the brainstem. Praeger Publishers, New York

Kerr FWL (1961) A mechanism to account for frontal headache in cases of posterior-fossa tumours. J Neurosurg 18:605–609

Kumar A, Patni AH, Charbel F (2002) The Chiari malformation and the neurotologist. Otol Neurotol 23:727–735

LaHaye PA, Batzdorf U (1988) Posttraumatic syringomyelia. West J Med 148:657–663

Milhorat TH, Mu HTM, LaMotte CC et al (1996) Distribution of substance P in the spinal cord of patients with syringomyelia. J Neurosurg 84:992–998

Milhorat TH, Chou MW, Trinidad EM et al (1999) Chiari I malformation redefined: clinical and radiographic findings for 364 symptomatic patients. Neurosurgery 44:1005–1017

Mueller DM, Oró JJ (2004) Prospective analysis of presenting symptoms among 265 patients with radiographic evidence of Chiari malformation type I with or without syringomyelia. J Am Acad Nurse Pract 16:134–138

Muhonen MG, Menezes AH, Sawin PD et al (1992) Scoliosis in pediatric Chiari malformations without myelodysplasia. J Neurosurg 77:69–77

Rekate HL (2010) Box: Pseudotumor and obesity, in Hayhurst C, Rowlands A, Rowe F. Idiopathic intracranial hypertension, chapter 19. In: Mallucci C, Sgouros S (eds) Cerebrospinal fluid disorders. Informa Healthcare, New York, pp 360–367

Ryken TC, Menezes AH (1994) Cervicomedullary compression in achondroplasia. J Neurosurg 81:43–48

Schmidek HH (1977) Neurological and neurosurgical sequelae of Paget's disease of bone. Clin Orthop 127:70–77

Sperling NM, Franco RA, Milhorat TH (2001) Otologic manifestations of Chiari I malformation. Otol Neurotol 22(5):678–681

Tabor EN, Batzdorf U (1996) Thoracic spinal pantopaque cyst and associated syrinx resulting in progressive spastic paraparesis: case report. Neurosurgery 39:1040–1042

Watson NF, Buchwald D, Goldberg J et al (2011) Is Chiari I malformation associated with fibromyalgia? Neurosurgery 68:443–449

Weig SG, Buckthal PE, Choi SK et al (1991) Recurrent syncope as the presenting symptom of Arnold-Chiari malformation. Neurology 41:1673–1674

Welch K, Shillito J, Strand R et al (1981) Chiari I "malformation" – an acquired disorder? J Neurosurg 55:604–609

Williams B (1981) Chronic herniation of the hindbrain. Ann R Coll Surg Engl 63(1):9–17

Williams B (1991) Pathogenesis of syringomyelia, chapter 4. In: Batzdorf U (ed) Syringomyelia: current concepts in diagnosis and treatment. Wiliams & Wilkins, Baltimore, pp 59–90

Yasui K, Hashizume Y, Yoshida M et al (1999) Age-related morphologic changes in the central canal of the human spinal cord. Acta Neuropathol (Berl) 97:253–259

Diagnostic Investigations

9

John Heiss

Contents

With Ayaz Khawaja and Juan Carlos Vera

J. Heiss
Surgical Neurology Branch, National Institute of
Neurological Disorders
and Stroke (NINDS), National Institutes of Health,
Bethesda, MD, USA
e-mail: heissj@ninds.nih.gov

9.1   Introduction

Anatomical MRI[1] of the brain and spine clearly identifies syringomyelia and associated conditions such as the Chiari I malformation, Chiari 0 malformation (Fig. 9.1) and intracranial masses that cause cerebellar tonsillar herniation, basilar invagination or a spinal tumour. The radiographic threshold for diagnosis of Chiari I malformation is tonsillar ectopia below the foramen magnum of 5 mm or more in adults (Barkovich et al. 1986) or 6 mm or more in children of age 10 years or younger (Mikulis et al. 1992). This threshold is often discrepant with clinical symptoms of Chiari I malformation, as 0.9 % of normal adults undergoing MRI studies of the brain in one study had tonsillar ectopia of at least 5 mm (Vernooij et al. 2007). Symptomatic Chiari I malformation is more reliably seen with greater ectopia, usually over 12 mm (Elster and Chen 1992). On the other hand, cervical or cervicothoracic syringomyelia identical to that seen with Chiari I malformation can occur with less than 5 mm of tonsillar ectopia (Milhorat et al. 1999), a condition referred to as "Chiari type 0 malformation" (Tubbs et al. 2001).

CSF pathway narrowing across the subarachnoid space at the level of foramen magnum, shortened posterior fossa bones, decreased posterior fossa height and caudal brainstem displacement can be noticed in both Chiari type 0 and 1 malformations (Bogdanov et al. 2004; Tubbs

---

[1] The use of this term, in this chapter, refers to static MR images.

G. Flint, C. Rusbridge (eds.), *Syringomyelia*,
DOI 10.1007/978-3-642-13706-8_9, © Springer-Verlag Berlin Heidelberg 2014, (outside the USA, 2014)

et al. 2001), suggesting a similar pathophysiological mechanism for both types of malformations, in which posterior fossa underdevelopment and caudal hindbrain displacement impair CSF dynamics and lead to syringomyelia development. Although phase-contrast cine MRI (Figs. 9.2 and 9.3) has helped clarify the pathophysiology of syringomyelia, anatomical MRI alone usually provides sufficient information to diagnose and make appropriate treatment decisions about syringomyelia (Enzmann and Pelc 1991; Heiss et al. 1999; Oldfield et al. 1994).

Primary spinal syringomyelia is suspected when anatomical MRI scanning detects syringomyelia in the absence of pathology at the craniocervical junction, particularly if there is a history of antecedent trauma or meningitis (Batzdorf 2005). Anatomical MRI can evaluate for a spinal deformity or an extramedullary tumour associated with this type of syringomyelia (Byun et al. 2010; Holly et al. 2000), but obstructions in the spinal subarachnoid space, caused by focal arachnoiditis or arachnoid cysts, may not be detected by anatomical MRI, and additional testing with myelography, CT myelography and phase-contrast cine MRI may be required (Fig. 9.4). Sometimes, syringomyelia is not associated with any imaging abnormality and may be declared idiopathic (Lee et al. 2002; Nakamura et al. 2009). This topic is dealt with in Chap. 12.

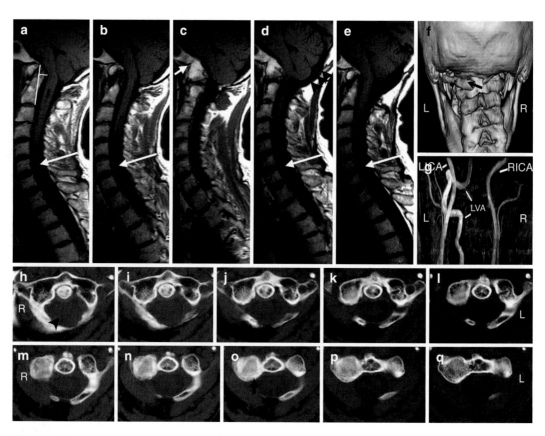

Fig. 9.1 Chiari 0 malformation and congenital atlanto-occipital fusion. T1-weighted midsagittal MRI in a 62-year-old woman with headache, dizziness and back pain (**a**) demonstrates that the cerebellar tonsils extend 4 mm inferior to the foramen magnum and that the odontoid is retroflexed 7 mm. A syrinx is seen (*long white arrows*, **a**, **b**). Fusion of the lateral mass of C1 and the occipital condyle is seen (*short white arrow*, **c**). MRI 3 months after suboccipital craniectomy, C1 laminectomy and duraplasty shows that a CSF space was created dorsal to the cerebellar tonsils (*black arrowheads*, **d**) and that the syrinx has resolved (*long white arrow*, **d**, **e**). Axial CT cuts (**h–q**) through the craniocervical junction demonstrate the foramen magnum (*black arrowhead*, **h**), vestigial right side of the arch of C1 (*black arrow*, **j–l**) and congenital atlanto-occipital fusion on the right side (**o**). Reconstructed 3-dimensional CT (**f**) confirms spina bifida occulta of the dorsal arch of C1 (*black arrow*). MR angiogram demonstrates a dominant left vertebral artery (LVA, **g**) and a normal left internal carotid artery (LICA) and RICA (right internal carotid artery)

a

Bipolar gradient creates a (+) phase change during inferior flow

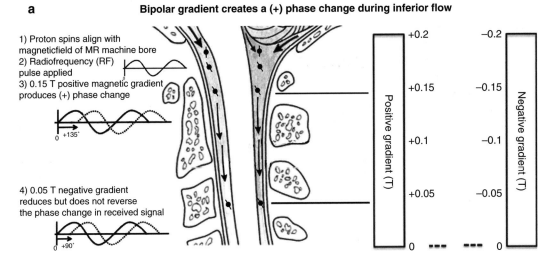

1) Proton spins align with magneticfield of MR machine bore
2) Radiofrequency (RF) pulse applied
3) 0.15 T positive magnetic gradient produces (+) phase change

4) 0.05 T negative gradient reduces but does not reverse the phase change in received signal

b

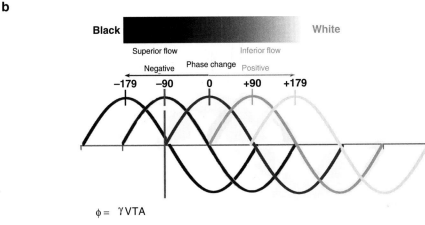

$$\phi = \gamma VTA$$

φ   Phase change
γ   Gyro magnetic ratio
V   Velocity
T   Time interval between lobes of bipolar gradient
A   Amplitude of gradient x time it is on

Fig. 9.2 Drawing of the craniocervical junction annotated to explain detection of CSF motion using phase-contrast cine MRI. In (**a**), protons in the water molecules of CSF align with the static magnetic field of the MRI machine (*1*). A radio-frequency pulse is delivered, which resonates with the protons (*2*). Two opposing magnetic field gradients, positive (*3*) and negative (*4*), are delivered. The inferior motion of the proton results in a greater positive than negative magnetic field being applied to the proton, resulting in a change in the phase of the radio-frequency signals that are released as the protons relax and realign with the static magnetic field. In (**b**), the phase change results in *black* (superior flow) and *white* (inferior flow) areas on the phase-contrast cine-MRI images. The intensity of phase changes is directly proportional to velocity

9.2   Plain Films

Plain radiographs are no longer routinely used to evaluate syringomyelia but may still detect an associated scoliosis and may identify skeletal deformity from spinal trauma that may be associated with post-traumatic syringomyelia (Rossier et al. 1985). Although plain films may also discover basilar invagination, they do not show the resulting effects on adjacent neural elements. Flexion-extension plain films of the cervical spine are still performed if instability or hypermobility of the craniovertebral junction or cervical spine is suspected.

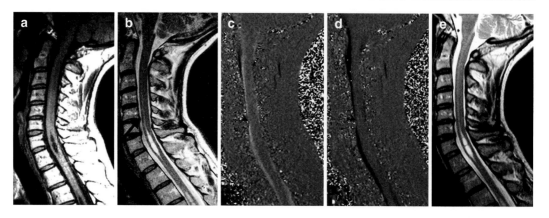

Fig. 9.3 Lack of syrinx fluid motion in a patient with stable cervical syrinx. A 41-year-old woman with moderate neck pain and no neurological deficit. T1-weighted and T2-weighted MRI (**a**, **b**) on presentation demonstrate mild central protrusion of the C5–6 intervertebral disc (*arrow*, **b**). Phase-contrast cine MRI during systole (**c**) or diastole (**d**) shows reduced CSF flow in the anterior subarachnoid space adjacent to the C5–6 disc protrusion (*arrowheads*) and absence of syrinx fluid motion. On re-evaluation 1 year later, neck pain persisted, but she remained free of neurological deficit. T2-weighted MRI at that time (**e**) demonstrates stable syrinx and disc size

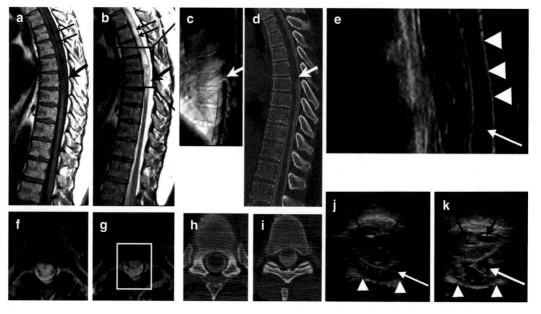

Fig. 9.4 A 63-year-old man with complaints of lower body numbness and tingling. Midsagittal T1-weighted (**a**) and T2-weighted MRI (**b**) demonstrates a thoracic syrinx (*thin black arrows*) and the dorsal subarachnoid space (*thick black arrow*). Axial T2-weighted MRI demonstrates expansion of the thoracic spinal cord by the syrinx (**f**) and signal changes in the dorsal subarachnoid space (**g**). A myelogram (**c**) demonstrates a block to the superior flow of contrast (*thick white arrow*) that proved incomplete on the CT-myelographic images (**d**, **h**, **i**). Note flat-tening of the dorsal surface of the spinal cord (**i**). Intraoperative ultrasonography in the lateral and axial planes (**e**, **j**, **k**) performed after laminectomy shows the dorsal dura (*white arrowheads*), an intricate web of membranes within the dorsal subarachnoid space typical of focal arachnoiditis (*white arrows*), and the multiple compartments of the syrinx (*thin, black arrows*). Lysis of adhesions and duraplasty resulted in stabilisation of symptoms and syrinx resolution (not shown)

9.3 Computerised Tomography (CT)

Computerised tomography is used when bony malformation, fracture or deformity is suspected in association with syringomyelia (Fig. 9.1). Contiguous two-dimensional CT images can be reformatted into a 3-dimensional volume, which can be examined in any plane to give a better understanding of the integrity of the bony elements of the spine and craniocervical junction. Such reconstructions can be used in complex cases to decide whether spinal instability is present or might be induced by a proposed surgical procedure. They can be used to plan the placement of instrumentation for fusion of unstable craniospinal or spinal segments.

9.4 Myelography

Myelography is performed by injecting a contrast medium into the spinal subarachnoid space and following its movement through the spinal canal, using fluoroscopy and capturing radiograms of the silhouette created around the spinal cord and nerve roots (Fig. 9.4). Water-soluble contrast media are presently used exclusively, and the use of both air- and oil-based contrast media in myelography has long been abandoned. This is because air produced inferior contrast and higher rate of headache and oil-based myelography can evoke spinal arachnoiditis. The development of myelography in the pre-CT, pre-MR era nevertheless makes for interesting reading and is the subject of Chap. 21.

Contrast medium is typically injected via lumbar puncture and advanced superiorly in the spinal subarachnoid space by tilting the fluoroscopy table. Because water-soluble contrast medium is a liquid solution that is denser than CSF, declining the myelography table to lower the head in relation to the lumbar spine results in the contrast moving superiorly in the subarachnoid space, outlining the conus medullaris, followed by the thoracic spinal cord, cervical spinal cord and cervicomedullary junction. A lesion completely obstructing the subarachnoid space prevents contrast from moving superiorly, thereby demarcating the inferior margin of the lesion. Lesions

associated with syringomyelia, however, usually, allow some contrast to pass, and the X-ray table can then be inclined, to run the contrast inferiorly once again, in order to outline the superior margin of the lesion. In cases in which CT myelography via lumbar puncture cannot define the superior margin of a spinal lesion, contrast can be injected additionally via cervical (C1–2) puncture and passed inferiorly to this level.

When myelography is followed immediately by a spinal CT scan, in the region of the partial or complete obstruction, images obtained provide greater spatial resolution and more conclusive identification of tonsillar ectopia associated with Chiari I malformation than provided by myelography (Grigorian and Lisianskii 1988; Yamada et al. 1981) (Fig. 9.4h, i). Thin-cut axial CT-myelographic images can then be reconstructed and viewed in any plane.

Myelography and CT myelography are still used in the diagnostic evaluation of patients with primary spinal syringomyelia in whom obstructive lesions cannot be identified using anatomical MRI or phase-contrast cine MRI (Fig. 9.4). In such cases, myelography often localises surgically remediable syringomyelia caused by a lesion, which partially or completely obstructs the subarachnoid space. Careful observation of dye movement during myelography is essential to localise a partial blockage of CSF flow by focal arachnoiditis, as CT-myelographic images in such cases may appear normal if dye passes the partial block and opacifies the subarachnoid space above a partial blockage (Mauer et al. 2008) (Fig. 9.4). CT myelography is often helpful in outlining arachnoid webs, pouches and cysts associated with syringomyelia and in demonstrating distortion of the spinal cord by these processes (Mallucci et al. 1997).

9.5 Magnetic Resonance Imaging (MRI)

9.5.1 The Physics of MRI

The human body is mostly made up of the elements hydrogen, carbon and oxygen, including 60 % as water and variable amounts of fat (lipids). The nucleus of each hydrogen atom is a proton, which is positively charged, has the quantum property of spin and has a magnetic moment. Placing protons in the static magnetic field of the MRI unit aligns the protons so they precess, or "wobble", about the main axis of the magnetic field. The precession frequency is directly proportional to the strength of the magnetic field according to the gyromagnetic ratio.[2] In magnetic resonance imaging, radio-frequency (RF) pulses, delivered at this specific precession frequency (the Larmor frequency), are absorbed by protons. After the RF pulse stops, the protons relax to their resting alignment by emitting the absorbed RF energy. The emitted RF signal varies according to the local tissue environment and various other physical parameters (e.g. T1 weighted, T2 weighted, diffusivity and proton density).

Three orthogonal magnetic field gradients (magnetic fields that change in intensity linearly over the body), known as the slice-select, phase-encoding and frequency-encoding gradients, are used to localise the received RF signal in space. These gradients alter the strength of the magnetic field over the body, and consequently, the Larmor frequency will vary across these regions. The bandwidth of RF delivered to the protons, in the imaged structure, must therefore be sufficient to span these frequencies. After applying the RF pulse, the relaxation of protons in the varying magnetic fields results in the emission of different frequencies of released RF energy from the imaged structure. These are used to encode the RF signal in three planes (X, Y and Z). The released RF signal is received by an antenna (coil), converted from analogue to digital form and then changed mathematically, using Fourier transformation, from an intensity-and-time function to an intensity-and-frequency function. A powerful computer analyses the digital signal and calculates intensity values for each spatial location in the imaging volume. It then creates and displays grey-scale images that represent the

magnetic resonance characteristics of normal and abnormal anatomical structures within the imaging volume (Hashemi et al. 2010).

Phase-contrast cine MRI of cerebrospinal fluid velocity is often referred to as a CSF flow study. This phase-contrast MRI technique delivers an RF pulse followed by sequential positive and negative magnetic gradients. These produce a net positive or negative phase change in the RF emission from moving protons but no net phase change from stationary protons (Fig. 9.2). The sign of the phase change (positive or negative) indicates the direction of fluid (proton) movement. The magnitude of the phase change indicates the velocity of moving fluid (Fig. 9.2b). Between 16 and 32 images are produced, displaying CSF velocity throughout the cardiac cycle, with each image being labelled with its temporal relation (ms) to the R wave of the electrocardiogram. When this set of images is viewed as a cine loop, the CSF oscillation, which repeats every cardiac cycle, is visualised, with CSF moving inferiorly during systole and superiorly during diastole (Enzmann and Pelc 1991) (Fig. 9.3c, d). Phase-contrast cine MRI can be used to identify regions of reduced CSF movement at the level of the foramen magnum or within the spine which may be associated with syrinx formation (Heiss et al. 1999; Oldfield et al. 1994).

9.5.2 Anatomical MRI

T1-weighted images are anatomically accurate and clearly identify fluid within a syrinx cavity and CSF pathways (Fig. 9.3a). Measurements of the width of the CSF channels are more accurate using T1-weighted, as compared with T2-weighted, imaging (Fig. 9.3b). Although uncommon, communications between the fourth ventricle and syrinx and between the subarachnoid space and syrinx may be detected with T1-weighted imaging (Beuls et al. 1996; Bogdanov et al. 2000, 2006). Postoperative T1-weighted MRI can also reveal the location of a shunt tip within a syrinx (Schwartz et al. 1999a).

The presence of an intramedullary tumour associated with a syrinx is detected by giving intravenous gadolinium contrast, which escapes

---

[2] The gyromagnetic ratio is equal to the precession frequency (measured in increments of 1,000 cycles/second, abbreviated as "MHz") divided by the magnetic field strength (Tesla, abbreviated as "T"). The gyromagnetic ratio for the proton of a hydrogen atom is 42.58 MHz/T, so in a 1 T MRI magnet, the precession (Larmor) frequency is 42.58 MHz; in a 3 T MRI magnet, the precession (Larmor) frequency is three times that or 127.74 MHz.

Table 9.1 Abnormal accumulations of water in CNS tissues

Increased pressure within a CSF space: e.g. transependymal movement of CSF from the lateral ventricles to the brain, caused by hydrocephalus

Opening of the blood-brain barrier or blood-spinal cord barrier: caused by an intra-axial brain tumor or intramedullary spinal tumor (vasogenic oedema)

Increased venous pressure: caused by an arteriovenous fistula or malformation

Cytotoxic oedema: fluid can accumulate within the intracellular space of the CNS when ischemia results in swelling of neural cells

from permeable tumour capillaries and produces high signal within the lesion.

T2-weighted imaging is more sensitive to the presence of excessive fluid within CNS tissues than is T1-weighted imaging. Fluid can form and expand both the extracellular and the intracellular spaces of the CNS (Table 9.1). T2-weighted imaging may detect, in particular, a "pre-syringomyelia" state, which is spinal cord oedema from a chronic condition. If left untreated, this may eventually result in syrinx formation (Fischbein et al. 1999; Jinkins et al. 1998; Levy et al. 2000).

Fast imaging employing steady state acquisition (FIESTA)[3] MRI produces high contrast between CSF and structures contained within the subarachnoid space, such as nerve roots. It uses short acquisition times to reduce motion artefacts (Chavez et al. 2005). It is particularly useful in studying syringomyelia, outlining arachnoid webs and cysts lying within the subarachnoid space.

Diffusion-weighted MRI (DWI) identifies diffusion of water molecules, which is less restricted within the extracellular than the intracellular space. This technique and its related sequences, diffusion tensor imaging (DTI) and fractional anisotropy (FA), have been used primarily as research tools in syringomyelia, to evaluate the integrity of white matter tracts (Roser et al. 2010a; Ries et al. 2000) and to identify injury in the spinal cord earlier than is possible with T1-weighted and T2-weighted images (Schwartz et al. 1999b). DWI of the spinal cord has lower resolution than brain DWI because of the smaller

size of the spinal cord and the artefacts created by CSF flow and cardiac and respiratory motion around the spinal cord (Clark et al. 2000). In a patient with multiple sclerosis, a large cervical syrinx and a stable neurological deficit, DTI confirmed preservation of the white matter tracts around the syrinx (Agosta et al. 2004). In a study comparing 28 patients, with cervical syringomyelia and sensory dysfunction, to 19 normal volunteers, the patients had lower fractional anisotropy, which correlated with loss of pain and temperature sensation in their hands and prolongation of their spinothalamic conduction time on electrophysiological studies (Hatem et al. 2009).

Other MRI studies are mostly of research interest. These include volume imaging, using extremely thin (1 mm thickness) MRI slices, to improve anatomical detail and appreciation of communications between the fourth ventricle and syrinx and between the subarachnoid space and syrinx.

9.5.3 MRI Flow Studies

Phase-contrast cine MRI measures CSF motion that arises from the brain pulsations that occur during the cardiac cycle (Fig. 9.5). Brain expansion during cardiac systole results in CSF being driven caudally, from the intracranial subarachnoid cisterns into the more compliant spinal subarachnoid compartment. Relaxation of the brain then results in the cephalad movement of CSF, back across the foramen magnum, during diastole. Syrinx fluid also moves during the cardiac cycle, in response to spinal CSF pressure waves and spinal cord motion.

Cine imaging can measure both CSF and syrinx fluid velocities in a defined region of interest. In patients with hindbrain-related syringomyelia, preoperative cine phase-contrast MRI demonstrates a reduction in CSF flow at the level of foramen magnum, in both Chiari 0 and Chiari I malformations. This improves after posterior fossa decompressive procedures (Iskandar et al. 1998) (Fig. 9.5). Progressive neurological symptoms are more likely when cine MRI demonstrates movement of syrinx fluid. Stable or absent symptoms are associated with lack of fluid flow within the syrinx (Tobimatsu et al.

---

[3] An equivalent sequence is constructive interference steady state – CISS.

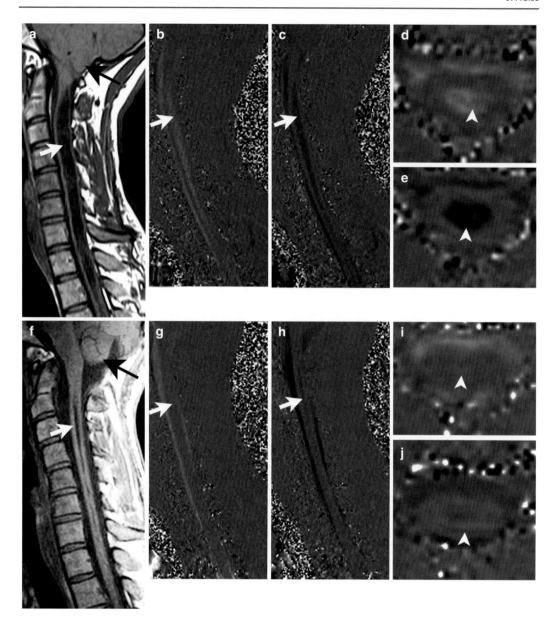

Fig. 9.5 Phase-contrast cine MRI. A 29-year-old woman with weakness, sensory loss and pain in both upper extremities. Before surgery, T1-weighted midsagittal MRI (**a**) shows the cerebellar tonsils (*black arrow*) to be located 11 mm below the foramen magnum, and a distended syrinx (*white arrow*) is present. Phase-contrast cine MRI in the midsagittal plane demonstrates flow in the syrinx (*white arrow*) in systole (**b**) and diastole (**c**).

Phase-contrast cine MRI in the axial plane confirms syrinx fluid motion (**d**, **e**, *arrowheads*). Three months after surgery, the cerebellar tonsils have ascended several millimetres (**f**, *black arrow*), and the syrinx has become much smaller (**f**, *white arrow*). Syrinx fluid velocity is decreased compared to before surgery (*white arrow*, **g**, **h**; *arrowheads*, **i**, **j**)

1991) (Fig. 9.3). Cine imaging can also be helpful in diagnosing spinal CSF flow obstructions in patients with primary spinal syringomyelia (Mauer et al. 2008) (Fig. 9.4).

9.6 MRI Protocols to Investigate Chiari and Syringomyelia

Radiographic evaluation of syringomyelia should include T1-weighted and T2-weighted MRI studies of the brain and entire spine, performed with and without contrast. Brain MRI will detect the presence of unsuspected hydrocephalus, which may contribute to the pathogenesis of some cases of syringomyelia (Krayenbuhl and Benini 1971), a posterior fossa mass producing tonsillar herniation, Chiari I malformation (Fig. 9.5) and basilar invagination. Lumbar spine MRI evaluates for cord tethering by the filum terminale, although the conus medullaris is usually in normal position in patients with Chiari I malformation (Milhorat et al. 2009; Royo-Salvador 1997). Tethering of the cervical or thoracic spinal cord has been associated with syringomyelia (Kitahara et al. 1995), and untethering of the spinal cord has been reported to result in syrinx resolution in these patients (Cusick and Bernardi 1995; Erkan et al. 1999; Levy 1999; Milhorat et al. 2009; Ragnarsson et al. 1986; Royo-Salvador 1997; Takahashi et al. 1999).

On T1-weighted and T2-weighted MRI, syringomyelia appears as a well-circumscribed intramedullary fluid-filled mass. In cases in which the cerebellar tonsils are in a normal position and the syrinx is located within the cervical or cervico-thoracic spinal cord, as in Chiari 0 malformation (Fig. 9.6) (Iskandar et al. 1998), FIESTA images should be obtained and examined closely for evidence of membranes occluding the foramen of Magendie or the subarachnoid space at the foramen magnum. Anatomical images should also be evaluated for narrowing of CSF pathways at the foramen magnum and reduced posterior fossa volume (Bogdanov et al. 2004). Phase-contrast cine MRI of the cervical spine in the sagittal plane may be performed, to confirm any narrowing of CSF pathways at the foramen magnum seen on anatomical MRI studies. Axial plane images are able

to measure CSF flow as well as velocity but have little clinical value because the length of their view of the subarachnoid space is restricted to the thickness of the axial sections.

On T1-weighted MRI, following intravenous administration of gadolinium contrast medium, enhancement within the spinal cord indicates the presence of an associated intramedullary tumour.

Certain findings on the spinal MRI predict more rapid neurological progression in patients with syringomyelia, particularly distension of the spinal cord by a syrinx of large diameter (over 5 mm) and the presence of associated spinal cord oedema (Levy 2000). On the other hand, a narrow syrinx that does not distend the spinal cord may no longer be associated with an active pathophysiological process and is less likely to cause neurological progression. Some patients, with long-standing symptoms of syringomyelia, will have a small-diameter syrinx and an atrophic spinal cord. In such cases, a previously distended syrinx has probably collapsed after a Chiari I malformation has spontaneously disimpacted at the foramen magnum or the syrinx has created a fistula to the spinal subarachnoid space (Santoro et al. 1993; Williams 1994). Prominence of the central canal of the spinal cord that does not distend the spinal cord is a normal anatomical variant, does not produce neurological deficit and does not require treatment (Holly and Batzdorf 2002).

In primary spinal syringomyelia of unknown aetiology, axial imaging of the spine using T2-weighted and FIESTA sequences may reveal previously undetected arachnoid cysts and arachnoid adhesions. If not, myelography and CT myelography may be required for diagnosis (Batzdorf 2005) (Fig. 9.4). Prior to injection of contrast medium, the intrathecal pressure should be measured and CSF obtained and sent to the clinical laboratory for analysis, including cell count and differential, protein, glucose, culture and sensitivity, cytology and a demyelination profile (Ravaglia et al. 2007; Waziri et al. 2007). These tests evaluate for inflammatory disease of the meninges (chronic meningitis) or spinal cord (inflammatory myelitis), which may themselves result in the development of syringomyelia. Pseudotumour cerebri (idiopathic or "benign"

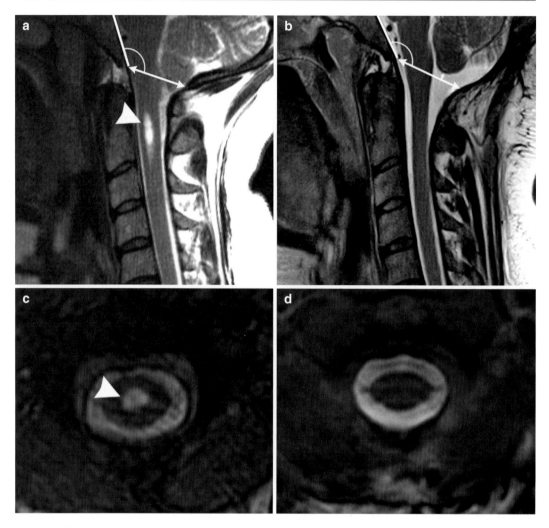

Fig. 9.6 Chiari 0 malformation causing headache. T2-weighted magnetic resonance imaging in a 35-year-old woman with occipital headache. Note Chiari 0 malformation with 3.0 mm of tonsillar ectopia before surgery (**a**). The CSF pathways at the foramen magnum are obliterated. Tonsillar ectopia resolved on MRI performed 1 year after craniocervical decompression and duraplasty (**b**), ascending 4 mm above its preoperative position. An associated small syrinx located in the C2 segment before surgery (*arrowhead*, **a**, **c**) resolved after surgery (**d**)

intracranial hypertension) could also be demonstrated, by the finding of elevated CSF pressure (Bret et al. 1986; Sullivan et al. 1988). A physiological block in CSF pressure transmission at the foramen magnum, or within the spinal canal, can be shown by Queckenstedt's jugular vein compression test (Heiss et al. 1999, 2012; Tachibana et al. 1992).

In rare cases, syringomyelia may not be associated with an imaging abnormality, and its cause is truly idiopathic (Lee et al. 2002; Nakamura et al. 2009). It has been reported that idiopathic

syringomyelia, with a small diameter that extends fewer than 3 vertebral levels, appears to have a good prognosis, with little chance of clinical or MRI progression if managed conservatively. In idiopathic syringomyelia without neurological deficit, MRI scans may be repeated in 1 year to verify that the syrinx size has not increased over time (Fig. 9.3). Idiopathic syringomyelia with a larger diameter and which extends beyond 4 vertebral levels generally will be accompanied by neurological progression and might be better treated surgically (Nakamura et al. 2009; Roser et al. 2010b). In such cases, intraoperative ultrasonographic imaging is performed (see below) after bone removal and exposure of the dura over the syrinx, to assess for previously undetected subarachnoid adhesions. If present, lysis of adhesions and duraplasty is performed (Fig. 9.4). If adhesions are not present, a syringo-subarachnoid shunt is inserted, with subsequent laboratory analysis of syrinx fluid, including cell count and differential, protein, glucose, culture and sensitivity and cytology.

To evaluate the radiographic outcome of previous surgical procedures for syringomyelia, MRI scanning can be repeated at 3–12 months after the surgical procedure. A prospective study of 29 patients with syringomyelia and Chiari type 1 malformation showed that, after successful craniocervical decompression surgery for Chiari I and syringomyelia, the cerebellar tonsils lose their conical shape, the CSF pathways expand at the foramen magnum, the syrinx becomes shorter and the cavity decreases to less than half of its pre-surgical diameter, in 86 % of patients by 6 months and in all patients by 2 years after surgery (Wetjen et al. 2008) (Figs. 9.1, 9.5 and 9.6). In another prospective study of 44 patients with Chiari I malformation, syringomyelia and scoliosis, 17 patients had complete syrinx resolution by 6 months after surgery; reduction in syrinx diameter and extent continued throughout the follow-up period of 6 years (Wu et al. 2011).

Patients with progressive weakness and/or sensory loss and persistent syrinx distension despite surgery should undergo targeted anatomical MRI, cine MRI and, if appropriate, myelography and CT myelography, to evaluate for a block in the CSF pathways that persisted or recurred after surgery. Failure of posterior fossa decompressive procedures to resolve syringomyelia associated with the Chiari I malformation has been reported to vary between 10 and 40 % (Matsumoto and Symon 1989). A prospective study examining the pathophysiology of persisting syringomyelia was performed in 16 patients whose syringomyelia did not resolve after craniocervical decompression (Heiss et al. 2010). Before re-exploration was undertaken, causes such as prominent retroflexion of the dens, basi-

lar invagination and hypermobility of the craniocervical junction were excluded (Aronson et al. 1991; Fenoy et al. 2008). Patients with persistent syringomyelia had significantly reduced width of the ventral and dorsal subarachnoid spaces at the level of foramen magnum, active pulsation of the cerebellar tonsils, mean tonsillar herniation of 12 mm, abnormally high CSF velocity across the foramen magnum, markedly reduced CSF flow across the dorsal subarachnoid space at the craniovertebral junction and reduced CSF compliance. Successful re-exploration surgery occurred in almost all patients, with significantly improved pressure transmission across the foramen magnum, reduced syrinx size and halted neurological progression. These findings support the use of anatomical MRI studies to measure the CSF pathway size at the foramen magnum in patients, whose syringes do not resolve after craniocervical decompression.

Imaging after a surgical procedure for primary spinal syringomyelia should establish if the procedure has opened the CSF pathways, reduced deformity and reduced the length and diameter of the syrinx (Byun et al. 2010; Holly et al. 2000). After successful laminectomy and duraplasty for primary spinal syringomyelia, the subarachnoid space expands dorsal to the spinal cord, and the syrinx diameter decreases dramatically (Batzdorf 2005; Heiss et al. 2012). If subarachnoid scarring extends over more than 3 spinal levels, opening of the subarachnoid space may be impossible. In these cases, shunting of syrinx fluid to the pleural or peritoneal space may be performed, and its effectiveness in reducing syrinx size can be assessed by anatomical MRI after surgery (Heiss et al. 2012; Hida et al. 1994).

9.7 Ultrasonography

Ultrasound uses a probe to deliver high-frequency pulses of sound waves into tissue and to receive sound waves that reflect off various anatomical structures. The ultrasound machine creates 2-dimensional images, based on the distance between the probe and underlying structures and the variable properties of these tissues to reflect and transmit sound waves. Ultrasonography clearly delineates interfaces between solid tissue and fluid, such as between the spinal cord and a syrinx cavity or between the cerebellar tonsils and the surrounding CSF (Wilberger et al. 1987).

Ultrasonography has been employed in an intraoperative setting in Chiari I malformation-associated syringomyelia, to monitor the pulsation of the cerebellar tonsils, brainstem and syrinx cavity. It has also been used in primary spinal syringomyelia, to identify the syrinx cavity and any associated subarachnoid septa or cysts that require dissection (Heiss et al. 1999, 2012; Oldfield et al. 1994) (Fig. 9.4e, j, k). Intraoperative ultrasonography provides real-time imaging that can be completed in a few minutes. It may also demonstrate several discrete syrinx cavities even though a single cavity was seen on preoperative MRI (Fig. 9.4). It can guide placement of a shunt within a syrinx and can evaluate for decompression of a syrinx after shunt placement (O'Toole et al. 2007). Some neurosurgeons advocate the use of intraoperative ultrasonography to measure the CSF space dorsal to the tonsils, after performing a suboccipital craniectomy. They use this to guide their decision to either (1) leave the dura alone, (2) excise or score the outer layer of dura or (3) open the dura and perform a duraplasty (Isu et al. 1993; Navarro et al. 2004; Yeh et al. 2006). Some investigators use colour Doppler ultrasonography before opening the dura, to decide if intra-arachnoidal dissection is necessary and, again after duraplasty, to assess if intradural intervention has resulted in increased CSF flow across the foramen magnum during the cardiac and respiratory cycles (Milhorat and Bolognese 2003). The use of 3D ultrasound has been reported to have some advantages over 2D ultrasound, including better registration of intraoperative ultrasonic images with MRI performed before surgery (Bonsanto et al. 2005).

9.8   Neurophysiological Studies

Somatosensory, motor and brainstem evoked potentials evaluate for abnormalities in the speed and amplitude of neural conduction through the somatosensory, motor and auditory pathways. These studies are not routinely used in evaluation of syringomyelia but may be useful in some circumstances, particularly as an aid to differential diagnosis. Detection of neurophysiological abnormalities may explain clinical symptoms of numbness and weakness that do not correspond with the size or location of the syrinx (Emery et al. 1998).

Median nerve sensory evoked potentials (SEP) are a sensitive indicator of cord pathology and can be used to screen for abnormal function of the somatosensory pathway in atypical cases of syringomyelia (Wagner et al. 1995). Upper limb somatosensory evoked potentials are frequently abnormal in patients with Chiari I malformation and syringomyelia, as is central somatosensory conduction time,[4] latency and amplitude (Anderson et al. 1986). Prolonged central motor conduction time measured after magnetic stimulation of the motor cortex has also been reported in post-traumatic syringomyelia prior to surgery. Central motor conduction time became much shorter after effective syringopleural shunting, which reduced the syrinx diameter (Robinson and Little 1990). Conditions affecting the peripheral nervous system, such as peripheral neuropathy and cervical radiculopathy, do not affect central conduction time (Anderson et al. 1986).

Posterior tibial somatosensory evoked potentials, motor evoked potentials and trigeminal sensory evoked potentials can also identify subclinical neurophysiological dysfunction in syringomyelia (Hort-Legrand and Emery 1999). Trigeminal sensory evoked potentials, for example, are frequently abnormal in patients with high cervical syringomyelia (Emery et al. 1998). Motor evoked potential abnormalities have been found in syringomyelia patients even in the absence of motor symptoms. Pain sensory evoked potentials (pain SEPs) using carbon dioxide laser stimulation of the skin and electrical SEPs have been used to quantify dissociative sensory loss in syringomyelia (Kakigi et al. 1991). The pain SEPs provided an objective mea-

---

[4] Central conduction time measures the time required for electrical signals to be transmitted through that segment of the somatosensory or motor pathway which lies with the central nervous system.

surement that correlated well with clinical findings and allowed evaluation of individual spinal cord segments. Pain SEPs improved after surgery that relieved compression (Kakigi et al. 1991), with improvement in SEPs usually preceding clinical improvement. Posterior tibial SSEP has been used along with neurological examination in surveillance of patients with stable syringomyelia (Morioka et al. 1992).

An improvement in brainstem auditory evoked potentials in Chiari I malformation in an intraoperative setting, after bone removal but before opening the dura, has been reported (Anderson et al. 2003; Zamel et al. 2009). Intraoperative SSEP has been used to monitor for dysfunction and possible harm to the dorsal columns during surgery (Wagner et al. 1995).

Conclusion

Anatomical MRI is a noninvasive method of diagnosing syringomyelia and discovering associated conditions, at the foramen magnum or within the spine, that create the milieu for syrinx formation. Progressive neurological dysfunction is most frequently seen with cavities of sufficient size to distend the spinal cord, whereas a normal neurological exam is expected with syringes of smaller diameter that do not distend the spinal cord (Bogdanov and Mendelevich 2002). Anatomical MRI scans can be used to follow syrinx size over time, both in patients with smaller-diameter syringes and normal neurological examinations and in patients who have undergone surgical treatment. Other imaging studies such as phase-contrast cine MRI, plain spinal films, myelography and CT myelography can be used to evaluate symptomatic patients if anatomical MRI is unable to detect an associated craniocervical or spinal lesion. Intraoperative ultrasonography provides real-time imaging of the subarachnoid space and can identify obstructive lesions, before opening the dura. Some neurosurgeons use the findings of intraoperative ultrasonography to tailor their surgical procedures for Chiari I malformation and syringomyelia. Evoked potentials may be used to provide an objective measure of dysfunction of the spinal cord and brainstem and to monitor electrophysiological changes that occur during surgery.

References

Agosta F, Rovaris M, Benedetti B et al (2004) Diffusion tensor MRI of the cervical cord in a patient with syringomyelia and multiple sclerosis. J Neurol Neurosurg Psychiatry 75:1647

Anderson NE, Frith RW, Synek VM (1986) Somatosensory evoked potentials in syringomyelia. J Neurol Neurosurg Psychiatry 49:1407–1410

Anderson RC, Emerson RG, Dowling KC et al (2003) Improvement in brainstem auditory evoked potentials after suboccipital decompression in patients with chiari I malformations. J Neurosurg 98:459–464

Aronson DD, Kahn RH, Canady A et al (1991) Instability of the cervical spine after decompression in patients who have Arnold-Chiari malformation. J Bone Joint Surg Am 73:898–906

Barkovich AJ, Wippold FJ, Sherman JL et al (1986) Significance of cerebellar tonsillar position on MR. AJNR Am J Neuroradiol 7:795–799

Batzdorf U (2005) Primary spinal syringomyelia. Invited submission from the joint section meeting on disorders of the spine and peripheral nerves, March 2005. J Neurosurg Spine 3:429–435

Beuls EA, Vandersteen MA, Vanormelingen LM et al (1996) Deformation of the cervicomedullary junction and spinal cord in a surgically treated adult Chiari I hindbrain hernia associated with syringomyelia: a magnetic resonance microscopic and neuropathological study. Case report. J Neurosurg 85:701–708

Bogdanov EI, Mendelevich EG (2002) Syrinx size and duration of symptoms predict the pace of progressive myelopathy: retrospective analysis of 103 unoperated cases with craniocervical junction malformations and syringomyelia. Clin Neurol Neurosurg 104:90–97

Bogdanov EI, Ibatullin MM, Mendelevich EG (2000) Spontaneous drainage in syringomyelia: magnetic resonance imaging findings. Neuroradiology 42: 676–678

Bogdanov EI, Heiss JD, Mendelevich EG et al (2004) Clinical and neuroimaging features of "idiopathic" syringomyelia. Neurology 62:791–794

Bogdanov EI, Heiss JD, Mendelevich EG (2006) The post-syrinx syndrome: stable central myelopathy and collapsed or absent syrinx. J Neurol 253:707–713

Bonsanto MM, Metzner R, Aschoff A et al (2005) 3D ultrasound navigation in syrinx surgery – a feasibility study. Acta Neurochir (Wien) 147:533–540; discussion 540–541

Bret P, Huppert J, Massini B et al (1986) Lumbo-peritoneal shunt in non-hydrocephalic patients. A review of 41 cases. Acta Neurochir (Wien) 80:90–92

Byun MS, Shin JJ, Hwang YS et al (2010) Decompressive surgery in a patient with posttraumatic syringomyelia. J Korean Neurosurg Soc 47:228–231

Chavez GD, De Salles AA, Solberg TD et al (2005) Three-dimensional fast imaging employing steady-state acquisition magnetic resonance imaging for stereotactic radiosurgery of trigeminal neuralgia. Neurosurgery 56:E628

Clark CA, Werring DJ, Miller DH (2000) Diffusion imaging of the spinal cord in vivo: estimation of the principal diffusivities and application to multiple sclerosis. Magn Reson Med 43:133–138

Cusick JF, Bernardi R (1995) Syringomyelia after removal of benign spinal extramedullary neoplasms. Spine (Phila Pa 1976) 20:1289–1293; discussion 1293–1294

Elster AD, Chen MY (1992) Chiari I malformations: clinical and radiologic reappraisal. Radiology 183:347–353

Emery E, Hort-Legrand C, Hurth M et al (1998) Correlations between clinical deficits, motor and sensory evoked potentials and radiologic aspects of MRI in malformative syringomyelia. 27 Cases. Neurophysiol Clin 28:56–72

Enzmann DR, Pelc NJ (1991) Normal flow patterns of intracranial and spinal cerebrospinal fluid defined with phase-contrast cine MR imaging. Radiology 178:467–474

Erkan K, Unal F, Kiris T (1999) Terminal syringomyelia in association with the tethered cord syndrome. Neurosurgery 45:1351–1359; discussion 1359–1360

Fenoy AJ, Menezes AH, Fenoy KA (2008) Craniocervical junction fusions in patients with hindbrain herniation and syringohydromyelia. J Neurosurg Spine 9:1–9

Fischbein NJ, Dillon WP, Cobbs C et al (1999) The "pre-syrinx" state: a reversible myelopathic condition that may precede syringomyelia. AJNR Am J Neuroradiol 20:7–20

Grigorian IuA, Lisianskii EI (1988) X-ray diagnosis of syringomyelia. Zh Vopr Neirokhir Im N N Burdenko 1:31–3

Hashemi RH, Bradley WGJ, Lisanti CJ (2010) MRI: the basics, 3rd edn. Lippincott Williams & Wilkins, Philadelphia

Hatem SM, Attal N, Ducreux D et al (2009) Assessment of spinal somatosensory systems with diffusion tensor imaging in syringomyelia. J Neurol Neurosurg Psychiatry 80:1350–1356

Heiss JD, Patronas N, DeVroom HL et al (1999) Elucidating the pathophysiology of syringomyelia. J Neurosurg 91:553–562

Heiss JD, Suffredini G, Smith R et al (2010) Pathophysiology of persistent syringomyelia after decompressive craniocervical surgery. Clinical article. J Neurosurg Spine 13:729–742

Heiss JD, Snyder K, Peterson MM et al (2012) Pathophysiology of primary spinal syringomyelia. J Neurosurg Spine 17(5):367–380. doi:10.3171/2012.8.SPINE11105

Hida K, Iwasaki Y, Imamura H et al (1994) Posttraumatic syringomyelia: its characteristic magnetic resonance imaging findings and surgical management. Neurosurgery 35:886–891; discussion 891

Holly LT, Batzdorf U (2002) Slitlike syrinx cavities: a persistent central canal. J Neurosurg 97:161–165

Holly LT, Johnson JP, Masciopinto JE et al (2000) Treatment of posttraumatic syringomyelia with extradural decompressive surgery. Neurosurg Focus 8:E8

Hort-Legrand C, Emery E (1999) Evoked motor and sensory potentials in syringomyelia. Neurochirurgie 45(Suppl 1):95–104

Iskandar BJ, Hedlund GL, Grabb PA et al (1998) The resolution of syringohydromyelia without hindbrain herniation after posterior fossa decompression. J Neurosurg 89:212–216

Isu T, Sasaki H, Takamura H et al (1993) Foramen magnum decompression with removal of the outer layer of the dura as treatment for syringomyelia occurring with Chiari I malformation. Neurosurgery 33:844–849; discussion 849–850

Jinkins JR, Reddy S, Leite CC et al (1998) MR of parenchymal spinal cord signal change as a sign of active advancement in clinically progressive posttraumatic syringomyelia. AJNR Am J Neuroradiol 19:177–182

Kakigi R, Shibasaki H, Kuroda Y et al (1991) Pain-related somatosensory evoked potentials in syringomyelia. Brain 114(Pt 4):1871–1889

Kitahara Y, Iida H, Tachibana S (1995) Effect of spinal cord stretching due to head flexion on intramedullary pressure. Neurol Med Chir (Tokyo) 35:285–288

Krayenbuhl H, Benini A (1971) A new surgical approach in the treatment of hydromyelia and syringomyelia. The embryological basis and the first results. J R Coll Surg Edinb 16:147–161

Lee JH, Chung CK, Kim HJ (2002) Decompression of the spinal subarachnoid space as a solution for syringomyelia without Chiari malformation. Spinal Cord 40:501–506

Levy LM (1999) MR imaging of cerebrospinal fluid flow and spinal cord motion in neurologic disorders of the spine. Magn Reson Imaging Clin N Am 7:573–587

Levy LM (2000) Toward an understanding of syringomyelia: MR imaging of CSF flow and neuraxis motion. AJNR Am J Neuroradiol 21:45–46

Levy EI, Heiss JD, Kent MS et al (2000) Spinal cord swelling preceding syrinx development. Case report. J Neurosurg 92:93–97

Mallucci CL, Stacey RJ, Miles JB et al (1997) Idiopathic syringomyelia and the importance of occult arachnoid webs, pouches and cysts. Br J Neurosurg 11:306–309

Matsumoto T, Symon L (1989) Surgical management of syringomyelia–current results. Surg Neurol 32:258–265

Mauer UM, Freude G, Danz B et al (2008) Cardiac-gated phase-contrast magnetic resonance imaging of cerebrospinal fluid flow in the diagnosis of idiopathic syringomyelia. Neurosurgery 63:1139–1144; discussion 1144

Mikulis DJ, Diaz O, Egglin TK et al (1992) Variance of the position of the cerebellar tonsils with age: preliminary report. Radiology 183:725–728

Milhorat TH, Bolognese PA (2003) Tailored operative technique for Chiari type I malformation using intraoperative color Doppler ultrasonography. Neurosurgery 53:899–905; discussion 905–906

Milhorat TH, Chou MW, Trinidad EM et al (1999) Chiari I malformation redefined: clinical and radiographic findings for 364 symptomatic patients. Neurosurgery 44:1005–1017

Milhorat TH, Bolognese PA, Nishikawa M et al (2009) Association of Chiari malformation type I and tethered cord syndrome: preliminary results of sectioning filum terminale. Surg Neurol 72:20–35

Morioka T, Kurita-Tashima S, Fujii K et al (1992) Somatosensory and spinal evoked potentials in patients with cervical syringomyelia. Neurosurgery 30:218–222

Nakamura M, Ishii K, Watanabe K et al (2009) Clinical significance and prognosis of idiopathic syringomyelia. J Spinal Disord Tech 22:372–375

Navarro R, Olavarria G, Seshadri R et al (2004) Surgical results of posterior fossa decompression for patients with Chiari I malformation. Childs Nerv Syst 20:349–356

O'Toole JE, Eichholz KM, Fessler RG (2007) Minimally invasive insertion of syringosubarachnoid shunt for posttraumatic syringomyelia: technical case report. Neurosurgery 61:E331–E332; discussion E332

Oldfield EH, Muraszko K, Shawker TH et al (1994) Pathophysiology of syringomyelia associated with Chiari I malformation of the cerebellar tonsils. Implications for diagnosis and treatment. J Neurosurg 80:3–15

Ragnarsson TS, Durward QJ, Nordgren RE (1986) Spinal cord tethering after traumatic paraplegia with late neurological deterioration. J Neurosurg 64:397–401

Ravaglia S, Bogdanov EI, Pichiecchio A et al (2007) Pathogenetic role of myelitis for syringomyelia. Clin Neurol Neurosurg 109:541–546

Ries M, Jones RA, Dousset V et al (2000) Diffusion tensor MRI of the spinal cord. Magn Reson Med 44:884–892

Robinson LR, Little JW (1990) Motor-evoked potentials reflect spinal cord function in post-traumatic syringomyelia. Am J Phys Med Rehabil 69:307–310

Roser F, Ebner FH, Maier G et al (2010a) Fractional anisotropy levels derived from diffusion tensor imaging in cervical syringomyelia. Neurosurgery 67:901–905

Roser F, Ebner FH, Sixt C et al (2010b) Defining the line between hydromyelia and syringomyelia. A differentiation is possible based on electrophysiological and magnetic resonance imaging studies. Acta Neurochir (Wien) 152:213–219; discussion 219

Rossier AB, Foo D, Shillito J et al (1985) Posttraumatic cervical syringomyelia. Incidence, clinical presentation, electrophysiological studies, syrinx protein and results of conservative and operative treatment. Brain 108(Pt 2):439–461

Royo-Salvador MB (1997) A new surgical treatment for syringomyelia, scoliosis, Arnold-Chiari malformation, kinking of the brainstem, odontoid recess, idiopathic basilar impression and platybasia. Rev Neurol 25:523–530

Santoro A, Delfini R, Innocenzi G et al (1993) Spontaneous drainage of syringomyelia. Report of two cases. J Neurosurg 79:132–134

Schwartz ED, Falcone SF, Quencer RM et al (1999a) Posttraumatic syringomyelia: pathogenesis, imaging, and treatment. AJR Am J Roentgenol 173:487–492

Schwartz ED, Yezierski RP, Pattany PM et al (1999b) Diffusion-weighted MR imaging in a rat model of syringomyelia after excitotoxic spinal cord injury. AJNR Am J Neuroradiol 20:1422–1428

Sullivan LP, Stears JC, Ringel SP (1988) Resolution of syringomyelia and Chiari I malformation by ventriculoatrial shunting in a patient with pseudotumor cerebri and a lumboperitoneal shunt. Neurosurgery 22:744–747

Tachibana S, Iida H, Yada K (1992) Significance of positive Queckenstedt test in patients with syringomyelia associated with Arnold-Chiari malformations. J Neurosurg 76:67–71

Takahashi Y, Tajima Y, Ueno S et al (1999) Syringobulbia caused by delayed postoperative tethering of the cervical spinal cord – delayed complication of foramen magnum decompression for Chiari malformation. Acta Neurochir (Wien) 141:969–972; discussion 972–973

Tobimatsu Y, Nihei R, Kimura T et al (1991) A quantitative analysis of cerebrospinal fluid flow in posttraumatic syringomyelia. Nihon Seikeigeka Gakkai Zasshi 65:505–516

Tubbs RS, Elton S, Grabb P et al (2001) Analysis of the posterior fossa in children with the Chiari 0 malformation. Neurosurgery 48:1050–1054; discussion 1054–1055

Vernooij MW, Ikram MA, Tanghe HL et al (2007) Incidental findings on brain MRI in the general population. N Engl J Med 357:1821–1828

Wagner W, Perneczky A, Maurer JC et al (1995) Intraoperative monitoring of median nerve somatosensory evoked potentials in cervical syringomyelia: analysis of 28 cases. Minim Invasive Neurosurg 38:27–31

Waziri A, Vonsattel JP, Kaiser MG et al (2007) Expansile, enhancing cervical cord lesion with an associated syrinx secondary to demyelination. Case report and review of the literature. J Neurosurg Spine 6:52–56

Wetjen NM, Heiss JD, Oldfield EH (2008) Time course of syringomyelia resolution following decompression of Chiari malformation Type I. J Neurosurg Pediatr 1:118–123

Wilberger JE Jr, Maroon JC, Prostko ER et al (1987) Magnetic resonance imaging and intraoperative neurosonography in syringomyelia. Neurosurgery 20:599–605

Williams B (1994) Spontaneous drainage in syringomyelia. J Neurosurg 80:949–950

Wu T, Zhu Z, Jiang J et al (2011) Syrinx resolution after posterior fossa decompression in patients with scoliosis secondary to Chiari malformation type I. Eur Spine J 21(6):1143–1150. doi:10.1007/s00586-011-2064-3

Yamada H, Kageyama N, Kato T et al (1981) The diagnosis of syringomyelia (author's transl). No Shinkei Geka 9:573–582

Yeh DD, Koch B, Crone KR (2006) Intraoperative ultrasonography used to determine the extent of surgery necessary during posterior fossa decompression in children with Chiari malformation type I. J Neurosurg 105:26–32

Zamel K, Galloway G, Kosnik EJ et al (2009) Intraoperative neurophysiologic monitoring in 80 patients with Chiari I malformation: role of duraplasty. J Clin Neurophysiol 26:70–75

Hindbrain-Related Syringomyelia

10

Jörg Klekamp

Contents

10.1 Anatomical Abnormalities

About one in every two patients with syringomyelia demonstrates pathology at the craniocervical junction. Any pathology in this region, which compromises the passage of cerebrospinal fluid (CSF), may lead to syringomyelia. The most common is the Chiari I malformation. Less common entities are basilar invagination, Chiari II malformation and foramen magnum arachnoiditis.

Hans Chiari described four varieties of malformations in his monograph (Chiari 1896). The most common is the type I, which is characterised by herniation of cerebellar tonsils into the spinal canal. In type II, the brainstem, the cerebellar tonsils and part of the vermis are displaced into the spinal canal. In type III, the features of type II are combined with an occipital meningoencephalocoele. Type IV is characterised by hypoplasia of the vermis. Chiari considered these abnormalities to be causally related to hydrocephalus. Modern imaging techniques and experimental studies, however, disclose a different aetiology.

10.1.1 Chiari I Malformation

It has been shown, in the majority of patients, that Chiari I malformation is a disorder related to a small posterior fossa volume, forcing the tonsils into the spinal canal (Stovner et al. 1993; Badie et al. 1995; Trigylidas et al. 2008; Nyland and Krogness 1978; Nishikawa et al. 1997; Boyles et al. 2006; Milhorat et al. 1999)

J. Klekamp
Department of Neurosurgery,
Christliches Krankenhaus Quakenbrück,
Quakenbrück, Germany
e-mail: j.klekamp@ckq-gmbh.de

G. Flint, C. Rusbridge (eds.), *Syringomyelia*,
DOI 10.1007/978-3-642-13706-8_10, © Springer-Verlag Berlin Heidelberg 2014

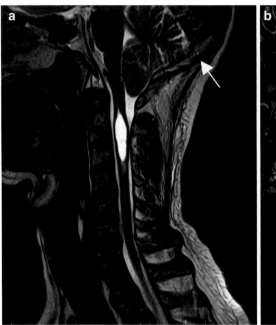
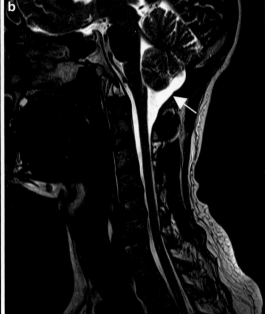

Fig. 10.1 (**a**) Preoperative T2-weighted MRI of a patient with Chiari I malformation. The image demonstrates a small posterior fossa, a slight caudal displacement of the tentorial insertion (*arrow*) and a syringomyelia at C2–C3. (**b**) The postoperative scan shows the decompression at the foramen magnum (*arrow*) with resolution of the syrinx

(Fig. 10.1). Marin-Padilla could demonstrate this effect in hamsters more than 30 years ago (Marin-Padilla and Marin-Padilla 1981). There may be a genetic disposition in some patients (Boyles et al. 2006; Milhorat et al. 1999; Tubbs et al. 2011). Not all Chiari I malformations are caused by a small posterior fossa, and they may develop after lumboperitoneal shunting (Payner et al. 1994; Chumas et al. 1993), birth trauma (Aghakhani et al. 1999; Hida et al. 1994; Williams 1977), arachnoid pathologies at the craniocervical junction (Aghakhani et al. 1999), posterior fossa arachnoid cysts (Galarza et al. 2010) or solid tumours in the posterior fossa (Klekamp et al. 1995).

Apart from a small posterior fossa volume, additional bony anomalies are common in Chiari I malformation and may involve the articulations at the craniocervical junction. Assimilations of the atlas to the occiput, basilar invaginations or Klippel-Feil syndromes may also be encountered (Kagawa et al. 2006; Tubbs et al. 2011; Smith et al. 2010). It is important to recognise that the compression of neural structures and CSF flow

obstruction are localised at the foramen magnum in all variants of Chiari I malformation although these may not be the only mechanisms responsible for the patients' symptoms. Instabilities of the craniocervical junction or upper cervical spine are important features to recognise in a significant proportion of Chiari I patients.

10.1.2 Basilar Invagination

Basilar invagination is defined as a protrusion of the odontoid peg into the foramen magnum (Fig. 10.2). A line between the posterior rim of the foramen and the hard palate constitutes Chamberlain's line. If the odontoid crosses this line for more than 2.5 mm, this is considered pathological. Basilar invagination may be associated with osteogenesis imperfecta, Hajdu-Cheney syndrome, Paget's disease (Menezes 2008b), Marfan's syndrome (Hobbs et al. 1997), Down's syndrome (Menezes 2008a) or rheumatoid arthritis (Krauss et al. 2010). The congenital form is caused by bony anomalies of the

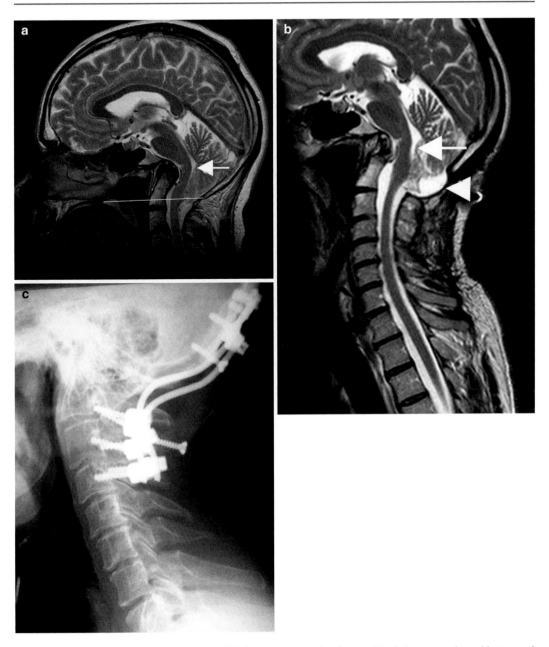

Fig. 10.2 (**a**) The preoperative T2-weighted MRI shows a Chiari I malformation associated with a profound basilar invagination and compression of the brainstem (*arrow*). The odontoid extends far above Chamberlain's line (*white horizontal line*). (**b**) The postoperative MRI demonstrates the result of a combined decompression with transoral resection of the dens (*arrow*) and posterior decompression (*arrowhead*) and fusion. (**c**) The postoperative lateral radiograph demonstrates the position of all implants and a good sagittal profile of the cervical spine

clivus, occipital bone, atlas and upper cervical vertebrae. The result of this altered anatomy is a gradual upward shifting of the upper cervical vertebrae towards the foramen magnum. The C1/2 intervertebral joints appear to play a major role for this effect as distraction of these joints may reverse the ventral compression by the odontoid peg (Jian et al. 2010; Goel 2004).

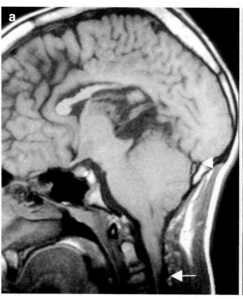
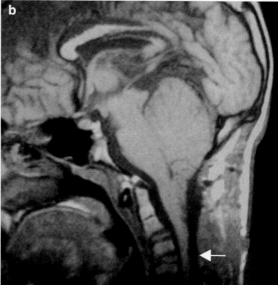

Fig. 10.3 (**a**) Preoperative T1-weighted MRI of a 14-year-old boy with a Chiari II malformation, demonstrating the enlarged foramen magnum with cerebellar tonsillar herniation to C3 (*arrow*). The tentorium inserts close to the posterior margin of the foramen magnum (*arrowhead*). (**b**) The postoperative image demonstrates the decompression of the upper cervical spine and discloses a kyphotic angulation at C3/4 (*arrow*)

10.1.3 Chiari II Malformation

In Chiari II malformation, the compression and cerebrospinal fluid flow obstruction occur in the upper spinal canal and not at the level of the foramen magnum. In contrast with Chiari I, the foramen magnum is enlarged in Chiari II, and the tonsils, the vermis and the brainstem are all herniated into the cervical canal (Fig. 10.3). Almost all patients with this malformation will also have a spinal myelomeningocoele. The pathophysiology of this malformation has been elegantly described by McLone and Knepper. Due to the spinal myelomeningocoele, CSF drains in utero into the amniotic fluid, resulting in a low intracranial pressure, which then inhibits the formation of a normally sized posterior fossa. The growth of the brain finally leads to herniation of cerebellar tonsils, vermis and brainstem into the spinal canal (McLone and Knepper 1989). As in the majority of Chiari I patients, the size of the skull forces the brain to grow towards the spinal canal in Chiari II. The major difference is the timing: in Chiari I, this effect takes place after birth, whereas in Chiari II the major pathological changes occur before birth with much graver consequences.

Support for this hypothesis comes from results of intrauterine operations on myelomeningoceles before the 26th week of gestation. If the spinal dysraphism could be closed successfully, then no Chiari II malformation developed (Danzer et al. 2011; Tulipan et al. 1999).

10.1.4 Foramen Magnum Arachnoiditis

Foramen magnum arachnoiditis is the only pathology at the craniocervical junction associated with syringomyelia without there being additional compression of brainstem or spinal cord (Fig. 10.4). Arachnoiditis at this level may be related to a previous episode of meningitis or trauma or other causes of haemorrhage (Klekamp et al. 2002; Appleby et al. 1969).

10.2   Neuroradiology

The diagnosis of Chiari I malformation should be straightforward these days, given the wide accessibility of magnetic resonance imaging

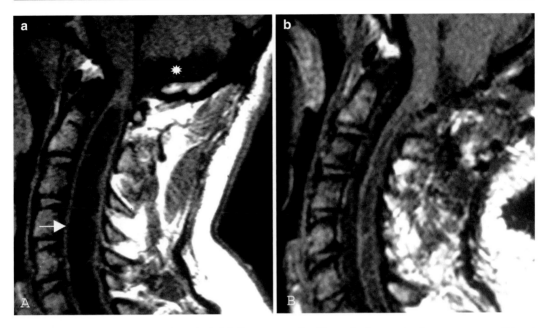

Fig. 10.4 (**a**) Preoperative T1-weighted MRI indicates foramen magnum arachnoiditis related to birth injury in a 29-year-old man with progressive tetraparesis. There is not a cerebellar tonsillar herniation, but there is an arachnoid pouch close to the foramen magnum (*) and a significant syrinx (*arrow*). (**b**) The postoperative MRI shows a collapse of the arachnoid pouch and the syrinx

(MRI) in western countries. To what extent tonsillar herniation may sometimes be seen as physiological and how neuroradiological criteria should be defined are, however, still a matter of controversy. A tonsillar herniation of more than 5 mm is widely considered pathological in adults (Aboulezz et al. 1985), but in young children, cerebellar growth causes a physiological herniation of the cerebellar tonsils. Conversely, in old age, atrophy of the brain may lead to tonsillar ascent (Mikulis et al. 1992). Tonsillar descent of less than 5 mm does not exclude the diagnosis of a Chiari I malformation (Milhorat et al. 1999), and in doubtful cases cardiac-gated cine MRI is very helpful to demonstrate a CSF flow obstruction and a clinically relevant herniation (Haughton et al. 2003; Panigrahi et al. 2004; Ellenbogen et al. 2000; Tubbs et al. 2007; Milhorat et al. 1999; Hofkes et al. 2007). Likewise neurophysiological examinations (Henriques Filho and Pratesi 2006) and neuro-otological evaluations (Kumar et al. 2002) have been proposed, as means of providing evidence of compression of the medulla oblongata or spinal cord.

In patients with Chiari I malformation, the radiological examination should include more than simply defining how far the tonsils are descended into the spinal canal. It is also important to consider the bony anatomy of the craniocervical junction. For example, is there evidence of anterior compression by the odontoid peg, i.e. basilar invagination (Fig. 10.2)? Is the atlas assimilated to the occiput? Are cervical segments fused, i.e. Klippel-Feil syndrome? If these anomalies are present, then instability of the craniocervical junction must be ruled out with flexion and extension studies, using either conventional radiography or CT imaging. The latter has the advantage of being able to visualise each of the different joints, in multiple planes and in both flexion and extension. In addition, sagittal and coronal reconstructions are particularly useful.

For all craniocervical pathologies, ventricular sizes should be evaluated. In Chiari I malformation, overt hydrocephalus is rare, but some degree of ventricular enlargement is not uncommon and was observed in 9 % of the author's series. With Chiari II malformation, on the other hand, hydrocephalus is almost ubiquitous.

In fact, it is uncommon for the neurosurgeon to encounter such a patient who has not already been managed with a ventricular shunt. If a Chiari II patient is evaluated because of new neurological symptoms, the first priority must be to assess the function of a previously implanted ventricular shunt. This requires a comparison of recent and old CT or MRI images, to look for changes of ventricular size that may indicate under- or over-drainage.

One important aspect for surgical planning in Chiari patients is the position of the tentorium, in relation to foramen magnum and the external occipital protuberance. Normally, the tentorium will insert at the level of this protuberance, and this indicates the position of the large intradural sinuses, such as the transverse sinus and the confluence of sinuses. In Chiari I patients, this tentorial insertion may be shifted by a centimetre or more towards the foramen magnum. When planning an occipital craniectomy, this must be taken into account and is even more important with regard to the dural incision. In Chiari II malformation, the foramen magnum is widened, and the tentorium usually inserts at the level of or very close to the foramen magnum (Fig. 10.3). For this reason, the suboccipital dura should not be incised in patients with a Chiari II malformation.

In patients with primary foramen magnum arachnoiditis, bony anomalies will not be apparent. The diagnosis is made by MRI and, in the absence of tonsillar herniation and brainstem or cervical cord compression, will require a cine MRI to demonstrate a CSF flow obstruction in the foramen magnum area. Such obstruction often involves the fourth ventricle exit foramina as well, and ventriculomegaly is common, being observed in half of the author's series of foramen magnum arachnoiditis. Another common feature of primary foramen magnum arachnoiditis is the formation of arachnoid cysts or pouches in the posterior fossa (Fig. 10.4).

Finally, the presence or absence of an associated syringomyelia or syringobulbia should be demonstrated as well as the entire extension of the cavity, to rule out additional abnormalities such as a tethered cord.

10.3 Clinical Presentation

With all craniocervical pathologies, clinical symptoms may evolve from different pathophysiological components. These may include hydrocephalus, compression of the brainstem and spinal cord, craniocervical instability, disturbances of brainstem or spinal cord blood flow, tethering mechanisms related to chronic arachnoiditis and CSF flow obstruction leading to syringomyelia. Clinical and radiological examinations therefore need to be analysed carefully, to identify the appropriate targets for treatment.

Considering all Chiari patients, it is interesting to note that the presentation is very much dependent on the age of the patient. In early childhood below age 2 years, signs of brainstem compression predominate, with apnoeic spells, cyanosis attacks and swallowing problems, whereas in later childhood scoliosis becomes the most common presenting sign. What are regarded as the more typical clinical features of a Chiari I malformation – occipital headaches, gait ataxia, sensory disturbances and motor weakness – are uncommon in children and are observed predominantly in adults (Rauzzino and Oakes 1995; Menezes et al. 2005) (Table 10.1). This age-related clinical profile can be explained by the postnatal growth of the cerebellum. At birth, most parts of the brain have reached about a third of their adult volume, but the cerebellum is the smallest part of the central nervous system, with just 15 % of its adult volume at this time; presumably, this serves to protect the brainstem during delivery. The adult volume of the cerebellum is reached late in the second year of life, indicating that the cerebellar volume increases by a factor of seven in that period (Klekamp et al. 1989). Therefore, if a Chiari malformation does become symptomatic before 2 years of age, dramatic presentations with respiratory problems are likely to be observed, something unknown in adult patients. Once the cerebellum is fully grown, the clinical course tends to be less dramatic and is characterised by slow progression.

As with every rule, however, there are exceptions. Minor traumas may cause acute symptoms in formerly asymptomatic patients with Chiari I

Table 10.1 Preoperative neurological symptoms (author's series)

Group	Occipital pain (%)	Neuropathic pain (%)	Hyperaesthesia (%)	Gait (%)	Motor power (%)	Sphincter function (%)	Swallowing difficulties (%)
Chiari I	79	50	71	62	40	16	20
Chiari II	25	19	64	100	67	92	22
FMA	74	39	83	78	83	48	15

The percentages given in this table represent the total number of patients presenting with a particular symptom

FMA foramen magnum arachnoiditis

malformation (Yarbrough et al. 2011; Murano and Rella 2006). In extremely rare cases, even sudden deaths have been reported (Wolf et al. 1998; Stephany et al. 2008; Agrawal 2008; Yoshikawa 2003). This raises questions as to whether asymptomatic children with Chiari I malformations should be allowed to participate in sport activities and whether prophylactic surgery for such patients is warranted. Chiari decompressions certainly cannot be considered to be no-risk procedures and are associated with a mortality of about 1 %. Given the fact that severe neurological deficits after minor trauma are extremely rare – no such instance was reported by a single patient in the author's series of more than 600 patients – it appears reasonable to leave decisions regarding timing of surgery and which sport activities can be pursued to the patients and their parents, without pressing them one way or the other.

In the author's series, patients with Chiari I presented with an average age of 43 ± 16 years, while those with Chiari II tended to be younger, at 17 ± 13 years. Compared to patients with a Chiari I malformation, patients with foramen magnum arachnoiditis presented at a similar age (37 ± 10 years) but with more severe neurological deficits (Table 10.1). Interestingly, this appeared not to hold for swallowing dysfunctions, which were more common with Chiari malformations, despite the significant scarring at the medulla oblongata level, which was present in all patients with foramen magnum arachnoiditis. The length of history was significantly longer for patients with arachnoiditis compared to Chiari patients (101 ± 96 months, compared to 71 ± 106 months for Chiari I and 26 ± 39 months for Chiari II).

10.4 Management

10.4.1 Chiari I Malformation

For all Chiari I patients, treatment of symptomatic hydrocephalus should be prioritised. Endoscopic third ventriculostomy is now preferred to traditional ventriculoperitoneal shunting as the first option for CSF diversion whenever patients present with clinical signs of raised intracranial pressure (Massimi et al. 2011).

Management options for arachnoid cysts include resection or fenestration (Fig. 10.5). Insertion of cyst shunts is not considered by the author due to their high failure rate. Treatment for Chiari I malformations due to solid masses requires tumour resection with foramen magnum duraplasty (Fig. 10.6).

For Chiari I hindbrain hernias, there is general agreement that surgical treatment should be reserved for symptomatic patients. In children, however, it may be unclear which complaints are linked to the malformation. It can also be a challenge to differentiate between physiological and pathological tonsillar descent, as revealed by MRI. In the absence of neurological symptoms or progressive scoliosis, the author does not recommend decompression for children with a Chiari I malformation, unless they demonstrate the typical occipital headache provoked by Valsalva-like manoeuvres, such as sneezing or coughing.

With all patients, it should be borne in mind that not every headache is due to tonsillar herniation, even when such an abnormality is present. Nor does the presence of syringomyelia constitute an indication for surgery in its own right, in children or adults alike. When neurological symptoms are present, however, surgery should

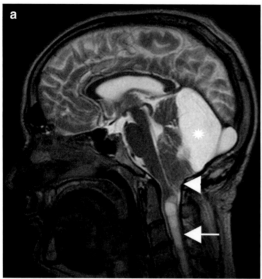
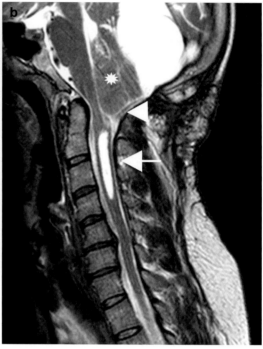

Fig. 10.5 (**a**) Preoperative T2-weighted MRI of a patient with syringomyelia (*arrow*) and a cerebellar tonsillar herniation (*arrowhead*) secondary to a large retrocerebellar arachnoid cyst (*). (**b**) The postoperative scan demonstrates a decrease in syrinx size (*arrow*) and a decompression at the foramen magnum (*arrowhead*). Despite large fenestration of the arachnoid cyst, the vermis has not changed its shape (*)

be recommended. As a general rule, progression of neurological symptoms occurs more rapidly than does enlargement of an underlying syrinx. The author has not observed enlargement of a syrinx in an asymptomatic patient with a Chiari I malformation.

Even though foramen magnum decompression is widely accepted as the treatment of choice for Chiari I malformation, there is no general agreement on how this operation should be performed (Schijman and Steinbok 2004; Haroun et al. 2000). Gardner's original operation consisted of a wide craniectomy of the posterior fossa and opening of the 4th ventricle in order to plug the obex with a piece of muscle. The dura was left open. He reported 5 mortalities after 74 such procedures (Gardner 1965). Similar mortality rates, as well as significant morbidity caused by manipulations at the obex (Williams 1978), led other surgeons to modify this operation. Guided by modern imaging techniques such as MRI in the 1980s and modern CT scanners, the anatomy of patients with Chiari I malformation

could be studied in much more detail than was previously possible. This led to less invasive procedures, such as leaving the arachnoid intact after dural opening (Logue and Edwards 1981), incising only the outer dural layer (Gambardella et al. 1998) or even restricting the operation to a purely bony decompression (James and Brant 2002). It should, of course, be the intention of every neurosurgeon to restrict any operation to its essential requirements in order to limit surgical morbidity, complications and discomfort for the patient but, at the same time, to do so without compromising the beneficial effects of the procedure.

The following account of a surgical technique describes the author's preferred method, as do subsequent accounts of operative techniques in this chapter. It should be noted, however, that there are many variations, and it is true to say that the only manoeuvre that all methods have in common is removal of bone from the occipital squama.

Surgery is performed in prone position. The decompression is limited to a foramen magnum decompression of 3–4 cm, together with removal

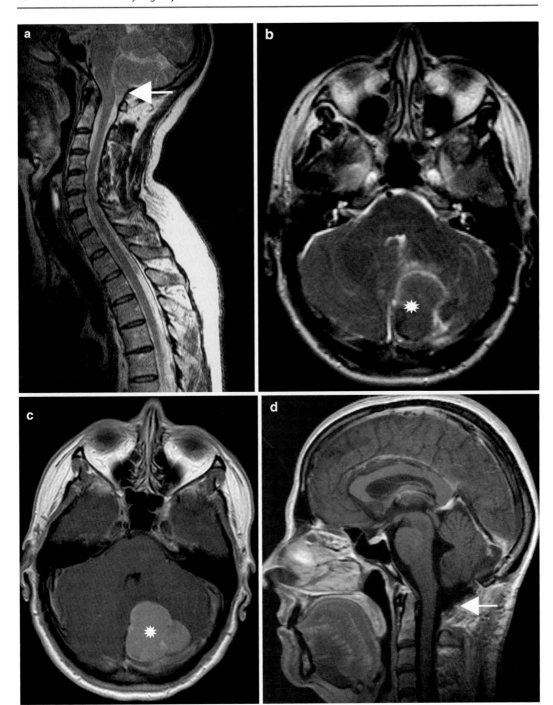

Fig. 10.6 (**a**) This preoperative T2-weighted MRI seems to demonstrate a typical Chiari I malformation (*arrow*). (**b**) The axial T2-weighted image indicates a lesion underneath the tentorium on the left side (*). (**c**) This turned out to be a large meningioma in T1 after contrast (*). (**d**) The postoperative T1-weighted scan with gadolinium shows a complete tumour removal and a decompressed foramen magnum (*arrow*)

of the posterior arch of the atlas. The atlanto-occipital membrane is coagulated and dissected off the dura, which is then incised in a Y-shape, under the microscope, and held open by sutures. Care should be taken to leave the arachnoid intact in order not to pull on and tear underlying bridging veins or small blood vessels supplying the spinal cord, brainstem or cerebellum. Leaving the arachnoid intact at this stage also avoids contamination of the subarachnoid cisterns with blood. Venous sinuses may be encountered upon opening the dura, in the midline or at the foramen magnum, and these will require suturing. The arachnoid should be examined for evidence of scar formation or adhesions to the cerebellum, brainstem or spinal cord. The arachnoid is then incised, starting below the cerebellar tonsils and continuing to an extent that allows these structures to be spread apart for inspection of the foramen of Magendie. For this purpose, the cerebellar tonsils are coagulated at their tips and medially. Resection of tonsils is advised against as this may risk injury to important blood vessels such as the posterior inferior cerebellar artery (PICA). If Magendie is patent and no arachnoid adhesions are detectable elsewhere, then no further intradural dissections need be performed. If the foramen is obstructed, then it should be opened by sharp dissection. In patients with severe arachnoid scarring, dissection will need to create at least a communication between the cranial and the spinal subarachnoid channels. In such instances, it may not always be possible to open Magendie without risking injury to important structures, such as the PICA. The dissection should not, in these circumstances, be carried out laterally, to avoid injury to perforating vessels of brainstem or spinal cord. A duraplasty is then inserted using alloplastic material. To avoid formation of adhesions between nervous tissue and the duraplasty or suture line, the graft is lifted off the cord by tenting sutures, which are fixed to muscle attachments laterally. Finally, the wound is closed, paying particular attention to the muscular layer in order to avoid CSF fistulas. Postoperatively, all patients should be supervised on the intensive care unit for at least 24 h before returning to the normal ward.

10.4.2 Basilar Invagination

In patients with additional basilar invagination, a combination of ventral and dorsal compression may be associated with instability of the craniocervical junction. These pathophysiological components may not, however, be relevant in all affected patients. Of a group of 53 patients with basilar invagination in the author's series, 35 were managed surgically. In 16 patients, there was neither a ventral compression by the odontoid nor craniocervical instability. These patients were managed with foramen magnum decompression for their Chiari malformation as the only procedure. In another 10 of the 35 patients, who demonstrated no clinical signs of ventral compression by the odontoid such as caudal cranial nerve deficits but either radiological evidence of craniocervical instability or assimilation of the atlas to the occiput, foramen magnum decompression was combined with craniocervical stabilisation. In the remaining 9 patients, ventral compression of the medulla oblongata had caused caudal cranial nerve dysfunctions. These patients underwent transoral resection of the odontoid, followed by posterior decompression and craniocervical fusion (Fig. 10.2) (Klekamp and Samii 2001).

Whenever the position of the odontoid leads to brainstem compression, the key elements of surgical treatment are distraction of the C1/2 intervertebral joints and C1/2 fusion. This distraction may reverse the ventral compression to a degree that no additional transoral resection of the odontoid is required. In the author's series, the decision for a transoral decompression was based on clinical signs of caudal cranial nerve deficits in the presence of compression of the medulla by the odontoid. Whether a transoral resection of the odontoid is obsolete (Goel and Shah 2009) or still required for patients with substantial and irreducible ventral compression (Smith et al. 2010) remains a controversial issue.

For craniocervical stabilisations, the implants need to be adjusted carefully to the abnormal anatomy. Precise planning is required to allow their safe fixation at the occipital bone as well as the allocation of the bone graft despite of the craniectomy required for foramen magnum decompression. All implants need to be covered completely by the muscular layer during closure, without too much strain being placed on soft tissues; otherwise, local discomfort or even CSF fistulas may result.

10.4.3 Chiari II Malformation

If clinical signs of hydrocephalus are present in Chiari II patients, treatment of the increased intracranial pressure has always the first priority. Endoscopic third ventriculostomy is again an optional alternative to ventriculoperitoneal shunts (Elgamal et al. 2011). In the literature, it has been stated in two large series that if the hydrocephalus has been managed successfully, then only a small minority of Chiari II patients require a decompression (Talamonti and Zella 2011; Rauzzino and Oakes 1995).

If one considers the pathophysiological considerations put forward by McLone (McLone and Knepper 1989) and the positive results obtained following intrauterine operations on foetuses (Danzer et al. 2011; Tulipan et al. 1999), Chiari II malformations are potentially preventable or reversible, if the decompression is carried out early enough in symptomatic patients with a sufficiently treated hydrocephalus. A number of studies have reported a benefit if decompression for Chiari II is performed as soon as neurological symptoms begin (Rauzzino and Oakes 1995; Teo et al. 1997; Pollack et al. 1992, 1996). Yet, there appears to be very little scientific evidence to support routine use of this approach for symptomatic infants (Tubbs and Oakes 2004). This may reflect the fact that, once severe brainstem dysfunctions are present, a decompression may not reverse established neurological deficits (Kirsch et al. 1968).

In the author's series, 42 patients presented with a Chiari II malformation. Surgical management was only recommended in 13 of these patients, when there was no evidence for ventricular shunt malfunction but a clear history of progressive brainstem or cervical cord dysfunction (Charney et al. 1987; Kirsch et al. 1968). Six were under 2 years of age, presenting with signs of central dysregulation. Three patients presented between 5 and 14 years of age (Fig. 10.3) and the remainder in adulthood, with progressive upper extremity dysfunction.

When operating for Chiari II malformation, the decompression must be undertaken at the spinal levels corresponding to the tonsillar descent, rather than at the foramen magnum, which is enlarged in this entity. Patients are operated in prone position. The exposure extends from the foramen magnum to the lowest lamina covering the herniated tonsils. After laminectomy of these segments, the atlanto-occipital membrane should be coagulated and dissected off the dura. The dural incision then starts at the level of the foramen magnum and extends over all levels involved. Then the arachnoid is opened. Dissection should be limited strictly to the midline in order to avoid injury to perforating vessels or caudal cranial nerves. It should be borne in mind that the brainstem is displaced caudally in these patients, taking with it important structures such as the PICA or caudal cranial nerves. As outlined for Chiari I operations, it is also desirable to open the foramen of Magendie in Chiari II patients, although this should be undertaken only if it can be performed safely. Coagulation of tonsils, which is a safe technique in Chiari I to gain access to Magendie, is not recommended in Chiari II as these are very often tightly adhered to the underlying brainstem and any such manoeuvre carries considerable risks. Arachnoid dissection should concentrate on creating a passage between the intracranial and spinal subarachnoid channels. Once that is achieved, a duraplasty should be inserted. As described for Chiari I surgery (above), the duraplasty is lifted off the cord by tenting sutures.

Laminectomies in this patient group carry a significant risk of producing postoperative kyphosis or swan-neck deformities (Lam et al. 2009) (Fig. 10.3). They should therefore be combined with posterior fusion, which can be achieved elegantly with lateral mass screws (Fig. 10.7).

10.4.4 Foramen Magnum Arachnoiditis

In the author's series, ventriculomegaly was more common in foramen magnum arachnoiditis compared to Chiari I malformations (52 % vs. 8.6 %). This implies that if a borderline tonsillar herniation is associated with ventricular dilatation, then arachnoiditis at the foramen magnum may well

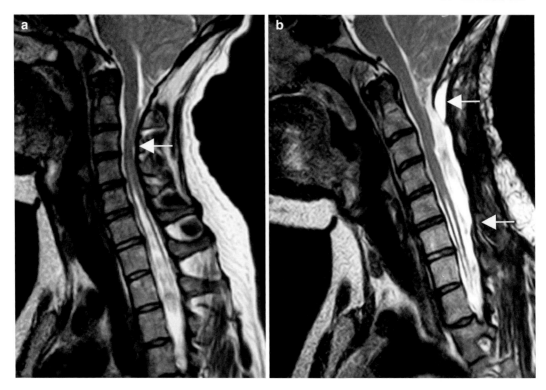

Fig. 10.7 (**a**) Preoperative T2-weighted MRI of an adult patient with Chiari II malformation presenting with progressive weakness of both hands. The image shows the tonsillar descent to C3 (*arrow*) with osteochondrosis and stenosis of the cervical spine at that level. (**b**) After bony decompression and duraplasty from C1 down to C5 (*arrows*), the enlarged subarachnoid space and decrease of the syrinx are apparent. To prevent a kyphotic deformity, a stabilisation was added with lateral mass screws. Postoperatively, she regained function in her hands

be present. Depending on the extent and severity of the arachnoiditis, surgical management may require CSF diversion, in addition to foramen magnum decompression.

When foramen magnum arachnoiditis is not diagnosed preoperatively, its presence, extent and severity must be determined after dural opening. Dural opening has to respect the arachnoid layer in such cases in order to avoid surgical morbidity related to vascular injuries in particular. Thereafter, the aim of surgery is to create a free CSF passage between the intracranial and spinal subarachnoid spaces. It is not advisable to dissect all arachnoid scarring off the spinal cord, medulla oblongata and cerebellar tonsils. On the contrary, such attempts are risky and simply lead to new adhesions and scar tissue formation. In foramen magnum arachnoiditis, the foramen of Magendie is always obstructed. A decision must therefore be made, intraoperatively, as to whether or not it can be opened safely. If important structures such as the PICAs are embedded in arachnoid scar tissue, then the risk may be too high. Some authors recommend placement of small catheters to provide an outflow for the 4th ventricle (Abe et al. 1995). However, even with ultrasound guidance, this remains a very risky manoeuvre, and the author has encountered patients with severe neurological deficits as a consequence of malpositioned catheters in this region. A safer strategy is to leave the foramen Magendie closed and place a supraventricular shunt. Indeed, because of such concerns, some surgeons have previously recommended limiting the management of foramen magnum arachnoiditis to ventricular shunting (Appleby et al. 1969).

10.5 Surgical Results and Complications

10.5.1 Chiari I Malformation

Two published analyses of foramen magnum decompressions gave extensive overviews on complications encountered during and immediately after surgery as well as delayed postoperative problems but did not provide any data (Menezes 1991; Mazzola and Fried 2003). When it comes to quantifying such complications, analysis of the literature shows enormous variations in reported figures. Not all studies seem to use the same standards when complications are analysed; how else can one explain figures of 2.4 % (Tubbs et al. 2011) and 37 % (Zerah 1999), both from series of more than 100 children, undergoing the same decompression procedure, carried out in respected institutions?

Tables 10.2 and 10.3 provide a literature overview, comparing complication rates, syrinx reduction rates and the frequency of surgical revisions, for different surgical decompression techniques for Chiari I. These include decompressions involving only bone removal, those with incision of the outer dural layer, those opening the dura completely and those where additional arachnoid dissection was performed.

The most common complication in the author's series was a CSF fistula, occurring in 6 % of cases overall but more often after revision surgeries than first operations (9 and 5.5 %, respectively). Use of autologous material for duraplasty was not associated with a lower rate for CSF fistulas compared to artificial materials although this is in contrast with the findings of other studies (Vanaclocha and Saiz-Sapena 1997). In order to limit the risk of a fistula, it is important to close the duraplasty with a tight running suture as well as ensure a good closure of the muscular layer, which appears to be the most effective barrier to CSF leakage. For that reason, the author does not use monopolar electrocautery for soft tissue dissection as this may cause significant damage to the muscular layers in particular. Leaving the arachnoid intact does not exclude fistulas because small lacerations and tears in this thin membrane are very common after dural opening. Nor does the additional use of tissue sealants appear to lower rates for fistulas (Parker et al. 2011).

Aseptic meningitis does seem to be related to the type of material used for duraplasty and was seen exclusively when lyophilised dura, fascia lata or galea had been used. To avoid any postoperative problems related to duraplasties, Bernard

Table 10.2 Literature review of the results of decompressions for Chiari I malformations, without dural opening

Authors	Group	N	Follow-up period	Peri- and postoperative complications	Syrinx size reduced	Recurrences/ deaths
Bony decompression only						
James and Brant (2002)	C	4	Not reported	None	Not reported	None
Hayhurst et al. (2008)	A, C	16	43 months[a]	27 %[a]	87 %[a]	25 %/none
McGirt et al. (2008b)	C	116	25 months	1 %	Not reported	7.8 %/none
Mutchnik et al. (2010)	A, C	56	Not reported	None	Not reported	12.5 %/none
Yilmaz et al. (2011)	A	24	Not reported	8.3 %	91.1 %	9.5 %/not reported
Bony decompression with outer dural decompression						
Gambardella et al. (1998)	A	8	Not reported	Not reported	88 %	12.5 %/none
Munshi et al. (2000)	A	11	Not reported	10 %	50 %	18.2 %/none
Navarro et al. (2004)	C	71	28 months[a]	5.6 %	65.7 %[a]	10.8 %/none
Limonadi and Selden (2004)	C	12	15.7 months	Not reported	No syrinx cases	Not reported
Caldarelli et al. (2007)	C	30	55 months	Not reported	50 %	6.7 %/none
Chauvet et al. (2009)	A	11	18 months	9.1 %	80 %	None

Abbreviations: *N* number of patients, *A* adults, *C* children
[a]Pooled data for different subgroups

Table 10.3 Literature review of the results of decompressions for Chiari I malformations, with dural opening

Authors	Group	N	Follow-up period	Peri- and postoperative complications	Syrinx size reduced	Recurrences/deaths
Bony decompression with arachnoid left intact and dura left open						
Di Lorenzo et al. (1995)	A	20	29 months	Not reported	100 %	15 %/none
Zerah (1999)	C	79	Not reported	37 %[a]	69 %[a]	1.6 %[a]/none
Bony decompression with arachnoid left intact and duraplasty						
Guyotat et al. (1998)	A, C	42	39 months	Not reported	58 %	50 %/4.7 %
Zerah (1999)	C	79	Not reported	37 %[a]	69 %[a]	1.6 %[a]/none
Munshi et al. (2000)	A, C	34	Not reported	42 %	100 %	None/none
Limonadi and Selden (2004)	C	12	14.8 months	8.3 %	100 %	Not reported
Navarro et al. (2004)	C	24	28 months[a]	42.1 %	65.7 %[a]	4.2 %/none
Galarza et al. (2007)	C	20	21 months[a]	8.3 %[a]	64[a]	Not reported
McGirt et al. (2008b)	C	140	29 months	3 %	Not reported	7.1 %/None
Wetjen et al. (2008)	A	29	36 months	Not reported	100 %	Not reported
Hoffman and Souweidane (2008)	A, C	40	11.4 months	CSF related 2.5 %	Not reported	5 %/None
Attenello et al. (2008)	C	49	41 months	10 %[a]	55 %[a]	10.2 %[a]/none
Sindou et al. (2002); Sindou and Gimbert (2009)	A	44	48 months	20.5 %	60 %	Not reported/none
Attenello et al. (2009)	C	27	Not reported	4 %	80 %	None Gore-Tex
Attenello et al. (2009)	C	40	Not reported	10 %	52 %	None Galea
Mutchnik et al. (2010)	A, C	64	Not reported	4.6 %	Not reported	3.1 %/none
Spena et al. (2010)	A	36	40 months	8.1 %	80.5 %	5.5 %/none
Yilmaz et al. (2011)	A	58	Not reported	12.1 %	84.2 %	Not reported
Valentini et al. (2011)	C	80	Not reported	6.3 %	91.5 %	6.3 %/none
Mottolese et al. (2011)	C	82	Not reported	18 %	Not reported	Not reported
Bony decompression with arachnoid opened and duraplasty						
Fischer (1995)	C	19	Not reported	26.3 %	93 %	Not reported
Vanaclocha and Saiz-Sapena (1997)	A	26	27 months	42.3 %	No syrinx cases	Not reported
Guyotat et al. (1998)	A, C	8	28 months	None	100 %	None
Aghakhani et al. (1999)	A	214	79 months	24 %	95 %	12.4 %/0.7 %
Zerah (1999)	C	105	Not reported	37 %[a]	69 %[a]	1.6 %[a]/none
Tubbs et al. (2003)	C	130	50 months	2.3 %	Not reported	6.9 %/none
Navarro et al. (2004)	C	14	28 months[a]	50 %	65.7 %[a]	28.6 %/none
Guo et al. (2007)	A, C	115	36 months	CSF 9.82–18.75 %	82–88 %	Not reported
Galarza et al. (2007)	C	40	21 months[a]	8.3 %[a]	64.3[a]	Not reported
Zhang et al. (2008)	A, C	234	Not reported	15.8 %[a]	66.5 %	Not reported/1.3 %[a]
Kumar et al. (2008)	A, C	87	34 months	17.2 %	Not reported	10.3 %/none
Aghakhani et al. (2009)	A	157	88 months	9.5 %	75.64 %	3.8 %/0.63 %
Zhang et al. (2011)	A, C	132	27 months	28 %	81.8 %	Not reported
Author's series[b]	A, C	203	52 months	19.2 %	87.9 %	5.9 %/1 %

Abbreviations: *N* number of patients, *A* adults, *C* children
[a]Pooled data for different subgroups
[b]Data for first decompressions with arachnoid opening and alloplastic material for duraplasty

Williams recommended against duraplasty. He favoured to suture the dura into the muscle and to close all soft tissues with tight sutures (Williams 1994). However, it has been claimed that omission of a duraplasty after arachnoid opening and dissection may predispose to severe arachnoiditis and recurrent CSF flow obstruction (Munshi et al. 2000).

Hydrocephalus is an important postoperative complication (Tubbs et al. 2003). In the author's series of 371 decompressions, it occurred after 3 % of decompressions within 30 days of surgery. An additional 2 of the 371 patients developed hydrocephalus months after the operation. An analysis of complications after posterior fossa surgery in general determined a rate of 4.6 % for postoperative hydrocephalus after 500 operations (Dubey et al. 2009). Most authors relate this problem to formation of subdural hygromas in the posterior fossa (Filis et al. 2009; Suzuki et al. 2011; Bahl et al. 2011; Marshman et al. 2005; Elton et al. 2002), but not all patients with postoperative hydrocephalus in the author's series demonstrated such collections. Whether or not postoperative ventriculomegaly needs surgical treatment should be based on the clinical course of the patient. The problem may resolve spontaneously (Marshman et al. 2005) or may require an intervention. Treatment options are either a ventriculoperitoneal shunt or a third ventriculostomy (Kandasamy et al. 2008).

Swallowing dysfunctions after craniovertebral decompression are related to surgical manipulations at or close to the obex and were observed early in 2.5 % of cases in the author's series, but this complication was not observed following application of the microsurgical dissection technique outlined above, which leaves the area of the obex and the fourth ventricular floor untouched.

The author's overall complication rate of 22 % is in line with those of several other studies (Zhang et al. 2011; Aghakhani et al. 1999; Guo et al. 2007; Fischer 1995; Kumar et al. 2008; Navarro et al. 2004; Zerah 1999; Aghakhani et al. 2009; Parker et al. 2011; Mottolese et al. 2011). This is a considerably higher complication rate than after bony decompression alone or following a decompression with incision of the outer

dura alone (McGirt et al. 2008b; Mutchnick et al. 2010; Navarro et al. 2004; Yilmaz et al. 2011; Chauvet et al. 2009; Limonadi and Selden 2004) (Table 10.2). As to whether leaving the arachnoid intact lowers the complication rate, the author's experience suggests that this is not the case. Furthermore, the same range of complication rates are reported in studies involving duraplasties, with or without arachnoid dissection (Guo et al. 2007; Tubbs et al. 2003, 2011; Zerah 1999; Zhang et al. 2008, 2011; Aghakhani et al. 1999; Sindou et al. 2002; McGirt et al. 2008b; Munshi et al. 2000; Sindou and Gimbert 2009). Yet other publications report considerably lower complication rates than the author's experience but, once again, independent of whether or not the arachnoid was opened (Mutchnick et al. 2010; McGirt et al. 2008b; Attenello et al. 2009; Spena et al. 2010; Yilmaz et al. 2011; Valentini et al. 2011; Tubbs et al. 2003; Aghakhani et al. 2009) (Table 10.3).

Decrease in syrinx size was observed in 81 % of 281 craniovertebral decompressions in the author's series. No change occurred in 15 and 3.7 % demonstrated a further expansion. The number of postoperative syrinx reductions was significantly greater after primary decompressions, as compared to secondary operations (85 and 72 %, respectively).

In the first postoperative year, improvements can be anticipated for all symptoms. The most profound effect will be seen with occipital pain, which almost always improves after surgery. In the author's series, there were no differences in short-term results between adults and children. Patients undergoing a revision usually had more severe preoperative motor deficits and gait disturbances, and these deficits improved only marginally with a secondary decompression. For all foramen magnum decompressions combined, 3 out of 4 of patients in the author's series considered their condition to have improved 3 months after surgery, while 1 in 5 reported no change, and 1 in 20 experienced a worsening of symptoms (Table 10.4).

Long-term results in the author's series were analysed with Kaplan-Meier statistics, to determine the rates at which patients experienced

Table 10.4 Postoperative results after 3 months for Chiari malformations and foramen magnum arachnoiditis (author's series)

Type	Chiari I first surgery (%)	Chiari I revision surgery (%)	Basilar invagination (%)	Chiari I all surgery (%)	Chiari II (%)	Foramen magnum arachnoiditis (%)
Improved	76.3	65.1	85	73.6	56	45
Unchanged	19.7	23.3	15	21.0	38	36
Worse	4.0	11.6	–	5.5	6	18

Table 10.5 Neurological recurrence rates for Chiari I malformations: Kaplan-Meier statistics

Group	5 years (%)	10 years (%)	P-value
First surgery	13.1	19.1	0.007
Revision surgery	34	34	
Adults	14.4	15.6	0.66
Children	11.8	–	
Arachnoid opened	13.5	14.7	0.023
Arachnoid not opened	34.1	–	
Artificial graft	10	11.5	0.022
Autologous graft	31.8	31.8	
Syringomyelia	13.8	15.2	0.61
No syringomyelia	15.5	15.5	
All	14.3	15.4	
Optimal first surgery	7	8.7	

neurological deterioration, compared with those maintaining a stable neurological status (Table 10.5). Overall, recurrences amounted to 14 % within 5 years and 15 % within 10 years. No significant differences were seen between adults and children or between patients with and without syringomyelia. Recurrence rates were, however, significantly lower for primary compared to revision operations. It is also interesting to note that recurrence rates were significantly higher after decompressions with duraplasties using autologous material, as compared with those using alloplastic materials.

When comparing results in the literature for different types of foramen magnum decompression, there is a lower frequency of complications in all types of procedures that leave the inner layer of the dura intact. This, however, is counterbalanced by a lower frequency of syrinx collapses and a higher frequency of patients experiencing a recurrence of symptoms and/or requiring revision surgery – if these data are reported (Tables 10.2 and 10.3). The two largest series where decom-

pression was restricted to a bony removal did not provide such numbers (McGirt et al. 2008b; Mutchnick et al. 2010). The largest series reporting on decompression with incisions of the outer dural layer reported rates for syrinx decrease of between 50 and 66 % (Caldarelli et al. 2007; Munshi et al. 2000; Navarro et al. 2004).

When it comes to opening the dura fully, series recommending a duraplasty but leaving the arachnoid intact once again often do not provide data for syrinx reductions (Mottolese et al. 2011; McGirt et al. 2008b; Mutchnick et al. 2010; Hoffman and Souweidane 2008). Studies do report syrinx reduction rates in the range of 50–60 % (Guyotat et al. 1997; Sindou et al. 2002; Attenello et al. 2009), although some smaller series observed a syrinx reduction in all their patients (Limonadi and Selden 2004; Wetjen et al. 2008; Munshi et al. 2000). Higher rates for postoperative improvements and syrinx reductions were found in 34 patients receiving duraplasties, as compared to 11 who underwent incisions of the outer dura (Munshi et al. 2000). A study comparing decompressions involving tonsillar coagulation and duraplasties, with decompressions confined to incision of the outer dura alone, found better results in the former group after a mean follow-up of 21 months, both in terms of clinical improvements and syrinx reductions (Galarza et al. 2007). This overview suggests but does not prove that postoperative syrinx reduction rates are lower after decompressions that do not open the arachnoid (Tables 10.2 and 10.3).

Looking on rates for postoperative revisions and recurrences, a study comparing results for 56 patients undergoing a pure bony decompression with 64 patients receiving duraplasty but without arachnoid opening concluded that the revision rate was higher in the former group (12.5 compared to 3.1 %), although the paper did not state the follow-up time (Mutchnick et al. 2010). A similar study on 82 patients reported a higher rate of revision after decompressions without duraplasty, compared to those with duraplasty – 9.5 and 3.6 %, respectively (Yilmaz et al. 2011). A meta-analysis from the literature of 582 patients came to the same conclusion (Durham and Fjeld-Olenec 2008). A study of results in children, however, concluded that decompression with incision of the outer dura gave comparable results to more invasive forms of decompression and avoided higher complication rates (Navarro et al. 2004). A report comparing results for 16 bony decompressions with 80 decompressions involving arachnoid dissection noted a lower recurrence rate after dura and arachnoid opening – 7.5 compared to 25 % after bony decompressions only (Hayhurst et al. 2008).

Some investigators have tried to tailor surgical steps for individual patients according to intraoperative ultrasound findings. A study to evaluate the effect of bony decompressions in children noted tonsillar pulsations and a sufficient subarachnoid space in 116 operations, so the dura was not opened. A duraplasty was performed without opening the arachnoid in a further 140 instances. Following this policy and at an average follow-up of 27 months, 15 % of children had a mild or moderate recurrence of symptoms, and another 7 % had severe symptom recurrence, requiring a revision surgery. Kaplan-Meier analyses showed a recurrence rate for headache of more than 40 % and a recurrence rate for brainstem and cranial nerve symptoms of more than 20 % within 80 months after surgery. A syrinx decrease was detected in 62 % of patients (McGirt et al. 2008b). Another group also modified their operative steps according to intraoperative ultrasonic CSF flow measurements and found arachnoid dissection necessary in the overwhelming majority of patients (Milhorat and Bolognese 2003). Others have also used ultrasound to establish an adequate decompression after bony removal but then restricted the operation to splitting the outer dural layer in only a minority of patients, who did not have a syrinx and where the tonsillar herniation was mild, not reaching C1. The majority of the 363 paediatric

patients underwent dural opening, arachnoid dissection, opening of the foramen of Magendie and duraplasty (Menezes et al. 2005). Neither set of authors gave any information on postoperative outcomes for their patients.

In summary, the outcome data as published in the literature for syrinx reduction and revision rates are considerably worse for limited decompressions when compared to those with arachnoid opening and duraplasty, in the author's and other similar series (Tables 10.2 and 10.3). Given the low morbidity rates of the technique described in this chapter and the much better long-term results for decompressions that involve at least a duraplasty, the author does not support methods of decompression that do not involve duraplasties.

This leaves the question of whether the arachnoid should be opened or not. In the author's series, the arachnoid was not opened in a subgroup of 24 Chiari I patients without syringomyelia because it appeared entirely normal after dural opening. In the long term, however, a significantly higher neurological recurrence rate[1] was observed for these patients compared to the other decompressions with arachnoid dissection (Table 10.5). So far, a few studies have analysed the influence of arachnoid changes on clinical symptoms and outcomes in Chiari I malformation. Some authors comment that severe arachnoid scarring is a sign of unfavourable long-term prognosis (Sakamoto et al. 1999; Aghakhani et al. 2009). However, there are little data on the frequency of arachnoid changes in Chiari I and even less information on their significance. One study found arachnoid scarring in 6 of 14 patients without and 19 of 51 patients with syringomyelia but made no statements as to whether this influenced the clinical outcome (Ellenbogen et al. 2000). Another found that patients with arachnoiditis showed more severe neurological signs before surgery and had a worse postoperative outcome than patients without arachnoid pathology (Aghakhani et al. 2009). In the author's series, severe arachnoid scarring was detected in 48 of

---

[1] The reappearance or progression of preoperative symptoms, or development of new neurological symptoms, related to the Chiari or the syrinx

371 decompressions (13 %). Severe scarring was significantly more common in secondary operations as compared to primary procedures (63 and 6 %, respectively). More data are available concerning patency of the foramen of Magendie. The foramen was obstructed in 12 % of 500 paediatric patients that were surgically managed for Chiari I (Tubbs et al. 2011). This group also emphasised in an earlier paper that such obstructions cannot be detected without arachnoid dissection (Tubbs et al. 2003). The foramen was found to be partially or completely obstructed in another study in 14 out of 105 children (Zerah 1999). In a third study, the foramen was obstructed in 7.4 %, with some arachnoid scarring at this level in 17 % of patients (Menezes et al. 2005). In the author's series, Magendie was obstructed in 33 % of patients. Again, this rate was significantly higher in revision as against primary surgeries (65 and 28 %, respectively). Again in the author's series, severe arachnoid scarring was associated with more severe preoperative neurological deficits, a lower frequency for syrinx reduction postoperatively and a higher frequency of long-term neurological deterioration.

These observations suggest that the arachnoid does play a role in the pathophysiology of Chiari I malformations at least for the formation and postoperative resolution of syringomyelia but also for the function of brainstem and spinal cord irrespective of a syrinx. Decompression techniques that do not address the arachnoid neglect a component that is relevant for a significant number of patients. Techniques that treat the arachnoid pathology can be expected to be associated with improved long-term results (Table 10.3). To settle this issue, however, a prospective study comparing postoperative results for decompressions with and without arachnoid dissection will be required.

10.5.2 Basilar Invagination

In the author's series of 35 operated patients, 30 patients with basilar invagination considered their condition improved following surgery, and 5 were unchanged 3 months postoperatively (Table 10.4). Four required further procedures

subsequently. Patients with basilar invagination treated by posterior decompression only require postoperative monitoring for evidence of instability. In one of the author's patients without preoperative evidence of craniocervical instability, postoperative MR scans demonstrated pannus formation around the odontoid peg and instability on functional X-rays about 6 months after decompression. A posterior fusion was necessary, which then led to neurological improvement. Among 9 patients treated by ventral and dorsal decompression and fusion, two revisions for late implant failures were required. Another patient in this group with a stable postoperative neurological status underwent a revision at another institution resulting in neurological worsening. Apart from these 4 patients, no subsequent operations were required or clinical recurrences detected in the group of patients with basilar invagination.

10.5.3 Chiari II Malformation

In the literature, good results have been reported for infants undergoing decompression before severe brainstem dysfunctions, such as bilateral vocal cord palsies, had developed, with success rates in the order of 80 % (Zerah 1999; Vandertop et al. 1992; Ishak et al. 1980; Teo et al. 1997; Pollack et al. 1996; Talamonti and Zella 2011). The author's series of six children under 2 years of age included four who presented as neonates with severe respiratory problems and two 1-year-old children who had cyanotic attacks when stressed or upon coughing. Following decompression, all infants showed improvement of respiratory functions, although one child still died, 17 months after surgery, due to recurrent respiratory problems. In children, radiological evidence of instability is common after decompressions and was found in 5 of 9 patients in one study addressing this problem, specifically. However, this appeared not to be clinically relevant as no clinical symptoms were related to it (Lam et al. 2009). Whether this conclusion still holds once these children have reached adulthood remains to be seen.

For adult patients with Chiari II malformation, few data exist in the literature. One study recommends a combination of decompression and stabilisation if surgery is required in this age group and reported good outcomes in 4 patients so treated (Rahman et al. 2009). Looking at short-term results for 7 older patients in the author's series undergoing 10 decompressions in total, 3 operations were followed by improvements, and 6 left the patients unchanged, while 1 patient considered his condition worsened within 3 months after decompression. In the longer term, the neurological status was stabilised in 4 of these 7 patients, requiring a total of 6 decompressions. The other 3 progressed despite 4 decompressions presumably related to compromised cervical stability. Therefore, a decompression for Chiari II malformation should be combined with a posterior fusion to prevent neurological deteriorations related to post-laminectomy deformities.

All patients with Chiari II malformations require a lifelong medical surveillance by neurologists, orthopaedic surgeons and neurosurgeons, to maintain as much quality of life and autonomy as possible.

10.5.4   Foramen Magnum Arachnoiditis

In the author's series, 10 patients with foramen magnum arachnoiditis underwent decompression at the foramen magnum. Five considered their condition improved 3 months after decompression, 3 were unchanged and 2 worsened (Table 10.4). In the long term, 6 clinical recurrences were detected. In this series, arachnoiditis had the worst prognosis among all pathologies at the foramen magnum, with only 33 % achieving a stable neurological status according to a Kaplan-Meier analysis. In the literature, no outcome data for a patient series treated by decompression exists.

10.6   Recurrences

This section will deal with surgical revisions for Chiari I malformations only. For Chiari II or foramen magnum arachnoiditis, the number requiring revision surgery was low in the author's series, and cases in the literature were discussed above.

10.6.1   Assessment

Once hydrocephalus is ruled out, the further evaluation of patients representing after a foramen magnum decompression must start with the clinical history. What symptoms were apparent before the previous decompression, and how did these symptoms respond to surgery? Was the neurology unchanged or improved, or did symptoms progress further without an interval of stable neurology? In the author's series of 107 patients presenting after a Chiari I foramen magnum decompression, 56 did not go on to a further surgical procedure, mainly because their neurological status either was stable or was considered unlikely to be stabilised by another intervention. Most of these patients not undergoing a revision presented because they were disappointed by the result of their initial decompression. Although many symptoms had improved and the syrinx had decreased in size, burning dysaesthesias persisted and proved extremely difficult to treat with analgesics in the great majority. It is certainly important to inform any patient, before any surgery, that dysaesthesias may not respond to an otherwise successful decompression. Indeed, such pains may even worsen following collapse of a syrinx (Milhorat et al. 1996). This phenomenon, however, was not observed in the author's series.

Progression of symptoms without an interval of clinical stability suggests an insufficient operation. In most instances, this will be related to an insufficient decompression; untreated features of an associated basilar invagination, such as anterior compression by the odontoid peg; or the result of craniocervical instability. In the majority of patients, however, the clinical history reveals a stable interval after foramen magnum decompression with or without improvement of preoperative symptoms. It should then be noted how and when the deterioration started. In the author's experience, the longer the interval of clinical stability before the deterioration began, the less likely the cause was related to the foramen magnum. The only clinical symptom, which always suggested a foramen magnum problem in these patients, was a recurrence of occipital headaches or swallowing dysfunctions.

As the next step, careful neuroradiological assessment is essential for these patients. First of all, the area of the previous operation needs to be evaluated, comparing pre- and postoperative MRI scans. There might be evidence of insufficient decompression or recurrent compression. It has been reported that new bone formation may cause recurrent compression (Zerah 1999; Aoki et al. 1995; Hudgins and Boydston 1995). An oversized craniectomy may result in cerebellar ptosis and medullary compression (Holly and Batzdorf 2001). The newly created artificial cisterna magna may not be of sufficient size. There may be a pseudomeningocoele pushing the dura anteriorly onto the cervicomedullary junction. MR imaging will also reveal whether there is basilar invagination with persistent anterior compression of the odontoid or if there is a precursor of craniocervical instability, such as an assimilated atlas, a Klippel-Feil syndrome of the upper cervical spine or pannus formation around the odontoid (Smith et al. 2010). Functional X-rays or CT scans should be part of the diagnostic workup in such patients to evaluate craniocervical stability.

Another important consideration is the postoperative course of a syrinx. If the syrinx is seen, radiologically, to have decreased after surgery and to have remained so, it was unlikely that any new symptoms were related to the foramen magnum, with the one exception that craniocervical instability still had to be ruled out. Next, a cardiac-gated cine MRI should be performed, to evaluate the CSF passage at the foramen magnum. This modality is the most sensitive method to detect or exclude arachnoid scarring and postoperative adhesions (Armonda et al. 1994; Bhadelia et al. 1995; Hofkes et al. 2007; McGirt et al. 2008a). If such a study demonstrates adequate CSF flow at the foramen magnum and the neuroradiological evaluation had excluded all the other above-mentioned possibilities, then the clinical deterioration was due to a mechanism or cause unrelated to the previous decompression.

In patients with syrinx shunts, the shunt catheter may have caused tethering of nerve roots or spinal cord leading to radicular or myelopathic symptoms, which are often provoked by neck or arm movements (Batzdorf et al. 1998). The MRI in these patients will show adherence of the cord to the dura at the level of the shunt.

If this, in turn, has been excluded, degenerative changes of the cervical spine should be evaluated. Many patients with a well-treated Chiari malformation and a collapsed syrinx demonstrate considerable spinal cord atrophy. MRI scans may then give the impression that a slight or moderate degree of cervical stenosis is not clinically relevant, but this is a dangerous assumption. Such patients have little functional reserve in their spinal cord, and any additional physical insult, even a minor one, may be enough to cause significant new deficits. It has even been suggested that Chiari patients may be particularly prone to the effects of degenerative problems of the cervical spine (Takeuchi et al. 2007). In particular, signs of hypermobility of cervical segments should be looked for by radiographs in ante- and retroflexion. Cervical fusion should be offered to patients with neurological deterioration despite a sufficiently treated Chiari I malformation but with signs of hypermobility in the cervical spine in functional studies. In the author's experience, such fusions may stabilise the neurological course of these patients.

10.6.2 Revision Surgery

Indications for revision surgery at the craniovertebral junction include untreated or new instability of the craniocervical junction, insufficient primary decompression or an obstruction of CSF flow, the latter related to arachnoid scarring or compression of the cisterna magna by a pseudomeningocoele (Fig. 10.8). In view of the poor response of Chiari-related syringomyelia to direct shunting, the author would not choose this treatment for patients after a failed primary decompression (Klekamp et al. 1996). Instead, if a syrinx reappears or does not regress in the first place, the reason for this must be established and treated at the level of the foramen magnum. This will require a revision with opening of the dura or duraplasty and then careful arachnoid dissection, to establish free outflow of CSF from the foramen

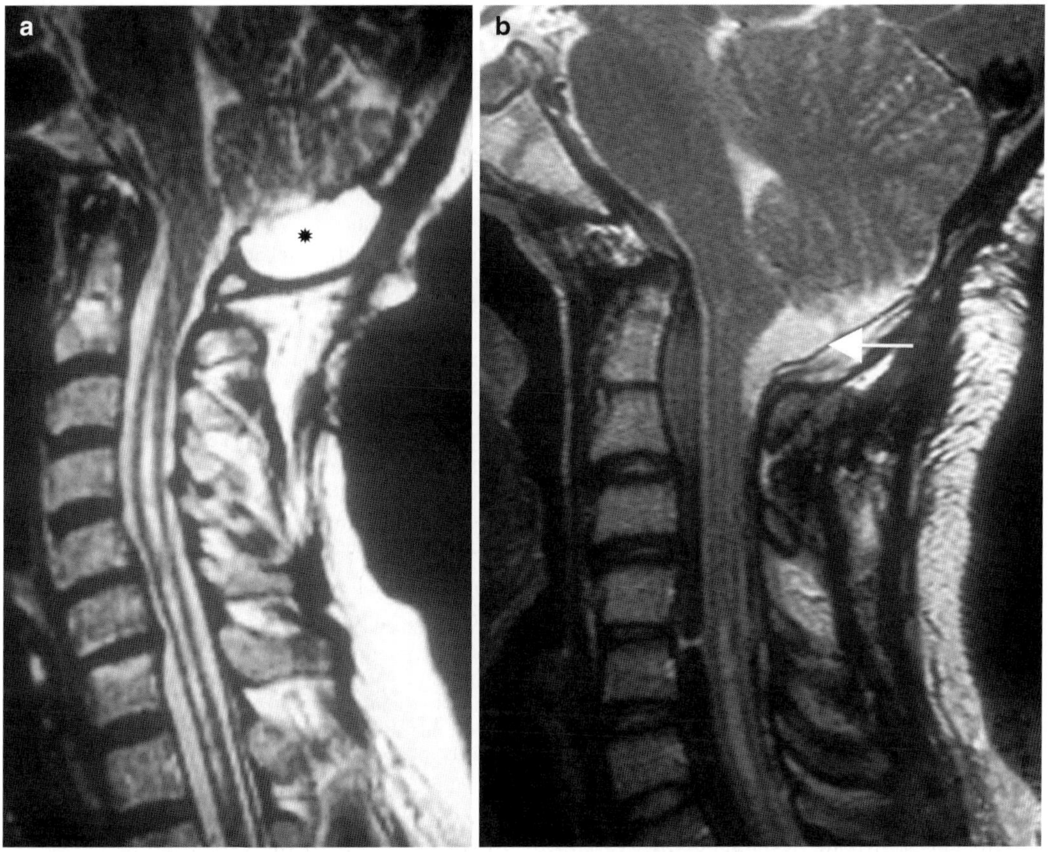

Fig. 10.8 (**a**) This preoperative T2-weighted MRI shows a situation after foramen magnum decompression for Chiari I malformation. C1 was not removed. A pseudomeningocoele developed (*), pushing the duraplasty anteriorly and resulting in CSF flow obstruction. Even though the syrinx had not enlarged, the patient complained of local discomfort and deteriorating gait. (**b**) After foramen magnum revision, with removal of C1 and exchange of the duraplasty, CSF flow is restored (*arrow*) and the patient improved

of Magendie. Several authors have mentioned the importance of opening Magendie during foramen magnum decompressions (Zerah 1999; Menezes et al. 2005; Tubbs et al. 2011) and particularly so during revisions (Sacco and Scott 2003; Tubbs et al. 2011). In some cases, such revisions may need to be combined with craniocervical fusion and even transoral resection of the odontoid. Severe arachnoid scarring related to surgical manoeuvres or postoperative meningitis is the most common feature in patients demonstrating a CSF flow obstruction, usually in the form of adhesions between dural graft and cerebellum or the spinal cord, although other factors may sometimes operate (Table 10.6) (Fig. 10.8) (Klekamp et al. 1996; Sakamoto et al. 1999; Ellenbogen

Table 10.6 Causes of postoperative cicatrix

Pseudomeningocoele pushing the graft anteriorly
Use of autologous graft material
Insufficient arachnoid dissection at primary surgery
Plugging the obex
History of meningitis

et al. 2000; Mazzola and Fried 2003; Rosen et al. 2003; Yanni et al. 2010; Pare and Batzdorf 1998). Leaving the arachnoid intact during the first decompression may also result in insufficient CSF flow postoperatively leading to a subsequent revision.

The more extensive and dense the arachnoid pathology, the less likely it is that a revision will produce a lasting benefit. Furthermore, the risk of secondary surgery is certainly higher than with primary decompressions. It is, therefore, very difficult to predict the outcome for a patient before revision surgery. Unless there is a history of meningitis or a clear description of severe arachnoid changes in the original operation notes, it is impossible to foresee exactly what will be discovered after reopening of the dura. A surgical strategy has to be adopted intraoperatively which improves CSF flow but minimises the risk of recurrent postoperative arachnoid scarring. Limiting the arachnoid dissection to the midline, with sharp transection of arachnoid adhesions obstructing the foramen of Magendie and the posterior spinal subarachnoid space, is all that is required. Blunt dissection or tackling arachnoid adhesions laterally carries the risk of damage to small perforating arteries and caudal cranial nerves and should be avoided. Finally, a spacious dura graft, using artificial material, provides reasonable protection against postoperative arachnoid scarring, which may otherwise cause another clinical recurrence. The realistic outlook for patients undergoing a foramen magnum revision is clinical stabilisation of the previously progressive course. Long-term results in the author's series, determined by Kaplan-Meier statistics, revealed a further recurrence rate of 1 in 3 within 5 years after foramen magnum revision (Table 10.5) (Klekamp et al. 2002).

References

Abe T, Okuda Y, Nagashima H et al (1995) Surgical treatment of syringomyelia. Rinsho Shinkeigaku 35(12):1406–1408

Aboulezz AO, Sartor K, Geyer CA et al (1985) Position of cerebellar tonsils in the normal population and in patients with Chiari malformation: a quantitative approach with MR imaging. J Comput Assist Tomogr 9(6):1033–1036

Aghakhani N, Parker F, Tadie M (1999) Syringomyelia and Chiari abnormality in the adult. Analysis of the results of a cooperative series of 285 cases. Neurochirurgie 45(Suppl 1):23–36

Aghakhani N, Parker F, David P et al (2009) Long-term follow-up of Chiari-related syringomyelia in adults: analysis of 157 surgically treated cases. Neurosurgery 64(2):308–315; discussion 315

Agrawal A (2008) Sudden unexpected death in a young adult with Chiari I malformation. J Pak Med Assoc 58(7):417–418

Aoki N, Oikawa A, Sakai T (1995) Spontaneous regeneration of the foramen magnum after decompressive suboccipital craniectomy in Chiari malformation: case report. Neurosurgery 37(2):340–342

Appleby A, Bradley WG, Foster JB et al (1969) Syringomyelia due to chronic arachnoiditis at the foramen magnum. J Neurol Sci 8(3):451–464

Armonda RA, Citrin CM, Foley KT et al (1994) Quantitative cine-mode magnetic resonance imaging of Chiari I malformations: an analysis of cerebrospinal fluid dynamics. Neurosurgery 35(2):214–223; discussion 223–224

Attenello FJ, McGirt MJ, Gathinji M et al (2008) Outcome of Chiari-associated syringomyelia after hindbrain decompression in children: analysis of 49 consecutive cases. Neurosurgery 62(6):1307–1313; discussion 1313

Attenello FJ, McGirt MJ, Garces-Ambrossi GL et al (2009) Suboccipital decompression for Chiari I malformation: outcome comparison of duraplasty with expanded polytetrafluoroethylene dural substitute versus pericranial autograft. Childs Nerv Syst 25(2):183–190

Badie B, Mendoza D, Batzdorf U (1995) Posterior fossa volume and response to suboccipital decompression in patients with Chiari I malformation. Neurosurgery 37(2):214–218

Bahl A, Murphy M, Thomas N et al (2011) Management of infratentorial subdural hygroma complicating foramen magnum decompression: a report of three cases. Acta Neurochir (Wien) 153(5):1123–1128

Batzdorf U, Klekamp J, Johnson JP (1998) A critical appraisal of syrinx cavity shunting procedures. J Neurosurg 89(3):382–388

Bhadelia RA, Bogdan AR, Wolpert SM et al (1995) Cerebrospinal fluid flow waveforms: analysis in patients with Chiari I malformation by means of gated phase-contrast MR imaging velocity measurements. Radiology 196(1):195–202

Boyles AL, Enterline DS, Hammock PH et al (2006) Phenotypic definition of Chiari type I malformation coupled with high-density SNP genome screen shows significant evidence for linkage to regions on chromosomes 9 and 15. Am J Med Genet A 140(24):2776–2785. doi:10.1002/ajmg.a.31546

Caldarelli M, Novegno F, Vassimi L et al (2007) The role of limited posterior fossa craniectomy in the surgical treatment of Chiari malformation Type I: experience with a pediatric series. J Neurosurg 106(3 Suppl):187–195

Charney EB, Rorke LB, Sutton LN et al (1987) Management of Chiari II complications in infants with myelomeningocele. J Pediatr 111(3):364–371

Chauvet D, Carpentier A, George B (2009) Dura splitting decompression in Chiari type 1 malformation: clinical experience and radiological findings. Neurosurg Rev 32(4):465–470

Chiari H (1896) Über Veränderungen des Kleinhirns, des Pons und der Medulla oblongata infolge congenitaler Hydrocephalie des Grosshirns. Denkschr Akad Wiss Wien 63:71–116

Chumas PD, Armstrong DC, Drake JM et al (1993) Tonsillar herniation: the rule rather than the exception after lumboperitoneal shunting in the pediatric population. J Neurosurg 78(4):568–573

Danzer E, Johnson MP, Adzick NS (2011) Fetal surgery for myelomeningocele: progress and perspectives. Dev Med Child Neurol 54(1):8–14

Di Lorenzo N, Palma L, Palatinsky E et al (1995) "Conservative" cranio-cervical decompression in the treatment of syringomyelia-Chiari I complex. A prospective study of 20 adult cases. Spine 20(23):2479–2483

Dubey A, Sung WS, Shaya M et al (2009) Complications of posterior cranial fossa surgery – an institutional experience of 500 patients. Surg Neurol 72(4):369–375

Durham SR, Fjeld-Olenec K (2008) Comparison of posterior fossa decompression with and without duraplasty for the surgical treatment of Chiari malformation Type I in pediatric patients: a meta-analysis. J Neurosurg Pediatr 2(1):42–49

Elgamal EA, El-Dawlatly AA, Murshid WR et al (2011) Endoscopic third ventriculostomy for hydrocephalus in children younger than 1 year of age. Childs Nerv Syst 27(1):111–116

Ellenbogen RG, Armonda RA, Shaw DW et al (2000) Toward a rational treatment of Chiari I malformation and syringomyelia. Neurosurg Focus 8(3):E6

Elton S, Tubbs RS, Wellons JC 3rd et al (2002) Acute hydrocephalus following a Chiari I decompression. Pediatr Neurosurg 36(2):101–104

Filis AK, Moon K, Cohen AR (2009) Symptomatic subdural hygroma and hydrocephalus following Chiari I decompression. Pediatr Neurosurg 45(6):425–428

Fischer EG (1995) Posterior fossa decompression for Chiari I deformity, including resection of the cerebellar tonsils. Childs Nerv Syst 11(11):625–629

Galarza M, Sood S, Ham S (2007) Relevance of surgical strategies for the management of pediatric Chiari type I malformation. Childs Nerv Syst 23(6):691–696

Galarza M, Lopez-Guerrero AL, Martinez-Lage JF (2010) Posterior fossa arachnoid cysts and cerebellar tonsillar descent: short review. Neurosurg Rev 33(3):305–314; discussion 314

Gambardella G, Caruso G, Caffo M et al (1998) Transverse microincisions of the outer layer of the dura mater combined with foramen magnum decompression as treatment for syringomyelia with Chiari I malformation. Acta Neurochir (Wien) 140(2):134–139

Gardner WJ (1965) Hydrodynamic mechanism of syringomyelia: its relationship to myelocele. J Neurol Neurosurg Psychiatry 28:247–259

Goel A (2004) Treatment of basilar invagination by atlantoaxial joint distraction and direct lateral mass fixation. J Neurosurg Spine 1(3):281–286

Goel A, Shah A (2009) Reversal of longstanding musculoskeletal changes in basilar invagination after surgical decompression and stabilization. J Neurosurg Spine 10(3):220–227

Guo F, Wang M, Long J et al (2007) Surgical management of Chiari malformation: analysis of 128 cases. Pediatr Neurosurg 43(5):375–381

Guyotat J, Bret P, Mottolese C et al (1997) Chiari I malformation with syringomyelia treated by decompression of the cranio-spinal junction and tonsillectomy. Apropos of 8 cases. Neurochirurgie 43(3):135–141

Guyotat J, Bret P, Jouanneau E et al (1998) Syringomyelia associated with type I Chiari malformation. A 21-year retrospective study on 75 cases treated by foramen magnum decompression with a special emphasis on the value of tonsils resection. Acta Neurochir (Wien) 140(8):745–754

Haroun RI, Guarnieri M, Meadow JJ et al (2000) Current opinions for the treatment of syringomyelia and Chiari malformations: survey of the Pediatric Section of the American Association of Neurological Surgeons. Pediatr Neurosurg 33(6):311–317

Haughton VM, Korosec FR, Medow JE et al (2003) Peak systolic and diastolic CSF velocity in the foramen magnum in adult patients with Chiari I malformations and in normal control participants. AJNR Am J Neuroradiol 24(2):169–176

Hayhurst C, Richards O, Zaki H et al (2008) Hindbrain decompression for Chiari – syringomyelia complex: an outcome analysis comparing surgical techniques. Br J Neurosurg 22(1):86–91

Henriques Filho PS, Pratesi R (2006) Abnormalities in auditory evoked potentials of 75 patients with Arnold-Chiari malformations types I and II. Arq Neuropsiquiatr 64(3A):619–623

Hida K, Iwasaki Y, Imamura H et al (1994) Birth injury as a causative factor of syringomyelia with Chiari type I deformity. J Neurol Neurosurg Psychiatry 57(3):373–374

Hobbs WR, Sponseller PD, Weiss AP et al (1997) The cervical spine in Marfan syndrome. Spine 22(9):983–989

Hoffman CE, Souweidane MM (2008) Cerebrospinal fluid-related complications with autologous duraplasty and arachnoid sparing in type I Chiari malformation. Neurosurgery 62(3 Suppl 1):156–160; discussion 160–161

Hofkes SK, Iskandar BJ, Turski PA et al (2007) Differentiation between symptomatic Chiari I malformation and asymptomatic tonsilar ectopia by using cerebrospinal fluid flow imaging: initial estimate of imaging accuracy. Radiology 245(2):532–540

Holly LT, Batzdorf U (2001) Management of cerebellar ptosis following craniovertebral decompression for Chiari I malformation. J Neurosurg 94(1):21–26

Hudgins RJ, Boydston WR (1995) Bone regrowth and recurrence of symptoms following decompression in the infant with Chiari II malformation. Pediatr Neurosurg 23(6):323–327

Ishak BA, McLone D, Seleny FL (1980) Intraoperative autonomic dysfunction associated with Arnold-Chiari malformation. Childs Brain 7(3):146–149

James HE, Brant A (2002) Treatment of the Chiari malformation with bone decompression without durotomy in children and young adults. Childs Nerv Syst 18(5):202–206

Jian FZ, Chen Z, Wrede KH et al (2010) Direct posterior reduction and fixation for the treatment of basilar invagination with atlantoaxial dislocation. Neurosurgery 66(4):678–687; discussion 687

Kagawa M, Jinnai T, Matsumoto Y et al (2006) Chiari I malformation accompanied by assimilation of the atlas, Klippel-Feil syndrome, and syringomyelia: case report. Surg Neurol 65(5):497–502; discussion 502

Kandasamy J, Kneen R, Gladstone M et al (2008) Chiari I malformation without hydrocephalus: acute intracranial hypertension managed with endoscopic third ventriculostomy (ETV). Childs Nerv Syst 24(12): 1493–1497

Kirsch WM, Duncan BR, Black FO et al (1968) Laryngeal palsy in association with myelomeningocele, hydrocephalus, and the Arnold-Chiari malformation. J Neurosurg 28(3):207–214

Klekamp J, Samii M (2001) Syringomyelia – diagnosis and treatment. Springer, Heidelberg

Klekamp J, Riedel A, Harper C et al (1989) Morphometric study on the postnatal growth of non-cortical brain regions in Australian aborigines and Caucasians. Brain Res 485(1):79–88

Klekamp J, Samii M, Tatagiba M et al (1995) Syringomyelia in association with tumours of the posterior fossa. Pathophysiological considerations, based on observations on three related cases. Acta Neurochir (Wien) 137(1–2):38–43

Klekamp J, Batzdorf U, Samii M et al (1996) The surgical treatment of Chiari I malformation. Acta Neurochir (Wien) 138(7):788–801

Klekamp J, Iaconetta G, Batzdorf U et al (2002) Syringomyelia associated with foramen magnum arachnoiditis. J Neurosurg Spine 97(3):317–322

Krauss WE, Bledsoe JM, Clarke MJ et al (2010) Rheumatoid arthritis of the craniovertebral junction. Neurosurgery 66(3 Suppl):83–95

Kumar A, Patni AH, Charbel F (2002) The Chiari I malformation and the neurotologist. Otol Neurotol 23(5):727–735

Kumar R, Kalra SK, Vaid VK et al (2008) Chiari I malformation: surgical experience over a decade of management. Br J Neurosurg 22(3):409–414

Lam FC, Irwin BJ, Poskitt KJ et al (2009) Cervical spine instability following cervical laminectomies for Chiari II malformation: a retrospective cohort study. Childs Nerv Syst 25(1):71–76

Limonadi FM, Selden NR (2004) Dura-splitting decompression of the craniocervical junction: reduced operative time, hospital stay, and cost with equivalent early outcome. J Neurosurg 101(2 Suppl):184–188

Logue V, Edwards MR (1981) Syringomyelia and its surgical treatment – an analysis of 75 patients. J Neurol Neurosurg Psychiatry 44(4):273–284

Marin-Padilla M, Marin-Padilla TM (1981) Morphogenesis of experimentally induced Arnold–Chiari malformation. J Neurol Sci 50(1):29–55

Marshman LA, Benjamin JC, Chawda SJ et al (2005) Acute obstructive hydrocephalus associated with infratentorial subdural hygromas complicating Chiari malformation Type I decompression. Report of two cases and literature review. J Neurosurg 103(4):752–755

Massimi L, Pravata E, Tamburrini G et al (2011) Endoscopic third ventriculostomy for the management of Chiari I and related hydrocephalus: outcome and pathogenetic implications. Neurosurgery 68(4): 950–956. doi:10.1227/NEU.0b013e318208f1f3

Mazzola CA, Fried AH (2003) Revision surgery for Chiari malformation decompression. Neurosurg Focus 15(3):E3

McGirt MJ, Atiba A, Attenello FJ et al (2008a) Correlation of hindbrain CSF flow and outcome after surgical decompression for Chiari I malformation. Childs Nerv Syst 24(7):833–840

McGirt MJ, Attenello FJ, Atiba A et al (2008b) Symptom recurrence after suboccipital decompression for pediatric Chiari I malformation: analysis of 256 consecutive cases. Childs Nerv Syst 24(11):1333–1339

McLone DG, Knepper PA (1989) The cause of Chiari II malformation: a unified theory. Pediatr Neurosci 15(1):1–12

Menezes AH (1991) Chiari I malformations and hydromyelia – complications. Pediatr Neurosurg 17(3): 146–154

Menezes AH (2008a) Specific entities affecting the craniocervical region: Down's syndrome. Childs Nerv Syst 24(10):1165–1168

Menezes AH (2008b) Specific entities affecting the craniocervical region: osteogenesis imperfecta and related osteochondrodysplasias: medical and surgical management of basilar impression. Childs Nerv Syst 24(10):1169–1172

Menezes AH, Greenlee JD, Donovan KA (2005) Honored guest presentation: lifetime experiences and where we are going: Chiari I with syringohydromyelia – controversies and development of decision trees. Clin Neurosurg 52:297–305

Mikulis DJ, Diaz O, Egglin TK et al (1992) Variance of the position of the cerebellar tonsils with age: preliminary report. Radiology 183(3):725–728

Milhorat TH, Bolognese PA (2003) Tailored operative technique for Chiari type I malformation using intraoperative color Doppler ultrasonography. Neurosurgery 53(4):899–905; discussion 905–906

Milhorat TH, Kotzen RM, Mu HT et al (1996) Dysesthetic pain in patients with syringomyelia. Neurosurgery 38(5):940–946; discussion 946–947

Milhorat TH, Chou MW, Trinidad EM et al (1999) Chiari I malformation redefined: clinical and radiographic findings for 364 symptomatic patients. Neurosurgery 44(5):1005–1017

Mottolese C, Szathmari A, Simon E et al (2011) Treatment of Chiari type I malformation in children: the experience of Lyon. Neurol Sci 32(Suppl 3):S325–S330

Munshi I, Frim D, Stine-Reyes R et al (2000) Effects of posterior fossa decompression with and without duraplasty on Chiari malformation-associated hydro-myelia. Neurosurgery 46(6):1384–1389; discussion 1389–1390

Murano T, Rella J (2006) Incidental finding of Chiari I malformation with progression of symptoms after head trauma: case report. J Emerg Med 30(3):295–298

Mutchnick IS, Janjua RM, Moeller K et al (2010) Decompression of Chiari malformation with and without duraplasty: morbidity versus recurrence. J Neurosurg Pediatr 5(5):474–478

Navarro R, Olavarria G, Seshadri R et al (2004) Surgical results of posterior fossa decompression for patients with Chiari I malformation. Childs Nerv Syst 20(5): 349–356

Nishikawa M, Sakamoto H, Hakuba A, Nakanishi N, Inoue Y (1997) Pathogenesis of Chiari malformation: a morphometric study of the posterior cranial fossa. J Neurosurg 86(1):40–47

Nyland H, Krogness KG (1978) Size of posterior fossa in Chiari type 1 malformation in adults. Acta Neurochir (Wien) 40(3–4):233–242

Panigrahi M, Reddy BP, Reddy AK et al (2004) CSF flow study in Chiari I malformation. Childs Nerv Syst 20(5):336–340

Pare LS, Batzdorf U (1998) Syringomyelia persistence after Chiari decompression as a result of pseudomeningocele formation: implications for syrinx pathogenesis: report of three cases. Neurosurgery 43(4):945–948

Parker SR, Harris P, Cummings TJ et al (2011) Complications following decompression of Chiari malformation Type I in children: dural graft or sealant? J Neurosurg Pediatr 8(2):177–183

Payner TD, Prenger E, Berger TS et al (1994) Acquired Chiari malformations: incidence, diagnosis, and management. Neurosurgery 34(3):429–434; discussion 434

Pollack IF, Pang D, Albright AL et al (1992) Outcome following hindbrain decompression of symptomatic Chiari malformations in children previously treated with myelomeningocele closure and shunts. J Neurosurg 77(6):881–888

Pollack IF, Kinnunen D, Albright AL (1996) The effect of early craniocervical decompression on functional outcome in neonates and young infants with myelodysplasia and symptomatic Chiari II malformations: results from a prospective series. Neurosurgery 38(4):703–710; discussion 710

Rahman M, Perkins LA, Pincus DW (2009) Aggressive surgical management of patients with Chiari II malformation and brainstem dysfunction. Pediatr Neurosurg 45(5):337–344

Rauzzino M, Oakes WJ (1995) Chiari II malformation and syringomyelia. Neurosurg Clin N Am 6(2):293–309

Rosen DS, Wollman R, Frim DM (2003) Recurrence of symptoms after Chiari decompression and duraplasty with nonautologous graft material. Pediatr Neurosurg 38(4):186–190

Sacco D, Scott RM (2003) Reoperation for Chiari malformations. Pediatr Neurosurg 39(4):171–178

Sakamoto H, Nishikawa M, Hakuba A et al (1999) Expansive suboccipital cranioplasty for the treatment of syringomyelia associated with Chiari malformation. Acta Neurochir (Wien) 141(9):949–960; discussion 960–961

Schijman E, Steinbok P (2004) International survey on the management of Chiari I malformation and syringomyelia. Childs Nerv Syst 20(5):341–348

Sindou M, Gimbert E (2009) Decompression for Chiari type I-malformation (with or without syringomyelia) by extreme lateral foramen magnum opening and expansile duraplasty with arachnoid preservation: comparison with other technical modalities (Literature review). Adv Tech Stand Neurosurg 34:85–110

Sindou M, Chavez-Machuca J, Hashish H (2002) Craniocervical decompression for Chiari type I-malformation, adding extreme lateral foramen magnum opening and expansile duroplasty with arachnoid preservation. Technique and long-term functional results in 44 consecutive adult cases – comparison with literature dat. Acta Neurochir (Wien) 144(10):1005–1019

Smith JS, Shaffrey CI, Abel MF et al (2010) Basilar invagination. Neurosurgery 66(3 Suppl):39–47

Spena G, Bernucci C, Garbossa D et al (2010) Clinical and radiological outcome of craniocervical osteo-dural decompression for Chiari I-associated syringomyelia. Neurosurg Rev 33(3):297–303; discussion 303–304

Stephany JD, Garavaglia JC, Pearl GS (2008) Sudden death in a 27-year-old man with Chiari I malformation. Am J Forensic Med Pathol 29(3):249–250

Stovner LJ, Bergan U, Nilsen G, Sjaastad O (1993) Posterior cranial fossa dimensions in the Chiari I malformation: relation to pathogenesis and clinical presentation. Neuroradiology 35(2):113–118

Suzuki F, Kitagawa T, Takagi K et al (2011) Subacute subdural hygroma and presyrinx formation after foramen magnum decompression with duraplasty for Chiari type 1 malformation. Neurol Med Chir (Tokyo) 51(5):389–393

Takeuchi K, Yokoyama T, Ito J et al (2007) Tonsillar herniation and the cervical spine: a morphometric study of 172 patients. J Orthop Sci 12(1):55–60

Talamonti G, Zella S (2011) Surgical treatment of CM2 and syringomyelia in a series of 231 myelomeningocele patients. Neurol Sci 32(Suppl 3):S331–S333

Teo C, Parker EC, Aureli S et al (1997) The Chiari II malformation: a surgical series. Pediatr Neurosurg 27(5):223–229

Trigylidas T, Baronia B, Vassilyadi M, Ventureyra EC (2008) Posterior fossa dimension and volume estimates in pediatric patients with Chiari I malformations. Childs Nerv Syst 24(3):329–336

Tubbs RS, Oakes WJ (2004) Treatment and management of the Chiari II malformation: an evidence-based review of the literature. Childs Nerv Syst 20(6):375–381

Tubbs RS, McGirt MJ, Oakes WJ (2003) Surgical experience in 130 pediatric patients with Chiari I malformations. J Neurosurg 99(2):291–296

Tubbs RS, Lyerly MJ, Loukas M et al (2007) The pediatric Chiari I malformation: a review. Childs Nerv Syst 23(11):1239–1250

Tubbs RS, Beckman J, Naftel RP et al (2011) Institutional experience with 500 cases of surgically treated pediatric Chiari malformation Type I. J Neurosurg Pediatr 7(3):248–256

Tulipan N, Hernanz-Schulman M, Lowe LH et al (1999) Intrauterine myelomeningocele repair reverses preexisting hindbrain herniation. Pediatr Neurosurg 31(3):137–142

Valentini L, Visintini S, Saletti V et al (2011) Treatment for Chiari 1 malformation (CIM): analysis of a pediatric surgical series. Neurol Sci 32(Suppl 3):S321–S324

Vanaclocha V, Saiz-Sapena N (1997) Duraplasty with freeze-dried cadaveric dura versus occipital pericranium for Chiari type I malformation: comparative study. Acta Neurochir (Wien) 139(2):112–119

Vandertop WP, Asai A, Hoffman HJ et al (1992) Surgical decompression for symptomatic Chiari II malformation in neonates with myelomeningocele. J Neurosurg 77(4):541–544

Wetjen NM, Heiss JD, Oldfield EH (2008) Time course of syringomyelia resolution following decompression of Chiari malformation Type I. J Neurosurg Pediatr 1(2):118–123

Williams B (1977) Difficult labour as a cause of communicating syringomyelia. Lancet 2(8028):51–53

Williams B (1978) A critical appraisal of posterior fossa surgery for communicating syringomyelia. Brain 101(2):223–250

Williams B (1994) A blast against grafts. Br J Neurosurg 8(3):275–278

Wolf DA, Veasey SP 3rd, Wilson SK et al (1998) Death following minor head trauma in two adult individuals with the Chiari I deformity. J Forensic Sci 43(6):1241–1243

Yanni DS, Mammis A, Ebersole K et al (2010) Revision of Chiari decompression for patients with recurrent syrinx. J Clin Neurosci 17(8):1076–1079

Yarbrough CK, Powers AK, Park TS et al (2011) Patients with Chiari malformation Type I presenting with acute neurological deficits: case series. J Neurosurg Pediatr 7(3):244–247

Yilmaz A, Kanat A, Musluman AM et al (2011) When is duraplasty required in the surgical treatment of Chiari malformation type I based on tonsillar descending grading scale? World Neurosurg 75(2):307–313

Yoshikawa H (2003) Sudden respiratory arrest and Arnold-Chiari malformation. Eur J Paediatr Neurol 7(4):191

Zerah M (1999) Syringomyelia in children. Neurochirurgie 45(Suppl 1):37–57

Zhang ZQ, Chen YQ, Chen YA et al (2008) Chiari I malformation associated with syringomyelia: a retrospective study of 316 surgically treated patients. Spinal Cord 46(5):358–363

Zhang Y, Zhang N, Qiu H et al (2011) An efficacy analysis of posterior fossa decompression techniques in the treatment of Chiari malformation with associated syringomyelia. J Clin Neurosci 18(10):1346–1349

Post-traumatic and Post-inflammatory Syringomyelia

11

Graham Flint

Contents

G. Flint
Department of Neurosurgery,
Queen Elizabeth Hospital,
University Hospitals Birmingham,
Birmingham, UK
e-mail: graham.flint@uhb.nhs.uk

11.1   Introduction

Most cases of syringomyelia resulting from pathology at the craniovertebral junction are not associated with a significant amount of local scar tissue formation. In contrast, the majority of cases of syringomyelia caused by obstruction elsewhere in the spinal canal have, as the primary underlying pathology, cicatrix within the leptomeninges. This condition is often referred to as arachnoiditis, but this is something of a misnomer because, when operating upon such conditions, we do not encounter active inflammation. Rather, we see mature scar tissue, which is the end result of an earlier inflammatory process.

The most common initiator of scar tissue formation is blood shed into the subarachnoid channels. Organisation of blood clot into scar tissue, anywhere in the body, is part of the normal healing process, but it can lead to problems when excessive adhesions form, be they in the peritoneal cavity, around a lumbar nerve root or within the spinal theca. The density and extent of this scar tissue varies, according to the underlying cause. In the spinal canal, causes include subarachnoid haemorrhage, from intracranial or intraspinal sources, intradural surgery and spinal trauma. The latter need not be particularly severe or even associated with spinal cord injury.

The second important cause of inflammation, with subsequent scar tissue formation, is infection, be this pyogenic, tuberculous or due to other microorganisms. A third cause, now only seen occasionally, is chemically induced meningitis,

G. Flint, C. Rusbridge (eds.), *Syringomyelia*,
DOI 10.1007/978-3-642-13706-8_11, © Springer-Verlag Berlin Heidelberg 2014

caused by radiographic contrast media. Finally, we sometimes encounter thin arachnoid webs, the origin of which is not always clear. Some may be congenital in origin, but others may have resulted from undiagnosed episodes of leptomeningeal inflammation, earlier in life.

What we do not know is just how frequently arachnoid scarring leads to the formation of syrinx cavities and how often such scar tissue exists without an associated syringomyelia. Neurosurgeons are unlikely to explore a cicatrised spinal canal in the absence of associated cord cavitation, so operative experience cannot answer these questions. Experience with spinal cord injuries suggests that syrinx cavities are generated in only a minority of cases, albeit not insignificant in number (see below). If we then assume that the various pathologies mentioned above will always be associated with some scar tissue formation, we must ask ourselves what other factors determine just when a syrinx will form.

There are other noninflammatory pathologies within the spinal canal, which can lead to syrinx formation. These include intramedullary tumours and dysraphic abnormalities, but this chapter is concerned with those post-arachnoiditic conditions that lead to syringomyelia. Idiopathic syringomyelia is also dealt with in a separate chapter, as is syringomyelia caused by fibrosis at the craniovertebral junction.

The filling mechanism underlying the formation of syringomyelia cavities is discussed in detail in Chap. 6. Suffice it to say here that the normal movement of CSF throughout the spinal canal depends upon there being an uninterrupted column of fluid, outside the cord, along the entire length of the spine. Interruption of this column results in abnormal dissipation of arterial and venous pressure waves, which pass up and down the spinal canal, with the result that fluid accumulates within the cord itself.

11.2 Post-traumatic Syringomyelia

This is the most commonly encountered variety of post-inflammatory syringomyelia (Fig. 11.1) although other forms share much in common with it, as regards pathogenesis and treatment

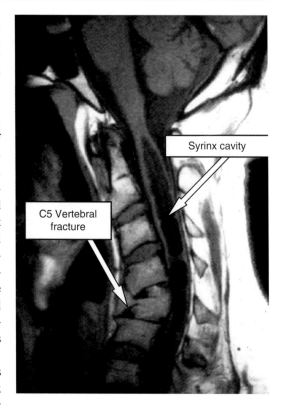

Fig. 11.1 Typical MR appearances of post-traumatic syringomyelia (Reproduced with kind permission of the Ann Conroy Trust)

options. It is generally assumed that post-traumatic syringomyelia cavities originate from local ischemic changes within the cord. Consequently, they are thought to represent "extracanalicular" syrinxes, rather than "hydromyelic" dilatations of the central canal (Milhorat et al. 1995a, b), although some histological studies suggest that post-traumatic syrinx cavities may not be entirely extracanalicular in origin (Reddy et al. 1989; Squier and Lehr 1994).

It is important to distinguish primary, post-traumatic cysts from true syringomyelia cavities. The former are more common and are seen on magnetic resonance imaging (MRI) scans in half of all spinal cord injury victims (Backe et al. 1991). They are the result of primary damage to the cord and are located at the level of the original injury. They are usually small and rounded or ovoid and do not produce a great deal in the way of cord expansion (Perrouin-Verbe et al. 1998). Post-traumatic syringomyelia, on the other hand, refers to propagating cavities, extending beyond the level of the original trauma. These develop as a secondary, delayed consequence of the original injury.

Post-traumatic syringomyelia is important in two respects. Whereas syringomyelia remains an uncommon condition in the community as a whole, it is very common in the population of spinal cord injury victims. Quoted figures vary, but even early estimates of about 5 % represent a significant incidence, more even than common medical disorders such as diabetes or asthma. Later publications give figures that are higher still, at around 20 %. These are based on both radiological surveys (Perrouin-Verbe et al. 1998; Squier and Lehr 1994; Wang et al. 1996) and post-mortem studies (Squier and Lehr 1994). The differences in these figures reflect the fact that earlier estimates were derived when MR imaging was carried out selectively, as indicated by the onset of new neurological symptoms (El Masry and Biyani 1996). The higher estimates also depend upon a definition of syrinx cavities as being those that extend two or more segments beyond the level of the original injury. If the definition stipulated three segments, then the incidence would fall back to single figures (Pearce 1995). A reasonable working rule, therefore, would be to say that up to one in five of all spinal cord injury victims develop anatomical syringomyelia and that at least 1 in 20 will develop symptoms.

The second point to note is that most victims of spinal cord injury already have to contend, in their day-to-day life, with significant neurological disability. The devastating transformation that spinal cord injury brings about in somebody's life is very apparent, and it is a cruel irony when the development of a post-traumatic syringomyelia cavity threatens the individual with further loss of independence. Yet most patients cope remarkably well, albeit requiring a good deal of support. They are often the least complaining of all the patients who come to our clinics. Few conditions in neurosurgery challenge our skills, as surgeons and as doctors, to the same extent.

11.2.1 Presentation

Most spinal cord injury patients living in economically privileged societies are currently offered regular surveillance of their neurological

Table 11.1 Common presenting features of post-traumatic syringomyelia

Symptoms
Increasing pain
Hyperhidrosis[a]
Increasing spasms
Loss of sensation
Loss of trunk control
Reduced dexterity
Altered bladder function
Autonomic dysreflexia
Signs
Ascending sensory level
Focal motor deficits
Loss of upper limb reflexes
Horner's syndrome

[a]Glasauer and Czyrny (1994), Stanworth (1982)

and general status. Their supervising units have a low threshold for carrying out MR imaging if problems develop. Indeed, there is a case for offering routine screening for all victims of spinal cord injury, looking specifically for post-traumatic syringomyelia (Sett and Crockard 1991). Syrinx cavities are now being detected with increasing frequency, often in patients with little in the way of new neurological symptoms.

Many patients do display clear indications of having developed a complication of their original spinal cord injury (Table 11.1). In most published series, pain is at the top of the list of presenting symptoms. The differential diagnosis of the symptoms of post-traumatic syringomyelia includes constipation, pressure sores and urinary tract infections, causing sweating attacks and spasms, and ulnar nerve palsies resulting from repeated pressure being placed on the elbows, during transfers. As with all forms of syringomyelia, there is a poor correlation between the size of the cavity and the magnitude of the clinical features.

An impressive feature of post-traumatic syringomyelia is the wide variation in the latent interval between the original spinal cord injury and the first onset of symptoms arising from the syrinx. The range extends from a few months to several decades. Attempts have been made to predict which spinal cord victims might go on to develop post-traumatic syringomyelia, and although individual studies have pointed to one factor or another (Table 11.2), there are currently

Table 11.2 Possible predictors of development of post-traumatic syringomyelia

Level	Cervical vs dorsal spine
Severity	Complete vs incomplete functional transection
	Displaced vs undisplaced fracture
Age	Older vs younger patients
Management	Conservative vs surgical management
	Fixation with or without bony decompression
References	Brodbelt and Stoodley (2003a), El Masry and Biyani (1996), Klekamp and Samii (2002), Levy et al. (1991), Vannemreddy et al. (2002)

For each proposed indicator listed here, the item underlined has been proposed as a possible indicator of increased likelihood of a spinal cord injury victim going on to develop post-traumatic syringomyelia

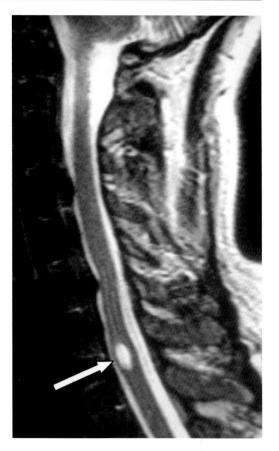

Fig. 11.2 Short, spindle-shaped cavity (*arrow*). Revealed during the course of investigation for pain and somatic sensory disturbances, following minor trauma, this could represent a small, post-traumatic syrinx or a pre-existing glioependymal cyst, rendered symptomatic by the injury

no reliable predictors. Lifelong surveillance remains the only safe option.

The generation of symptoms and neurological deficits probably relates, in part at least, to hydraulic pressure within the syrinx, leading to local ischemia, as well as stretching of decussating fibres and long tracts (Milhorat et al. 1997; Young et al. 2000). The magnitude and duration of raised pressure may account for whether or not these clinical features are reversible. Another mechanism is tethering, leading to traction on the cord during normal movement of the spinal column. Release of tethering may, in some cases, be at least as important as collapse of the syrinx, when it comes to gaining some clinical improvement (Ragnarsson et al. 1986). It has also been suggested that leptomeningeal fibrosis may lead to cord ischemia, but it is difficult to substantiate or refute such suggestions.

11.2.2 Syringomyelia Following Minor Trauma

A particular category of lesions is that of cavities detected following relatively minor injuries, such as whiplash or a fall. Victims may complain, often after an interval, of a variety of neurological symptoms, yet there may be no accompanying physical signs. MR imaging is carried out, sooner or later, and the sort of lesion revealed may consist of a short, spindle-shaped intramedullary cavity, without any associated abnormality at the craniovertebral junction and without any obvious obstruction elsewhere in the spinal canal (Fig. 11.2). Not uncommonly, medicolegal experts become involved and discussions centre on whether the cyst was caused by the accident or was pre-existing. Questions arise as to whether it is a true syrinx or something else, such as a glioependymal cyst. The latter are well documented as intracranial lesions but also occur within the spinal cord. Radiologically, they are usually short but relatively plump in size, being quite well defined but not enhancing with contrast injection

(Robertson et al. 1991; Saito et al. 2005). Legal debate continues as to whether, irrespective of its nature, the cavity was rendered symptomatic by the injury or was simply an incidental finding, having nothing to do with the claimant's symptoms. Onset of symptoms immediately after the injury suggests a pre-existing cavity, rendered symptomatic by the event. Delayed onset suggests that the cavity was caused by the trauma (Barnett 1973). To declare that the presence of a syrinx bears no relationship to a prior injury, or to suggest that neurological symptoms do not arise from the lesion, ignores the temporal association between the injury and detection of the syrinx. This legal issues are discussed in more detail in Chap. 18, but it is fair to say that there is little in the literature to guide an expert witness, beyond the fact that any series of post-traumatic syringomyelia cases may well include a significant number where the initial trauma was moderate and where no neurological deficits were evident at the time (Klekamp and Samii 2002; LaHaye and Batzdorf 1988).

11.3 Subarachnoid Haemorrhage

Relative to the overall incidence of subarachnoid haemorrhage, the occurrence of spinal arachnoid adhesions, as a complication, is low (Augustijn et al. 1989; Tjandra et al. 1989). The incidence of syrinx formation, as a further sequel, is distinctly rare, although cavities can develop following both intracranial and intraspinal subarachnoid haemorrhage (Siddiqi et al. 2005). What determines why and when this complication occurs is unknown. It may be that, if a patient remains recumbent for any period, after a subarachnoid haemorrhage, blood products pool on the spinal canal.

Clearly, any intradural surgical procedure carried out on the spine will result in some blood and tissue products being shed into the canal. This can result in formation of arachnoid adhesions, potentially resulting in syringomyelia. Once again, such complications are rare (Cusick and Bernardi 1995; Klekamp et al. 1997).

11.4 Contrast Media

Prior to the advent of MR scanning, the principal means of investigating the spinal canal and its contents was by myelography. Originally, this involved the use of oil-based contrast media although, subsequently, water-soluble agents were developed. Once injected into the spinal canal, this oily material would not be absorbed, and in some cases, an arachnoiditic reaction followed. Once these effects were recognised, it became the normal practice to aspirate as much of the contrast medium as possible, after the radiological study was completed. Some patients, nevertheless, developed meningeal fibrosis, with disabling consequences. A curious aspect of the problem was why only a minority of people developed this complication. One suggestion was that the inflammatory response depended upon a synergistic reaction between the contrast medium and something else, such as blood or even powder from surgical gloves.

Although largely a matter of historical interest these days, newly diagnosed cases of syringomyelia still present, occasionally, in somebody who underwent myelography, with an oil-based contrast medium, many years ago (Tabor and Batzdorf 1996).

11.5 Post-tuberculous Syringomyelia

Spinal cord involvement is a recognised complication of tuberculosis, and as with tuberculosis anywhere in the nervous system, different pathological manifestations are seen. These include acute inflammation and oedema of the cord, intramedullary abscesses and intramedullary or intradural granuloma formation (Muthukumar and Sureshkumar 2007). The most common consequence, however, is late adhesive arachnoiditis. Despite this, syringomyelia is a relatively uncommon sequel. Even surgeons who deal with a lot of cases of syringomyelia are unlikely to see many tuberculosis-related syrinxes, and most reports in the literature relate to no more than a handful of patients (Kaynar et al. 2000; Moghtaderi et al. 2006; Schon and Bowler 1990).

Most cases present at an interval, after the underlying infection has been treated. As with post-traumatic syringomyelia, this latent interval can vary widely from case to case. Early presentation has also been described and the assumption is that acute cord inflammation is the underlying mechanism rather than arachnoid adhesions (Daif et al. 1997; Fehlings and Bernstein 1992).

Post-tuberculous adhesions are likely to be extensive, making the creation of a conduit all but impossible in most cases. It is in this type of syringomyelia that direct shunting may be a preferred option.

11.6   Other Infections

Syringomyelia is also recognised as an occasional complication of other infections involving the spinal cord. Organisms which have been reported include Listeria (Nardone et al. 2003), Cryptococcus (McLone and Siqueira 1976), Syphilis (Bulundwe et al. 2000; Mebrouk et al. 2011) and Candida (Phanthumchinda and Kaoropthum 1991). Syringomyelia is also occasionally seen in association with previous epidural inflammatory pathology (Klekamp et al. 1997). All these examples are much less common than post-tuberculous cases. It should, nevertheless, be part of the routine history taking, in all cases of syringomyelia where the cause is not immediately apparent, to enquire about a past history of meningitis, spinal trauma, head injury and subarachnoid haemorrhage.

11.7   Arachnoid Webs and Cysts

When we consider what might happen as a consequence of obstruction to CSF flow within the spinal canal, we might reasonably predict a build-up of fluid on the outside of the cord rather than the more usual finding of syrinx formation. Indeed, we do sometimes see such external, "hydraulic compression" of the cord, in association with arachnoid webs (Fig. 11.3). Such webs, as well as cysts (or pouches), may be congenital lesions or may arise as the result of earlier haemorrhage (Thines et al. 2005) or arachnoiditis from other causes (Gnanalingham et al. 2006; Gopalakrishnan et al. 2010). The obstruction caused by such webs may also result in syrinx formation (Mallucci et al. 1997). The likely mechanism, once again, is that normal arterial and venous pressure waves are not dissipated normally down the spinal canal, leading to creation of the syrinx cavity (Brodbelt and Stoodley 2003a, b; Holly and Batzdorf 2006). The syrinx is the more obvious abnormality on imaging and a careful search should be made to identify the web. Indeed, there may be occasions when it is only revealed at the time of surgical exploration.

When an operation is planned, the surgeon must realise that the lesion might be an arachnoid cyst rather than a simple web. The myelopathy, be this due to the pressure within the cyst or from a resulting syrinx, might not be relieved unless both the upper and lower limits of the cyst are broached.

11.8   Surgical Management

Compared with operations for hindbrain-related syringomyelia, surgery for cavities caused by spinal arachnoid fibrosis does not yield results that are as good overall. Indeed, this category of syringomyelia is one of the most difficult conditions that neurosurgeons are called upon to treat, at least in terms of gaining consistent results. It is not surprising, therefore, that various techniques have been described over the years (Edgar and Quail 1994). Further, not all syrinx cavities progress relentlessly (Anderson et al. 1986) and it is certainly the author's experience that many seem to enter a state of "hydrodynamic equilibrium" (see also Chap. 2). For all these reasons, surgical intervention should be reserved for those cases that show clear evidence of neurological deterioration. Not surprisingly, most published series include significant numbers of patients who do not go on to surgical intervention.

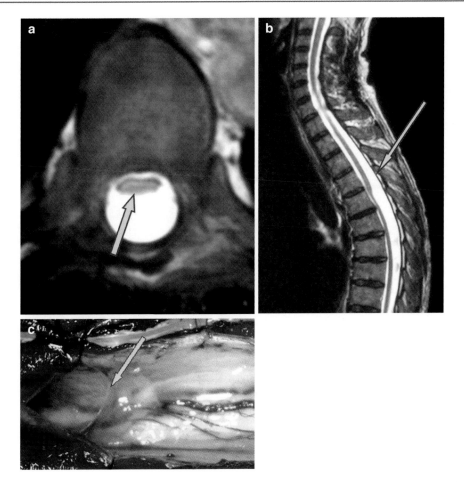

Fig. 11.3 Spinal arachnoid webs. (**a**) T2-weighted MRI, transverse section: the cord is clearly compressed flat, in the anterior half of the spinal canal (*arrow*). (**b**) T2-weighted sagittal MRI: the same feature is evident in the sagittal plane, where the level of the focal point of obstruction to CSF flow is very evident (*arrow*). (**c**) Operative appearances of the lesion. With the dura opened, a free edge forms along the dorsal aspect of the web (*arrow*). Extending anterior to this can be seen the thin membrane, which occupies the full cross-sectional area of the thecal sac

Table 11.3 Treatment options

| Creation of a conduit for CSF flow |
| Direct drainage of the syrinx cavity |
| Lowering the overall CSF pressure |
| Conservative management |

11.8.1 Creation of a CSF Conduit

There are, broadly speaking, three types of surgical manoeuvre that we can offer to a patient with syringomyelia (Table 11.3). Clearly, it makes sense to treat the underlying cause if possible. So, when we can identify a focal point of obstruction to CSF movement, the logical approach is to try and relieve that blockage and create a new conduit for CSF flow. This is, of course, a major operation, involving the removal of several laminae, and it requires microsurgical technique for the intradural part of the procedure. In most cases of post-traumatic syringomyelia, the scar tissue encountered is relatively limited in extent, and breaking it down is not unduly difficult. The offending cicatrix is clearly recognisable by its typical milky-white appearance and can be readily distinguished from normal, translucent arachnoid. Dissection dorsal and dorsolateral to the cord

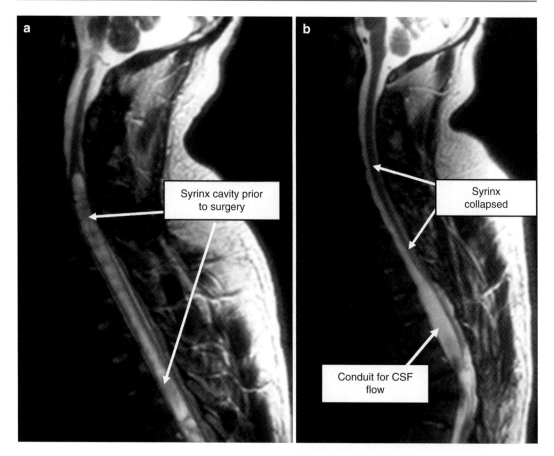

Fig. 11.4 Effective surgery for post-traumatic syringomyelia. Laminectomy, with release of intradural adhesions and creation of an artificial conduit for CSF flow, can produce very rewarding anatomical results, with arrest of clinical deterioration and sometimes recovery of lost function. (**a**) Prior to surgery. (**b**) Following laminectomy, release of scar tissue and creation of pseudomeningocoele, to act as an artificial conduit for CSF flow

will eventually result in it falling anteriorly, into the spinal canal. At this point, the syrinx has usually collapsed and the cord may begin to pulsate. It is unnecessarily hazardous for the dissection to be carried anteriorly, although opinions vary as to the value of dividing dentate ligaments. The exposure also needs to be of sufficient length to allow free, rhythmic movement of CSF, up and down the spinal canal.

The anatomical results from this sort of surgery can be very satisfying (Fig. 11.4). The problem is that blood products and muscle proteins, which are inevitably "spilt" into the laminectomy site, may go on to organise into scar tissue once more, and this leads to recurrent obstruction of the spinal subarachnoid channels (Fig. 11.5). Early postoperative imaging is, therefore, of

limited value; it is very likely to show a reduction in the volume of the syrinx, but this by no means guarantees long-term anatomical improvement. If, however, the cavity remains collapsed at 6 months and beyond, then it is likely that a good result will have been achieved in the long term, in anatomical terms at least and probably in terms of function as well.

How the dura is handled is likely to have a major influence on the success or otherwise of this operation. With craniovertebral decompression for hindbrain-related syringomyelia, we have discussions about dural opening – full, partial or not at all – reduction or excision of cerebellar tonsils, use of dural grafts and the role of cranioplasty. We have similar debates about the best methods of exposure and closure, when it

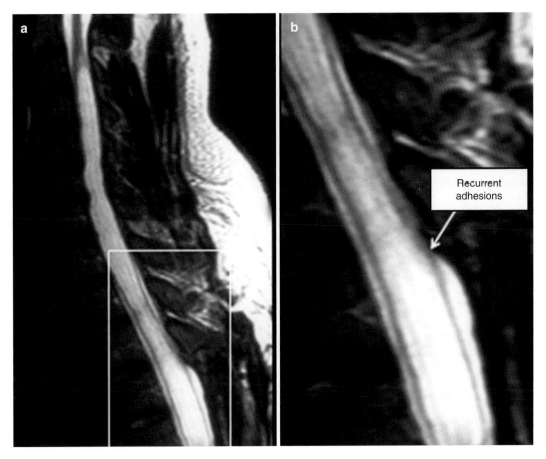

Fig. 11.5 Recurrence of syringomyelia after laminectomy. (**a**) Despite the initial operative creation of a good conduit for CSF flow, the syrinx cavity has refilled after an interval. (**b**) The *enlarged inset* from "a" reveals that recurrent adhesions at the upper aspect of the laminectomy have once again obstructed normal CSF flow

comes to operating for post-arachnoiditic syringomyelia. Dural patch grafts might be expected to limit the amount of blood and muscle products entering the spinal theca, from the surrounding tissue planes. This, we might expect, would lessen the amount of postoperative scar tissue formation. Many surgeons therefore feel more comfortable reconstituting the thecal sac, usually augmenting its volume at the same time by suturing in place a patch graft. Autografts are readily obtained from nearby muscle fascia, but synthetic materials are now preferred by most surgeons, mainly because they provoke less in the way of postoperative adhesions. The risk, however, with any form of patch graft, is that CSF may leak around its edges and collect extradurally. This may lead to a build-up of hydrostatic pressure,

which pushes the graft onto the cord. This can encourage adhesions to develop between the graft and the cord. This constricting effect becomes more pronounced as healing progresses and defeats the object of opening up CSF channels in the first place. The resultant obstruction to CSF flow may be worse than preoperatively, leading to refilling of the syrinx. Many surgeons therefore make a point of hitching the dural patch graft upwards, to try to prevent such adhesions forming. The author's preference has been to leave the dura widely open, using lateral retaining sutures. With a good closure of the long paraspinal muscles, a pseudomeningocoele forms between the short muscles and this provides a conduit for CSF flow. It is important to pay close attention to the cranial and caudal aspects of the thecal opening,

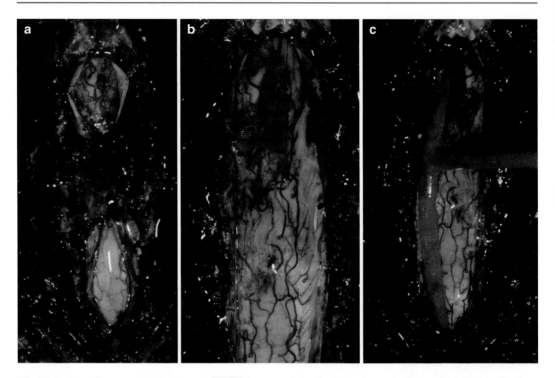

Fig. 11.6 Operative exposure of post-traumatic syringomyelia. (**a**) Initial dural opening, above and below the level of intradural fibrosis. Note the relative anaemia of the cord in the lower part of the exposure, caused by tension within the syrinx cavity. (**b**) Following completion of the dural opening and release of arachnoid adhesions. The syrinx has collapsed and the cord is now better perfused. (**c**) Optional placement of a soft tube, to allow drainage of blood-stained CSF, for 48 h after surgery

taking care to suture up the dura under the laminae at the upper and lower aspects of the exposure, to ensure that adhesions do not form at these sites. Leaving the dura open also provides an opportunity for placement of temporary subdural stents or drains (Williams and Page 1987). A soft drainage tube, left in place for no more than 48 h, not only serves as a stent but also allows CSF to "auto-irrigate" the subarachnoid channels and drain blood products away (Fig. 11.6). One study did note, however, a higher syrinx recurrence rate if the dura was left open in this way, although the difference between the two groups did not reach statistical significance (Klekamp et al. 1997).

11.8.2 Direct Syrinx Drainage

If the attempt to create a conduit fails, or is not suitable for some other reason, then the option of draining the syrinx is available. Indeed, this was a principal means of treatment for some years,

and results were considered to be reasonable (Tator et al. 1982; Williams and Page 1987). About half of the patients treated by direct drainage of the syrinx will obtain useful relief (Batzdorf et al. 1998; Sgouros and Williams 1995). The method, however, has a number of drawbacks. In the first place, a myelotomy is required, with an incision through the dorsal columns. Some loss of proprioception is almost inevitable, and this is often more disabling for patients than one might expect, despite the individual retaining good motor power. Further, septa within larger syrinx cavities may obstruct passage of the shunt tubing. The concern then is that the cavity will not drain adequately although, in truth, this is not always a problem. The main difficulty with syrinx drainage tubes is that, in common with all shunt systems, there is a distinct likelihood that they will eventually block. Even if a shunt continues to function and the syrinx remains collapsed, there is a chance that a new cavity may form alongside, simply because the

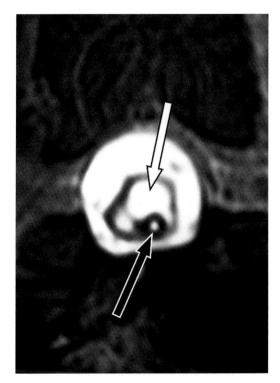

Fig. 11.7 Formation of new syrinx cavity following insertion of a syringopleural shunt. This example shows a syrinx which was initially drained effectively, after placement of a syringo-peritoneal shunt (*black arrow*). Unfortunately, the return of symptoms at a later date heralded the formation of a new cavity (*white arrow*), indicating that the underlying filling mechanism had not been disabled by the surgery

Table 11.4 CSF receptacles for direct drainage of syrinx cavities

Pleural cavity
Peritoneal cavity
Spinal subarachnoid channels
Via shunt tubing
Cord transection
Terminal ventriculostomy

underlying filling mechanism has not been disabled (Fig. 11.7).

Direct drainage requires the surgeon to choose carefully the optimum site for insertion of the shunt tubing. Lower down the cord is preferable to higher up, provided that the conus is avoided. As to the circumferential point of entry, a myelotomy away from the median sulcus may be preferable because a midline incision risks damage to dorsal columns on both sides. If one leg is already affected more than the other, then it makes sense for the myelotomy to be placed on the same side. Appearances at surgery will, of course, have a major influence. If the syrinx presents under the pia at one location, with no intervening neural tissue, then this will be the preferred point of entry. As regards the size of catheter used, it might be supposed that bigger is better, but some surgeons prefer smaller catheters (Lohlein et al.

1990; Tator et al. 1982). Either way, it is sensible to anchor the tube to the pia, to prevent displacement.

Creation of a conduit and direct drainage may be combined. The exposure required to insert a drainage tube into a syrinx may well involve microdissection and arachnolysis, sufficient in its own right to create an adequate channel for CSF flow. Equally, a surgeon may elect to drain the syrinx as a supplementary manoeuvre to creating a conduit. Whereas the shunt may not function indefinitely, it may keep the syrinx cavity collapsed sufficiently long for the deep layers of the wound to heal, with the CSF channels remaining open. Thus, the planned primary procedure may have been different in each case but the end result is the same.

Several "receptacles" are available to receive the contents of a drained syrinx cavity (Table 11.4). We cannot be dogmatic as regards whether to use the peritoneum, the pleura or the spinal subarachnoid channels. The latter are preferred by many and are often the easiest to access. A syringo-subarachnoid shunt may certainly function adequately in a case with localised fibrosis, but with more extensive fibrosis, such as seen with postinfective syringomyelia, an extra-spinal receptacle may be better. The pleural cavity is convenient when operating with the patient in the prone position, but some surgeons prefer the peritoneum, on the basis that absorption is probably more reliable in the long term. A dual system of drainage can sometimes be effected by bringing the tubing out from the syrinx and along the spinal subarachnoid channels, with side holes cut in this section, before routing the distal end to its extra-spinal receptacle (Brodbelt and Stoodley 2003a, b). A potential drawback is development of low-pressure headaches, necessitating the subsequent placement of an anti-siphon device.

It is worth remembering that syringo-subarachnoid drainage can also be achieved by cord transection and terminal ventriculostomy. The former manoeuvre sounds rather drastic, especially when explained to patients. Many spinal cord injury victims understandably hold on to hopes that techniques for inducing spinal cord regeneration may be developed in their lifetime. Whilst, however, there is little prospect of such advancements in treatment, it would be wrong to leave a completely paraplegic individual to develop progressive upper limb motor and sensory deficits, for the sake of a procedure which could both drain the syrinx and untether the cord, with beneficial results (Durward et al. 1982; Ewelt et al. 2010; Kasai et al. 2008; Laxton and Perrin 2006). Terminal ventriculostomy may be an option in those occasional cases where the syrinx passes right down to the tip of the conus (Williams and Fahy 1983).

Finally, it is worth noting that percutaneous drainage of a syrinx cavity is perfectly feasible, as a test of whether or not a patient's symptoms might respond to surgery. Relief of symptoms may last for several months and the method may therefore have therapeutic value, in those considered unsuitable for surgery (Levy et al. 1991; Sudheendra and Bartynski 2008).

11.8.3 Lowering CSF Pressure

The third surgical option is to lower the pressure throughout the CSF pathways as a whole, using a theco-peritoneal shunt (Bret et al. 1986; Vassilouthis et al. 1994; Vengsarkar et al. 1991). This strategy may be adopted when the other methods cannot be carried out or fail in the first place. If there is hydrocephalus associated with the syringomyelia, then shunting of the ventricles is the more appropriate first procedure. This may well lead to collapse of the syrinx as well, obviating the need for further procedures (McLone and Siqueira 1976).

Lowering CSF pressure is, for the most part, empirically based, but one can propose a reasonable theoretical explanation for any

response seen. A length of silastic tubing, inserted above the blockage in the spinal canal and fed round to the peritoneal cavity (a theco-peritoneal shunt), may reduce hydrostatic tension within the theca and lessen the magnitude of arterial and venous pressure waves within the enclosed column of CSF. The forces driving CSF into the syrinx will, as a result, be reduced. A similar shunt system but with the shunt tube placed below the obstruction may act differently, by inducing mass flow of interstitial water through the cord, leading to reduction in hydrostatic pressure within the syrinx. Lumboperitoneal shunts, inserted below the blockage, should normally take the form of an unvalved tube, in order to maximise the flow of interstitial fluid. Shunts placed above the blockage need a flow-regulating device, either terminal slit valves or apparatus designed to compensate for changes in posture.

Success rates are always likely to be limited with this form of treatment. Operative risks, however, are generally low, particularly with a lumboperitoneal shunt. This is a relatively minor procedure, not needing extensive laminectomy and not requiring myelotomy. About a third of patients treated with lumboperitoneal shunts are likely to improve, with reduction in syrinx size in some of cases (Oluigbo et al. 2010). This simple procedure may be suitable for frail patients, those who do not wish to undergo major surgery or those in whom a conduit or shunt has failed.

11.8.4 Omental Grafts

Based on its angiogenic properties and capacity to induce outgrowth of neurites in cell culture, vascularised omental pedicles have been used in an attempt to promote functional recovery in victims of spinal cord injury. Whilst radiographic changes may follow and some subjective improvements have been reported, objective evidence of any real value for this procedure is lacking (Clifton et al. 1996). The author's experience of reexploring one such case revealed an anaemic cord and extensive fibrosis, of a degree that could only increase the likelihood of syrinx formation.

11.8.5 Skeletal Stability and Alignment

Most patients with post-traumatic syringomyelia who come to surgery will long since have fused the skeletal elements in their spinal column. Concern about post-laminectomy instability is, therefore, usually unfounded, but if the vertebral injury has not healed adequately, it will obviously need to be managed appropriately. In such cases, a surgeon may prefer to achieve stability with a preliminary operation, prior to opening up the CSF channels posteriorly. This may well involve an anterior decompression and fusion, which raises the question as to whether correction of any extradural narrowing of the spinal canal could lead to decompression of the syrinx. It has been reported that syringomyelia may be more likely to develop if the diameter of the spinal canal is severely compromised by a bony injury (Perrouin-Verbe et al. 1998), and improvement in function has been recorded following anterior extradural decompression, although such procedures may need to be supplemented by posterior intradural surgery (Holly et al. 2000). This latter finding is not surprising, given that the pathology underlying post-traumatic syringomyelia consists of leptomeningeal fibrosis.

A related consideration is the role of surgery at the time of the original injury, in particular decompression and stabilisation of the vertebral column. Although of value in allowing early mobilisation of the patient, particularly when damage is confined to the skeletal elements of the spine, there are potential drawbacks when the cord is injured. In the early stages after injury, the spinal cord is in a very unstable physiological state. It is particularly vulnerable to falls in blood pressure that may accompany general anaesthesia or episodes of hypoxia and sepsis that may follow surgery. Further, any damage to the theca, occurring during surgery, may increase the likelihood of intradural adhesion formation and obstruction of the CSF pathways. Vertebral instability can almost always be handled, instead, by external forms of immobilisation. On the other hand, it is fair to argue that prolonged recumbency may lead to stasis of blood products shed into the spinal CSF channels, thereby increasing the chances of local scar tissue formation. The role of early surgical intervention, as a means of preventing the formation of post-traumatic syringomyelia, remains unclear (Bonfield et al. 2010).

11.8.6 Radiological Localisation

With most cases of post-traumatic syringomyelia, the level to target is obvious, being the site of the original injury, which in most cases will be marked by the bony injury. It is here that the cicatrix will be encountered, whether the syrinx cavity has since propagated in a cephalad direction, a caudal direction or both. In cases without bony injury, there may be MR features to guide the surgeon, such as focal compression or distortion of the cord. Constructive interference steady-state (CISS) or fast imaging employing steady-state acquisition (FIESTA) sequences may demonstrate an arachnoid web, which may not have been apparent on routine T2 sequences (Fig. 11.8). Cine MRI may reveal restricted CSF flow. When no such clues are present, then comparison of images taken at intervals may show progressive longitudinal enlargement of the syrinx. This will usually be in one direction, away from the point of obstruction to CSF flow, which will therefore be at the "static" end of the cavity (Klekamp and Samii 2002). This rule is not infallible, especially in cases that may have propagated in both directions by the time of initial diagnosis. Other clues are that cavities tend to be largest close to the site of obstruction and that turbulence may be seen inside the syrinx, close to its point of origin. Finally, there may be clinical clues, in the form of localising features noted at the time of the patient's initial presentation.

CT myelography may still have a role to play, if other investigations prove negative. With advances in MR technology, however, the likely additional yield from myelography is now quite low. The clinician may, therefore, reasonably declare "MR-negative" cases as being idiopathic

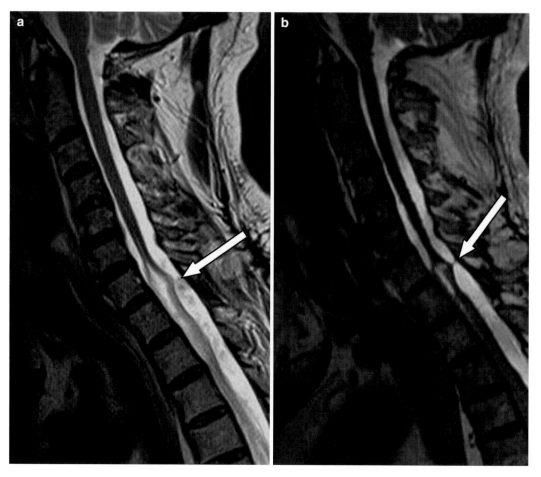

Fig. 11.8 The value of constructive interference steady-state (CISS) imaging. (**a**) Standard T2-weighted sagittal MRI shows turbulence in the CSF dorsal to the cord and oedema within the cord (*arrow*) but no clear underlying obstruction to CSF flow. (**b**) CISS sequences reveal an arachnoid web dorsal to the cord (*arrow*)

and manage them as such, by shunting the syrinx or lowering the overall CSF pressure. There may, occasionally, be a case for surgical exploration of a syringomyelia cavity, looking for a focal point of scar tissue formation, in the absence of prior radiological identification.

Finally, it is worth noting that intraoperative ultrasound may be a useful tool, to help locate the syrinx cavity, if it is not immediately obvious under the operating microscope (Aschoff et al. 1993; Lee et al. 2001; Schwartz et al. 1999).

11.8.7 Outcome and Prognosis

The natural history of syringomyelia in general is poorly defined. Deterioration is not inevitable in all cases. It would be reasonable to suggest that 50 % of patients experience functional decline and 50 % remain stable. Spontaneous collapse of a syrinx cavity is rare (Vinas et al. 2001) as is clinical progression to a state of quadriplegic helplessness, something which is feared by many patients. Post-arachnoiditic syringomyelia is probably no different in these respects, although sudden deterioration may occasionally follow episodes such as a bout of coughing or a period of straining (Balmaseda et al. 1988). Ageing will, of course, exacerbate the effects of any existing neurological disability, including any caused by syringomyelia.

Results following surgery for post-arachnoiditic syringomyelia are inconsistent and not all of the aims will be achieved (Table 11.5). Many patients may need to undergo more than one procedure (Klekamp et al. 1997). Difficulties

Table 11.5 Aims of treatment

Prevention of progressive motor deterioration
Relief of pain
Control of sensory disturbances
Reduction of sweating and spasms
Restoration of lost function

relate in part to the narrow calibre of the canal in the thoracic region, as opposed to the wider "funnel-shaped" morphology of the cranioverte-bral junction. More important is the extent of fibrosis that has developed, and outcome following surgery is inversely proportional to this, which in turn is largely dependent upon the underlying pathology. Focal arachnoid webs may be relatively straightforward to treat, but extensive post-tuberculous adhesions present a considerable challenge.

Whilst collapse of the syrinx is always an encouraging result following surgery, it will not always predict a good functional result. Nor does failure of the syrinx to collapse mean that no gain will follow. In either case, improvement in function is seldom substantial. Even so, modest gains, or simply just the arrest of deterioration, may be of great benefit to a patient, who may well already bear a substantial physical disability. In this respect, a patient's perception may better reflect functional outcome than might attempts at objective assessment (Falci et al. 2009; Kramer and Levine 1997; Ushewokunze et al. 2010). Figures vary from one series to another, but it would be reasonable to quote figures of roughly one third of patients improving, one third stabilising and one third continuing to deteriorate (Sgouros and Williams 1996; Ushewokunze et al. 2010).

Regrettably, most publications on the outcome of surgery for syringomyelia do not adhere to any standards of data presentation. Klekamp and Samii have stressed the value of Kaplan-Meier analyses, as the only meaningful way of presenting outcome data (Klekamp and Samii 2002).

11.8.8 Pain Control

Of all the symptoms of syringomyelia, pain is perhaps the most difficult to control (Milhorat et al. 1996). Published results suggest very variable responses to surgery, but this may reflect a failure, on the part of authors, to differentiate between pains of different types or to use standard nomenclature. Pain induced by Valsalva manoeuvres is likely to be caused by transient rises in intra-syrinx pressure and can be expected to improve if the cavity collapses after surgery. Likewise, pain caused by movement may be related to cord tethering and may well improve if the cord is adequately released at surgery. Pain which is not modified by such influences and which has the characteristics of central, neuropathic pain will very likely persist, despite an anatomically successful operation (Klekamp and Samii 2002).

11.9 Summary

Syringomyelia remains an uncommon disorder and cases caused by leptomeningeal fibrosis are relatively rare. Post-traumatic syringomyelia, however, is very common amongst the population of spinal cord injury victims, with an incidence of about one in five and producing symptoms in 1 in 20 patients. The condition can cause significant additional disability, and surveillance should be the norm for all spinal cord injury patients. Surgery is not mandatory in all cases as many syrinx cavities remain stable for many years. Further, the outcome following surgery for post-traumatic as well as other forms of post-arachnoiditic syringomyelia is variable and cannot be predicted in an individual case. The major determinant of outcome is the extent of scar tissue that has formed, which limits surgical options in some circumstances, such as post-tuberculous syringomyelia.

Broadly speaking, there are four management options: (1) release of the scar tissue and creation of an artificial conduit for normal CSF movement; (2) direct drainage of the syrinx cavity into the pleura, peritoneum or elsewhere in the spinal canal; (3) lowering of the overall CSF pressure with a thecal or ventricular shunt; and (4) conservative management. Of the surgical options, the first is the best in terms of maintaining a good long-term result. Unfortunately, it is not always possible to achieve, in which case one of the other methods may be appropriate. Management must be tailored to the individual patient and his or her circumstances. It should be made clear that any functional improvement following surgery is likely to be limited. At the same time, even modest gains, or simply the arrest of deterioration, may be very welcome from the patient's perspective.

References

Anderson N, Willoughby E, Wrightson P (1986) The natural history of syringomyelia. Clin Exp Neurol 22:71–80

Aschoff A, Albert F, Mende U et al (1993) Intra-operative sonography in syringomyelia–technique, results, limitations. Acta Neurochir (Wien) 123(3–4):176

Augustijn P, Vanneste J, Davies G (1989) Chronic spinal arachnoiditis following intracranial subarachnoid haemorrhage. Clin Neurol Neurosurg 91(4):347–350

Backe H, Betz R, Mesgarzadeh M et al (1991) Post-traumatic spinal cord cysts evaluated by magnetic resonance imaging. Paraplegia 29:607–612

Balmaseda MT Jr, Wunder JA, Gordon C et al (1988) Posttraumatic syringomyelia associated with heavy weightlifting exercises: case report. Arch Phys Med Rehabil 69(11):970–972

Barnett H (1973) Syringomyelia consequent on mild to moderate trauma. In: Barnett HJM, Foster J, Hudgson P (eds) Syringomyelia. W B Saunders, London, p 318

Batzdorf U, Klekamp J, Johnson J (1998) A critical appraisal of syrinx cavity shunting procedures. J Neurosurg 89:382–388

Bonfield CM, Levi AD, Arnold PM et al (2010) Surgical management of post-traumatic syringomyelia. Spine 35:S245–S258

Bret P, Huppert J, Massini B et al (1986) Lumbo-peritoneal shunt in non-hydrocephalic patients. Acta Neurochir (Wien) 80(3):90–92

Brodbelt AR, Stoodley MA (2003a) Post-traumatic syringomyelia: a review. J Clin Neurosci 10:401–408

Brodbelt AR, Stoodley MA (2003b) Syringomyelia and the arachnoid web. Acta Neurochir 145(8):707–711

Bulundwe KK, Myburgh CJ, Gledhill RF (2000) Syringomyelia complicating syphilitic spinal meningitis: a case report. Eur J Neurol 7:231–236

Clifton GL, Donovan WH, Dimitrijevic MM et al (1996) Omental transposition in chronic spinal cord injury. Spinal Cord 34(4):193–203

Cusick JF, Bernardi R (1995) Syringomyelia after removal of benign spinal extramedullary neoplasms. Spine 20(11):1289

Daif AK, Al Rajeh S, Ogunniyi A et al (1997) Syringomyelia developing as an acute complication of tuberculous meningitis. Can J Neurol Sci 24(1):73

Durward QJ, Rice GP, Ball MJ et al (1982) Selective spinal cordectomy: clinicopathological correlation. J Neurosurg 56(3):359–367

Edgar R, Quail P (1994) Progressive post-traumatic cystic and non-cystic myelopathy. Br J Neurosurg 8:7–22

El Masry W, Biyani A (1996) Incidence, management, and outcome of post-traumatic syringomyelia. In memory of Mr Bernard Williams. J Neurol Neurosurg Psychiatry 60(2):141

Ewelt C, Stalder S, Steiger HJ et al (2010) Impact of cordectomy as a treatment option for posttraumatic and non-posttraumatic syringomyelia with tethered cord syndrome and myelopathy. J Neurosurg Spine 13:193–199

Falci SP, Indeck C, Lammertse DP (2009) Posttraumatic spinal cord tethering and syringomyelia: surgical treatment and long-term outcome. J Neurosurg Spine 11:445–460

Fehlings M, Bernstein M (1992) Syringomyelia as a complication of tuberculous meningitis. Can J Neurol Sci 19(1):84

Glasauer FE, Czyrny JJ (1994) Hyperhidrosis as the presenting symptom in post-traumatic syringomyelia. Paraplegia 32:423–429

Gnanalingham KK, Joshi SM, Sabin I (2006) Thoracic arachnoiditis, arachnoid cyst and syrinx formation secondary to myelography with Myodil, 30 years previously. Eur Spine J 15:661–663

Gopalakrishnan CV, Mishra A, Thomas B (2010) Iophendylate myelography induced thoracic arachnoiditis, arachnoid cyst and syrinx, four decades later. Br J Neurosurg 24:711–713

Holly LT, Batzdorf U (2006) Syringomyelia associated with intradural arachnoid cysts. J Neurosurg Spine 5(2):111–116

Holly L, Johnson JP, Masciopinto JE et al (2000) Treatment of posttraumatic syringomyelia with extradural decompressive surgery. Neurosurg Focus 8:E8

Kasai Y, Kawakita E, Morishita K et al (2008) Cordectomy for post-traumatic syringomyelia. Acta Neurochir 150:83–86

Kaynar MY, Kocer N, Gencosmanoglu BE et al (2000) Syringomyelia–as a late complication of tuberculous meningitis. Acta Neurochir 142:935–938

Klekamp J, Samii M (2002) Syringomyelia: diagnosis and treatment. Springer, Berlin/Heidelberg

Klekamp J, Batzdorf U, Samii M et al (1997) Treatment of syringomyelia associated with arachnoid scarring caused by arachnoiditis or trauma. J Neurosurg 86:233–240

Kramer KM, Levine AM (1997) Posttraumatic syringomyelia: a review of 21 cases. Clin Orthop Relat Res 334:190–199

LaHaye P, Batzdorf U (1988) Posttraumatic syringomyelia. West J Med 148:657–663

Laxton AW, Perrin RG (2006) Cordectomy for the treatment of posttraumatic syringomyelia. J Neurosurg Spine 4(2):174–178

Lee TT, Alameda GJ, Camilo E et al (2001) Surgical treatment of post-traumatic myelopathy associated with syringomyelia. Spine 26(24S):S119

Levy R, Rosenblatt S, Russell E (1991) Percutaneous drainage and serial magnetic resonance imaging in the diagnosis of symptomatic posttraumatic syringomyelia: case report and review of the literature. Neurosurgery 29:429–433

Lohlein A, Paeslack V, Aschoff A (1990) Cystic degeneration following severe spinal trauma. Clinical observations in 30 patients. Neurosurg Rev 13(1):41–44

Mallucci C, Stacey R, Miles J et al (1997) Idiopathic syringomyelia and the importance of occult arachnoid webs, pouches and cysts. Br J Neurosurg 11:306–309

McLone DG, Siqueira EB (1976) Post-meningitic hydrocephalus and syringomyelia treated with a ventriculoperitoneal shunt. Surg Neurol 6:323–325

Mebrouk Y, Chraa M, McMaughey C et al (2011) Syringomyelia associated with syphilitic spinal meningitis: real complication or possible association? Spinal Cord 49:757–760

Milhorat TH, Capocelli AL Jr, Anzil AP et al (1995a) Pathological basis of spinal cord cavitation in syringomyelia: analysis of 105 autopsy cases. J Neurosurg 82:802–812

Milhorat TH, Johnson RW, Milhorat RH et al (1995b) Clinicopathological correlations in syringomyelia using axial magnetic resonance imaging. Neurosurgery 37:206–213

Milhorat TH, Kotzen RM, Mu H et al (1996) Dysesthetic pain in patients with syringomyelia. Neurosurgery 38(5):940

Milhorat TH, Capocelli AL Jr, Kotzen RM et al (1997) Intramedullary pressure in syringomyelia: clinical and pathophysiological correlates of syrinx distension. Neurosurgery 41(5):1102

Moghtaderi A, Alavi-Naini R, Rahimi-Movaghar V (2006) Syringomyelia: an early complication of tuberculous meningitis. Trop Doct 36:254–255

Muthukumar N, Sureshkumar V (2007) Concurrent syringomyelia and intradural extramedullary tuberculoma as late complications of tuberculous meningitis. J Clin Neurosci 14:1225–1230

Nardone R, Alessandrini F, Tezzon F (2003) Syringomyelia following Listeria meningoencephalitis: report of a case. Neurol Sci 24(1):40–43

Oluigbo CO, Thacker K, Flint G (2010) The role of lumboperitoneal shunts in the treatment of syringomyelia. J Neurosurg Spine 13(1):133–138

Pearce JM (1995) Post-traumatic syringomyelia. J Neurol Neurosurg Psychiatry 58:520

Perrouin-Verbe B, Lenne-Aurier K, Robert R et al (1998) Post-traumatic syringomyelia and post-traumatic spinal canal stenosis: a direct relationship: review of 75 patients with a spinal cord injury. Spinal Cord 36(2):137

Phanthumchinda K, Kaoropthum S (1991) Syringomyelia associated with post-meningitic spinal arachnoiditis due to Candida tropicalis. Postgrad Med J 67(790): 767–769

Ragnarsson TS, Durward QJ, Nordgren RE (1986) Spinal cord tethering after traumatic paraplegia with late neurological deterioration. J Neurosurg 64(3):397–401

Reddy KK, Del Bigio MR, Sutherland GR (1989) Ultrastructure of the human posttraumatic syrinx. J Neurosurg 71:239–243

Robertson DP, Kirkpatrick JB, Harper RL et al (1991) Spinal intramedullary ependymal cyst. J Neurosurg 75(2):312–316

Saito K, Morita A, Shibahara J et al (2005) Spinal intramedullary ependymal cyst: a case report and review of the literature. Acta Neurochir 147(4):443–446

Schon F, Bowler J (1990) Syringomyelia and syringobulbia following tuberculous meningitis. J Neurol 237(2): 122–123

Schwartz ED, Falcone SF, Quencer RM et al (1999) Posttraumatic syringomyelia: pathogenesis, imaging, and treatment. Am J Roentgenol 173:487–492

Sett P, Crockard HA (1991) The value of magnetic resonance imaging (MRI) in the follow-up management of spinal injury. Spinal Cord 29(6): 396–410

Sgouros S, Williams B (1995) A critical appraisal of drainage in syringomyelia. J Neurosurg 82:1–10

Sgouros S, Williams B (1996) Management and outcome of posttraumatic syringomyelia. J Neurosurg 85: 197–205

Siddiqi F, Hammond R, Lee D et al (2005) Spontaneous chronic spinal subdural hematoma associated with spinal arachnoiditis and syringomyelia. J Clin Neurosci 12:949–953

Squier MV, Lehr R (1994) Post-traumatic syringomyelia. J Neurol Neurosurg Psychiatry 57(9):1095

Stanworth PA (1982) The significance of hyperhidrosis in patients with post-traumatic syringomyelia. Paraplegia 20:282–287

Sudheendra D, Bartynski WS (2008) Direct fluoroscopic drainage of symptomatic post-traumatic syringomyelia: a case report and review of the literature. Interv Neuroradiol 14:461–464

Tabor EN, Batzdorf U (1996) Thoracic spinal Pantopaque cyst and associated syrinx resulting in progressive spastic paraparesis: case report. Neurosurgery 39: 1040–1042

Tator CH, Meguro K, Rowed DW (1982) Favorable results with syringosubarachnoid shunts for treatment of syringomyelia. J Neurosurg 56(4):517–523

Thines L, Khalil C, Fichten A et al (2005) Spinal arachnoid cyst related to a nonaneurysmal perimesencephalic subarachnoid hemorrhage: case report. Neurosurgery 57(4):E817

Tjandra J, Varma T, Weeks R (1989) Spinal arachnoiditis following subarachnoid haemorrhage. Aust N Z J Surg 59(1):84–87

Ushewokunze SO, Gan YC, Phillips K et al (2010) Surgical treatment of post-traumatic syringomyelia. Spinal Cord 48:710–713

Vannemreddy S, Rowed D, Bharatwal N (2002) Posttraumatic syringomyelia: predisposing factors. Br J Neurosurg 16(3):276–283

Vassilouthis J, Papandreou A, Anagoustaras S (1994) Theco-peritoneal shunt for posttraumatic syringomyelia. J Neurol Neurosurg Psychiatry 57:755–756

Vengsarkar US, Panchal VG, Tripathi PD et al (1991) Percutaneous theco-peritoneal shunt for syringomyelia. J Neurosurg 74(5):827–831

Vinas FC, Pilitsis J, Wilner H (2001) Spontaneous resolution of a syrinx. J Clin Neurosci 8:170–172

Wang D, Bodley R, Sett P et al (1996) A clinical magnetic resonance imaging study of the traumatised spinal cord more than 20 years following injury. Spinal Cord 34(2):65–81

Williams B, Fahy G (1983) A critical appraisal of terminal ventriculostomy for the treatment of syringomyelia. J Neurosurg 58(2):188–197

Williams B, Page N (1987) Surgical treatment of syringomyelia with syringopleural shunting. Br J Neurosurg 1:63–80

Young WF, Tuma R, O'Grady T (2000) Intraoperative measurement of spinal cord blood flow in syringomyelia. Clin Neurol Neurosurg 102:119–123

Idiopathic Syringomyelia

12

Anil Roy

Contents

12.1 Introduction

Although no precise definition of idiopathic syringomyelia exists, the general consensus is that the term applies to a syrinx not associated with Chiari I malformation, spinal cord tumour, post-traumatic or infectious adhesive arachnoiditis (Bogdanov et al. 2004; Mauer et al. 2008; Nakamura et al. 2009; Roser et al. 2010; Struck and Haughton 2009) or other obstruction to cerebrospinal flow (CSF) detected by imaging studies. Given the high prevalence of MRI in the routine evaluation of back and neck pain, incidental discovery of idiopathic syringomyelia is becoming more common (Roser et al. 2010; Nakamura et al. 2009). Although syringomyelia can be associated with a clinical centromedullary syndrome, with predominantly sensory symptoms such as pain and temperature insensitivity, in many cases it is an incidental finding. We present here a broad overview of the topic referencing much of the work from our recent review on the subject (Roy et al. 2011).

The underlying pathophysiology of idiopathic syringomyelia is unclear and probably multifactorial. Few studies directly address this topic, although it has been hypothesised that the underlying filling mechanisms for idiopathic syringomyelia may be similar to those which operate with Chiari malformation type 1 (Bogdanov et al. 2004; Heiss et al. 2012). A study comparing patients with idiopathic syringomyelia, people with Chiari malformation type 1 and controls found similar morphometric abnormalities in

A. Roy
Department of Neurosurgery,
Emory University School of Medicine,
Atlanta, GA, USA
e-mail: akroy2@emory.edu

G. Flint, C. Rusbridge (eds.), *Syringomyelia*,
DOI 10.1007/978-3-642-13706-8_12, © Springer-Verlag Berlin Heidelberg 2014

both the idiopathic syringomyelia and the Chiari type one patients (Bogdanov et al. 2004). This included similar shortening of the posterior fossa and a reduction in ventral CSF space, although the dorsal CSF space was significantly smaller in Chiari type 1 patients. Syrinx diameter was also found to be significantly larger in Chiari malformation type 1 patients (5.5 ± 4.7 mm versus 2.7 ± 1.9 mm). This study posits that a posterior fossa with decreased compliance promotes the development of pulsatile CSF subarachnoid pressure waves aiding in the development of syringomyelia. Abnormal CSF flow velocities have been reported in idiopathic syringomyelia patients, raising the possibility of similarities in flow patterns at the foramen magnum in both Chiari type 1 and idiopathic syringomyelia patients (Struck and Haughton 2009). The idea of similar morphometric abnormalities in idiopathic syringomyelia and Chiari malformation type 1 seems to follow the reasoning by Klekamp (2002), who questions if a true idiopathic syrinx actually exists. A report on two patients with idiopathic syringomyelia postulated that subtle micro trauma may have been contributory (Porensky et al. 2007). In summary, the available evidence strongly suggests that a thorough anatomical investigation is required before labelling a patient as truly idiopathic.

12.2 Imaging and Classification

By the very meaning of the term, idiopathic syringomyelia does not have an underlying anatomical abnormality readily seen on imaging. With the benefit of modern imaging, however, we can, more often than not, find a structural abnormality. Increased peak CSF flow velocities have been reported in idiopathic syringomyelia (Struck and Haughton 2009). A small posterior fossa and narrow CSF spaces have been reported in idiopathic syringomyelia (Bogdanov et al. 2004). A series of four patients with idiopathic syringomyelia were all documented as having a 'tight cisterna magna', referring to the cisterna magna being impacted by the tonsils (Kyoshima et al. 2002). In a study looking at 10 patients, with apparently idiopathic syringomyelia, subsequent

CT myelography revealed obstruction to CSF flow in nine of them (Mallucci et al. 1997). Those patients who subsequently underwent laminectomy and release of arachnoid adhesions or webs fared much better than those who were treated with direct shunting of the syrinx. Another reported patient had a T2–C5 syrinx, together with a spinal intradural arachnoid cyst extending between T6 and T3, which was revealed by aqueous myelography. After laminectomy and collapse of the cyst, the patient improved (Clifton et al. 1987). A study looking at 125 patients with idiopathic syringomyelia, using cardiac-gated, phase-contrast CSF flow studies, found blockage of flow in 33 patients (Mauer et al. 2008). The most common level of blockage was T6. In 8 of these 33 patients, the evidence of CSF flow blockage was unequivocal, and yet CT myelography revealed a blockage in only 2 of these cases. The authors concluded that conventional myelography is not a useful tool in the diagnosis of idiopathic syringomyelia and that cardiac-gated CSF flow studies should suffice.

Idiopathic syringomyelia may be subdivided into localised versus extended cavities, with localised being described as being under three vertebrae in length and extended as stretching behind four or more vertebrae. The localised variant, which may simply represent an enlargement of the central canal, usually has milder symptoms and can be treated conservatively (Nakamura et al. 2009). Numerous other classification systems delineate terms such as hydromyelia, simple hydromyelia, syringomyelia and syringohydromyelia (see Chap. 20) (Kyoshima et al. 2002), but it is unclear whether these terms aid in the diagnostic or management process.

Variants of syringomyelia referred to as dilated or persisting central canals, or hydromyelia, are based on the concept that the central canal normally involutes with aging and is often not easily seen on imaging. Holly and Batzdorf (2002) looked at 32 patients with slitlike syrinx cavities, which they referred to as asymptomatic persistent central canal. Their study found symmetrically enlarged, central-placed cavities within the spinal cord, with a mean diameter of 2 mm (range 1–5 mm) and with no enhancement seen after intravenous gadolinium. Interestingly, however, 10 of these 32 patients did give a history of trauma, even though the study did not classify them as being post-traumatic. Half of the patients in this study also had alternate diagnostic explanations for their symptoms. The authors therefore argued that that these slitlike syrinx cavities do not represent true syringomyelia and are possibly even different from a pre-syrinx-like state. Yet, in the literature, there is no uniformity regarding this opinion. For example, Roser et al. (2010) differentiated hydromyelia, which they refer to as simply a dilated central canal, from idiopathic syringomyelia which, they point out, is accompanied by different clinical and radiological signs. In particular, they portend that patients with hydromyelia (dilated central canal) have no neurological deficits and mainly present with pain, which could be radicular, burning or musculoskeletal; a constellation of symptoms is similar to those described by Holly and Batzdorf. They further suggest that hydromyelia (dilated central canal) is a congenital condition which, in the setting of trauma, could develop into syringomyelia. It is difficult to determine, based on these studies, if slitlike syringes, hydromyelia (dilated central canal) and idiopathic syringomyelia are truly different entities or simply a continuum on a spectrum.

A wide variety of syringes is also seen in association with spinal cord pathology, including various inflammatory conditions or lesions compressing the subarachnoid space (Heiss et al. 2012). The specific pathologies are varied in nature and include delayed reactions to meningitis, extramedullary tumours, osteophytes and herniated intervertebral discs.

12.3 Presentation

With noncommunicating syringomyelia, symptoms can include spastic weakness of the lower extremities, paraesthesias, dysaesthesias and segmental sensory loss (Milhorat et al. 1995a, b). The pace of neurological deterioration in syringomyelia may be rapid initially but slows down after neurological signs become well established (Bogdanov and Mendelevich 2002). In Chiari 0 patients with syringomyelia, presenting symptoms include scoliosis, headaches and neck, back or leg pain (Chern et al. 2011). With idiopathic syringomyelia, the most common presenting symptom is pain, followed by paraesthesias, numbness and unnoticed hand injuries, but it is also not uncommon for patients to present with long tract signs (Mallucci et al. 1997). Although syringomyelia symptoms are classically described as pain and temperature insensitivity in a cape-like distribution, few of our own patients and indeed few of the studies reviewed actually demonstrated this (Roy et al. 2011). Although we did find an overall increased syrinx diameter in the two operated cases, the relevance is unclear given the few cases we have. In a population of 48 children with idiopathic syringomyelia, symptoms that led to the diagnosis of this condition fell into five groups: scoliosis, cutaneous marker/developmental anomaly,[1] pain, neurological findings and screening/incidental findings (Magge et al. 2011).

With idiopathic syringomyelia, it is difficult to correlate the presenting symptoms with the location of the syrinx (Roy et al. 2011). Specifically, regarding the issue of pain, there does not appear to be any correlation between syrinx size or location and the pain (Magge et al. 2011). Even when we can attempt to localise the symptoms, patients may actually have comorbid symptoms, from degenerative changes of the spine and musculoskeletal complaints, which require separate medical evaluation. Thus, it is important to stress that idiopathic syringomyelia is commonly an incidental, asymptomatic finding. Non-specific symptoms, such as pain, may result from other causes and be coincidental to the finding of the syrinx.

12.4 Management

Table 12.1 provides a review of the key literature regarding idiopathic syringomyelia. Only some of the details for each study are included, and some of the patients, in some of the series, were eventually found to have other structural

---

[1] The original paper does not clarify further the meaning of these terms.

Table 12.1 Summary of papers reporting cases of idiopathic syringomyelia

Authors and year	Type	Number of patients (sex)	Age (mean)	Location	Symptoms	Treatment	Outcomes	Follow-up period
Ataizi et al. (2007)	Case report	1 (F)	28	C5–T1	Neck and back pain	Conservative (patient refused surgery)	Resolution of pain Spontaneous collapse of syrinx	16 months
Bogdanov et al. (2004) (Note 1)	Cross-sectional	17 (2 F, 15 M)	49	Cervical	Segmental sensory loss Pyramidal signs Muscle atrophy	Not applicable	Not applicable	Not applicable
Chen et al. (2004)	Case report	1 (F)	19	C2–C6	Proximal upper limb weakness Diminished pain and temperature sensation	Suboccipital craniectomy + C1 and C3–C5 laminectomies	Improved strength Sensory deficit unchanged Syrinx reduced	12 months
Chern et al. (2011)	Retrospective case series	15 (6 F,9 M)	11	Multiple	Scoliosis Headache Neck pain	Suboccipital craniectomy + C1 laminectomy	Resolved – 4 Improved – 6 Stable – 3 Worse – 1	12–75 months
Holly and Batzdorf (2002) (Note 2)	Prospective study	32 (14 F, 18 M)	40	Cervical (16 cases) Thoracic (12 cases) Cervical-thoracic (4 cases)	Mechanical spinal pain Radicular pain Numbness	Anterior fusion C6–C7 (1 patient) Conservative (31 patients)	Improved – 6 Unchanged – 19 Worse – 7	6–110 months (mean 38)
Jinkins and Sener (1999)	Case series	3 (2 F, 1 M)	27	Lumbar Cervical Thoracic	Low back pain Headache	Conservative	Stable with resolution of pain in 2 patients	2–4 years (mean 3)
Kastrup et al. (2001)	Case report	1 (F)	61	C1–conus	Burning pain	Carbamazepine	Subsequent collapse of syrinx Symptoms unchanged	8 years
Kyoshima et al. (2002) (Note 3)	Retrospective case series	4 (3 F, 1 M)	38	Whole or near whole cord	Impaired touch and pain sensation Weakness Hypoalgesia	Craniocervical decompression	Improved symptoms in all Syrinx decreased in all but 1 case	2.5–11 years (mean 8)
Lin et al. (2006)	Case report	1 (M)	35	T2–T9	Leg weakness Reduced touch and pinprick	T6–T8 laminectomy + shunt (syringosubarachnoid)	JOA score [a] improved from 10 to 14 at day 30 post-op	30 days

Magge et al. (2011)	Retrospective case series	48 (30 F,18 M)	10	2–17 levels; mostly thoracic	Scoliosis, Cutaneous stigmata Leg or back pain (neurological symptoms were judged to be incidental)	Shunt (syringosubarachnoid) (1 patient) Fenestration of syrinx (1 patient) Conservative (remainder)	Operated cases: weakness and worsened gait (1st case) No change (2nd case)	Clinical: 3–56 months (mean 15.5) Radiographic: 2–64 months (mean 23.8)
Mallucci et al. (1997)	Retrospective case series	10 (2 F, 8 M)	48	Not described	Sensory disturbance weakness	Laminectomy and excision of web/cyst, Shunt (syringosubarachnoid) (2 patients)	Improved symptoms and syrinx reduced except for the 2 shunted cases	Not described
Mauer et al. (2008) (Note 1)	Prospective case series	125 (76 F,49 M)	36	1–18 levels not clearly defined	No surgery: Pain + sensory impairment With surgery: Bowel/bladder dysfunction, gait problems Paralysis	Arachnoid scar or web resection (10 patients) Conservative (115 patients)	Surgery: 4 improved, rest stabilised Conservative: outcomes not described	Not described
Nakamura et al. (2009)	Retrospective case series	15 (4 F, 11 M)	45	Localised C3–T2 (12 cases) Extended C1–T8 (3 cases)	Upper limb numbness Neck pain, 3pts extended: also progressive upper limb weakness	Conservative (12 patients) Shunt (syringosubarachnoid) (3 patients)	Conservative: no changes Surgical cases: reduced syrinx and mean JOA [a] decreased	7–20 years (mean 10)
Porensky et al. (2007)	Case report	2 (M)	43y and 44y	T1–T2 and C5–T5	Ataxia Neck pain Progressive left leg paresis, pinprick deficit on right leg	Laminectomy, lysis of adhesions + duraplasty	Reduced syrinx and asymptomatic (1st case) Refilled syrinx and unchanged neurology (2nd case)	1 year and 7 months
Roser et al. (2010)	Prospective case series	40 (25 F, 15 M)	37	Cervical (23 %) Thoracic (51 %) Cervical-thoracic (25 %)	Pain or dysaesthesias in limbs	Conservative	No radiological changes Neurologically stable	6–93 months (mean 36.9)
Struck and Haughton (2009) (Note 1)	Retrospective case series	8 (4 F,4 M)	12	Lower cervical or thoracic	Scoliosis Headache Back pain Extremity numbness, family history Nausea and vomiting	Posterior fossa decompression (4 patients) Conservative (4 patients)	Surgical cases: decreased symptoms in all Reduction of syrinx in 1 case	Not described

Notes: (1) Imaging studies. (2) 10 patients had a history of trauma. (3) Technically not idiopathic since a tight cisterna magna is a definite lesion (Roy et al. 2011)
M male, *F* female
[a] *Japanese Orthopaedic Association spondylotic myelopathy score*

anomalies. A large number of treatment options are discussed, including posterior fossa and foramen magnum decompression, laminectomy, lysis of adhesions, syrinx fenestration and syringosubarachnoid, syringoperitoneal and syringopleural shunting. Recent studies have emphasised the importance of improving CSF flow dynamics, regardless of the treatment strategy employed (Bogdanov et al. 2004; Kyoshima et al. 2002; Lee et al. 2002; Nakamura et al. 2009).

Surgical treatment should be reserved for clearly symptomatic patients, with progression on serial clinical and radiological examination. The majority of the patients in our own series were conservatively managed. We caution against the automatic tying of symptoms to the syrinx and proceeding with surgical management, since the symptoms may be purely coincidental, as mentioned above. A nonoperative approach is perfectly justifiable when a patient is either asymptomatic or experiences relatively mild symptoms. Surgical management may not offer much utility, with cases either worsening or showing no changes clinically (Magge et al. 2011). The frequency of follow-up MRI may be dictated by symptomatology.

Historically, shunting strategies have been employed for idiopathic syringomyelia and have led to clinical and radiological improvement. However, some studies have reported a variety of complications, including shunt failure, syrinx relapse, catheter tip migration and comorbidities from mechanical damage to cord tissue (Batzdorf et al. 1998; Sgouros and Williams 1995). Shunts may not be an effective solution in preventing the progress of syringomyelia, given the subsequent gliosis that can follow within the cord (Mallucci et al. 1997). We believe that shunting should be used as a measure of last resort, when no aetiology is evident after repeated imaging studies and surgical exploration does not reveal any pathology around the site of the syrinx.

In the case where the aetiology is clearly evident, such as a tight cisterna magna or small posterior fossa, craniocervical decompression is the best option for restoring CSF flow dynamics. An overly wide suboccipital craniectomy can, however, lead to cerebellar ptosis (Holly and Batzdorf 2002). The key to successful management is a wider opening to the foramen magnum but not the posterior fossa (Kyoshima et al. 2002). If CSF flow obstruction originates from spinal subarachnoid pathology such as a cyst, web or scar, treatment should be targeted towards decompressing the spinal subarachnoid space and reconstituting flow. This is illustrated by the two patients in our series that underwent surgical treatment. There is no clear evidence on precisely what such decompression and reconstruction should include. Laminectomy followed by scar, web or cyst resection has been commonly employed in other studies (Clifton et al. 1987; Lee et al. 2002; Mallucci et al. 1997) and has been used with good results in our published series (Roy et al. 2011). In the event of no evidence of any anatomical abnormality, in the setting of progressive neurological dysfunction attributable to a syrinx, surgical exploration is a reasonable option with a shunt as the last resort.

We have combined evidence on idiopathic syringomyelia and our experience into an algorithm (Fig. 12.1), to assist in the decision-making process. In most cases of incidental, asymptomatic findings, clinical review and imaging as indicated should be sufficient. For the more challenging symptomatic cases, the key focus is to resolve CSF flow problems since most of the evidence points to disrupted flow dynamics, leading to the development of syringomyelia.

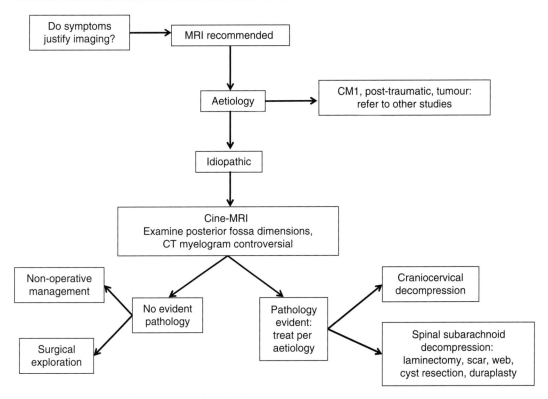

Fig. 12.1 Management algorithm for idiopathic syringomyelia. Indications for imaging include progressive deterioration in signs or symptoms (Roy et al. 2011)

Conclusion

Idiopathic syringomyelia is a pathological entity where no overt aetiology is evident for a syrinx. As imaging technology develops, increasing numbers of apparently idiopathic syringomyelia are being attributed to CSF flow abnormalities. Most incidental cases of idiopathic syringomyelia can be successfully managed using conservative approaches. With regard to surgical options, for continued progression of symptoms, syrinx shunting is generally a less-favoured approach as it does not resolve the underlying aetiology and is associated with high failure rates. A particular challenge to the neurosurgeon is surgical treatment of the patient with worsening symptoms but with no overt aetiology for their syrinx, even after a complete diagnostic workup, including flow studies. While we recommend surgical exploration in these cases, future studies will, hopefully, reveal a more systematic approach for these patients.

References

Ataizi S, Canakci Z, Baloglu M et al (2007) Spontaneously resorbed idiopathic syringomyelia: a case report. Turk Neurosurg 17(4):247–250

Batzdorf U, Klekamp J, Johnson JP (1998) A critical appraisal of syrinx cavity shunting procedures. J Neurosurg 89(3):382–388. doi:10.3171/jns.1998.89.3.0382

Bogdanov EI, Mendelevich EG (2002) Syrinx size and duration of symptoms predict the pace of progressive myelopathy: retrospective analysis of 103 unoperated cases with craniocervical junction malformations and syringomyelia. Clin Neurol Neurosurg 104(2):90–97

Bogdanov EI, Heiss JD, Mendelevich EG et al (2004) Clinical and neuroimaging features of "idiopathic" syringomyelia. Neurology 62(5):791–794

Chen JK, Chen CH, Lee CL, Chen TW, Weng MC, Huang MH (2004) Acute idiopathic syringomyelia: a case report. Kaohsiung J Med Sci 20(8):404–409

Chern JJ, Gordon AJ, Mortazavi MM et al (2011) Pediatric Chiari malformation Type 0: a 12-year institutional experience. J Neurosurg Pediatr 8(1):1–5. doi:10.3171/2011.4.PEDS10528

Clifton AG, Ginsberg L, Webb WJ et al (1987) Idiopathic spinal arachnoid cyst and syringomyelia. Br J Radiol 60(718):1023–1025

Heiss JD, Snyder K, Peterson MM et al (2012) Pathophysiology of primary spinal syringomyelia. J Neurosurg Spine 17(5):367–380. doi:10.3171/2012. 8.SPINE111059

Holly LT, Batzdorf U (2002) Slitlike syrinx cavities: a persistent central canal. J Neurosurg 97(2 Suppl):161–165

Jinkins JR, Sener RN (1999) Idiopathic localized hydromyelia: dilatation of the central canal of the spinal cord of probable congenital origin. J Comput Assist Tomogr 23(3):351–353

Kastrup A, Nagele T, Topka H (2001) Spontaneous resolution of idiopathic syringomyelia. Neurology 57(8):1519–1520

Klekamp J (2002) The pathophysiology of syringomyelia – historical overview and current concept. Acta Neurochir (Wien) 144(7):649–664. doi:10.1007/s00701-002-0944-3

Kyoshima K, Kuroyanagi T, Oya F et al (2002) Syringomyelia without hindbrain herniation: tight cisterna magna. Report of four cases and a review of the literature. J Neurosurg 96(2 Suppl):239–249

Lee JH, Chung CK, Kim HJ (2002) Decompression of the spinal subarachnoid space as a solution for syringomyelia without Chiari malformation. Spinal Cord 40(10):501–506. doi:10.1038/sj.sc.3101322

Lin JW, Lin MS, Lin CM et al (2006) Idiopathic syringomyelia: case report and review of the literature. Acta Neurochir Suppl 99:117–120

Magge SN, Smyth MD, Governale LS et al (2011) Idiopathic syrinx in the pediatric population: a combined center experience. J Neurosurg Pediatr 7(1): 30–36. doi:10.3171/2010.10.PEDS1057

Mallucci CL, Stacey RJ, Miles JB et al (1997) Idiopathic syringomyelia and the importance of occult arachnoid webs, pouches and cysts. Br J Neurosurg 11(4): 306–309

Mauer UM, Freude G, Danz B et al (2008) Cardiac-gated phase-contrast magnetic resonance imaging of cerebrospinal fluid flow in the diagnosis of idiopathic syringomyelia. Neurosurgery 63(6):1139–1144. doi:10.1227/01.NEU.0000334411.93870.45; discussion 1144

Milhorat TH, Capocelli AL Jr, Anzil AP et al (1995a) Pathological basis of spinal cord cavitation in syringomyelia: analysis of 105 autopsy cases. J Neurosurg 82(5):802–812. doi:10.3171/jns.1995.82.5.0802

Milhorat TH, Johnson RW, Milhorat RH et al (1995b) Clinicopathological correlations in syringomyelia using axial magnetic resonance imaging. Neurosurgery 37(2):206–213

Nakamura M, Ishii K, Watanabe K et al (2009) Clinical significance and prognosis of idiopathic syringomyelia. J Spinal Disord Tech 22(5):372–375. doi:10.1097/BSD.0b013e3181761543

Porensky P, Muro K, Ganju A (2007) Nontraumatic cervicothoracic syrinx as a cause of progressive neurologic dysfunction. J Spinal Cord Med 30(3):276–281

Roser F, Ebner FH, Sixt C et al (2010) Defining the line between hydromyelia and syringomyelia. A differentiation is possible based on electrophysiological and magnetic resonance imaging studies. Acta Neurochir (Wien) 152(2):213–219. doi:10.1007/s00701-009-0427-x; discussion 219

Roy AK, Slimack NP, Ganju A (2011) Idiopathic syringomyelia: retrospective case series, comprehensive review, and update on management. Neurosurg Focus 31(6):E15. doi:10.3171/2011.9.FOCUS11198

Sgouros S, Williams B (1995) A critical appraisal of drainage in syringomyelia. J Neurosurg 82(1):1–10. doi:10.3171/jns.1995.82.1.0001

Struck AF, Haughton VM (2009) Idiopathic syringomyelia: phase-contrast MR of cerebrospinal fluid flow dynamics at level of foramen magnum. Radiology 253(1):184–190. doi:10.1148/radiol.2531082135

Paediatric Perspectives

13

Jerry Oakes and Dominic Thompson

Contents

With Shane Tubbs and Melandee Brown

J. Oakes (✉)
Department of Neurosurgery, Children's Hospital of
Alabama, Birmingham, AL, USA
e-mail: jerry.oakes@childrensal.org

D. Thompson
Department of Neurosurgery, Great Ormond Street
Hospital for Children NHS Trust, London, England, UK
e-mail: thompd@gosh.nhs.uk

13.1 Introduction

In the paediatric population, the diagnosis of syringomyelia is most commonly associated with hindbrain hernias (Chiari malformations). In this chapter, syringomyelia that accompanies the pathology of Chiari I and Chiari II malformations will be discussed. Syringomyelia may also be encountered in cases without frank tonsillar ectopia but with noted crowding of the cisterna magna. This so-called Chiari 0 will also be reviewed. The relationship between syringomyelia, hindbrain hernia and scoliosis will also be addressed.

Hindbrain malformations were first studied in detail in the 1890s, by Hans Chiari. He described three types of herniation, as well as cases of hypoplasia or complete aplasia of the cerebellum and tentorium cerebelli – the Chiari IV malformation (Soleau et al. 2008).

The three types of hindbrain herniation share a common pathophysiology that involves the loss of free movement of cerebrospinal fluid (CSF) out of the fourth ventricle and into the cervicomedullary subarachnoid cisterns. An understanding of the pressure gradients that develop between the intraventricular and largely intracranial space and the subarachnoid channels surrounding the cervicomedullary junction allows for an appreciation of the developmental differences between the Chiari I and Chiari II malformations. It is this pressure gradient that is also thought to be responsible for the development of the syringomyelia that frequently accompanies these conditions (Attenello et al. 2008; Ball and Dayan 1972).

G. Flint, C. Rusbridge (eds.), *Syringomyelia*,
DOI 10.1007/978-3-642-13706-8_13, © Springer-Verlag Berlin Heidelberg 2014

13.2 Chiari I Malformation and Syringomyelia

The more common Chiari I malformation is classically defined as caudal displacement of the cerebellar tonsils 5 mm or more below the foramen magnum. Affected individuals are distinguished from Chiari II patients by the normal location and appearance of the brainstem and caudal displacement of the cerebellar tonsils, rather than the vermis. The true incidence of tonsillar herniation is not known, but a review of radiological images of over 22,000 patients reported it to be 1 in 130 (Meadows et al. 2000). A more recent series, based on a review of MRI images of 5,248 patients under the age of 20, found the incidence of Chiari I malformation to be 1 in 102 (Tubbs et al. 2011)

13.2.1 Presentation

Although Chiari I malformation more often presents symptomatically in early adult life, the widespread use of magnetic resonance imaging (MRI) has led to increased recognition of this disorder in children (Meadows et al. 2000). At the same time, given this increasing frequency of radiological diagnosis of Chiari I malformation, care must be taken to differentiate between patients with recognisable symptoms and individuals with symptoms that are unrelated to the finding of tonsillar herniation on imaging. Patients with Chiari I malformation may present with a variety of complaints, ranging from headache and neck pain to symptoms of myelopathy and brainstem compression. The most common presentation is one of pain in the occipital region or upper cervical spine that is exacerbated by Valsalva or tussive manoeuvres. In infants and non-verbal children, headache may be signalled by generalised irritability and neck grabbing. With headaches that are not Valsalva-related and pain that is remote from the occipital-cervical junction, it is unlikely that the symptoms are attributable to the presence of a Chiari I malformation (Soleau et al. 2008).

More unusual presentations of Chiari I malformations include features of brainstem compression, cranial nerve dysfunction or cerebellar signs. Symptoms of brainstem dysfunction include tongue atrophy, down-beat nystagmus and isolated abducens nerve palsies. Symptomatic lower cranial nerve dysfunction has been reported to occur in 12–25 % of patients, the most common symptoms including dysphagia, gagging or chronic emesis and sleep apnoea (Soleau et al. 2008). In a recent series, however, fewer than 10 % of patients presented with cranial nerve deficits and 5 % presented with central apnoea, confirmed by a sleep study (Tubbs et al. 2011). Rarely, patients may present with an acute crisis, and in another series of 500 patients, three presented with symptoms of dysphagia, anisocoria and hemiparesis that progressed rapidly over 2–3 days (Tubbs et al. 2011). Three other reported cases presented with abrupt onset of severe symptoms, two following mild head injury (Massimi et al. 2011).

Clinical myelopathy can result from direct compression of the upper cord, by the herniated cerebellar tonsils, or can be due to the presence of a syrinx. Loss of pain and temperature sensation in the upper extremities, with preservation of light touch and proprioception, in a Chiari I patient, should alert the examiner to the presence of an accompanying syringomyelia. Scoliosis in a Chiari I patient may also signal the presence of a syrinx. Patients with a left convex thoracic curve, abnormal or absent abdominal reflexes or complaints of non-dermatomal pain should also raise the suspicion of an underlying syrinx (Soleau et al. 2008). Syringomyelia has been described as affecting between 35 and 75 % of patients with Chiari I malformation (Attenello et al. 2008). In one series of 500 patients, who underwent surgery for Chiari I malformation, 57 % were found to have syringomyelia. Syrinx cavities were most commonly located in the cervicothoracic cord, followed by the cervical cord, lumbar cord and brainstem. A surprising 39 % of patients had holocord syringes (Tubbs et al. 2011).

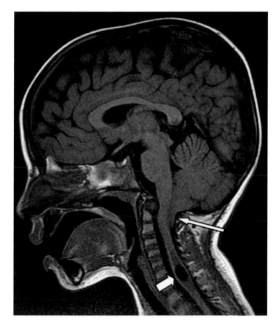

Fig. 13.1 Sagittal T1-weighted MRI. Note the Chiari I malformation (*long arrow*) and cervical syrinx (*short arrow*)

13.2.2 Imaging

Conventional computerised tomography (CT) is sometimes the imaging modality that leads to the initial diagnosis of Chiari I malformation. The radiologist may identify characteristic crowding of the foramen magnum, although the axial plane of the standard head CT makes it difficult to appreciate fully the extent of the hindbrain herniation. Sagittal reconstructions of the source data may be helpful, but CT imaging alone is inadequate in evaluating a patient for the presence of a syrinx or Chiari malformation.

On magnetic resonance imaging (MRI), Chiari I malformation is characterised by significant herniation of the cerebellar tonsils through the foramen magnum. An associated cervical, cervical thoracic or holocord syrinx may also be found (Figs. 13.1 and 13.2). The herniated cerebellar tonsils also often lose their rounded appearance and become peglike (Fig. 13.3). They frequently lead to obliteration of the retrocerebellar subarachnoid space (Aitken et al. 2009). Although extension of one or both tonsils 5 mm

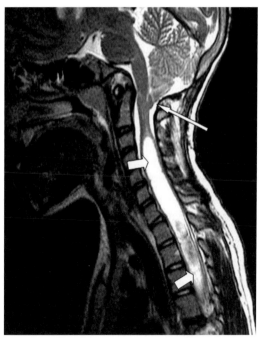

Fig. 13.2 Sagittal T2-weighted MRI. Note the Chiari I malformation (*long arrow*) and holocord syrinx (*short arrows*)

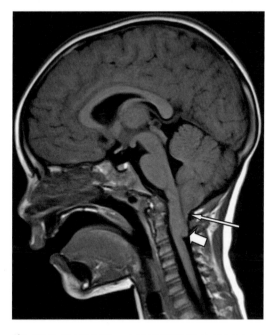

Fig. 13.3 Sagittal T1-weighted MRI. Note the pointed cerebellar tips (*long arrow*) often seen in the Chiari I malformation and elongation of the brainstem (*short arrow*)

below the foramen magnum is sufficient for a radiological diagnosis, these findings should be considered in conjunction with the patient's symptoms. Patients that do not have symptoms or syringomyelia, even when the MR imaging is impressive, can be managed conservatively with observation (Soleau et al. 2008). The presence of syringomyelia will, however, lead the practitioner towards surgical intervention even in the presence of minimal symptoms (Oakes 1991).

Patients suspected of having Chiari I malformation should also undergo imaging of the brain, as a small percentage of patients will be found to have associated hydrocephalus, nearly one in ten cases in one large series. Those with untreated hydrocephalus should have this addressed, prior to any decompressive procedure at the craniovertebral junction, and those patients with an already shunted hydrocephalus should have the functioning of the shunt confirmed.

Other radiographic abnormalities are seen in association with the Chiari I malformation, including retroverted odontoid process which was found in 24 % of operative Chiari I patients in one series. Other reported associations include scoliosis (18 %), atlanto-occipital fusion (8 %), Klippel-Feil anomaly (3 %) and basilar invagination (3 %) (Tubbs et al. 2011). Plain flexion-extension radiographs of the cervical spine are helpful in resolving the question of spinal instability and can further delineate the extent of the bony abnormalities. The presence of significant basilar invagination should alert the practitioner to the possible need for an anterior decompression, prior to a posterior decompression (Oakes 1991).

Cine-MRI may be used to assess flow across the foramen magnum. Some authors find it a valuable tool in decision making, whilst others find that its usefulness is dependent upon the software used to process the acquired sequences (Soleau et al. 2008; Ventureyra et al. 2003).

13.2.3 Surgical Intervention

Surgical manoeuvres in the paediatric Chiari I patient include bony decompression of the

posterior fossa, usually with exploration and decompression of the fourth ventricular outlet. In most cases this necessitates removal of the posterior arch of C1 as well, with excision of the subadjacent fibrous band and duraplasty. Coagulation or partial resection of the herniated tonsils may be necessary, if they obstruct fourth ventricular outflow or in the event that a re-operation is needed due to failure of the syrinx to collapse after the initial procedure.

Controversy exists regarding the necessity for duraplasty in the treatment of Chiari I malformation. A small retrospective study of 11 adult patients, who underwent bone only decompression, with removal of the posterior arch of C1, found that eight of the patients had improvement in their symptoms. Seven of these patients also had syringomyelia, and three had radiological decrease in the size of their cavities and improvement in their symptoms. All three of these patients also had increased posterior fossa volume on post-operative imaging (Munshi et al. 2000). A study of brainstem auditory evoked potentials in 11 paediatric patients, before and after duraplasty, found that no additional improvement was noted following this manoeuvre (Anderson et al. 2003). Intraoperative ultrasound has been employed in an effort to identify patients who might benefit from duraplasty, in addition to bony decompression (McGirt et al. 2008; Yeh et al. 2006). A retrospective study of 256 paediatric patients stratified the success rates of bone only decompression versus duraplasty, according to the extent of tonsillar herniation. In children with tonsillar herniation caudal to C1, suboccipital decompression alone was associated with a twofold increase in the risk of symptom recurrence, when compared with those children who also underwent duraplasty. Children who had tonsillar herniation rostral to C1 had equivalent outcomes when undergoing duraplasty or bone only decompression (McGirt et al. 2008).

A large retrospective review of 500 surgically treated paediatric Chiari I patients, of whom 285 also had syringomyelia, found that 12 % of this latter group had an arachnoid veil occluding the fourth ventricular outlet. Fifteen patients in total required re-operation, 13 for persistent syringes and two for persistent Valsalva-related headache. One of the latter, two improved following re-operation with duraplasty. Of the 13 patients with persistent syrinx, 11 had resolution of their hydromyelia with re-operation and tonsillar coagulation. The two patients that did not improve following re-operation enjoyed some decrease in their syrinx size following subsequent placement of syringopleural shunts (Tubbs et al. 2011).

Some authors have noted an association between duraplasty and a higher complication rates (Navarro et al. 2004). Others have noted a small but significant correlation between duraplasty and longer hospitalisations (Yeh et al. 2006). Other authors report low complication rates but including transient acute hydrocephalus and extra-axial subdural collections (Elton et al. 2002). Other complications include direct vascular or neural injury, bleeding from dural venous sinuses, CSF leak, meningitis and pseudomeningocoele formation. Sagging or slumping of the cerebellum may also be encountered, in the setting of overly generous craniectomy and dural grafting. In this case, a partial cranioplasty, with revisional duraplasty, to create a cerebellar 'sling', can be effective in supporting the herniated cerebellum (Holly and Batzdorf 2001). Bone regrowth at the foramen magnum and at the site of the C1 bone removal has been reported in young children and infants (Aoki et al. 1995).

13.2.4 Response to Cervicomedullary Decompression

A review of 49 paediatric patients operated on for Chiari I and syringomyelia observed that just over half had radiological improvement in their syringomyelia during a mean follow-up period of 41 months. The median time until radiological improvement was 14 months following surgery. The same proportion of children enjoyed symptomatic improvement with a median time to improvement of 4 months (Attenello et al. 2008).

A series of 500 operated paediatric patients, of which 57 % had syringomyelia, included a re-operation rate of 3 %, mostly for persistent syrinx. Posterior fossa decompression was sufficient in relieving symptoms in 80 % of patients at the time of the first operation and in 95 % of patients following a second operation. In the 13 patients with persistent syringomyelia, all but two improved with re-exploration alone. The two patients who did not improve following re-operation underwent placement of syringopleural shunts, but given the success rates of re-operation, the authors have almost completely abandoned the practice of syrinx shunting (Tubbs et al. 2011). In this same series, an arachnoid veil was found to be obstructing the outlet of the fourth ventricle in 12 % of patients with syringomyelia. Thirty patients in the series underwent placement of stents, passing from the fourth ventricle into the subarachnoid space. These patients were less likely to have resolution of their syringomyelia, although this may be because patients selected for stent placement had unfavourable anatomical features.

13.3 Chiari II Malformation and Syringomyelia

The Chiari II malformation is characterised by caudal displacement of the cerebellar vermis, brainstem and fourth ventricle below the level of the foramen magnum (Fig. 13.4). It occurs exclusively in association with myelodysplasia. In the United States, the historical prevalence of myelomeningocoele is cited as one to two per 1,000 live births, but the advent of prenatal screening and increased awareness of the need for maternal folic acid supplementation has decreased the prevalence to between 2 and 4.6 cases per 10,000 births (Honein et al. 2001; Piatt 2010), although regional variations in prevalence do exist (Shurtleff 2004). The frequency of syringomyelia in Chiari II patients varies between different reports, from 40 to 80 %, and was documented in 20 out of 26 (3 in 4) autopsy cases of young children born with myelomeningocoele (Piatt 2004). The true incidence may, in fact, be underestimated because some pre-existing but undiagnosed cavities may collapse, following shunting of hydrocephalus in infancy.

Fig. 13.4 Sagittal T1-weighted MRI. An adult patient with Chiari II malformation

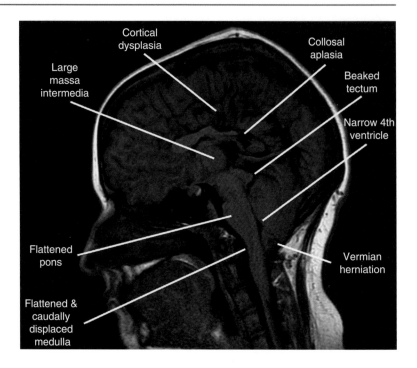

Cortical dysplasia

Collosal aplasia

Large massa intermedia

Beaked tectum

Narrow 4th ventricle

Flattened pons

Vermian herniation

Flattened & caudally displaced medulla

Syringomyelia cavities are often found in the lower cervical and upper thoracic cord and may be missed on routine cranial imaging. Low lumbar syrinx cavities are rare but are frequently associated with rapidly progressive scoliosis and are less likely to respond to ventricular shunting (Piatt 2004). Spinal arachnoid cysts may also be found in association with Chiari II malformation.

Biopsy specimens of the cyst walls, when analysed by electron microscopy, have demonstrated the presence of axons which suggests that some of these cysts are actually formed by dorsal rupture of eccentrically located syringes (Heinz et al. 1992).

There also appears to be an association between untreated or partially treated hydrocephalus and syringomyelia. A study of 18 Chiari II patients with progressive myelopathy, who underwent radionucleotide ventriculography, demonstrated the accumulation of tracer in the syrinx cavities of the 14 patients with untreated hydrocephalus (Batnitzky et al. 1976). These observations underscore the need to confirm the presence of a functioning shunt in Chiari II patients with shunted hydrocephalus that present with syringes.

13.3.1 Presentation of Chiari II

Patients with Chiari II malformations present at birth with myelomeningocoele. The outlook for this population is somewhat restricted, and historically, approximately one third of the neonates with symptoms of brainstem dysfunction did not survive beyond infancy. Survival has, however, increased with prompt ventricular shunting, shunt revision when needed and posterior fossa decompression when appropriate (Talamonti et al. 2007). Overall, some 20–30 % of Chiari II patients will become symptomatic from their hindbrain herniation at some point in their lifetime.

Clinical presentation varies in different age groups. Infants and neonates can present with apnoea, inspiratory stridor, dysphagia, bradycardia and opisthotonus. The dysphagia may be severe enough to necessitate placement of a gastrostomy tube. When present at birth, such symptoms suggest hypoplasia or aplasia of brainstem nuclei and often predict a poor prognosis. More commonly, symptoms begin within the first few months of life and when they are seen in a previously well infant attention should first be given to normalisation of the intracranial pressure through shunt placement or shunt revision if necessary (Holinger et al. 1978; Soleau et al. 2008). Feeding and swallowing difficulties are the most common presenting symptoms for infants at risk and were found in 59–71 % of symptomatic Chiari II patients in one series (Pollack et al. 1992b). Infants may present with weak suck and prolonged feeding times, and they may demonstrate weight loss and failure to thrive, as their physical growth outpaces their ability to meet their nutritional needs. Breathing difficulties are the most dangerous symptom in Chiari patients and have been reported to occur in between 29 and 76 % of patients (Rauzzino and Oakes 1995). Inspiratory stridor is the result of bilateral tenth nerve paresis, with weakness of the vocal cord abductors. It may be caused by direct traction on the tenth nerve or by damage to the dorsal motor nuclei, secondary to micro-haemorrhage or compressive ischemia (Benjamin et al. 2009; Linder and Lindholm 1997; Rauzzino and Oakes 1995). One series observed that all infants began with normal swallowing and feeding that progressively deteriorated (Pollack et al. 1992b). In these cases, they found that feeding problems preceded respiratory difficulties and were a recognisable warning sign. In another publication, the same group found that all neonates that underwent surgical decompression, prior to the development of bilateral vocal cord paralysis, demonstrated some improvement in neurological function following surgery (Pollack et al. 1992a).

Older children more commonly have symptoms of spinal cord compromise, and the syringomyelia associated with Chiari II malformation behaves in a manner similar to that seen in Chiari I patients. Classic presentation is with lower motor neuron features in the arms and upper motor neuron findings in the legs. These include atrophy of the small muscles of the hands, together with disassociated sensory loss. Progressive enlargement of the syrinx cavity leads to loss of the ability to perform fine motor tasks, and fasciculation and loss of tendon reflexes may be evident in the upper limbs. Further expansion of the syrinx may impede descending corticospinal tracts, such that patients who were previously ambulatory may report a history of increasing falls, coming on over months or years.

Syringobulbia, or expansion of the syrinx into the brainstem, will manifest itself as dysfunction in multiple brainstem nuclei, which may wrongly be attributed to the underlying Chiari II malformation. Neurogenic athropathies may also be present. Back pain and scoliosis (see below) may also be the initial presenting complaints.

Changes in bowel or bladder function, however, should prompt imaging to exclude a tethered cord (Rauzzino and Oakes 1995). Headache and posterior cervical neck pain are also common and may be due to the distortion of the descending fibres of the spinal trigeminal tract or the upper cervical roots.

13.3.2 Imaging Chiari II

Radiographic assessment of patients with Chiari II malformation can begin with plain films of the cervical spine. Flexion and extension views can be used to assess for cervical instability. The posterior arch of C1 is incomplete in up to 70 % of cases and may be replaced by a compressive band of periosteal tissue. Full spine radiographs permit assessment of scoliosis, segmentation errors and other occult dysraphisms. Rarely, split cord malformation, with a bony median septum, may be identified on plain films (Rauzzino and Oakes 1995).

CT images are inadequate for studying the pathology of hindbrain herniation, but head CT imaging is helpful in evaluating ventricular size and can provide an objective measurement of the adequacy of ventricular shunting, although surgical exploration remains the 'gold standard' for the determination of the adequacy of shunt function.

MRI is the diagnostic tool of choice in evaluating patients with suspected Chiari malformations. The hallmark of the Chiari II malformation is the elongation and caudal displacement of the cerebellar vermis, medulla and lower brainstem, below the foramen magnum. In up to 70 % of

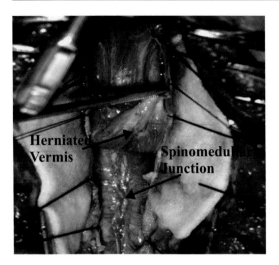

Fig. 13.5 Operative view of the Chiari II malformation

Chiari II patients, a medullary kink may be identified. Elongation of the fourth ventricle into the upper cervical cord is also a common finding. The cerebellum of Chiari II patients is smaller than normal and is contained in a hypoplastic posterior fossa with obliterated retrocerebellar CSF spaces (Fig. 13.5). The tentorium cerebelli has a low insertion and can also be hypoplastic, allowing the cerebellum to tower above it. Other frequently observed cerebellar findings include persistent foetal location with extension around the midbrain into the cerebellopontine cisterns and cerebellar dysplasias and heterotopias (Rauzzino and Oakes 1995).

13.3.3 Surgery for Chiari II Malformations

The surgical management of Chiari II malformation generally consists of bony decompression followed by some form of dural expansion manoeuvre. Prior to any posterior fossa decompression, however, patients with questionable shunt function should first undergo shunt revision. This approach can sometimes avoid the need for posterior fossa surgery because reducing the downward pressure on the cerebellum may lead to resolution of symptoms. Obtaining effective ventricular drainage may also lead to collapse

of the syrinx, without recourse to major posterior fossa surgery. On the other hand, ignoring an active hydrocephalus and performing a craniovertebral decompression may sometimes lead to a potentially dangerous exacerbation of a hydrocephalus that was previously in a state of hydrodynamic equilibrium.

Reference to pre-operative MRI assists in the localisation of the vermian herniation, a medullary kink, the fourth ventricle and a low-lying torcular Herophilus and transverse sinus. For patients with a large foramen magnum, occipital craniectomy may not be required. If the torcular is low-lying, care must be taken to avoid inadvertent entry into the major venous sinuses, which could lead to dangerous blood loss. Care must be taken to distinguish the medullary kink from the cerebellar vermis, and intraoperative ultrasonography may be useful in this regard (Tubbs and Oakes 2004). In Chiari II patients, the choroid plexus usually retains its embryonic extraventricular location and marks the caudal end of the fourth ventricle.

Unlike with Chiari I malformations, adequate decompression of the Chiari II hindbrain hernia requires that the decompression should extend to the level of the displaced posterior fossa content. The herniated brainstem, unlike the cerebellar tonsils, cannot be delivered upwards or coagulated (Fig. 13.6). The fourth ventricular outlet should be identified and widely opened, and it is often necessary to develop several tissue planes, before the floor of the fourth ventricle can be clearly identified. Misidentification of anatomical landmarks or excessive tissue manipulation can result in damage to at-risk parts of the medulla or lower pons. Dense adhesions and hypervascularity may be encountered at points of compression or traction, making identification and dissection of these structures more difficult.

13.3.4 Surveillance

Early surgical therapy may prove to be life saving for symptomatic Chiari II patients, when the symptoms are attributable to brainstem

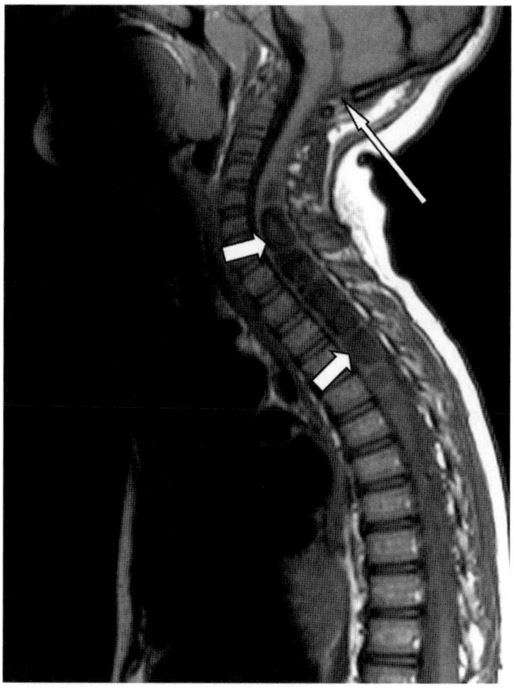

Fig. 13.6 Sagittal T1-weighted MRI of the Chiari 0 malformation. Note the absence of cerebellar tonsillar herniation (*long arrow*) and large cervicothoracic syrinx (*short arrows*) that resolved following posterior fossa decompression

13.4 Chiari 0

The term Chiari 0 malformation has been used to describe a subset of patients with syringomyelia and without cerebellar tonsillar ectopia but with observed 'crowding' of the posterior fossa (Tubbs et al. 2001; Weprin and Oakes 2001). These patients do not have caudal displacement of their cerebellar tonsils, beyond that which is considered to be within the normal anatomical range (Soleau et al. 2008). Analysis of the posterior fossa in these patients has, however, demonstrated that they have caudal displacement of their brainstems, with a low-lying obex and a hypoplastic posterior fossa (Weprin and Oakes 2001). These patients are considered to have impaired circulation of CSF at the outlet of the fourth ventricle and across the craniovertebral junction. In addition, those that come to surgery are often found to have barriers to free egress of CSF. The first published series described five patients with syringomyelia but without hindbrain herniation. They all underwent posterior fossa decompression that entailed a suboccipital craniectomy, removal of the posterior arch of C1 and duraplasty. Additionally, the patients underwent lysis of adhesions, opening of the fourth ventricular veil (if present) and partial resection of one of the cerebellar tonsils. Four patients had resolution of their symptoms post-operatively, and all went on to display a diminution in the size of their syringes (Iskandar et al. 1998).

dysfunction. For infants and neonates who present with respiratory distress and stridor, the timing of decompression is important. Beyond this age group, approximately 10 % of patients who survive will have late symptoms of brainstem dysfunction (Talamonti et al. 2007). Continued well-child surveillance and family education can therefore help to ensure that late presentations of brainstem compression do not go unrecognised. The importance of having a functioning shunt in this patient population should again be stressed. Obstructive apnoea, which can have a mortality rate as high as 60 %, can be reversed by an optimally functioning shunt (Cochrane et al. 1991; Hesz and Wolraich 1985; Soleau et al. 2008).

The extensive laminectomy required to decompress a Chiari II malformation increases the risk of delayed cervical instability, and the patients should undergo post-operative cervical spine evaluation (Oakes 1991).

13.5 Scoliosis

There is a particularly marked association between scoliosis and syringomyelia in children. One review identified scoliosis in 4 out of 5 syringomyelia patients under 20 years of age, compared with 1 in 6 older patients (Isu et al. 1990). Scoliosis is the presenting feature of syringomyelia in as many as two thirds of children (Isu et al. 1992). Features that alert an orthopaedic surgeon to the possibility of such underling cord pathology include male sex and curves that are convex to the left; idiopathic curves are more commonly convex to the right and have a predilection for girls. The presence of neurological symptoms and signs as well as rapid progression of a curve also suggest a neurogenic aetiology. Extensive cord cavitations, comprising 50 % or more of the cross-sectional diameter of the cord, are more likely to experience progression of their scoliosis.

Our understanding of the pathophysiological mechanisms underlying the association between syringomyelia and scoliosis is limited. A syrinx cavity is rarely symmetrical in its transverse dimensions, so there is usually asymmetrical impairment of function in the anterior horn cells. The assumption is that the resultant imbalance in the innervation to the axial musculature results in progressive spinal curvature. Alternatively, abnormal intramedullary pressure may interfere with postural tonic reflexes (Eule et al. 2002). It is generally accepted in veterinary medicine that scoliosis occurs secondary to dorsal grey column damage and disruption of proprioceptive information coming from Golgi tendon organs (see Chap. 14). In animal models, sectioning dorsal roots can be followed by development of scoliosis (Alexander et al. 1972; Liszka 1961; MacEwen 1973), although paraspinal muscle dissection and laminectomy may play a role in the development of scoliosis in these animals. It is important to bear in mind that syrinx cavities may have diverse aetiologies (e.g. post infectious, and post traumatic) and in some instances neurological damage and spinal innervation may be compromised by mechanisms other than, or in addition to the syrinx. Additionally, in the paediatric population congenital vertebral malformations are common and may co-exist with syrinx cavities however the causal relationship between these two entities is by no means clear. That there is a causal relationship between syringomyelia and scoliosis is now generally accepted and supported by many studies (Bertran et al. 1989; Muhonen et al. 1992), however, it is not always clear whether a syrinx is the cause of or a consequence of a scoliosis. Greitz argued that the spinal subarachnoid pressure is lower adjacent to a syrinx, as a result of the Bernoulli principle (Greitz 2006). This states that an increase in fluid velocity, as might occur where the subarachnoid space is narrowed (as for example at the apex of a scoliotic curve), is accompanied by a decrease in the pressure exerted by that fluid. This drop in CSF

Table 13.1 Clinical associations between Chiari malformation, syringomyelia and scoliosis

Chiari with syrinx and scoliosis
Idiopathic syrinx with scoliosis
Chiari with scoliosis but no syrinx

pressure increases the pressure gradient between the spinal cord parenchyma and subarachnoid space, with the result that fluid is drawn from the cord capillary bed into the parenchyma, initiating formation of a syrinx. If we apply this reasoning to a case of scoliosis, then it is possible that the spinal curvature might compromise the streamline flow of CSF in the subarachnoid channels and, thereby, encourage the accumulation of fluid within the substance of the cord. Furthermore, an idiopathic syrinx can also occur in the absence of scoliosis, the finding of syringomyelia in association with a scoliosis may be simply coincidence.

The issue of the Chiari I malformation adds a further dimension, and trying to unravel the interaction between hindbrain hernia, syringomyelia and scoliosis is challenging, particularly as regards which is the primary anomaly and which component of this triad should receive our initial attention. Three scenarios that are commonly encountered in paediatric neurosurgical practice (Table 13.1).

13.5.1 Scoliosis and Chiari-Related Syringomyelia

The increasing trend for all paediatric scoliosis patients to be evaluated with MRI has resulted in the identification of a variety of intraspinal anomalies, of which syringomyelia is the most common (Diab et al. 2011; Lewonowski et al. 1992). Further, the term syrinx is frequently used to cover a spectrum of appearances, ranging from short segments of hydromyelia, that may be little more than focal dilatations of the central canal, through to larger intramedullary fluid collections, more consistent with classical syringomyelia. Chiari-related syringomyelia is the most commonly seen association with scoliosis in the paediatric population. A series of 500 paediatric Chiari I malformations reported a syrinx to be present in 57 % and scoliosis in 18 % of cases (Tubbs et al. 2011)

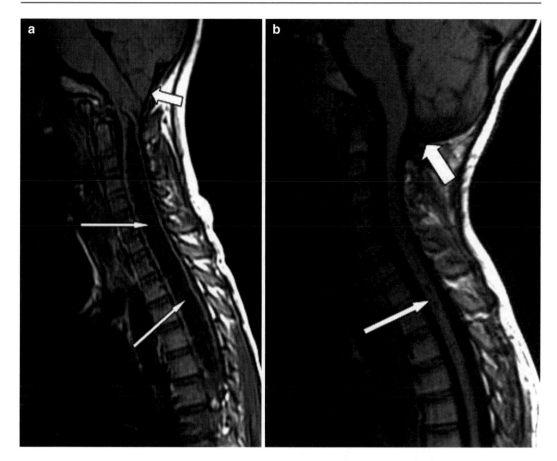

Fig. 13.7 Sagittal T1-weighted MRI scans, before and after craniovertebral decompression. (**a**) Showing syringomyelia (*narrow arrows*) and a Chiari I malformation (*broad arrow*) in a child presenting with scoliosis. (**b**) Following foramen magnum decompression and duraplasty (*broad arrow*), there has been resolution of the syr-inx (*narrow arrow*). There has also been some improvement in the sagittal alignment of the spinal column. This is revealed by scrutiny of the lower part of the images, where the midline of the lower vertebral bodies lies outside the plane of the image before surgery, whereas they lie in the midsagittal plane after surgery

Abnormal CSF flow in the region of the foramen magnum can also lead to syringomyelia formation, in the absence of Chiari malformation – the Chiari 0 condition (Klekamp et al. 2002; Kyoshima et al. 2002). As with syringomyelia associated with Chiari I and II malformations, scoliosis may coexist. In some of these cases, foramen magnum decompression and intradural exploration can result in improvement in the syrinx (Fig. 13.7) (Goel and Desai 2000; Iskandar et al. 1998). The scoliosis may improve as well, and in one series of 15 children with Chiari 0, eight had scoliosis and foramen magnum decompression led to the curve improving in four cases and stabilising in another three (Chern et al. 2011).

13.5.2 Scoliosis and Idiopathic Syringomyelia

The natural history of idiopathic syringomyelia in the paediatric population seems to be benign. In a study of 48 children with an idiopathic syrinx, followed over a 2½ year period, 9 out of 10 either improved or remained clinically stable and asymptomatic. Almost all of these cavities also remained stable radiologically or reduced in size (Magge et al. 2011). In those children who had a scoliosis as well, neither the site nor size of the syrinx correlated with the severity or progression of the scoliosis. In another study of children with apparently idiopathic scoliosis, neither the presence of syringomyelia nor Chiari had any bearing on the eventual outcome of the scoliosis surgery (Diab et al. 2011). Orthopaedic surgeons are, however, likely to continue screening scoliosis children because associated bony malformations, such as hemivertebrae or other structural anomalies increase the chance of scoliosis surgery being required (Magge et al. 2011).

13.5.3 Scoliosis and Chiari Without Syringomyelia

Occasionally, in the investigation of scoliosis, MRI will reveal a Chiari I malformation but no demonstrable syrinx. This was the case in 2 of 22 patients in one study (Brockmeyer et al. 2003). It has been suggested that direct compression on the cervicomedullary junction, by the impacted cerebellar tonsils, might interfere with spinal cord function, providing the impetus to initiate and then propagate the scoliosis (Brockmeyer 2011).

13.5.4 Treatment

A number of reasons have been put forward to justify treating syringomyelia in the child presenting with scoliosis (Table 13.2). It is important to emphasise that the following discussion pertains to the effect of syrinx treatment on the scoliosis. Clearly, there may be concomitant neurological indications to treat a syrinx, and neurological features may improve or stabilise after syrinx drainage procedures, despite there being no demonstrable benefit in terms of scoliosis progression (Farley et al. 1995).

Numerous articles support the assertion that scoliosis can be improved or at least stabilised by treating the underlying syringomyelia (Brockmeyer et al. 2003; Eule et al. 2002; Isu

Table 13.2 Suggested reasons for treating syringomyelia associated with scoliosis

Favourably influences the natural history of the scoliosis?
Safer subsequent correction of the scoliosis?
Tonsillar herniation represents a risk under anaesthesia?

et al. 1992; Krieger et al. 2011; Muhonen et al. 1992; Nohria and Oakes 1990; (Ozerdemoglu et al. 2003). This approach, however, needs qualification. Age, for example, seems to be a pertinent factor, and scoliosis is more likely to improve after syrinx treatment in young children compared with adolescents and young adults (Brockmeyer et al. 2003; Ozerdemoglu et al. 2003). The severity of the deformity may also influence the outcome, with curves less than 40° often being halted by early posterior fossa decompression, whereas more severe curves are less likely to improve (Eule et al. 2002). There may also be other aetiological factors influencing outcome, besides the syrinx itself. Congenital scoliosis and scoliosis associated with myelomeningocoele will, for example, have a much lower chance of improvement following treatment of an accompanying syrinx (Ozerdemoglu et al. 2003). The surgical procedure used to treat the syrinx is also likely to be important. After the foramen magnum decompression, the proportion of patients in whom scoliosis improves or is stabilised ranges widely, from 25 % to more than 80 % (Brockmeyer et al. 2003; Eule et al. 2002; Muhonen et al. 1992; Sengupta et al. 2000). The success rate of direct syrinx drainage procedures on the evolution of scoliosis is considerably less. In one group of four patients, progression of the curve was seen in all, in spite of syringe-arachnoid shunting (Phillips et al. 1990). Such variable results may, of course, reflect differences in the severity of the scoliosis pre-operatively, as well as the child's age at the time of surgery.

Another commonly quoted argument in favour of treatment of a syrinx, prior to correction of a scoliosis, is that its decompression makes subsequent correction of the scoliosis safer. The presence of syringomyelia could increase the risk of neurological complications of scoliosis surgery in various ways. The syrinx might make the spinal cord more vulnerable to direct injury, the spinal cord vasculature might be compromised or adhesions around the spinal cord might make it vulnerable to traction forces (Phillips et al. 1990). Evidence to support such assertions is, however, weak and largely stems from case reports and anecdotal experience (Huebert and MacKinnon 1969; Noordeen et al. 1994; Nordwall and Wikkelso 1979). In one study neurological complications were seen in 3 out of 38 patients whose scoliosis was treated without prior syrinx treatment, compared with 1 out of 37 patients where there had been prior intervention to treat syrinx (Ozerdemoglu et al. 2003). In a large multicentre study of idiopathic adolescent scoliosis, 1 in 10 patients who were screened with MRI were found to have an abnormality of the neuraxis. Anomalies included Chiari malformation in 1 in 3 cases and syrinx in 2 out of 3 cases (Diab et al. 2011). None of these patients received neurosurgical intervention prior to scoliosis surgery, and there was no increased morbidity observed in these children. This suggests that, in the absence of symptoms, syringomyelia cavities do not require treatment as a prelude to treating the scoliosis. More recent and larger studies have also shown how benign idiopathic syringomyelia can be and have questioned the dogma that syrinx treatment is essential, to reduce the risk of spinal orthopaedic surgery (Diab et al. 2011 ; Magge et al. 2011). This being so, we may also conclude that there is no role for surgical treatment of Chiari malformation in scoliosis patients when there is no associated syrinx or when there are no symptoms arising from the Chiari itself. When a syrinx is detected, then, unless it is unduly large or there are associated clinical symptoms or signs in addition to the scoliosis, then surgical treatment of the syrinx may, once again, not be needed.

With the scoliosis child facing up to corrective surgery, questions may be raised as to the safety of anaesthesia in the presence of a Chiari malformation. For the otherwise asymptomatic patient, there is no clear evidence to support the assertion that compression of the brainstem at the foramen magnum, by the herniated cerebellar tonsils, represents a risk under anaesthesia. Chiari I malformations can, however, be associated bony anomalies at the craniovertebral junction and can then, occasionally, cause bulbar dysfunction. This may lead to problems such as central respiratory disturbance, vocal cord paresis and reduced pharyngeal sensation. Whilst these disturbances may well be of anaesthetic relevance, it is diffi-

cult, in the absence of clear clinical symptoms of bulbar compromise, to identify an evidence base to support posterior fossa decompressive surgery, solely to ameliorate an anaesthetic risk.

13.6 Summary

Chiari malformations share the common pathology of impaired cerebrospinal fluid circulation through the foramen magnum. Children with symptomatic Chiari malformations and accompanying syringomyelia should be managed by first treating elevated intracranial pressure if present, followed by adequate bony decompression of the cerebellum and brainstem with intradural exploration and duraplasty. With this approach, the vast majority of patients will have resolution of their pre-operative symptoms, diminution of their syrinx and sustained clinical stability.

The interplay between syrinx, Chiari and scoliosis is complex, and the evidence base to guide neurosurgical management in these cases is incomplete and sometimes conflicting. It is clear that there are some patients in whom neurosurgical intervention to decompress a Chiari malformation and improve a syrinx will beneficially affect the natural history of scoliosis, particularly when that intervention is performed at young age and at an early stage in the evolution of the spinal deformity. There are, however, many instances in which a Chiari or a syrinx is identified, simply as a result of screening with MRI and here the need to intervene with a neurosurgical procedure should be evaluated critically. The risks of Chiari or syrinx surgery are not insignificant, and any surgical risk needs particular justification in the case of a neurologically asymptomatic patient. On the basis of current evidence, it is not possible to define rigorous criteria to guide patient selection for surgery. Perhaps more appropriate is a recommendation that scoliosis patients harbouring an abnormality of the neuraxis receive a comprehensive, individualised evaluation, by a neurosurgeon, looking carefully for additional symptoms or signs, which together strengthen the argument for a neurosurgical procedure.

References

Aitken LA, Lindan CE, Sidney S et al (2009) Chiari type I malformation in a pediatric population. Pediatr Neurol 40(6):449–454

Alexander MA, Bunch WH, Ebbesson SO (1972) Can experimental dorsal rhizotomy produce scoliosis? J Bone Joint Surg 54(7):1509–1513

Anderson RC, Emerson RG, Dowling KC et al (2003) Improvement in brainstem auditory evoked potentials after suboccipital decompression in patients with chiari I malformations. J Neurosurg 98(3):459–464

Aoki N, Oikawa A, Sakai T (1995) Spontaneous regeneration of the foramen magnum after decompressive suboccipital craniectomy in Chiari malformation: case report. Neurosurgery 37(2):340–342

Attenello FJ, McGirt MJ, Gathinji M et al (2008) Outcome of Chiari-associated syringomyelia after hindbrain decompression in children: analysis of 49 consecutive cases. Neurosurgery 62(6):1307–1313; discussion 1313

Ball MJ, Dayan AD (1972) Pathogenesis of syringomyelia. Lancet 2(7781):799–801

Batnitzky S, Hall PV, Lindseth RE et al (1976) Meningomyelocele and syringomyelia. Some radiological aspects. Radiology 120(2):351–357

Benjamin JR, Goldberg R, Malcolm W (2009) Neonatal vocal cord paralysis. NeoReviews 10:e494–e501

Bertran SL, Drvaric DM, Roberts JM (1989) Scoliosis in syringomyelia. Orthopaedics 12(2):335–337

Brockmeyer D (2011) Editorial. J Neurosurg Pediatr 7:22–23

Brockmeyer D, Gollogly S, Smith JT (2003) Scoliosis associated with Chiari 1 malformations: the effect of suboccipital decompression on scoliosis curve progression: a preliminary study. Spine 28(22):2505–2509

Chern JJ, Gordon AJ, Mortazavi MM et al (2011) Pediatric Chiari malformation type 0: a 12-year institutional experience. J Neurosurg Pediatr 8(1):1–5

Cochrane DD, Adderley R, White CP et al (1991) Apnea in patients with myelomeningocele. Pediatr Neurosurg 16(4–5):232–239

Diab M, Landman Z, Lubicky J et al (2011) Use and outcome of MRI in the surgical treatment of adolescent idiopathic scoliosis. Spine 36(8):667–671

Elton S, Tubbs RS, Wellons JC 3rd et al (2002) Acute hydrocephalus following a Chiari I decompression. Pediatr Neurosurg 36(2):101–104

Eule JM, Erickson MA, O'Brien MF et al (2002) Chiari I malformation associated with syringomyelia and scoliosis: a twenty-year review of surgical and nonsurgical treatment in a pediatric population. Spine 27(13):1451–1455

Farley FA, Song KM, Birch JG et al (1995) Syringomyelia and scoliosis in children. J Pediatr Orthop 15(2):187–192

Goel A, Desai K (2000) Surgery for syringomyelia: an analysis based on 163 surgical cases. Acta Neurochir 142(3):293–301; discussion 301–392

Greitz D (2006) Unraveling the riddle of syringomyelia. Neurosurg Rev 29(4):251–263; discussion 264

Heinz R, Curnes J, Friedman A et al (1992) Exophytic syrinx, an extreme form of syringomyelia: CT, myelographic, and MR imaging features. Radiology 183(1):243–246

Hesz N, Wolraich M (1985) Vocal-cord paralysis and brainstem dysfunction in children with spina bifida. Dev Med Child Neurol 27(4):528–531

Holinger PC, Holinger LD, Reichert TJ et al (1978) Respiratory obstruction and apnea in infants with bilateral abductor vocal cord paralysis, meningomyelocele, hydrocephalus, and Arnold-Chiari malformation. J Pediatr 92(3):368–373

Holly LT, Batzdorf U (2001) Management of cerebellar ptosis following craniovertebral decompression for Chiari I malformation. J Neurosurg 94(1):21–26

Honein MA, Paulozzi LJ, Mathews TJ et al (2001) Impact of folic acid fortification of the US food supply on the occurrence of neural tube defects. JAMA 285(23):2981–2986

Huebert HT, MacKinnon WB (1969) Syringomyelia and scoliosis. J Bone Joint Surg Br 51(2):338–343

Iskandar BJ, Hedlund GL, Grabb PA et al (1998) The resolution of syringomyelia without hindbrain herniation after posterior fossa decompression. J Neurosurg 89(2):212–216

Isu T, Iwasaki Y, Akino M et al (1990) Syringomyelia associated with a Chiari I malformation in children and adolescents. Neurosurgery 26(4):591–596; discussion 596–597

Isu T, Chono Y, Iwasaki Y et al (1992) Scoliosis associated with syringomyelia presenting in children. Childs Nerv Syst 8(2):97–100

Klekamp J, Iaconetta G, Batzdorf U et al (2002) Syringomyelia associated with foramen magnum arachnoiditis. J Neurosurg 97(3 Suppl):317–322

Krieger MD, Falkinstein Y, Bowen IE et al (2011) Scoliosis and Chiari malformation type I in children. J Neurosurg Pediatr 7(1):25–29

Kyoshima K, Kuroyanagi T, Oya F et al (2002) Syringomyelia without hindbrain herniation: tight cisterna magna. Report of four cases and a review of the literature. J Neurosurg 96(2 Suppl):239–249

Lewonowski K, King JD, Nelson MD (1992) Routine use of magnetic resonance imaging in idiopathic scoliosis patients less than eleven years of age. Spine 17(6 Suppl):S109–S116

Linder A, Lindholm CE (1997) Laryngologic management of infants with the Chiari II syndrome. Int J Pediatr Otorhinolaryngol 39(3):187–197

Liszka O (1961) Spinal cord mechanisms leading to scoliosis in animal experiments. Acta Med Pol 2:45–63

MacEwen GD (1973) Experimental scoliosis. Clin Orthop Relat Res 93:69–74

Magge SN, Smyth MD, Governale LS et al (2011) Idiopathic syrinx in the pediatric population: a combined center experience. J Neurosurg Pediatr 7(1): 30–36

Massimi L, Della Pepa GM, Tamburrini G et al (2011) Sudden onset of Chiari malformation type I in previously asymptomatic patients. J Neurosurg Pediatr 8(5):438–442

McGirt MJ, Attenello FJ, Datoo G et al (2008) Intraoperative ultrasonography as a guide to patient selection for duraplasty after suboccipital decompression in children with Chiari malformation type I. J Neurosurg Pediatr 2(1):52–57

Meadows J, Kraut M, Guarnieri M et al (2000) Asymptomatic Chiari type I malformations identified on magnetic resonance imaging. J Neurosurg 92(6):920–926

Muhonen MG, Menezes AH, Sawin PD et al (1992) Scoliosis in pediatric Chiari malformations without myelodysplasia. J Neurosurg 77(1):69–77

Munshi I, Frim D, Stine-Reyes R et al (2000) Effects of posterior fossa decompression with and without duraplasty on Chiari malformation-associated hydromyelia. Neurosurgery 46(6):1384–1389; discussion 1389–1390

Navarro R, Olavarria G, Seshadri R et al (2004) Surgical results of posterior fossa decompression for patients with Chiari I malformation. Childs Nerv Syst 20(5):349–356

Nohria V, Oakes WJ (1990) Chiari I malformation: a review of 43 patients. Pediatr Neurosurg 16(4–5): 222–227

Noordeen MH, Taylor BA, Edgar MA (1994) Syringomyelia. A potential risk factor in scoliosis surgery. Spine 19(12):1406–1409

Nordwall A, Wikkelso C (1979) A late neurologic complication of scoliosis surgery in connection with syringomyelia. Acta Orthop Scand 50(4):407–410

Oakes WJ (1991) Chiari malformations and syringomyelia in children. In: Neurosurgical operative atlas, vol 1. The American Association of Neurological Surgeons, Park Ridge, pp 59–65

Ozerdemoglu RA, Transfeldt EE, Denis F (2003) Value of treating primary causes of syrinx in scoliosis associated with syringomyelia. Spine 28(8):806–814

Phillips WA, Hensinger RN, Kling TF Jr (1990) Management of scoliosis due to syringomyelia in childhood and adolescence. J Pediatr Orthop 10(3): 351–354

Piatt JH Jr (2004) Syringomyelia complicating myelomeningocele: review of the evidence. J Neurosurg 100 (2 Suppl Pediatrics):101–109

Piatt JH Jr (2010) Treatment of myelomeningocele: a review of outcomes and continuing neurosurgical considerations among adults. J Neurosurg Pediatr 6(6): 515–525

Pollack IF, Pang D, Albright AL et al (1992a) Outcome following hindbrain decompression of symptomatic Chiari malformations in children previously treated with myelomeningocele closure and shunts. J Neurosurg 77(6):881–888

Pollack IF, Pang D, Kocoshis S et al (1992b) Neurogenic dysphagia resulting from Chiari malformations. Neurosurgery 30(5):709–719

Rauzzino M, Oakes WJ (1995) Chiari II malformation and syringomyelia. Neurosurg Clin N Am 6(2):293–309

Sengupta DK, Dorgan J, Findlay GF (2000) Can hindbrain decompression for syringomyelia lead to regression of scoliosis? Eur Spine J 9(3):198–201

Shurtleff DB (2004) Epidemiology of neural tube defects and folic acid. Cerebrospinal Fluid Res 1(1):5

Soleau S, Tubbs RS, Oakes JW (2008) Chiari malformations. In: Pollack I, Adelson P, Albright L (eds) Principles and practice of pediatric neurosurgery. Thieme Medical Publishers, New York, pp 217–232

Talamonti G, D'Aliberti G, Collice M (2007) Myelomeningocele: long-term neurosurgical treatment and follow-up in 202 patients. J Neurosurg 107 (5 Suppl):368–386

Tubbs RS, Oakes WJ (2004) Treatment and management of the Chiari II malformation: an evidence-based review of the literature. Childs Nerv Syst 20(6): 375–381

Tubbs RS, Elton S, Grabb P et al (2001) Analysis of the posterior fossa in children with the Chiari 0 malformation. Neurosurgery 48(5):1050–1054; discussion 1054–1055

Tubbs RS, Beckman J, Naftel RP et al (2011) Institutional experience with 500 cases of surgically treated pediatric Chiari malformation type I. J Neurosurg Pediatr 7(3):248–256

Ventureyra EC, Aziz HA, Vassilyadi M (2003) The role of cine flow MRI in children with Chiari I malformation. Childs Nerv Syst 19(2):109–113

Weprin BE, Oakes WJ (2001) The chiari malformations and associated syringomyelia. In: McLone DG (ed) Pediatric neurosurgery: surgery of the developing nervous system. W.B. Saunders Co, Philadelphia, pp 214–235

Yeh DD, Koch B, Crone KR (2006) Intraoperative ultrasonography used to determine the extent of surgery necessary during posterior fossa decompression in children with Chiari malformation type I. J Neurosurg 105(1 Suppl):26–32

Veterinary Aspects

14

Clare Rusbridge

Contents

C. Rusbridge
Fitzpatrick Referrals, Eashing,
Godalming, Surrey, UK

Faculty of Health and Medical Sciences,
School of Veterinary Medicine, University of Surrey,
Guildford, Surrey, UK
e-mail: neurovet@virginmedia.com

14.1 Introduction

Since the increase in availability of magnetic resonance imaging (MRI), syringomyelia is an increasingly common diagnosis in veterinary medicine (Parker et al. 2011; Rusbridge et al. 2006). The most common cause in the dog is Chiari-like malformation, a condition analogous to Chiari I malformation in humans (Cappello and Rusbridge 2007). The suffix 'like' is added because there are some important features distinguishing Chiari-like malformation from Chiari I malformation in humans, namely, that dogs and cats do not have cerebellar tonsils, and the condition is not dependant on the size of cerebellar vermis herniation (Fig. 14.1).

14.2 Pathophysiology

Chiari-like malformation is characterised by disparity in volume between the caudal cranial fossa and its contents, so that the cerebellum and brainstem are herniated into or through the foramen magnum. Brachycephalicism and miniaturisation are risk factors for Chiari-like malformation (Schmidt et al. 2011). The condition is most commonly reported in toy breed dogs, in particular Cavalier King Charles spaniels, King Charles spaniels, Griffon Bruxellois, Affenpinschers, Yorkshire terriers, Maltese, Chihuahuas, Pomeranians and Papillons. Partly because of its popularity as a pet, the Cavalier King Charles spaniel is overrepresented (Fig. 14.2). Chiari-like

G. Flint, C. Rusbridge (eds.), *Syringomyelia*,
DOI 10.1007/978-3-642-13706-8_14, © Springer-Verlag Berlin Heidelberg 2014

Fig. 14.1 Midline sagittal T2-weighted MRI images from 8-month-old (*top*) and 8-year-old (*bottom*) Cavalier King Charles spaniels with Chiari-like malformation and syringomyelia. The 8-year-old dog is asymptomatic and syringomyelia was identified as part of a programme of screening breeding stock. The 8-month-old dog has a more obvious cerebellar vermis herniation (*arrow*) and a holocord syrinx (*asterisk*). This dog had clinical signs of neuropathic pain including phantom scratching of the shoulder region

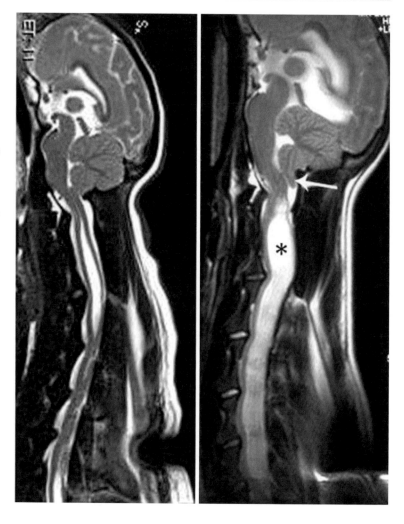

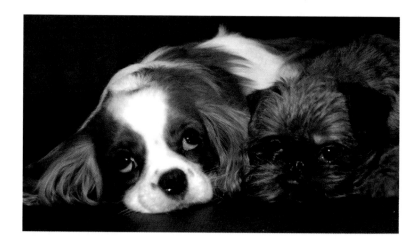

Fig. 14.2 *Left*: Cavalier King Charles Spaniel. *Right*: Griffin Bruxellois (Picture courtesy of Henny van de Berg)

Table 14.1 Comparison between features of Crouzon syndrome and the breed standard for the Griffon Bruxellois

Features	Crouzon syndrome (branchial arch syndrome)	Breed standard Griffon Bruxellois
Skull	Brachycephaly (short and broad head)	Broad head, with rounded and often domed skull Head large in comparison to body
Ears	Low-set ears and high prevalence of ear canal malformations	Semi-erect, high set, the smaller the better
Eyes	Exophthalmos (bulging eyes due to shallow eye sockets after early fusion of surrounding bones)	Large[a] and wide spaced eyes
	Hypertelorism (greater than normal distance between the eyes)	Showing white in the corner of eyes (lateral strabismus) considered desirable by some
	Lateral strabismus	
Nose	Psittichorhina (beak-like nose)	Nose placed between the eyes and as short as possible
Chin	Concave face and protruding chin because of insufficient growth of the upper jaw (hypoplastic maxilla)	Lower jaw curves upwards and should protrude beyond the upper jaw

When the descriptions of some craniosynostosis syndromes associated with Chiari type 1 malformation, e.g. Crouzon syndrome, are compared to the breed standard of some breeds, there is a disturbingly similarity. Selection for a smaller dog and brachycephalic head shape is undoubtedly a contributing factor to canine Chiari-like malformation and syringomyelia. However, it is not the only explanation as Chiari-like malformation is uncommon in some brachycephalic breeds such as Japanese Chin, Pugs and Pekinese. These breeds are less predisposed because, although these dogs have small volume skulls, the brain is also smaller volume and there is no overcrowding in the caudal region of the caudal cranial fossa. In selecting for certain skull and facial characteristics, show breeders are unwittingly selecting for craniosynostosis

[a]Large eyes desired by some breeders appear larger because there is less orbital coverage (larger palpebral aperture) rather than the eyeball being bigger

malformation may also be seen in cats and is again more common in brachycephalic varieties such as the Persian.

Brachycephaly in dogs and cats is a consequence of selecting for juvenile characteristics of flattened face and a 'domed' or 'apple' head (Stockyard 1941). This rounding of the top of the skull is actually bony compensation for basicranial shortening and in reality breeders are actually selecting for craniosynostosis (Table 14.1). Brachiocephalic breeds have early closure of the spheno-occipital synchondrosis, and in Cavalier King Charles spaniels, this closure occurs even earlier (Schmidt et al. 2013). Dog breeders generally strive to produce dogs which adhere strictly to a breed standard.[1] Many breed standards were formulated in the nineteenth or early twentieth century, and registered pedigree dogs can be traced back to foundation stock from this time. Closed stud books ensure that no new genetic material is introduced. Only a small subset of each generation of dogs is used for breeding, and certain males produce a disproportionate number of offspring. This means that many breeds have very small effective population sizes and little genetic diversity. Although this has the advantage of ensuring the desirable appearance, it also means that spontaneous deleterious mutations can become widespread in a population. In addition, to improve success in the show ring, breeders may select for more extreme variations of the breed standard, which may be predisposed to disease and or discomfort (Fig. 14.3).

Brain size is not necessary correlated with body weight in domestic dogs; the ratio of brain size to body weight is larger in miniature compared to large breeds (Roberts et al. 2010). Brachycephalic dogs have considerable brain reorganisation, with the longitudinal axis of the brain adopting a more ventral orientation and the

---

[1]Written guidelines for the appearance, movement and temperament of a dog, which is the template used by breeders to produce typical specimens of the breed and the tool of the judge for assessing dogs in the show ring. In the UK the Kennel Club was founded in 1873 and took ownership of the breed standards drafted by the early dog breeders.

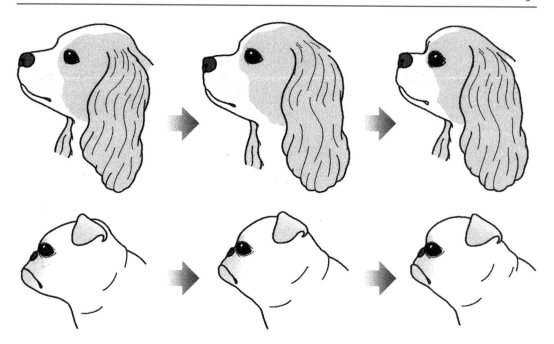

Fig. 14.3 How the Cavalier King Charles spaniel (*top*) and Griffon Bruxellois (*bottom*) head shapes have altered since the 1980s (*left*). A tendency to breed with dogs that are at the extremes of breed standards, or that display characteristics that are slightly bigger, better or more ostentatious than the dogs currently enjoying success in the show ring, will gradually produce dogs that are increasingly extreme. The modern Cavalier King Charles spaniel (*upper right*) typically has a shorter nose, a more pronounced 'stop' (i.e. a more acute angle between the skull and the nasal bone near the eyes), wider spacing between the eyes with the top of the head being broader and more domed. The modern Griffon Bruxellois (*lower right*) often has a shorter muzzle with a more domed skull with a more an 'open face', i.e. eyes that are larger and wider apart giving the dog a more appealing expression (Picture concept and expert opinion from Mrs Lee Pieterse 'Statuesque' Kennel, Sydney Australia, ANKC judge for all Toys and Terriers)

olfactory lobe shifting to a more ventral position (Roberts et al. 2010). Chiari-like malformation in the dog is characterised by extreme brachycephalism (Schmidt et al. 2011) combined with a disproportionately large brain (Cross et al. 2009).

The characteristics of Chiari-like malformation have been most studied in the Cavalier King Charles spaniel where the condition is almost ubiquitous within the breed (Knowler et al. 2011). Compared to some brachycephalic dog breeds, the Cavalier King Charles spaniel has a shorter braincase in relation to width (Schmidt et al. 2011), and compared to Cavalier King Charles spaniels without syringomyelia, syringomyelia-affected Cavalier King Charles spaniels have a shallower and smaller volume caudal cranial fossa (Carrera et al. 2009; Driver et al. 2010a). In the Griffon Bruxellois, Chiari-like malformation is characterised by shortening of the basicranium and supraoccipital bone, with a compensatory lengthening of the cranial vault, especially the parietal bone (Fig. 14.4) (Rusbridge et al. 2009). It has been suggested that, as the skull base is shortened, the developing forebrain is accommodated by lengthening of the other skull bones; however, insufficiency of the caudal cranial fossa bones (basioccipital and supraoccipital) means there is inadequate space for the hindbrain.

The relative size of the brain is also important. The absolute and relative volume of the cavalier King Charles spaniel skull is similar to other brachycephalic toy dog breeds, but cavalier King Charles spaniels have a greater ditto volume of parenchyma within the caudal cranial fossa. Their brain parenchymal volume is approximately equal to that of the Labrador Retriever, a mesaticephalic breed which is two to three times the weight of the Cavalier King Charles spaniel (Cross et al. 2009). There is a relationship between this mismatch in skull and brain volume and the development of syringomyelia. Cavalier King Charles spaniels with early-onset syringomyelia have a

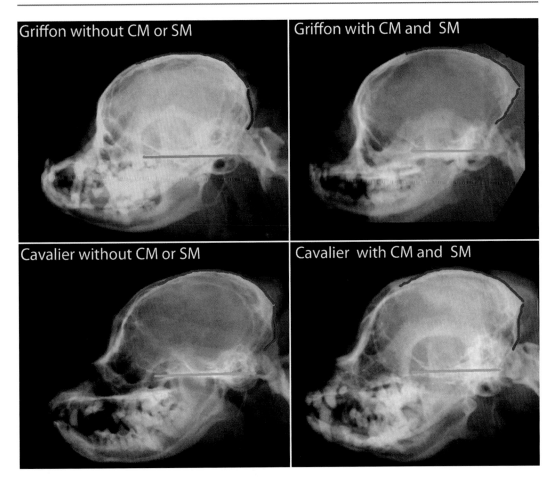

Fig. 14.4 Skull comparisons between Cavalier King Charles spaniels and Griffon Bruxellois with and without Chiari-like malformation or syringomyelia. *Red* approximates outline of parietal and inter parietal bone. *Blue* approximates outline of supraoccipital bone. *Green* approximates the basicranium. Note that with Chiari-like malformation (CM) and syringomyelia (SM), the basicranium shortens. In addition the supraoccipital bone is shorter and straighter, and there is an apparent compensatory lengthening of the parietal bone

larger volume of parenchyma within a smaller caudal cranial fossa compared to older Cavalier King Charles spaniels with Chiari-like malformation only (Driver et al. 2010a, b). This suggests that Chiari-like malformation with syringomyelia is characterised by shortened skull and a lack of coordinated growth of the brain and skull, with a comparatively oversized brain. Moreover, further investigation has shown that Cavalier King Charles spaniels have relatively increased cerebellar volume compared to other breeds and that increased cerebellar volume in Cavalier King Charles spaniels is linked to the development of syringomyelia (Shaw et al. 2012). In addition increased cerebellar volume in Cavalier King Charles spaniels is correlated with increased

crowding of the cerebellum in the caudal part of the caudal cranial fossa (Shaw et al. 2012).

The caudal cranial fossa can be subdivided into three regions, according to their bony walls. The caudal region is bounded by the occipital bones, the middle region by the squamous portion of the temporal bone and the rostral region by the tentorium cerebelli. Cavaliers have a strong relationship between hindbrain volume and rostral part of the caudal cranial fossa volume and a weak relationship between hindbrain volume and caudal part of the caudal cranial fossa volume. In Labrador retrievers and other small breed dogs, this relationship is reversed. This suggests that small breed dogs and Labrador retrievers compensate for variations in hindbrain volume by modifying the growth of the occipital skull. However, in the Cavalier King Charles spaniel, increased cerebellar size is not accommodated by increased occipital bone development and consequently the tentorium cerebelli compensates by bulging in a rostral direction (Shaw et al. 2013). In Cavalier King Charles spaniels with syringomyelia, the angle of the tentorium cerebelli is larger (Carrera et al. 2009). Increase in the angle of the tentorium is also reported in humans with Chiari-like malformation I (Sekula et al. 2005). The overcrowding in the caudal part of the caudal cranial fossa alters cerebrospinal fluid (CSF) dynamics. A phase-contrast cine MRI study indicated that obstruction to CSF flow at the foramen magnum is common in Cavalier King Charles spaniels (Cerda-Gonzalez et al. 2009b). The presence and severity of syringomyelia were positively associated with turbulent flow and jet particularly at the level of the C2–C3 intervertebral disc space. A higher peak CSF flow velocity at the level of the foramen magnum, combined with a lower CSF flow velocity at the level of the C2–C3 intervertebral disc, predicts a higher likelihood of development of a syrinx (Cerda-Gonzalez et al. 2009b). Additionally, in Cavalier King Charles spaniels, ventricle dimensions are positively correlated with syrinx width, supporting the theory that the clinical manifestations of Chiari-like malformation are related to CSF disturbances (Driver et al. 2010a).

14.3 Clinical Signs

Prevalence of syringomyelia is very high in some breeds but not all dogs are symptomatic. In a questionnaire study of all 6-year-old Danish Cavalier King Charles spaniels, the prevalence of dogs expressing signs consistent with syringomyelia was found to be 15.4 % (personal communication in an email from Dr. Mette Berendt 24th November 2011 mbe@life.ku.dk). By contrast MRI of asymptomatic 6-year-old Cavalier King Charles spaniels found a syringomyelia prevalence of 70 % (Parker et al. 2011). The most

important and consistent clinical sign of Chiari-like malformation with syringomyelia is neuropathic pain, arising from damage and dysfunction of the central nervous system and disruption of the balance between nociceptive input and descending regulatory control from the brainstem. Owners may present dogs with signs of spinal pain and may describe spontaneous vocalisation, especially when the dog stands up, jumps or when it is picked up. Sleeping with the head in unusual positions and/or disrupted sleep may be reported (Fig. 14.5). Neuropathic pain can also manifest as allodynia, i.e. signs of discomfort from a non-noxious stimulus, such as touch or wearing a collar, or presumed dysaesthesia, which in the dog can manifest as phantom scratching (Fig. 14.6) or occipital/facial/ear rubbing (Rusbridge and Jeffery 2008). Signs may be exacerbated by excitement and exercise; it is thought because of increased systolic pulse pressure.

Pain is positively correlated with syrinx transverse width and symmetry on the vertical axis, i.e. dogs with a wider asymmetrical syrinx are more likely to experience discomfort, and dogs with a narrow symmetrical syrinx may be asymptomatic (Fig. 14.7) (Rusbridge et al. 2007). However, some dogs with Chiari-like malformation alone express signs of pain; for example, ear/back of skull rubbing, with vocalisation. Histopathological studies of syringomyelia in Cavalier King Charles spaniels found that dogs that expressed signs of pain had an asymmetrical syrinx, with profound alteration of dorsal horn laminar structure (Fig. 14.8) and reduced expression of pain-related neuropeptide substance P and calcitonin gene-related peptide (Hu et al. 2011a). Glial and fibrous proliferation was also associated with expression of clinical signs (Hu et al. 2011b). In symptomatic dogs the syrinx cavity margin is defined by a layer of condensed collagenous tissue, together with small blood vessels with abundant surrounding collagen (Fig. 14.9). Proliferative astrocytes (glial scar) adjacent to the cavity are common. In contrast, the histopathological appearance for asymptomatic Cavalier King Charles spaniels is

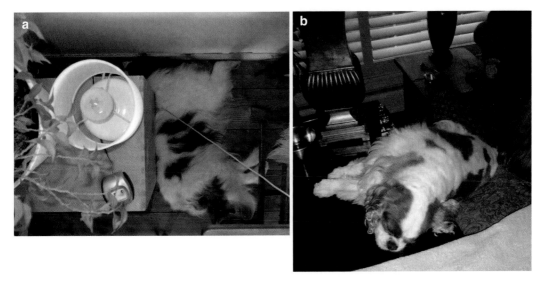

Fig. 14.5 (**a**) Cavalier King Charles spaniel with Chiari-like malformationand syringomyelia This dog routinely slept with his head dorsiflexed and wedged behind a solid object (Picture courtesy of Ms P Persson). (**b**) Cavalier King Charles spaniel with Chiari-like malformation and syringomyelia. This dog slept with her hindquarters lower than her head and with her head on a cooler surface. To achieve this, her head is on a wooden table and her hindquarters are balanced on a cushion and the back of a sofa (Picture courtesy of Mrs S Smith)

Fig. 14.6 'Phantom scratching' in a Cavalier King Charles spaniel. This is typically unilateral and to the neck and shoulder region. Here the scratching left hind limb can be seen as a blur (*arrow*). The dog does not make skin contact. This behaviour can be elicited or exacerbated by excitement, exercise, touch and wearing of neck collars and harnesses (Picture courtesy of Ms J Harrison, Passionate Productions)

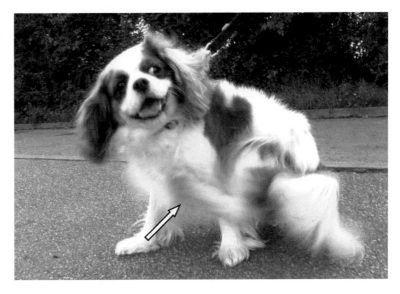

characterised by focal spongiosis, rarefaction and oedema, giving the neural tissue adjacent to the cavity a spongy appearance (Hu et al. 2011b).

Neuropathic pain has an important impact on an individual's quality of life and neurobehaviour (Gustorff et al. 2008), and a recent study in syringomyelia-affected Cavalier King Charles span- iels found an association between the degree of neuropathic pain and fear-/anxiety-related behavioural changes (Rutherford et al. 2012). Dogs with higher neuropathic pain scores were more likely to act fearfully when approached by an unfamiliar person (stranger-directed fear), when in unfamiliar situations or when sudden loud noises occurred, e.g. thunderstorms (nonsocial

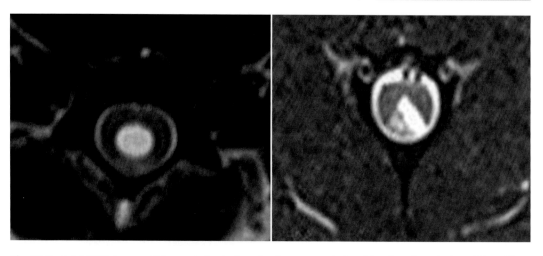

Fig. 14.7 Axial T2W images of the cervical spinal cord from dogs with asymptomatic (*left*) and symptomatic (*right*) syringomyelia. The syrinx in the symptomatic dog is asymmetrical and involves the spinal cord dorsal horn area. NB images are orientated according to the 'human' not the veterinary convention

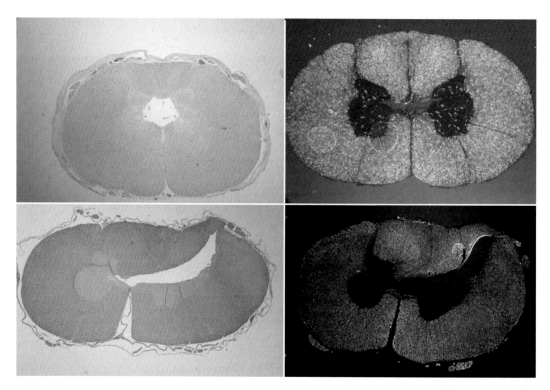

Fig. 14.8 Dark field (*left*) and haematoxylin and eosin (*right*) histopathology sections of cervical spinal cord from Cavalier King Charles spaniels with asymptomatic (*top*) and symptomatic (*bottom*) syringomyelia. The syrinx in the symptomatic dog is asymmetrical, and loss of grey matter from the dorsal horn is evidence. In both dogs the central canal ependyma is lost (Picture courtesy of Drs Hilary Hu and Fernando Constantino-Casas)

fear). Dogs were more attached ('clingy') to the owners (attachment behaviour) and appeared to be more 'afraid' when left alone (separation-

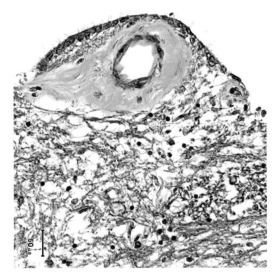

Fig. 14.9 Histopathology sections of cervical spinal cord stained with Masson's Trichrome stain from a symptomatic Cavalier King Charles spaniel with syringomyelia. In close proximity to the syrinx cavity, there are often an increased large number of small blood vessels, both arterial and venous suggestive of angiogenesis. These vessels are often surrounded by a copious amount of collagenous material with markedly thickened tunica media (suggestive of hypertrophy) (Picture courtesy of Drs Hilary Hu and Fernando Constantino-Casas)

related behaviour). Additionally, dogs increased their attention-seeking behaviour and were more excitable in positive, reward-associated situations (excitability) (Rutherford et al. 2012). Cavalier King Charles spaniels with higher neuropathic pain score also showed decreased willingness to exercise and were more likely to have disturbed sleep (Rutherford et al. 2012).

Dogs with a wide syrinx and dorsal grey column damage are also more likely to have cervical torticollis and cervicothoracic scoliosis (Fig. 14.10). This is thought to be due to asymmetrical damage of the dorsal grey column, over a number of spinal cord segments, resulting in an imbalance of afferent proprioceptive information from the cervical neuromuscular spindles (Rusbridge et al. 2007; Van Biervliet et al. 2004). Syringomyelia may result in other neurological deficits, such as thoracic limb weakness and muscle atrophy (due to ventral horn cell damage) and pelvic limb ataxia and weakness (due to white matter damage or involvement of the lumbar spinal cord by the syrinx) (Rusbridge et al. 2006). Cavalier King Charles spaniels with Chiari-like malformation only, or Chiari-like malformation with syringomyelia, may also have subtle gait abnormalities, relating to cerebellar or spinocerebellar tract dysfunction. Investigation is ongoing to establish if these are acquired, for

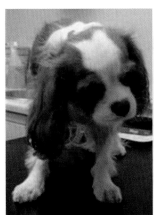
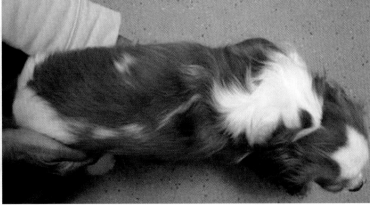

Fig. 14.10 A 2-year-old female Cavalier King Charles spaniel with cervicothoracic scoliosis and torticollis as a consequence of syringomyelia

example, secondary to compression, or if they represent a developmental cerebellar abnormality (personal communication in an email from Dr. Holger Volk 26th June 2012 hvolk@rvc.ac.uk).

There is a high incidence of epilepsy in dogs with Chiari-like malformation, especially in Cavaliers King Charles spaniels. In one report, 32 % of the study population had seizures (Lu et al. 2003), and in a long-term study of 48 Cavalier King Charles spaniels, with syringomyelia-associated neuropathic pain and where dogs with a history of seizures had been excluded from the original cohort, 12.5 % of the study population developed epilepsy in the follow-up period (Plessas et al. 2012). Consequently it has been suggested that there may be an association between Chiari-like malformation and epilepsy in the dog. An association has also been suggested in humans, but again it is unclear whether the association is coincidental (Granata and Valentini 2011). It is important to exclude the possibility of 'drop attacks', i.e. paroxysmal attacks of collapse, with or without loss of consciousness, abnormal extensor posturing and varying degrees of respiratory compromise, that are commonly associated with structural lesions of the cerebellum (Granata and Valentini 2011). In the Cavalier King Charles spaniel, it is also important to exclude the possibility of episodic collapse[2] (Forman et al. 2012). A recent study compared ventricle size and caudal cranial fossa overcrowding and found no significant difference between Cavalier King Charles spaniels with Chiari-like malformation and seizures and those with Chiari-like malformation and other clinical signs but not seizures (Driver et al. 2013).

[2] This autosomal recessive-inherited paroxysmal exertion-induced dyskinesia is characterised by hypertonicity and abnormal posturing, usually occurring after exercise or periods of excitement. It is due to a 16 kb deletion encompassing the first three exons of the brevican gene (BCAN). Brevican is one of the central nervous system-specific members of the hyaluronan-binding chondroitin sulphate proteoglycan family. It is important in the organisation of the nodes of Ranvier in myelinated large diameter axons, and disruption of this region results in a delay in axonal conduction (Forman et al. 2012). Dogs can be screened for the disorder with a DNA test.

Electroencephalogram evaluation, performed in three epileptic dogs, suggested paroxysmal abnormalities were mainly located over the frontal and temporal regions. Similar changes have been reported in humans with seizures and Chiari type I malformation (Elia et al. 1999). Further study is required to investigate if there is a connection between Chiari-like malformation and epilepsy. Vestibular dysfunction, facial nerve paralysis and deafness may also be seen, but, as with epilepsy, no direct relationship has been proven and this association may also be circumstantial.

14.4   Surgical Management

Medical and surgical treatment options exist for dogs with Chiari-like malformation with syringomyelia, and a possible approach to management is illustrated in Fig. 14.11. The main treatment objective is pain relief. The most common surgical management is craniocervical decompression, establishing a CSF pathway via the removal of part of the supraoccipital bone and dorsal arch of C1 (Vermeersch et al. 2004; Rusbridge 2007). Depending on the surgeon, this may be combined with a durotomy, with or without patching with a suitable graft material and with or without a cranioplasty, using titanium mesh or other prosthesis (Dewey et al. 2005, 2007). Craniocervical decompression surgery is successful in reducing pain and improving neurological deficits in approximately 80 % of cases, and approximately 45 % of cases may have a satisfactory quality of life 2 years post-operatively. However, surgery may not adequately address the factors leading to syringomyelia, and the syrinx appears persistent in the majority of cases (Dewey et al. 2005, 2007; Rusbridge 2007; Vermeersch et al. 2004). The clinical improvement is probably attributable to improvement in CSF flow through the foramen magnum. A syringosubarachnoid shunting procedure using a five French equine ocular lavage catheter has also been described. Clinical improvement in approximately 80 % of cases was reported, but there was no evidence of long-term syrinx resolution on

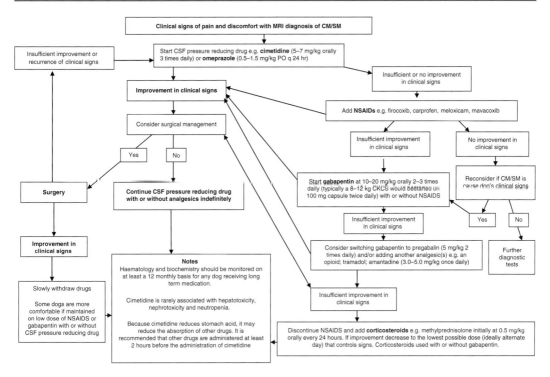

Fig. 14.11 Treatment algorithm for Chiari-like malformation and syringomyelia

post-operative MRI and dogs still expressed signs of neuropathic pain post-operatively (Motta and Skerritt 2012).

14.5 Medical Management

Due to the persistence of syringomyelia and/or spinal cord dorsal horn damage, it is likely that the post-operative patient will require continuing medical management for pain relief. Also, in the majority of canine patients, medical management alone is chosen for financial reasons or owner preference. There are three main drugs used for treatment of Chiari-like malformation with syringomyelia: drugs that reduce CSF production (cimetidine or omeprazole), analgesics (nonsteroidal anti-inflammatory drugs and antiepileptic drugs that have analgesic properties), and corticosteroids. As yet there are no scientific studies to prove the efficacy of these drugs in the management of neuropathic pain in dogs, and recommended management is based on anecdotal evidence only.

14.5.1 Drugs Reducing Cerebrospinal Fluid Production

In experimental models and using a ventriculo-cisternal perfusion technique, omeprazole reduces canine CSF production by 26 % (Javaheri et al. 1997). Although omeprazole is a specific inhibitor of H(+)-K(+)-activated ATPase, it is not clear if this is the mechanism by which it reduces CSF production (Lindvall-Axelsson et al. 1992). Cimetidine has been shown to be superior to ranitidine to reducing CSF production in an experimental cat model. The mechanism of action is proposed to be competitive inhibition of the histamine effect on H2 receptors located on the choroid plexus epithelial cell or by a direct effect on the capillaries of the choroid plexus (Naveh et al. 1992). However, there is also evidence that histamine may act physiologically by increasing the electrical activity of vasopressin-secreting neurons (Armstrong and Sladek 1985). Vasopressin reduces blood flow to the choroid plexus, thereby decreasing CSF production

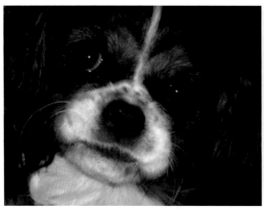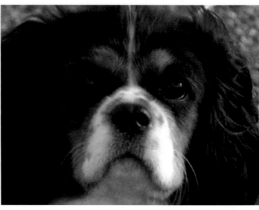

Fig. 14.12 A 2-year-old female Cavalier King Charles spaniel before (*left*) and after (*right*) medication with cimetidine. The image on the left shows 'pain face', i.e. a grimace suggesting discomfort. In contrast the dog's expression on the right is more relaxed (Picture courtesy of Ms T Ledger)

(Faraci et al. 1990). The usefulness of omeprazole or cimetidine on Chiari-like malformation, with or without syringomyelia, is unclear. It is often prescribed in the hope that this may limit disease progression, a variable that is difficult to assess in a scientific study of clinical cases. Some owners report a significant improvement in clinical signs of pain (Fig. 14.12). Adverse effects from these drugs are infrequently reported. Cimetidine retards P450 oxidative hepatic metabolism so caution is advised if using this preparation concurrently with other drugs metabolised by the liver, and with both cimetidine and omeprazole, periodic monitoring of haematology and serum biochemistry is advised. Absorption of gabapentin may be reduced with concurrent cimetidine administration so it has been advised that gabapentin is given 2 h before the cimetidine. An untried alternative may be gabapentin enacarbil, which is a prodrug of gabapentin, stable in gastrointestinal contents and absorbed throughout the intestinal tract by high-capacity nutrient transporters (Lal et al. 2010). It has been suggested that chronic hypergastrinaemia, caused by omeprazole, may increase the risk of gastric carcinomas, at least in laboratory rodent models, but this has not been reported in any other species (Hagiwara et al. 2011; Chapman et al. 2011).

Use of diuretics such as acetazolamide and furosemide for management of Chiari-like

malformation and syringomyelia has also been described (Rusbridge et al. 2000; Rusbridge and Jeffery 2008). The use of acetazolamide is often limited by adverse effects, including lethargy, abdominal pain and bone marrow suppression (Rusbridge et al. 2000). Furosemide may not be ideal in toy breed dogs that also have a high likelihood of mitral valve disease (Lewis et al. 2011) and where the most common cause of death is congestive heart failure (Adams et al. 2010). Furosemide can result in significant increase in plasma aldosterone concentration and renin activity in healthy dogs (Pedersen 1996). This early activation of the renin-angiotensin-aldosterone system might be deleterious in an animal predisposed to heart disease (Connell et al. 2008). Moreover, long-term use of diuretics can lead to a diuretic-resistant state, which necessitates the use of higher doses, further activating the renin-angiotensin-aldosterone system (Parrinello et al. 2011).

14.5.2 Analgesics

Anecdotally, nonsteroidal anti-inflammatory drugs (NSAIDS), e.g. meloxicam, carprofen, firocoxib and mavacoxib, can be useful in management of Chiari-like malformation and syringomyelia. NSAIDS are inhibitors of Cyclooxygenase-1 and/or Cyclooxygenase-2 and suppress inflammatory pain by reducing generation of prostanoids, in particular prostaglandin E2. Prostaglandin E2 also contributes to the genesis of neuropathic pain (Kawabata 2011). However, monotherapy with NSAIDs is unlikely to provide sufficient analgesia, especially if there has been damage to the spinal cord dorsal column. Therefore, in these situations, the addition of antiepileptic drugs with an anti-allodynic effect is recommended (Rusbridge and Jeffery 2008). Gabapentin and pregabalin modulate voltage-gated calcium channels resulting in a reduction of glutamate and substance P release and can be effective for neuropathic pain syndromes (Tremont-Lukats et al. 2000). Anecdotally, pregabalin is most efficacious for treating Chiari-like malformation and syringomyelia in dogs, but gabapentin can also be useful and is more economic. In severe cases that still have clinical signs, despite polypharmacy, the addition of opioids, tramadol or amantadine can be useful. It should be borne in mind that, with the exception of NSAIDs, there are no licenced oral analgesics in veterinary medicine.

14.5.3 Corticosteroids

Corticosteroids are believed to provide long-term pain relief because of their ability to inhibit the production of phospholipase-A-2 (Nolan 2000) and to inhibit the expression of multiple inflammatory genes coding for cytokines, enzymes, receptors and adhesion molecules (Barnes 1998). Corticosteroids are also reported to reduce sympathetically mediated pain (Gellman 2000) and decrease substance P expression (Wong and Tan 2002). Anecdotally, oral drugs such as methylprednisolone and prednisolone provide relief for some dogs with syringomyelia and can also be useful where there are significant neurological deficits, but adverse effects limit their usefulness for long-term therapy (Rusbridge et al. 2000).

14.6 Progression and Prognosis

The clinical signs of Chiari-like malformation and syringomyelia are often progressive. A recent long-term study, over a mean of 39 ± 14.3 months, found that approximately three-quarters of Cavalier King Charles spaniels with Chiari-like malformation and syringomyelia-associated neuropathic pain will deteriorate when managed medically, whereas one quarter remain static or improved (Plessas et al. 2012). However, despite this progression, all the owners of the alive dogs in this study reported that their dog's quality of life was not severely compromised (Plessas et al. 2012). Fifteen percent of dogs were euthanased because of severe neuropathic pain. Morphometric values (volume of the caudal cranial fossa, parenchyma within the caudal cranial fossa and the sizes of the ventricles and syringes) were not correlated with prognosis. As discussed above, dogs with higher neuropathic pain scores are more likely to have fear-related behaviour, which can have a negative impact on the owner-perceived quality of life of a dog (Rutherford et al. 2012). Interestingly, obesity is also positively correlated with a reduced quality of life but not greater neuropathic pain. Obesity has an influence on the health and the quality of life in animals as it does in humans (German et al. 2012). In humans there is also a known association between increasing body mass index and CSF disorders such as idiopathic intracranial hypertension; however, it has not been established if the obesity is the cause or effect of this disease (Hannerz and Ericson 2009).

Some authors have suggested that early surgical intervention may improve prognosis, but robust studies evaluating this hypothesis have not been performed (Dewey et al. 2005). In addition, surgery does not necessarily improve long-term prognosis as 25–47 % of the operated dogs have recurrence or deterioration of the clinical signs within 0.2–3 years after surgery (Dewey et al. 2005, 2007; Rusbridge 2007). However, it should be remembered that it is probable that the groups of surgically managed cases contain dogs with more severe clinical signs so a valid comparison between medical and surgical management cannot be made at this time.

Fig. 14.13 Pseudorosettes of ependymocytes clustered around a core of fibrovascular tissue (Picture courtesy of Drs Hilary Hu and Fernando Constantino-Casas)

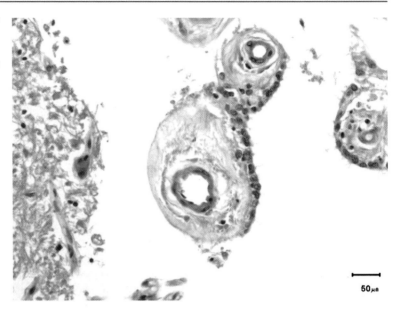

50 μs

14.7 Learning About the Pathogenesis of Syringomyelia from Observations in Dogs

There are many poorly understood features of canine Chiari-like malformation and syringomyelia, including the pathogenesis of the syrinx and the precise origin of the pain. Pathological observations suggest that in the Cavalier King Charles spaniels, development of syringomyelia is related to increased central canal pressure. Central canal dilatation is typically the first change observed on MRI (Rusbridge et al. 2006), and disrupted integrity of the ependyma is a universal feature, regardless of clinical status (Hu et al. 2011b). Moreover there is an absence of pathological changes to suggest that fluid is drawn into the parenchyma from blood vessels or the subarachnoid space. For example, we do not see an accumulation of pools of fluid within the parenchyma, distant from the central canal. However, there is evidence of increased intra-canal pressure, in the form of tissue responses that would increase mechanical strength (Hu et al. 2011b). It has been demonstrated, in a contusion model of chronic

spinal cord injury, that ascending central canal dilation occurs following injury and that expansion of the central canal lumen beyond a critical diameter corresponds with ependymal cell ciliary loss, together with thinning and a decrease in cell proliferation in the ependymal region.[3] Normally, ependymal cells form a pseudostratified monolayer of epithelium that regulates fluid and electrolyte balance between the CSF and neuropil and also plays an important role in cellular signalling and wound repair in the spinal cord (Radojicic et al. 2007). In addition to ependymal disruption, pseudorosettes of ependymocytes may be observed, clustered around a core of fibrovascular tissue (Fig. 14.13), a finding also described by others (Williams and Weller 1973; Attar et al. 2005).

The normal histology of the central canal has been studied in the German shepherd (Marin-Garcia et al. 1995). There is functional communication between the central canal and the

---

[3] The ependymal region contains stem cells which proliferate in response to injury and have the potential to generate new neurons and glial cells in adulthood (Attar et al. 2005; Hugnot and Franzen 2011).

subarachnoid space at the terminal ventricle.[4] This probably constitutes one of the drainage pathways of the cerebrospinal fluid. Some researchers are of the opinion that the spinal cord itself produces extracellular fluid, whose egress towards the subarachnoid space or central canal depends on the pressure differential between the two compartments (Radojicic et al. 2007). Even in very old dogs, the spinal cord central canal reaches the tip of the filum terminale and remains patent (Marin-Garcia et al. 1995). Occasional communication of syrinx cavities with the spinal subarachnoid space, at the level of the filum terminale, has been demonstrated in an experimental model of canine syringomyelia (Williams and Bentley 1980). Although loss of ependymal integrity and central canal dilation is observed in adult Cavalier King Charles spaniels, studies of neonatal cervical spinal cords found increased ependymal cell counts, in addition to reduced height of the grey commissure, in other words the central grey matter above the central canal. The central canal diameter was considered normal (Giejda et al. 2012). Whether this ultrastructural change is involved in the pathogenesis of syringomyelia is unclear, but temporary increase in ependymal cell numbers has been observed as an early change in a contusion model of chronic spinal cord injury (Radojicic et al. 2007).

Dogs from breeds predisposed to Chiari-like malformation and syringomyelia, which are intended for breeding purposes, are often MRI-screened for the disease. This allows observations of early preclinical stages of these disorders. The earliest change is a central canal dilatation,

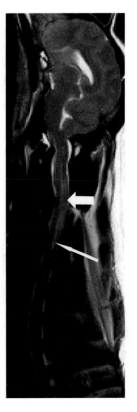

Fig. 14.14 Midline sagittal T2-weighted MRI images from a 3-year-old Cavalier King Charles spaniel. There is a central canal dilatation particularly in the C2–C5 region (*narrow arrow*) and a presyrinx in the dorsal C2 and C3 spinal cord (*broad arrow*)

in particular in the C2/C3 region. Another common early change is spinal cord oedema or the presyrinx state (Fig. 14.14). In some dogs this appears to be associated with clinical signs of neuropathic pain, with histopathological changes in the spinal cord dorsal horn. In the Cavalier King Charles spaniel, syringomyelia tends to develop first within the C2–C4, T2–T4 and T12–L2 spinal cord segments (Fig. 14.15). These are areas where the subarachnoid space narrows and/or there is a change in the angulation of the vertebral canal. According to the Venturi effect, increased fluid velocity through a narrowed flow channel decreases hydrostatic pressure in the fluid, meaning that there may be a tendency for the spinal cord to be 'sucked' outward in these regions which may be a contributory factor in

---

[4] The terminal ventricle (ventriculus terminalis, or fifth ventricle) is an enlargement of spinal cord central canal within or near the filum terminale. In many species, and possibly some humans, there is a functional communication between this dilated central canal and the subarachnoid space. In humans the terminal ventricle is visible in the foetus and children but is usually absent in adults. There is evidence suggesting that the cerebrospinal fluid in the central canal may facilitate non-synaptic neural transmission or clear waste products and particulate matter from the parenchyma (so called 'sink' function) (Storer et al. 1998).

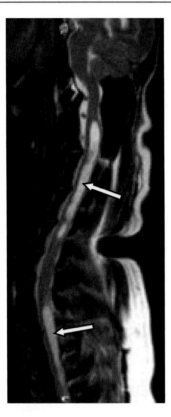

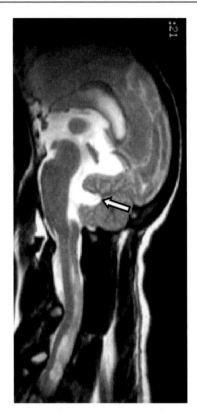

Fig. 14.15 Midline sagittal T2-weighted MRI images from a 6-year-old Cavalier King Charles spaniel. Syringomyelia typically develops in the cranial cervical and cranial thoracic spinal cord (*arrows*)

Fig. 14.16 Midline sagittal T2-weighted MRI image from a Griffon Bruxellois with syringomyelia but without Chiari-like malformation. This dog also has a small quadrigeminal cyst and ventriculomegaly of in particular the fourth ventricle (*arrow*)

syrinx development (Rusbridge et al. 2006). Development of holocord syrinx is characterised by 'joining up' of the cervical, thoracic and lumbar syringes and will typically extend from C2 to L4 (the conus medullaris is at the level of the L6 vertebrae in most dogs and there are seven lumbar vertebrae). In clinically affected dogs, it is important to image the entire spinal cord to determine the extent of disease. One study demonstrated that 76 % of dogs with a syrinx at C1–C4 also had a syrinx in the C5–T1 and T2–L2 regions and 49 % had a syrinx in the L3–L7 region (Loderstedt et al. 2011).

14.7.1 Idiopathic Syringomyelia

Another question in the pathogenesis of syringomyelia in toy breeds is the mechanism of development of syringomyelia when there

is not an obvious Chiari-like malformation and/ or marked foramen magnum obstruction (Fig. 14.16). This observation has led to the suggestion of alternative hypotheses for syringomyelia pathogenesis, such as the role of intracranial hypertension (Rusbridge et al. 2009). This hypothesis has also been suggested in humans with achondroplasia – a condition also characterised by a small skull base (Moritani et al. 2006). It has been postulated that only a small abnormal gradient of static pressure across the cerebral mantle is sufficient to produce ventricular dilatation (Levine 2004). In humans, it has been demonstrated that venous narrowing at the jugular foramina associated with a small skull base can lead to elevated venous pressure (Cinalli et al. 2005; Di Rocco et al. 2011). This impairs CSF absorption, resulting in communicating hydrocephalus (Moritani et al. 2006). It has also been proposed that in humans, herniation of the cerebellum and brainstem in craniosynostosis is not just a consequence of the anatomical deformity and small posterior fossa but also because of intracranial hypertension (Di Rocco et al. 2011; Thompson et al. 1997). Recently it has been demonstrated that Cavalier King Charles spaniels with syringomyelia have significantly smaller volume jugular foramina than Cavalier King Charles spaniels without syringomyelia (Schmidt et al. 2012a).

14.7.2 Conditions Associated with Chiari-Related Syringomyelia in the Dog

Occipital dysplasia, i.e. widened foramen magnum, is commonly associated with Chiari-like malformation and syringomyelia (Rusbridge and Knowler 2006). There is evidence to suggest that this is an acquired condition as the size of the foramen magnum increases significantly between serial MRI scans in Cavalier King Charles spaniels (Driver et al. 2013). The length of the cerebellar herniation also increases, suggesting that there is resorption of bone as a consequence of overcrowding of the caudal cranial fossa (Driver et al. 2012). Other abnormalities of the craniocervical regions, which may be seen in dogs with Chiarilike malformation and syringomyelia, are atlantoaxial subluxation (Stalin et al. 2008), dens abnormalities (Bynevelt et al. 2000) and atlantooccipital overlapping, similar to basilar invagination in humans (Cerda-Gonzalez et al. 2009a; Marino et al. 2012) (Fig. 14.17). It is common for there to be bony or ligamentous dorsal impingement of the spinal canal at the C1/C2 junction, and it is possible that this may contribute to the pathogenesis of syringomyelia, by either compression of the subarachnoid space and/or the spinal cord (Marino et al. 2012) (Fig. 14.17). Brachycephalic dogs are also predisposed to quadrigeminal cysts (Matiasek et al. 2007). By occupying space within an already crowded caudal cranial fossa, this may aggravate the obstruction at the foramen magnum and increase the likelihood of syringomyelia developing, although most quadrigeminal cysts are incidental findings (Fig. 14.16).

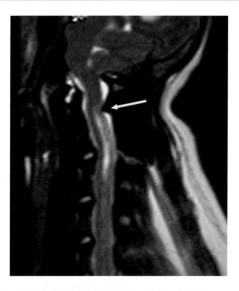

Fig. 14.17 Midline sagittal T2-weighted MRI image from a Cavalier King Charles spaniel with atlantoaxial overlapping and dorsal compression of the spinal canal by the dorsal arch of C1 (*arrow*). The syringomyelia appears to start at the level of spinal cord impingement

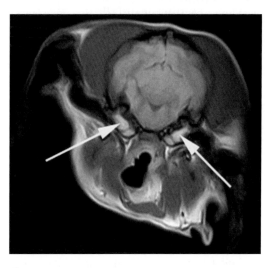

Fig. 14.18 Transverse T1-weighted MRI scan at the level of the tympanic bullae in a Cavalier King Charles spaniel with bilateral otitis media with effusion (*arrows*)

Cavalier King Charles spaniels with Chiarilike malformation are predisposed to otitis media with effusion[5] (Fig. 14.18). This may be in part

---

[5] Otitis media with effusion is often referred to as 'glue ear' and is characterised by thick or sticky fluid behind the eardrum in the middle ear but no ear infection. In the Cavalier King Charles spaniel, it is also sometimes referred to as primary secretary otitis media or PSOMs.

due to skull conformation but is also significantly associated with greater thickness of the soft palate and reduced nasopharyngeal aperture (Hayes et al. 2010). This is associated with conductive hearing loss of 10–33 dB in affected dogs (Harcourt-Brown et al. 2011) and anecdotally may be associated with discomfort. After flushing of the dog's external auditory meatus, some owners report reduction in signs suggesting ear discomfort. A similar situation is common in humans, and most patients with syndromic and complex craniosynostosis have recurrent otitis media with effusion, causing episodes of conductive hearing loss throughout their lives (de Jong et al. 2011).

In addition to Chiari-like malformation and syringomyelia, the Cavalier King Charles spaniel breed has a high prevalence of other disorders, such as mitral valve disease (40.6 % prevalence) (Serfass et al. 2006), macrothrombocytopaenia, a platelet disorder due to a mutation in the gene-encoding beta1-tubulin (46 % prevalence) (Pedersen et al. 2002), and a tendency towards systemic fibrosis, resulting in multiple organ dysfunction and in particular pancreatic disorders (Watson et al. 2007). Investigation of possible common causal mechanisms in these diverse conditions is ongoing.

14.8 Learning About Neuropathic Pain from Observations in Dogs

As a natural-occurring model, dogs present a valuable resource for understanding and managing both Chiari-like malformation, with or without syringomyelia, and central neuropathic pain in humans. Unlike laboratory rodent models, dogs are higher mammals exposed to similar environmental conditions as humans, for example, variable diet and exercise. They are expected to enjoy an active lifestyle with a life expectancy of 10 years or more. Central neuropathic pain is an important and disabling but under-researched problem in human medicine (Finnerup 2008).

The majority of clinical trials for drugs licenced for treatment of neuropathic pain are in groups of humans with peripheral neuropathic pain, such as post-herpetic neuralgia (Argoff 2011) and diabetic neuropathy (Chong and Hester 2007). Although providing useful information, these trials are not necessarily applicable to patients with central neuropathic pain. Therefore, ongoing clinical trials in these much-loved pets may provide paramount information about managing syringomyelia in humans.

Chronic neuropathic pain is often associated with affective disorders, such as depression and anxiety (Wetering et al. 2010). However, because of the complex nature of mood disorders, investigating an association or attributing a subtle behavioural change to neuropathic pain is difficult. Dogs suffering from chronic pain may also have negative mental states, and there is ongoing investigation as to whether this affects cognitive bias, i.e. the tendency to make systematic decisions in certain circumstances based on cognitive factors, rather than evidence.

14.9 Genetic Factors and Breeding Advice

The high prevalence, within one closely related population, suggests that syringomyelia is inherited in the dog and studies in the Cavalier King Charles spaniel have shown it to be a complex trait, with a moderately high heritability ($h2 = 0.37 \pm 0.15$ standard error) (Lewis et al. 2010). Syringomyelia has a varying age of onset – there is 46 % prevalence in asymptomatic breeding Cavalier King Charles spaniels – but prevalence increases with age and may be as high as 70 % in dogs over 6 years of age (Parker et al. 2011). Since the early 2000s, it has been recommended that dogs of breeds predisposed to Chiari-like malformation and/or syringomyelia be MRI-screened at least twice in their lifetime. Breeding recommendations based on syringomyelia status and ages were formulated in 2006. These guidelines concentrated on removing dogs with early-onset syringomyelia from the breeding pool whilst maintaining genetic diversity (Cappello and Rusbridge 2007). Early results from this breeding programme indicated that offspring without syringomyelia were more common when the parents were both clear of syringomyelia (syringomyelia-free; Cavalier King Charles spaniels 70 %, Griffon Bruxellois 73 %). Conversely offspring with syringomyelia were more likely when both parents had syringomyelia (syringomyelia affected; Cavalier King Charles spaniels 92 %, Griffon Bruxellois 100 %). A mating of one syringomyelia-free parent with an syringomyelia-affected parent was risky for syringomyelia affectedness with 77 % of Cavalier King Charles spaniels and 46 % of Griffon Bruxellois offspring being syringomyelia affected (Knowler et al. 2011).

In the UK, from January 2012, there has been a British Veterinary Association/Kennel Club Canine Health Scheme to MRI-screen potential breeding stock for Chiari-like malformation and/or syringomyelia. MRI images are assessed by two scrutineers and graded for severity for both Chiari-like malformation and syringomyelia and, as syringomyelia is a late-onset condition, the age of onset. Results are also submitted to a central database, in order to generate estimated breeding values. An estimated breeding value is statistical, numerical estimate of an individual's true breeding value for a trait(s), based on the diagnostic or screening test results of the individual and their close relatives. This is a systematic way of combining available health information on a breed-wide scale and the estimated breeding values for Chiari-like malformation, and syringomyelia can be combined with those for other genetic diseases (e.g. mitral valve dysplasia in the Cavalier King Charles spaniels). Estimated breeding values are limited to the genetic liabilities and do not include environmental influences subsequent to birth. Using an estimated breeding value system will provide breeders with accurate information about puppies from birth and allow them to select mates with the lowest risk for disease-affected offspring, whilst maintaining genetic diversity.

As an accurate estimated breeding value, database may take some time to compile; the recommended breeding guidelines have been revised (more details are available at http://www.veterinary-neurologist.co.uk/).

References

Adams VJ, Evans KM, Sampson J et al (2010) Methods and mortality results of a health survey of purebred dogs in the UK. J Small Anim Pract 51(10):512–524. doi:10.1111/j.1748-5827.2010.00974.x

Argoff CE (2011) Review of current guidelines on the care of postherpetic neuralgia. Postgrad Med 123(5):134–142. doi:10.3810/pgm.2011.09.2469

Armstrong WE, Sladek CD (1985) Evidence for excitatory actions of histamine on supraoptic neurons in vitro: mediation by an H1-type receptor. Neuroscience 16(2):307–322

Attar A, Kaptanoglu E, Aydin Z et al (2005) Electron microscopic study of the progeny of ependymal stem cells in the normal and injured spinal cord. Surg Neurol 64(Suppl 2):S28–S32. doi:10.1016/j.surneu.2005.07.057

Barnes PJ (1998) Anti-inflammatory actions of glucocorticoids: molecular mechanisms. Clin Sci (Lond) 94(6):557–572

Bynevelt M, Rusbridge C, Britton J (2000) Dorsal dens angulation and a Chiari type malformation in a Cavalier King Charles Spaniel. Vet Radiol Ultrasound 41(6):521–524

Cappello R, Rusbridge C (2007) Report from the Chiari-Like Malformation and Syringomyelia Working Group round table. Vet Surg 36(5):509–512. doi:10.1111/j.1532-950X.2007.00298.x

Carrera I, Dennis R, Mellor DJ et al (2009) Use of magnetic resonance imaging for morphometric analysis of the caudal cranial fossa in Cavalier King Charles Spaniels. Am J Vet Res 70(3):340–345. doi:10.2460/ajvr.70.3.340

Cerda-Gonzalez S, Dewey CW, Scrivani PV et al (2009a) Imaging features of atlanto-occipital overlapping in dogs. Vet Radiol Ultrasound 50(3):264–268

Cerda-Gonzalez S, Olby NJ, Broadstone R et al (2009b) Characteristics of cerebrospinal fluid flow in Cavalier King Charles Spaniels analyzed using phase velocity cine magnetic resonance imaging. Vet Radiol Ultrasound 50(5):467–476

Chapman DB, Rees CJ, Lippert D et al (2011) Adverse effects of long-term proton pump inhibitor use: a review for the otolaryngologist. J Voice 25(2):236–240. doi:10.1016/j.jvoice.2009.10.015

Chong MS, Hester J (2007) Diabetic painful neuropathy: current and future treatment options. Drugs 67(4):569–585

Cinalli G, Spennato P, Sainte-Rose C et al (2005) Chiari malformation in craniosynostosis. Childs Nerv Syst 21(10):889–901. doi:10.1007/s00381-004-1115-z

Connell JM, MacKenzie SM, Freel EM et al (2008) A lifetime of aldosterone excess: long-term consequences of altered regulation of aldosterone production for cardiovascular function. Endocr Rev 29(2):133–154. doi:10.1210/er.2007-0030

Cross HR, Cappello R, Rusbridge C (2009) Comparison of cerebral cranium volumes between cavalier King Charles spaniels with Chiari-like malformation, small breed dogs and Labradors. J Small Anim Pract 50(8):399–405. doi:10.1111/j.1748-5827.2009.00799.x

de Jong T, Toll MS, de Gier HH et al (2011) Audiological profile of children and young adults with syndromic and complex craniosynostosis. Arch Otolaryngol Head Neck Surg 137(8):775–778. doi:10.1001/archoto.2011.115

Dewey CW, Berg JM, Barone G (2005) Foramen magnum decompression for treatment of caudal occipital malformation syndrome in dogs. J Am Vet Med Assoc 227(8):1270–1275, 1250–1251

Dewey CW, Marino DJ, Bailey KS et al (2007) Foramen magnum decompression with cranioplasty for treatment of caudal occipital malformation syndrome in dogs. Vet Surg 36(5):406–415. doi:10.1111/j.1532-950X.2007.00286.x

Di Rocco C, Frassanito P, Massimi L et al (2011) Hydrocephalus and Chiari type I malformation. Childs Nerv Syst 27(10):1653–1664. doi:10.1007/s00381-011-1545-3

Driver CJ, Rusbridge C, Cross HR et al (2010a) Relationship of brain parenchyma within the caudal cranial fossa and ventricle size to syringomyelia in cavalier King Charles spaniels. J Small Anim Pract 51(7):382–386. doi:10.1111/j.1748-5827.2010.00952.x

Driver CJ, Rusbridge C, McGonnell IM et al (2010b) Morphometric assessment of cranial volumes in age-matched Cavalier King Charles spaniels with and without syringomyelia. Vet Rec 167(25):978–979. doi:10.1136/vr.c4109

Driver CJ, De Risio L, Hamilton S et al (2012) Changes over time in craniocerebral morphology and syringomyelia in cavalier King Charles spaniels with Chiari-like malformation. BMC Vet Res 8(1):215. doi:10.1186/1746-6148-8-215

Driver CJ, Chandler K, Walmsley G et al (2013) The association between Chiari-like malformation, ventriculomegaly and seizures in cavalier King Charles spaniels. Vet J 195:235–237. doi:10.1016/j.tvjl.2012.05.014

Elia M, Biondi R, Sofia V et al (1999) Seizures in Chiari I malformation: a clinical and electroencephalographic study. J Child Neurol 14(7):446–450

Faraci FM, Mayhan WG, Heistad DD (1990) Effect of vasopressin on production of cerebrospinal fluid: possible role of vasopressin (V1)-receptors. Am J Physiol 258(1 Pt 2):R94–R98

Finnerup NB (2008) A review of central neuropathic pain states. Curr Opin Anaesthesiol 21(5):586–589. doi:10.1097/ACO.0b013e32830a4c11

Forman OP, Penderis J, Hartley C et al (2012) Parallel mapping and simultaneous sequencing reveals deletions in BCAN and FAM83H associated with discrete inherited disorders in a domestic dog breed. PLoS Genet 8(1):e1002462. doi:10.1371/journal.pgen.1002462

Gellman H (2000) Reflex sympathetic dystrophy: alternative modalities for pain management. Instr Course Lect 49:549–557

German AJ, Holden SL, Wiseman-Orr ML et al (2012) Quality of life is reduced in obese dogs but improves after successful weight loss. Vet J 192(3):428–434. doi:10.1016/j.tvjl.2011.09.015

Giejda A, Veal J, Volk H et al (eds) (2012) Spinal cord analysis in the Neonatal Cavalier King Charles Spaniel 25th annual symposium of the European College of Neurology, Ghent, 14–15 Sept 2012.

Granata T, Valentini LG (2011) Epilepsy in type 1 Chiari malformation. Neurol Sci 32(Suppl 3):S303–S306. doi:10.1007/s10072-011-0697-y

Gustorff B, Dorner T, Likar R et al (2008) Prevalence of self-reported neuropathic pain and impact on quality of life: a prospective representative survey. Acta Anaesthesiol Scand 52(1):132–136. doi:10.1111/j.1399-6576.2007.01486.x

Hagiwara T, Mukaisho K, Nakayama T et al (2011) Long-term proton pump inhibitor administration worsens atrophic corpus gastritis and promotes adenocarcinoma development in Mongolian gerbils infected with Helicobacter pylori. Gut 60(5):624–630. doi:10.1136/gut.2010.207662

Hannerz J, Ericson K (2009) The relationship between idiopathic intracranial hypertension and obesity. Headache 49(2):178–184. doi:10.1111/j.1526-4610.2008.01240.x

Harcourt-Brown TR, Parker JE, Granger N et al (2011) Effect of middle ear effusion on the brain-stem auditory evoked response of Cavalier King Charles Spaniels. Vet J 188(3):341–345. doi:10.1016/j.tvjl.2010.05.018

Hayes GM, Friend EJ, Jeffery ND (2010) Relationship between pharyngeal conformation and otitis media with effusion in Cavalier King Charles spaniels. Vet Rec 167(2):55–58. doi:10.1136/vr.b4886

Hu HZ, Rusbridge C, Constantino-Casas F et al (2011a) Distribution of substance P and calcitonin gene-related peptide in the spinal cord of Cavalier King Charles Spaniels affected by symptomatic syringomyelia. Res Vet Sci 93(1):318–320. doi:10.1016/j.rvsc.2011.08.012

Hu HZ, Rusbridge C, Constantino-Casas F et al (2011b) Histopathological investigation of syringomyelia in the Cavalier King Charles spaniel. J Comp Pathol 146(2–3):192–201. doi:10.1016/j.jcpa.2011.07.002

Hugnot JP, Franzen R (2011) The spinal cord ependymal region: a stem cell niche in the caudal central nervous system. Front Biosci 16:1044–1059

Javaheri S, Corbett WS, Simbartl LA et al (1997) Different effects of omeprazole and Sch 28080 on canine cerebrospinal fluid production. Brain Res 754(1–2): 321–324

Kawabata A (2011) Prostaglandin E2 and pain–an update. Biol Pharm Bull 34(8):1170–1173

Knowler SP, McFadyen AK, Rusbridge C (2011) Effectiveness of breeding guidelines for reducing the prevalence of syringomyelia. Vet Rec 169(26):681. doi:10.1136/vr.100062

Lal R, Sukbuntherng J, Luo W et al (2010) Clinical pharmacokinetic drug interaction studies of gabapentin enacarbil, a novel transported prodrug of gabapentin, with naproxen and cimetidine. Br J Clin Pharmacol 69(5):498–507. doi:10.1111/j.1365-2125.2010.03616.x

Levine DN (2004) The pathogenesis of syringomyelia associated with lesions at the foramen magnum: a critical review of existing theories and proposal of a new hypothesis. J Neurol Sci 220(1–2):3–21. doi:10.1016/j.jns.2004.01.014

Lewis T, Rusbridge C, Knowler P et al (2010) Heritability of syringomyelia in Cavalier King Charles spaniels. Vet J 183(3):345–347. doi:10.1016/j.tvjl.2009.10.022

Lewis T, Swift S, Woolliams JA et al (2011) Heritability of premature mitral valve disease in Cavalier King Charles spaniels. Vet J 188(1):73–76. doi:10.1016/j.tvjl.2010.02.016

Lindvall-Axelsson M, Nilsson C, Owman C et al (1992) Inhibition of cerebrospinal fluid formation by omeprazole. Exp Neurol 115(3):394–399

Loderstedt S, Benigni L, Chandler K et al (2011) Distribution of syringomyelia along the entire spinal cord in clinically affected Cavalier King Charles Spaniels. Vet J 190(3):359–363. doi:10.1016/j.tvjl.2010.12.002

Lu D, Lamb CR, Pfeiffer DU et al (2003) Neurological signs and results of magnetic resonance imaging in 40 cavalier King Charles spaniels with Chiari type 1-like malformations. Vet Rec 153(9):260–263

Marin-Garcia P, Gonzalez-Soriano J, Martinez-Sainz P et al (1995) Spinal cord central canal of the German shepherd dog: morphological, histological, and ultrastructural considerations. J Morphol 224(2):205–212. doi:10.1002/jmor.1052240209

Marino DJ, Loughin CA, Dewey CW et al (2012) Morphometric features of the craniocervical junction region in dogs with suspected Chiari-like malformation determined by combined use of magnetic resonance imaging and computed tomography. Am J Vet Res 73(1):105–111. doi:10.2460/ajvr.73.1.105

Matiasek LA, Platt SR, Shaw S et al (2007) Clinical and magnetic resonance imaging characteristics of quadrigeminal cysts in dogs. J Vet Intern Med 21(5): 1021–1026

Moritani T, Aihara T, Oguma E et al (2006) Magnetic resonance venography of achondroplasia: correlation of venous narrowing at the jugular foramen with hydrocephalus. Clin Imaging 30(3):195–200. doi:10.1016/j.clinical.2005.10.004

Motta L, Skerritt GC (2012) Syringosubarachnoid shunt as a management for syringohydromyelia in dogs. J Small Anim Pract 53(4):205–212. doi:10.1111/j.1748-5827.2011.01185.x

Naveh Y, Kitzes R, Lemberger A et al (1992) Effect of histamine H2 receptor antagonists on the secretion of cerebrospinal fluid in the cat. J Neurochem 58(4): 1347–1352

Nolan AM (2000) Pharmacology of analgesic drugs. In: Flecknell PA, Waterman-Pearson A (eds) Pain management in animals. W.B. Saunders, London, pp 21–52

Parker JE, Knowler SP, Rusbridge C et al (2011) Prevalence of asymptomatic syringomyelia in Cavalier King Charles spaniels. Vet Rec 168(25):667. doi:10.1136/vr.d1726

Parrinello G, Torres D, Paterna S (2011) Salt and water imbalance in chronic heart failure. Intern Emerg Med 6(Suppl 1):29–36. doi:10.1007/s11739-011-0674-8

Pedersen HD (1996) Effects of mild mitral valve insufficiency, sodium intake, and place of blood sampling on the renin-angiotensin system in dogs. Acta Vet Scand 37(1):109–118

Pedersen HD, Haggstrom J, Olsen LH et al (2002) Idiopathic asymptomatic thrombocytopenia in Cavalier King Charles Spaniels is an autosomal recessive trait. J Vet Intern Med 16(2):169–173

Plessas IN, Rusbridge C, Driver CJ et al (2012) Long-term outcome of Cavalier King Charles spaniel dogs with clinical signs associated with Chiari-like malformation and syringomyelia. Vet Rec 171(20):501. doi:10.1136/vr.100449

Radojicic M, Nistor G, Keirstead HS (2007) Ascending central canal dilation and progressive ependymal disruption in a contusion model of rodent chronic spinal cord injury. BMC Neurol 7:30. doi:10.1186/1471-2377-7-30

Roberts T, McGreevy P, Valenzuela M (2010) Human induced rotation and reorganization of the brain of domestic dogs. PloS ONE 5(7):e11946. doi:10.1371/journal.pone.0011946

Rusbridge C (2007) Chiari-like malformation with syringomyelia in the Cavalier King Charles spaniel: long-term outcome after surgical management. Vet Surg 36(5): 396–405. doi:10.1111/j.1532-950X.2007.00285.x

Rusbridge C, Jeffery ND (2008) Pathophysiology and treatment of neuropathic pain associated with syringomyelia. Vet J 175(2):164–172. doi:10.1016/j.tvjl.2006.12.007

Rusbridge C, Knowler SP (2006) Coexistence of occipital dysplasia and occipital hypoplasia/syringomyelia in the cavalier King Charles spaniel. J Small Anim Pract 47(10):603–606.doi:10.1111/j.1748-5827.2006.00048.x

Rusbridge C, MacSweeny JE, Davies JV et al (2000) Syringohydromyelia in Cavalier King Charles spaniels. J Am Anim Hosp Assoc 36(1):34–41

Rusbridge C, Greitz D, Iskandar BJ (2006) Syringomyelia: current concepts in pathogenesis, diagnosis, and treatment. J Vet Intern Med 20(3):469–479

Rusbridge C, Carruthers H, Dube MP et al (2007) Syringomyelia in cavalier King Charles spaniels: the relationship between syrinx dimensions and pain. J Small Anim Pract 48(8):432–436. doi:10.1111/j.1748-5827.2007.00344.x

Rusbridge C, Knowler SP, Pieterse L et al (2009) Chiari-like malformation in the Griffon Bruxellois. J Small Anim Pract 50(8):386–393. doi:10.1111/j.1748-5827.2009.00744.x

Rutherford L, Wessmann A, Rusbridge C et al (2012) Questionnaire-based behaviour analysis of Cavalier King Charles spaniels with neuropathic pain due to Chiari-like malformation and syringomyelia. Vet J 194(3):294–298. doi:10.1016/j.tvjl.2012.05.018

Schmidt MJ, Neumann AC, Amort KH et al (2011) Cephalometric measurements and determination of general skull type of Cavalier King Charles Spaniels. Vet Radiol Ultrasound 52(4):436–440. doi:10.1111/j.1740-8261.2011.01825.x

Schmidt MJ, Ondreka N, Rummel C et al (2012a) Volume reduction of the jugular foramina in Cavalier King Charles Spaniels with syringomyelia. BMC Vet Res 8(1):158. doi:10.1186/1746-6148-8-158

Schmidt MJ, Volk H, Klingler M, Failing K, Kramer M, et al (2013) Comparison of closure times for cranial base synchondroses in mesaticephalic, brachycephalic, and Cavalier King Charles Spaniel dogs. Vet Radiol Ultrasound 54:497–503

Sekula RF Jr, Jannetta PJ, Casey KF et al (2005) Dimensions of the posterior fossa in patients symptomatic for Chiari I malformation but without cerebellar tonsillar descent. Cerebrospinal Fluid Res 2:11. doi:10.1186/1743-8454-2-11

Serfass P, Chetboul V, Sampedrano CC et al (2006) Retrospective study of 942 small-sized dogs: prevalence of left apical systolic heart murmur and left-sided heart failure, critical effects of breed and sex. J Vet Cardiol 8(1):11–18. doi:10.1016/j.jvc.2005.10.001

Shaw TA, McGonnell IM, Driver CJ et al (2012) Increase in cerebellar volume in Cavalier King Charles Spaniels with Chiari-like malformation and its role in the development of syringomyelia. PloS ONE 7(4):e33660. doi:10.1371/journal.pone.0033660

Shaw TA, McGonnell IM, Driver CJ et al (2013) Caudal cranial fossa partitioning in Cavalier King Charles spaniels. HA Volk Veterinary Record 172(13):341–341

Stalin CE, Rusbridge C, Granger N et al (2008) Radiographic morphology of the cranial portion of the cervical vertebral column in Cavalier King Charles

Spaniels and its relationship to syringomyelia. Am J Vet Res 69(1):89–93. doi:10.2460/ajvr.69.1.89

Stockyard CR (1941) The genetic and endocrinic basis for differences in form and behaviour. In: Anatomical memoirs. Wistar Institute of Anatomy and Biology, Philadelphia

Storer KP, Toh J, Stoodley MA et al (1998) The central canal of the human spinal cord: a computerised 3-D study. J Anat 192(Pt 4):565–572

Thompson DN, Harkness W, Jones BM et al (1997) Aetiology of herniation of the hindbrain in craniosynostosis. An investigation incorporating intracranial pressure monitoring and magnetic resonance imaging. Pediatr Neurosurg 26(6):288–295

Tremont-Lukats IW, Megeff C, Backonja MM (2000) Anticonvulsants for neuropathic pain syndromes: mechanisms of action and place in therapy. Drugs 60(5):1029–1052

Van Biervliet J, de Lahunta A, Ennulat D et al (2004) Acquired cervical scoliosis in six horses associated with dorsal grey column chronic myelitis. Equine Vet J 36(1):86–92

Vermeersch K, Van Ham L, Caemaert J et al (2004) Suboccipital craniectomy, dorsal laminectomy of C1, durotomy and dural graft placement as a treatment for syringohydromyelia with cerebellar tonsil herniation in Cavalier King Charles spaniels. Vet Surg 33(4):355–360. doi:10.1111/j.1532-950X.2004.04051.x

Watson PJ, Roulois AJ, Scase T et al (2007) Prevalence and breed distribution of chronic pancreatitis at postmortem examination in first-opinion dogs. J Small Anim Pract 48(11):609–618. doi:10.1111/j.1748-5827.2007.00448.x

Wetering EJ, Lemmens KM, Nieboer AP et al (2010) Cognitive and behavioral interventions for the management of chronic neuropathic pain in adults–a systematic review. Eur J Pain 14(7):670–681. doi:10.1016/j.ejpain.2009.11.010

Williams B, Bentley J (1980) Experimental communicating syringomyelia in dogs after cisternal kaolin injection. Part 1. Morphology. J Neurol Sci 48(1):93–107

Williams B, Weller RO (1973) Syringomyelia produced by intramedullary fluid injection in dogs. J Neurol Neurosurg Psychiatry 36(3):467–477

Wong HK, Tan KJ (2002) Effects of corticosteroids on nerve root recovery after spinal nerve root compression. Clin Orthop Relat Res 403:248–252

Pregnancy

15

James van Dellen

Contents

J. van Dellen
Department of Neurosurgery, Queen Elizabeth
Hospital, Birmingham, UK

BUPA Cromwell Hospital, London, UK
e-mail: james.vandellen@uhb.nhs.uk

15.1   Introduction

Chiari malformations, with or without an associated syrinx, as well as syringomyelia from other causes, are frequently first diagnosed in women of a childbearing age. Consequently, many such patients develop justifiable concerns with respect to pregnancy, labour and delivery (Table 15.1). Thoughts about starting a family may also raise questions about possible inheritance of the condition, and genetic aspects of Chiari are therefore covered within Chap. 5 of this monograph. Chiari malformation is also one of the central nervous system abnormalities that can be diagnosed with confidence in the prenatal period, and ultrasonography may be used if there is particular concern about the unborn child, on the part of the mother or the obstetrician (Bianchi et al. 2000; Iruretagoyena et al. 2010).

15.2   Pathophysiology

Symptoms of Chiari develop as a result of compression of the medulla and upper spinal cord and disturbance of cerebrospinal fluid (CSF) flow through foramen magnum. The typical Chiari headache is an intense occipital pain or a more

Table 15.1 Common concerns about Chiari and syringomyelia that arise during pregnancy

Is a normal vaginal delivery safe?
Can a spinal or epidural anaesthetic be used?
Are any offspring likely to be affected as well?

G. Flint, C. Rusbridge (eds.), *Syringomyelia*,
DOI 10.1007/978-3-642-13706-8_15, © Springer-Verlag Berlin Heidelberg 2014

generalised, 'explosive' headache, usually triggered by Valsalva-like manoeuvres such as coughing or physical activity. A study of 19 Chiari I patients analysed the triggers of their headaches: ten suffered from headaches lasting an average of 11 min, brought on by coughing, sneezing, laughing, sexual activity or other physical efforts. Eight patients had classical occipital headaches but six described frontal pain (Martins et al. 2010).

The pathophysiology of these symptoms probably centres on the pressure differences between the spine and intracranial compartments that come about during and immediately after Valsalva manoeuvres. The possible mechanisms by which disordered flow of CSF through the foramen magnum results in formation of syringomyelia cavities are discussed in Chap. 6. The pathophysiology of Chiari II is likely to be more complex than with Chiari I, but similar mechanisms are likely to operate in the generation of symptoms, although the additional effect of hydrocephalus, in further exacerbating the downward displacement of brainstem structures, has to be borne in mind.

15.3 Valsalva

When a person carries out moderately forceful exhalation against a closed airway (Valsalva manoeuvre), the resultant rise in intrathoracic pressure affects venous return, cardiac output, arterial pressure and heart rate. These effects can occur when the thoracic and abdominal muscles are strongly contracted, such as when a person strains while having a bowel movement or when lifting a heavy weight. Both actions are usually accompanied by involuntary breath holding. The normal physiological response in Valsalva occurs in clear phases. An initial rise in intrathoracic pressure forces blood out of the pulmonary circulation and into the left atrium. At the same time return of systemic blood to the right atrium is impeded. As a consequence the cardiac output is reduced and stroke volume falls. When forced exhalation ceases the pressure on the chest is released, allowing the major intrathoracic vessels

to re-expand. Venous blood can also once more enter the heart and exit into these vessels and so cardiac output increases. The pressure changes have a direct effect, positive and negative, on the pressures and blood flow in the unvalved spinal and cerebral venous structures.

During labour, pushing down involves a series of particularly prolonged Valsalva manoeuvres. An inevitable concern, therefore, is whether or not labour might aggravate or complicate the anatomy or pathophysiology of a Chiari and/or an associated syrinx cavity. Theoretically, at worst, there is a potential risk of brainstem compression from forced impaction of the tonsils. At the very least, pressure rises might be expected to aggravate any preexisting symptoms, and they might even cause deterioration in the patient's neurological state. Spinal or epidural anaesthetics could also introduce new variables into the events of labour for Chiari or syringomyelia patients (Nel et al. 1998). The concerns relate to possible dural puncture and then CSF egress and also physical and pressure alterations in the epidural compartment. Abnormal CSF pressures might influence the effectiveness of the anaesthetic. Inadvertent or intended puncture, in the case of a spinal anaesthetic, of the lumbar theca might, in turn, affect intracranial or intraspinal pressures.

15.4 Effects of Pain

In addition to the effects of Valsalva, both the uterine contractions and the pain that they generate are also likely to increase CSF pressure, both inside the cranium and the spinal canal. Measuring the CSF pressure in normal patients during labour has revealed considerable elevations when pain is intense. Pressures may be as high as 70 cm H_2O, which is more than three times the upper limit of normal (Mueller and Oro 2005).

15.5 Uncertainties

Yet, despite the recognition that syringomyelia and Chiari symptoms, in particular headaches, get worse with straining and exertion, we know relatively little about the consequences of pregnancy, labour and delivery, in terms of precipitation, worsening or even improvement of maternal symptoms and signs. Nor do we know whether or not a sudden or repeated episodes of a 'high venous pressure' event can cause the formation of a syrinx in the first place, but there are clear episodes in some patient's clinical histories where this may be considered to have been possible, and such episodes may certainly be considered to have possibly aggravated a preexisting syrinx state if La Place's law is operative. There is, however, no report of such events occurring during pregnancy, labour or delivery.

There is, unfortunately, very little literature and virtually no research to guide either the patients or their obstetricians and anaesthetists on the appropriate management of the Chiari or syringomyelia during pregnancy and labour. Reliable scientific data on the consequences, or potential interactions, of the physiological or interventional events occurring during pregnancy and labour are not available. There is no clear guidance at all in the literature, whether from large studies or case reports which specifically highlight or clearly identify common or uniform problems or pathological sequelae with a normal, or assisted, vaginal delivery and the use of epidural or intrathecal anaesthesia in patients with Chiari or syringomyelia. Nor, indeed, has there been any evidence to demonstrate increased safety or benefit conferred on pregnant mother with these conditions, by employing a Caesarean section.

Neurosurgeons are, nevertheless, frequently asked to advise on what is the best or safest mode of delivery for Chiari and syringomyelia patients. Is a vaginal delivery safe or is a Caesarean section necessary? Is a 'supported' delivery, with an epidural, or possibly even a spinal anaesthetic, permissible?

15.6   Literature Review

Women who are diagnosed with Chiari sometimes report that previous pregnancies or births first triggered the onset of their symptoms, or made them worse. One large series of 364 Chiari patients reported 16 female patients who identified pregnancy as an event precipitating their symptoms (Milhorat et al. 1999). Some women, already diagnosed with Chiari, reported that their symptoms became slightly worse during the pregnancy but then resolved spontaneously and fairly quickly after delivery. A further paradox is that in some cases patients' symptoms actually got better during the pregnancy, for periods at least (Mueller and Oro 2005). Equally, many women, when first diagnosed with Chiari, have already completed pregnancies successfully without having experienced any aggravation of their symptoms.

What publications exist on this subject consist mainly of single case reports, without detailed reference or scientific justification for decisions taken and advice given. There are reports of women with Chiari or syringomyelia undergoing elective Caesarean sections (Castello et al. 1996; Daskalakis et al. 2001), the stated reason for this management decision being the fear that the straining and pushing during delivery would aggravate the Chiari or syringomyelia state One of the earliest reports of Chiari or syringomyelia 'complicating' pregnancy and delivery was that of a woman who presented with worsening of her neurological symptoms and who went on to have a Caesarean section (Baker and Stoll 1948). Other published case studies have concluded that, with 'proper' management, a normal uncomplicated delivery is possible, without aggravating Chiari or syringomyelia symptoms. Unfortunately, in these different reports, 'proper' varied from a normal vaginal delivery to an elective Caesarean section. Vaginal delivery in a Chiari patient has certainly been documented (Parker et al. 2002), and, clearly, it is unlikely that this report represents the first or only patient who has been managed in this way. Indeed, an earlier case was of a woman who underwent a successful operative vaginal delivery, without voluntary maternal expulsive efforts; there were no adverse consequences. A more recent case report was of the successful vaginal delivery, under epidural anaesthesia, in a mother who had Chiari and sickle cell anaemia (Newhouse and

Kuczkowski 2007). In another study, of twelve mothers, delivering thirty babies in total, three underwent Caesarean section. Six deliveries were facilitated with epidural anaesthesia and three with spinal anaesthetic (Chantigian et al. 2002). In another group of six patients, only one had a Caesarean section, this under intrathecal anaesthesia. Another two of these six women had epidural anaesthesia for delivery, with no reported related symptoms (Mueller and Oro 2005). A further questionnaire, sent two of seven women with Chiari, who had all completed their pregnancies, revealed that four mothers had received an epidural anaesthetic and that six had undergone vaginal deliveries. There were no Chiari-related complications during delivery. Five women, however, had benefited from foramen magnum decompressive surgery before their vaginal delivery.

15.7   Recommendations

Unfortunately, even when all reports are combined, the number of cases commented upon is still too few for us to be able to draw definitive conclusions (Chantigian et al. 2002; Mueller and Oro 2005). Based on what literature there is, there appears to be no convincing evidence that vaginal delivery aggravates a syringomyelia or Chiari state. We can draw reassurance from the case reports of patients with untreated Chiari or syringomyelia who have delivered vaginally without any complications or concerns.

Despite this, when faced with the question of delivery management in Chiari or syringomyelia patients, most neurosurgeons have usually tended to 'play safe' and recommended a Caesarean section. Even so, patients should at least have been given the benefit of a full discussion, with their obstetrical team, neurosurgeon or neurologist, as to the benefits of a section, as against a normal vaginal delivery. Clearly, if the patient with Chiari or syringomyelia develops worsening neurological symptoms during a trial of normal vaginal delivery, then moving on to a Caesarean section may well be the safest and quickest route to follow.

There is no evidence to suggest that a patient who has previously undergone an adequate decompression of a Chiari malformation is in a situation different from that of a 'normal' patient and that she cannot or should not have a normal vaginal delivery. If the foramen magnum has been adequately decompressed in a patient with Chiari, and any associated syringomyelia cavity has subsequently collapsed, there is no reason to avoid a normal vaginal delivery or to impose a Caesarean section upon this mother.

There is no evidence to generate anxiety concerning the use of an epidural anaesthetic during labour. A spinal anaesthetic, with its dural breach and resultant changes in CSF pressure, might at first appear to be inadvisable on the grounds that it could aggravate the craniospinal pressure dissociation in a patient with an untreated Chiari malformation (Nel et al. 1998). The method has, however, been employed without complication in a patient with a corrected Chiari (Landau et al. 2003).

15.8   Summary

All in all, in considering this topic at this time, it is clear that important data elements are missing and there is obviously scope for future research (Table 15.2). This information should not prove impossible to collate, and it constitutes essen-

Table 15.2 Missing data elements regarding mothers with Chiari and/or syringomyelia

How many were symptomatic and had been diagnosed before their pregnancies?
How many, who were diagnosed after the birth, had their symptoms at the time of their pregnancies?
How many, who were diagnosed after the birth, were symptom-free at the time of their pregnancies?
For each of the above:
How many underwent Caesarean section and if so, why?
How many were given a spinal or epidural anaesthetic?
How many completed a normal vaginal delivery?
Then, for each of these:
How many subsequently suffered first onset or exacerbation of existing symptoms?
How many subsequently experienced improvements in their symptoms?

tial data, if rational and scientific recommendations are to be made, to aid patients with Chiari or syringomyelia and to advise obstetricians and midwives with respect to pregnancy and labour. At present, however, in terms of providing general advice, we can suggest the following guidelines:

- In patients with proven and untreated Chiari malformation, with or without syringomyelia, and in cases of syringomyelia from other causes, care should be taken to avoid any factor that may significantly elevate intracranial or intrathecal pressure.
- In this regard the importance of pain in labour, as a cause of considerable increases in CSF pressure, should be borne in mind. Effective pain management would appear to be important in reducing CSF pressure. There is, however, no evidence to favour general over regional anaesthesia for pain relief.
- No uniform recommendations are possible with respect to a particular mode of delivery as there is no current scientific or literature support to indicate that any mode of delivery, in terms of Chiari or syringomyelia, treated or untreated, is safer or less likely to cause harm than another.
- Decisions made should therefore be interdisciplinary and inclusive of all the parturition practitioners – obstetrician, neurosurgeon and/or neurologist, anaesthetist and midwife – and in full discussion with the patient. Discussions should accurately reflect and recognise the current, limited state of knowledge on this subject.
- The mother who develops, during pregnancy or delivery, severe Valsalva headaches or other neurological symptoms, which might point to a Chiari or syringomyelia state, should be investigated as soon as practicable after the birth.

References

Baker JT, Stoll J Jr (1948) Report of a case of syringomyelia complicating pregnancy. Bull Sch Med Univ Md 32(4):163–165

Bianchi DW, Crombleholme TM et al (2000) Fetology: diagnosis and management of the fetal patient. McGraw-Hill, New York

Castello C, Fiaccavento M, Vergano R et al (1996) Syringomyelia and pregnancy. Report of a clinical case and review of the literature. Minerva Ginecol 48:253–257

Chantigian RC, Koehn MA, Ramin KD et al (2002) Chiari I malformations in parturients. J Clin Anesth 14(3):201–205

Daskalakis GJ, Katsetos CN, Papageorgiou IS et al (2001) Syringomyelia and pregnancy-case report. Eur J Obstet Gynecol Reprod Biol 97:98–100

Iruretagoyena JI, Trampe B, Shah D (2010) Prenatal diagnosis of Chiari malformation with syringomyelia in the second trimester. J Matern Fetal Neonatal Med 23:184–186

Landau R, Giraud R, Delrue V et al (2003) Spinal anesthesia for cesarean delivery in a woman with a surgically corrected type I Arnold Chiari malformation. Anesth Analg 97(1):253–255

Martins HA, Ribas VR, Lima MD et al (2010) Headache precipitated by Valsalva maneuvers in patients with congenital Chiari I malformation. Arq Neuropsiquiatr 68(3):406–409

Milhorat TH, Chou MW, Trinidad EM et al (1999) Chiari I malformation redefined: clinical and radiographic findings for 364 symptomatic patients. Neurosurgery 44(5):1005–1017

Mueller DM, Oro J (2005) Chiari I malformation with or without syringomyelia and pregnancy: case studies and review of the literature. Am J Perinatol 22:67–70

Nel MR, Robson V, Robinson PN (1998) Extradural anaesthesia for Caesarean section in a patient with syringomyelia with Chiari type I anomaly. Br J Anaesth 80:512–515

Newhouse BJ, Kuczkowski KM (2007) Uneventful epidural labour analgesia and vaginal delivery in a parturient with Arnold-Chiari malformation type I and sickle cell disease. Arch Gynecol Obstet 275:311–313

Parker JD, Broberg JC, Napolitano PG (2002) Maternal Arnold-Chiari type I malformation and syringomyelia: a labour management dilemma. Am J Perinatol 19:445–450

Pain Management

16

Jan Keppel Hesselink

Contents

With Clare Rusbridge

J.K. Hesselink
Department of Molecular Pharmacology,
University of Witten/Herdecke, Witten, Germany
e-mail: jan@neuropathie.nu

16.1 Introduction

Neuropathic pains associated with syringomyelia are often refractory to conventional analgesic therapy, with most patients obtaining, at best, only partial relief of symptoms. There is still a tendency to treat these pains with one analgesic, or two in combination, but the pathogenesis of neuropathic pain is complex and multifactorial, so this approach is often unsuccessful. To make matters worse, there is scant scientific literature on which to base best management.

Most physicians follow a hierarchy of treatments for chronic neuropathic pain, starting with monotherapy or a combination of agents such as opioids, serotonin-noradrenaline uptake inhibitors, tricyclic antidepressants, anticonvulsants, cannabinoids and topical analgesics. Such compounds are often combined with non-pharmacological treatments like transcutaneous electrical nerve stimulation, percutaneous electrical nerve stimulation and supportive interventions such as cognitive and physical therapies.

G. Flint, C. Rusbridge (eds.), *Syringomyelia*,
DOI 10.1007/978-3-642-13706-8_16, © Springer-Verlag Berlin Heidelberg 2014

If patients do not respond to these approaches, then interventional procedures can be considered, such as nerve blockade, dorsal cord stimulation and intrathecal drug delivery systems. Beyond these methods there is invasive neuromodulation, such as spinal cord stimulation. Unfortunately, some patients never achieve adequate pain control, despite all such measures.

In this chapter, our current understanding of the mechanisms causing neuropathic pain and the nonsurgical therapy of syringomyelia are reviewed. Limitations of therapy are discussed, together with likely future directions for treatment. Non-pharmacological treatments, such as acupuncture, complementary medicine, cognitive therapy and neurostimulation, are also considered.

16.2 Neuropathic Pain in Syringomyelia

Clinical features of syringomyelia are diverse, but common signs include sensory deficits such as reduced thermoalgesic sensitivity, often presenting in conjunction with neuropathic pain. There is, however, much clinical variability between individual cases, ranging from asymptomatic patients, through those with mild, chronic pains to individuals with extreme and intractable pain (Tables 16.1 and 16.2). Pain in syringomyelia is often unilateral: with cervicodorsal cavities it is commonly located in the hand, shoulder, thorax or neck; in patients with dorsolumbar syringomyelia, the pain is usually in the lower limb (Attal and Bouhassira 2006). In posttraumatic syringomyelia, months or years may elapse, from the initial injury up until the onset of pain (Attal and Bouhassira 2006). Pain associated with syringomyelia may vary in intensity, and periods of both exacerbation and remission are common. Suboccipital headache is frequent and is often described as being oppressive in nature, the intensity being influenced by the sufferer's posture or their intracranial pressure. If intracranial pressure rises, such as after Valsalva manoeuvres, coughing, sneezing and defecation, both the headache and the neck pain can intensify. On the other hand, the headache might have a more

Table 16.1 Sensory symptoms in syringomyelia

Specific and nonspecific pains (*see* Table 16.2)
Hypoaesthesia: reduced sense of touch or sensation or a partial loss of sensitivity to sensory stimuli
Hypoalgesia or *hypalgesia*: decreased sensitivity to painful stimuli
Hyperpathia or *hyperalgesia*: an excessively painful response to a mildly painful stimulus, such as a slight prick
Paraesthesia: abnormal but not unpleasant sensations, for example, tingling
Dysaesthesia: unpleasant abnormal sensations often described as a sensation of burning, pins and needles and stretching of the skin
Allodynia: a painful response to a non-painful stimulus, such as light touch
Vasoconstriction or *vasodilatation*
Hyperhidrosis or *anhidrosis*
Piloerection or *loss of piloerection*
Trophic changes, e.g. pale glossy skin with a sensation of coldness

Table 16.2 Pain-related symptoms in syringomyelia

Headache
Valsalva induced
Suboccipital
Retro-orbital
Generalised, nonspecific headache
Trigeminal pain
Orofacial pains
Neck pain
Segmental pain
Radicular pain
Back pain
Neuropathic arthropathy pains
Leg pain

nonspecific character and seem similar to a tension headache. Neck pain is frequent and characterised by an absence of accompanying radicular arm pain. It may be associated with a continuous burning, deep-seated discomfort in the shoulders, the nape of the neck, the chest or the upper limbs. Some symptoms such as hyperalgesia,[1] allodynia[2] and segmental and radicular pains can

---

[1] Increased sensitivity and lowered threshold to painful stimuli.

[2] Pain in response to something that would not typically cause pain, such as a light touch or contact with clothing.

be anatomically related to the injured neurons or territory innervated by the injured segment. There can also be spread of these symptoms to adjacent, noninjured segments or even to involve the entire body. Other symptoms, such as trophic changes,[3] are linked to the global influence of the lesion on autonomic nervous system function (Soria et al. 1989; Milhorat et al. 1996). Features such as hyperhidrosis or hypohidrosis may occur as isolated symptoms of syringomyelia, without any other associated neurological features, or they may be part of the autonomic hyperreflexia syndrome.[4] They may also be a manifestation of a developing posttraumatic syringomyelia (Sudo et al. 1999).

Scoliosis, when seen in relation to syringomyelia, presumably relates to degeneration of motor neurons innervating the spinal muscles. Once initiated, progression of the curve can occur without further motor neuron degeneration. The resulting deformity can generate discomfort of mechanical origin, in addition to the pain arising from the syrinx itself.

Following surgery for Chiari malformation, with or without syringomyelia, patients frequently enjoy a significant improvement in their quality of life (Gautschi et al. 2011; Falci et al. 2009). Headache and neck pain may diminish, as may symptoms attributable to compression of the brain stem, such as dysphagia, ataxia, nystagmus and diplopia. In contrast, symptoms directly attributable to a syrinx cavity, including pain, scoliosis, and loss of sensitivity, are the least likely to improve.

There is no clear and simple relationship between the anatomical extent of a syrinx cavity and the symptoms and signs it creates. Nor is it possible to distinguish, just by looking at their MR scans, between patients who will and those who will not develop neuropathic pain, even when this imaging is combined with electro-physiological assessments of nociceptive and non-nociceptive pathways (Hatem et al. 2010). On the other hand, higher-average daily pain intensities do correlate with greater structural damage to the spinal cord. Further, patients experiencing both spontaneous and evoked pain have less severe structural damage to the cord than do patients with spontaneous pain alone, who tend to have more severe spinal cord damage (Hatem et al. 2010).

16.3 Pain Pathophysiology and Treatment Targets

Neuropathic pain, in its various forms, is thought to result from a number of interrelated phenomena:
1. Peripheral[5] and central sensitisation[6]
2. Hyperexcitability of central nociceptive neurons
3. Altered gene expression
4. Spontaneous neuronal activity
5. Disinhibition
6. Abnormal sprouting and cellular connectivity[7]
7. Neuronal cell death

In general, we can describe the progression of acute pain into chronic neuropathic pain as taking place in five steps. Drugs based on different mechanisms of action can be used to target each step.

1. *Activation of Glutamate Receptors*
   Glutamate transmitter release results in increased activation of spinal receptors and increased neuronal excitability. Release of the

---

[3] Atrophic changes of the skin which becomes thin, shiny and smooth. Hair growth may be increased, especially in early stages, or it may be decreased.

[4] Autonomic hyperreflexia can occur in spinal cord-injured individuals with spinal lesions above level T6 and is characterised by paroxysmal hypertension, throbbing headaches, profuse sweating, flushing of the skin above the level of the lesion, bradycardia and anxiety.

[5] A reduction in threshold and an increase in responsiveness of peripheral nociceptive neurons.

[6] An increase in the excitability of nociceptive neurons within the central nervous system.

[7] Neuroplasticity—the process by which neurons compensate for injury and disease and adjust their activities in response to new situations or to changes in their environment. Central nervous system reorganisation occurs by processes such as 'axonal sprouting' in which axons sprout nerve endings and connect with other nerve cells, forming new neural pathways.

glutamate is calcium channel dependent. Analgesics such as gabapentin and pregabalin target these altered calcium channels and inhibit their function.

2. *Activation of the N-methyl-D-aspartate (NMDA) Receptor*

In the spinal cord, release of peptides and glutamate activates the NMDA receptor, which, in concert with other spinal systems, generates a persistent pain state. Wind-up[8] and long-term potentiation[9] are key processes related to chronic activation of NMDA receptors. Wind-up is induced by C-fibre and A-delta fibre inputs and, once produced, enhances all responses, including those from low-threshold inputs. If the peripheral sensory input declines, there might be a slow return of neuronal responses back to baseline, so blocking such peripheral drives should attenuate central sensitisation. Unfortunately, in some cases chronic pain does not cease, most probably because of glial activation (see below). Long-term potentiation is a longer-lasting version of wind-up, where high-frequency C-fibre input produces chronic excitability, an event that persists even though the input is terminated. Ketamine blocks the NMDA receptor complex, and use of NMDA antagonists has been a useful tool for demonstration of NMDA receptor-mediated hypersensitivity in patients with neuropathic and complex regional pain syndrome pains (Azari et al. 2010).

3. *Temporal Summation (Wind-up and Further Wind-Up)*

If the nociceptive input continues, neuronal responses remain elevated, resulting in a cascade of detrimental neuronal overactivity. By this process weak stimuli may evoke pain, if repeated or if their duration is prolonged.

4. *Glial Activation (See Below)*

5. *Cortical Reorganisation (See Below)*

Spinal cord neurons that become hyperexcitable, as a result of the mechanisms described above, show reduced thresholds to normal sensory inputs, greater evoked responses to such input, increased receptive field sizes[10] and ongoing stimulus-independent activity. These processes are all important factors in the pathogenesis of allodynia, hyperalgesia and spontaneous pain. Overactive neurons in the central nervous system can be inhibited via drugs that target neural cells directly such as antidepressants, antiepileptics, GABAergic agonists (benzodiazepines) and opioids. A common feature of these drugs is that their targets are ion channels and receptors on nerve endings (synapses).

16.4 The Role of Glial Cells in Neuropathic Pain

Virchow (1821–1902) first described and depicted glia as gelatinous material giving structural support to the nerve cells. In 1894 Franz Nissl described the morphological changes seen in glial cells following spinal cord injury, regarding these as a biological response to promote nerve repair. These days we are increasingly aware of other roles played by the glial cells, including in the development of neuropathic pain. Until recently development of new analgesics and treatment of neuropathic pain has focused on neuronal targets. The vital role played by glial and inflammatory cells has been overlooked but is now a fast-emerging area of research (Bulanova and Bulfone-Paus 2010). A concept, which the author refers to as 'the hexapartite synapse', describes six interconnecting elements that play a functional role in neurotransmission of pain (Fig. 16.1). The hexapartite synapse consists of two neurons making synaptic contact, a microglial cell, an astrocyte, a T-cell lymphocyte and a mast cell. All these

---

[8] Wind-up pain is a mechanism leading to chronic pain via the constant bombardment of the second-order neurons in the dorsal horn of the spinal cord.

[9] Long-term potentiation (LTP) is a long-lasting enhancement in signal transmission between two neurons as a consequence of stimulation.

[10] The receptive field of a sensory neuron is a term originally coined by the famous neurophysiologist Sherrington to describe an area of the body surface where a stimulus alters the firing of that neuron. In neuropathic pain, repetitive painful stimulation results in an expansion of the receptive fields.

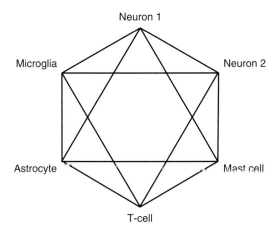

Fig. 16.1 The hexapartite synapse. Six cellular elements play a functional role in the genesis and maintenance of neuropathic pain: two neurons, a microglia cell, an astrocyte, a mast cell and a T lymphocyte. The non-neuronal cells play an underestimated role in neuropathic pain, and failure to deal with this is one of the major reasons for unsatisfactory control of neuropathic pain

neuronal and non-neuronal cells function as a unit, and non-neuronal cells can influence the generation of electric impulses. The familiar paradigm of one afferent and one efferent neuron with a synapse in between is obsolete, and consequently therapies that only target the neuron are likely to be inadequate (Fields 2009; Keppel Hesselink 2011).

Damage to the sciatic nerve in rats causes astrocytes in the dorsal horn of the spinal cord to increase in volume and to multiply, a pivotal factor in the development of neuropathic pain (Garrison et al. 1991). Low-grade inflammation also develops in the spinal cord dorsal horn and along the pain pathways to the thalamus, as well as further upstream, as far as the parietal cortex (Saade and Jabbur 2008). A consequence of this neuro-inflammation is glial cell activation, especially of the microglia (Aldskogius 2011; Gao and Ji 2010a). This activation also takes place in central pain (Wasserman and Koeberle 2009). Activated microglia and astrocytes then release many irritant molecules such as proinflammatory cytokines, including interleukins, chemokines and tumour necrosis factor (TNF)-alpha, which contribute to chronic pain states. Hyperactive neurons produce comparable compounds, such

as growth factors which in turn activate spinal cord microglia and astrocytes, and a vicious circle emerges, where both cell types wind up each other and neuropathic pain is both initiated and maintained (Graeber 2010). In the rat spinal cord, astrocytes are responsive to the pain neurotransmitter substance P (Marriott et al. 1991). There is an intimate interaction between neuronal and non-neuronal cells. For example, following nerve cell injury, certain enzymes are activated, such as c-Jun N-terminal kinase in spinal cord astrocytes, leading to the expression and release of monocyte chemotactic protein-1 (MCP-1). Monocyte chemotactic protein-1 is a cytokine which increases pain sensitivity via direct activation of NMDA receptors in the spinal cord. c-Jun N-terminal kinase plays a key role in the body's response to stressful stimuli such as inflammatory signals and changes in levels of reactive oxygen species. c-Jun N-terminal kinase activity regulates several important cellular functions, including cell growth, differentiation, survival and apoptosis, and pharmacological inhibition of c-Jun N-terminal kinase attenuates neuropathic pain in animal models (Wang et al. 2011). In addition to spinal wind-up phenomena like these, cortical reorganisation adds to the complexity of the central sensitisation processes (Dimcevski et al. 2007). The term cortical reorganisation refers to the functional changes that occur in parts of the brain. An extensive network of brain regions often referred to as the 'pain matrix' frequently show abnormalities on functional imaging studies in chronic pain states, and changes in the motor and sensory homunculus have also been described (Henry et al. 2011).

There are currently five major neurobiological pathways known to activate microglia (Fig. 16.2) (Smith 2010).

1. *Fractalkine* (also known as chemokine (C-X3-C motif) ligand 1 or neurotactin) is a chemokine[11] produced by a variety of cells, including neuronal and glial cells. It induces microglia chemotaxis. Microglia are the

---

[11] Chemotactic cytokines are small proteins capable of inducing chemotaxis (migration) of nearby responsive cells such as microglia.

Fig. 16.2 Microglia-activating pathways. There are many targets to inhibit overactive glia in neuropathic pain

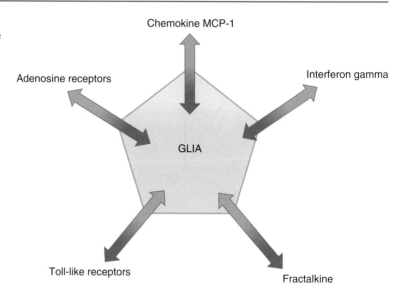

only central nervous system (CNS) cells that express the fractalkine receptors, which are upregulated in pain states. Upon activation, microglia secrete proinflammatory mediators such as prostaglandins, proteases, cytokines (TNF-alpha, interleukin-1 beta, interleukin-6) and excitatory amino acids, whose receptors are expressed on dorsal horn neurons. It is speculated that it is by this process that microglia alter sensory neuronal activity (Owolabi and Saab 2006).

2. *Interferon gamma* (INF-γ) is a cytokine with antiviral, immunoregulatory and antitumour properties. Interferon gamma alters transcription in up to 30 genes producing a variety of physiological and cellular responses. After becoming activated with INF-γ, microglia release further interferon gamma which activates more microglia and initiates a cytokine-induced activation cascade, rapidly activating all nearby microglia.

3. *Monocyte chemotactic protein-1* (MCP-1) is also known as chemokine (C-C motif) ligand 2 (CCL2) or small inducible cytokine A2. Monocyte chemotactic protein induces monocyte, macrophage, basophil and mast cell migration and is synthesised by monocytes, macrophages, dendritic cells and astrocytes (Deshmane et al. 2009). This cytokine contributes to the pathogenesis of monocyte-dependent tissue injury, and release is

triggered by increasing NMDA concentrations (Szaflarski et al. 1998). The consequence of increased MCP-1 concentrations and upregulation of the chemokine receptor CCR2 and MCP-1/CCL2 is an enhanced and prolonged persistent pain state (White and Wilson 2008; Gao and Ji 2010b).

4. *Toll-like receptors* (TLR) are membrane-spanning receptors that have a pivotal role in the innate immune response[12] in particular cellular activation and cytokine production in response to microbes. In the CNS TLR4 is expressed exclusively by the microglia, and TLR4 mRNA expression is significantly increased in experimental neuropathic pain states (Smith 2010) (Fig. 16.3).

5. *P2X receptors* (receptors for the nucleotide adenosine). Nucleotides that are released and leaked from cells are involved in cell-to-cell communication in physiological and pathophysiological conditions (Smith 2010). The upregulation of P2X4 receptor in microglia appears to be an important process in contributing to neuropathic pain (Smith 2010).

It is increasingly recognised that these phenomena play a central role in neuropathic pain.

---

[12] The innate immune system (nonspecific immune system) is the body's first line of defence and comprises the cells that recognise and respond to pathogens in a generic way and defend the host from infection by organisms.

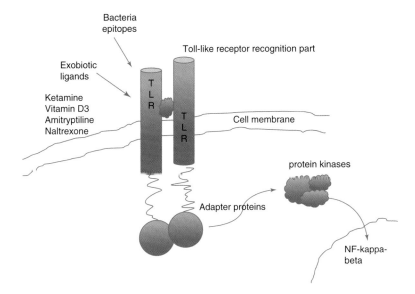

Fig. 16.3 Toll-like receptors. The Toll-like receptors are membrane-spanning receptors (named TLR1 to TLR13). The receptors function as dimers, and after activation, for instance, by an analgesic drug, Toll-like receptors recruit adapter molecules within the cytoplasm of cells to propagate a signal leading to the induction in the nucleus of certain key genes or the suppression of other genes that orchestrate the inflammatory response and chronic pain states. Toll-like receptors can be found on mast cells, glia and many immune-competent cells as well as on neurons. These receptors might play an important role in glia modulation by drugs such as ketamine, propofol, vitamin D3 or low-dose opiate antagonists such as naltrexone

Gliopathic or asteropathic pain may become new synonyms for neuropathic pain, and glia-modulating drugs may become a new class of neuropathic pain drugs (Ohara et al. 2009). Other non-neuronal targets, for instance, gap junctions and connections,[13] are still in an early phase of research and development. These new non-neuronal targets will also lead, hopefully, to additional avenues of pain medication (Wu et al. 2012).

16.5 Traditional Pharmacological Therapies

Most outcome studies looking at the treatment of neuropathic pain are focused on painful peripheral polyneuropathies, especially diabetic and postherpetic neuralgias. Studies of central neuropathic pain are few in number, largely because it is laborious to recruit sufficient patients for entering into clinical trials. There is therefore little data on nonsurgical management of neuropathic pain secondary to Chiari malformation and syringomyelia and certainly no methodologically sound outcome studies. The literature is confined to anecdotal recommendations, case reports and series with small patient numbers. In addition, the majority of the animal models used in drug trials are not representative of the real-life situation for human patients. The only comparable animal models relevant to syringomyelia are some breeds of toy dog, especially Cavalier King Charles Spaniels (see Chap. 14), which have a high prevalence of syringomyelia (Knowler et al. 2011). The opportunities that this model may represent have not yet been realised, with only a few unpublished clinical trials having taken place.

Drawing conclusions about what is the most effective therapy is even more difficult when one has to take into account the many differences in study design (Table 16.3).

Whilst our understanding of neuropathic pain-generating mechanisms has grown considerably, this has not been translated into a similar improvement in treatment efficacy, and most

---

[13] Gap junctions are channels between cells allowing a direct connection between the cytoplasm and allowing passage of molecules and ions. One gap junction channel is composed of two connections (or hemichannels).

Table 16.3 Variations in study design between different trials

Population differences
Race
Sex
Age
Patient numbers
Power calculations
Estimated magnitude of effect
Number of subjects included
Number of subjects dropping out
Trial duration
Inclusion and exclusion criteria
Pain intensity
Outcome measures

neuropathic pain patients are still left with insufficient pain relief (Finnerup et al. 2010). Clear insights into why some patients are nonresponders remain absent. Given the high variability in intensity, severity and location of symptoms, each patient must receive an individualised treatment plan.

The analgesics most often used for treatment of spinal cord injury-related pain are nonsteroidal anti-inflammatory drugs (NSAIDs), acetaminophen (paracetamol) and non-opioid muscle relaxants, such as baclofen and tizanidine. Generally, these analgesics are not prescribed by pain physicians but are purchased by patients themselves or prescribed by general practitioners. As single agents, or in combination, they are, unfortunately, ineffective in many spinal cord injury patients (Cardenas and Jensen 2006). They also have potential risks due to gastrointestinal, renal and hepatic toxicity, especially with prolonged use and higher dosage.

From the perspective of most pain specialists, antidepressants, antiepileptics and opioids are the best established and most commonly used adjuvant analgesics. Most have similar equivalent efficacy, with a number needed to treat[14] (NNT) of 3–6, but the adverse effect profiles differ (Finnerup et al. 2010).

16.5.1 Tricyclic Antidepressants

Tricyclic antidepressants such as amitriptyline and nortriptyline have 'dirty'[15] pharmacology, which is perhaps the reason for their efficacy in pain states with complex pathophysiology. Pharmacologically dirty drugs, which bind to multiple receptors, tend to be more effective for neuropathic pain but have more potential adverse effects. The therapeutic effect of the classical tricyclic antidepressants is mediated by their inhibition of the reuptake of noradrenaline and of serotonin. However, they also interact with the muscarinic acetylcholine receptor, the histamine-1 receptor, the alpha-1 adrenergic receptor and sodium ion channels (Pancrazio et al. 1998). The more receptors that are triggered, then the greater the biological effect. If only one receptor in a complicated network is influenced, then this impact will ultimately be neutralised. If multiple sites are affected, then the network is more likely to be broken and for longer. There have been some anecdotal reports that tricyclic antidepressants are effective for neuropathic pain following spinal cord injury in the presence of depressive symptoms and less effective in patients not suffering from signs of depression (Attal et al. 2009; Rintala et al. 2007).

Tricyclic antidepressants are mostly metabolised by cytochrome P450 2D6 (CYP2D6); therefore drug interactions and high serum concentrations can occur, as this hepatic enzyme plays an important role in the metabolism of many different drugs and compounds. The same dose can result in 10- to 30-fold variation in serum concentration between different patients. Patients who metabolise the drug slowly may sometimes develop a toxic serum concentration following just a single oral dose or, rarely, even after topical application. At the same time, even a small amount of amitriptyline can have a positive effect. For example, 10 mg amitriptyline before bedtime may improve sleep and decrease nocturnal pains.

---

[14] The NNT is defined as the number of patients that need to be treated, in a clinical trial, for one to benefit, as compared with the control group (Laupacis et al. 1988). The ideal NNT is 1, where every patient improves with treatment and no one improves with control. The higher the NNT, the less effective is the treatment.

---

[15] Drugs that bind to many molecular targets or receptors with a wide range of effects and possibly negative side effects. Novel drugs tend to be 'cleaner' and have a more selective action with fewer adverse reactions. There may, however, be advantages in using drugs that exhibit multireceptor activity, and, depending on the perspective, sometimes these drugs are referred to as 'enriched'.

16.5.2 Serotonin Antagonist and Reuptake Inhibitors

Serotonin antagonist and reuptake inhibitors are a class of drugs, most commonly prescribed for depression, which act by antagonising serotonin receptors and/or inhibiting the reuptake of serotonin, norepinephrine or dopamine. Additionally, most also act as alpha1-adrenergicreceptor antagonists. Examples of this class of drugs include venlafaxine, duloxetine and trazodone. Compared to tricyclic antidepressants, SARIs have a more selective action, and as they are cleaner in their receptor affinities, there are fewer histaminergic and muscarinergic adverse effects. Whether this theoretical advantage translates into better tolerability for neuropathic pain has not been substantiated in comparison trials. Compared to amitriptyline, serotonin antagonist and reuptake inhibitors have a higher NNT and are therefore less efficacious for neuropathic pain. A recent trial compared duloxetine and pregabalin for patients with diabetic peripheral neuropathic pain, who had inadequate pain control following gabapentin monotherapy. Duloxetine was not superior to pregabalin as a monotherapy, and there was no synergistic effect with combination therapy. On the contrary, the efficacy of the combination was less than the efficacy of duloxetine alone. In addition, adverse effects such as nausea, insomnia, hyperhidrosis and decreased appetite were more common with duloxetine than pregabalin (Tanenberg et al. 2011).

16.5.3 Antiepileptic Drugs

Carbamazepine seems to be effective for peripheral neuropathic pain but has not been subjected to a clinical trial lasting longer than 4 weeks (Wiffen et al. 2011b). In patients with central, post-stroke pain, there was no difference in efficacy between amitriptyline and carbamazepine (Selph et al. 2011).

Gabapentin and pregabalin target the alpha-2-delta subunit of the voltage-dependent calcium channel. The efficacy of both is comparable, but due to the higher affinity of pregabalin for the receptor, a lower dose is required to achieve optimal analgesia. Gabapentinoids have been evaluated specifically in spinal cord injury pain, with positive effects (Vranken et al. 2008; Tai et al. 2002; Levendoglu et al. 2004). A Cochrane review investigating gabapentin in randomised trials for acute, chronic or cancer pain concluded that gabapentin was superior to placebo in 14 of 29 studies (Moore et al. 2011). Patients taking gabapentin can expect to have at least one adverse event (66 %), and some will withdraw because of such effects (12 %). Common side effects include dizziness (21 %), somnolence (16 %), peripheral oedema (8 %) and gait disturbance (9 %). To date, no head-to-head comparison studies are available for clinicians to determine whether one of these drugs is superior for central neuropathic pain (Tzellos et al. 2008). These studies are not popular to conduct and are very rarely, if ever, sponsored by the manufacturer.

Benzodiazepines may inhibit some of the ectopic activity[16] in peripheral nerves following nerve injury and consequently may be used in the management of neuropathic pain, but efficacy has never been proven in well-controlled trials (Reddy and Patt 1994). There are a few old reports, from small, open-label trials,[17] where clonazepam was successfully used to treat burning mouth syndrome and trigeminal neuralgia (Smirne and Scarlato 1977; Court and Kase 1976). It is not uncommon for clonazepam to be used for spinal cord injury pain, but supportive data is lacking. Doses of up to 8 mg of clonazepam often result in marked drowsiness, so, typically, a lower dose of up to 2 mg is used. Although not supported by enough data, sometimes one may want to explore the usefulness of clonazepam in central neuropathic pain, especially in case of muscle spasms.

Lamotrigine initially appeared promising in animal models of peripheral neuropathic pain and perhaps more effective than compounds such as carbamazepine and gabapentin (Chogtu et al.

---

[16] After nerve injury, spontaneous neuronal ectopic activity may occur, leading to more pain.

[17] Open-label trials are clinical trials where both the participant and the researchers know what treatment is being administered. They may be randomised, e.g. comparing two treatments, but are generally not controlled, i.e. there is no placebo group.

2011). Clinical trials have not, however, been convincing, and there is no solid evidence supporting the use of this drug in neuropathic pain (Selph et al. 2011).

A number of antiepileptic drugs have been investigated and have shown no efficacy for pain management in patients after spinal cord injury. These include valproic acid and its sodium salt (Drewes et al. 1994; Gill et al. 2011), levetiracetam (Finnerup et al. 2009) and lamotrigine (Wiffen et al. 2011a). Compounds such as phenytoin, topiramate and carbamazepine have not been studied in post spinal cord injury pain.

For spinal cord pain and post-spinal cord injury neuropathic pain, there is enough evidence to support the use of gabapentin and pregabalin (Ahn et al. 2003; Siddall et al. 2006; Putzke et al. 2002). Evidence to support the use of other antiepileptic drugs is less substantial, and results of long-term studies have not yet been published (Eisenberg et al. 2007).

16.5.4 Opioids

Opioids have been used for pain management for thousands of years and are mentioned in pivotal medical texts of the ancient world. They were used extensively for chronic pain management and palliative care in the nineteenth and early twentieth century. In the 1970s and 1980s, opioids were not considered useful for the management of neuropathic pain, and one definition of neuropathic pain was that which was unresponsive to opioids (Arner and Meyerson 1988). This view, which was founded on results from small, mostly short duration and uncontrolled trials, is no longer held. Even so, trials of opioid use in central neuropathic pain are still scarce. Tramadol and tapentadol have been evaluated in peripheral neuropathic pain conditions, but the efficacy in central neuropathic pain states is not widely tested. One relatively small but randomised trial does, however, support their use in post-spinal cord injury pain (Norrbrink and Lundeberg 2009).

A study comparing methadone to placebo, for neuropathic pain, demonstrated evidence of analgesic effect at a dose of 20 mg/day but not at a dose of 10 mg/day (Cherny 2011). Methadone

does have several distinct advantages over other opioids, particularly as it has no active metabolites. Classic opioids like morphine, oxycodone and fentanyl are broken down into metabolites that are 'hyperalgesic', that is, molecules that can cause pain when they accumulate under conditions of chronic administration. This means that patients taking opioids may experience more pain or even allodynia, a phenomenon referred to as opioid-induced hyperalgesia Consequently, methadone is a good alternative when intolerable adverse effects from another opioid limit further dose escalation. Often a much lower dose is required than would be expected from equianalgesic conversion tables. In addition, methadone is comparatively inexpensive, and with chronic use, the long duration of analgesia allows less-frequent dosing than is required with other opioids. Methadone is therefore often regarded as a logical choice for controlling malignant and non-malignant chronic pain (Portenoy and Foley 1986) although this view is not universally held, partly because of the risk of fatal overdose. Some recommend that methadone should not be the first-choice drug for pain and nor should it be used in opioid-naive patients (Terpening and Johnson 2007). Nor is there a clear consensus on the appropriate interval for dosing of methadone with recommended intervals ranging from 3 to 24 h (Ripamonti et al. 1997). The duration of analgesia following a single dose of methadone is 4–6 h. One study in which patients controlled their own dosing interval, at a fixed 10 mg dose, showed that after a week of repeated dosing, the initial 3- to 7-h interval lengthened to an average of 10 h (Sawe 1986). The recommended starting dose in an opioid-naive patient is 2.5 mg orally every 8 h. Frail elderly patients may require a lower initial dose, and 2.5 mg orally, once daily, has been suggested (Toombs and Kral 2005).

There is some limited data supporting intravenous use of opioids (oxycodone) for spinal cord injury patients with anticonvulsant refractory neuropathic pain (Barrera-Chacon et al. 2011). A 3-month follow-up prospective, multicentre study, following 54 patients, concluded that oxycodone, in combination with anticonvulsants, decreased pain intensity and diminished the impact of pain on physical activity and sleep.

However, half of the patients showed at least one treatment-related adverse event, with constipation being the most frequent, in one-third of patients.

16.5.5 NMDA Receptor Antagonists

Ketamine is an anaesthetic drug and an N-methyl-D-aspartate (NMDA) receptor antagonist. It also inhibits pain by a number of other routes, including depression of the Toll-like receptor 3 pathway, via certain ion channels and downregulating activated glia (Hayashi et al. 2011; Mei et al. 2011a, b). Ketamine is an old drug which has been in clinical practice for nearly 40 years and may have a valuable role in management of refractory neuropathic pain patients (Cohen et al. 2011; Truin et al. 2011; Zhou et al. 2011). The effective dose for analgesia is much lower than that required for anaesthesia. This is thought to be due to a second mechanism of action, most likely via the Toll-like receptors on the glia (Mei et al. 2011b).

The usefulness of ketamine, delivered via a patient-controlled intravenous delivery system, has been reported in a single patient with cervical syringomyelia (Cohen and DeJesus 2004). The regime used resulted in a significant lessening of the pain, permitting a reduction in opioid dosage (Cohen and DeJesus 2004). It has also been reported that relative short courses (4 days) of intravenous ketamine infusion could trigger long periods (11 weeks) of decreased pain in complex regional pain syndrome type I (Sigtermans et al. 2009). The intravenous preparation can also be given orally, sublingually or rectally or as a spray for intranasal delivery.

16.5.6 Other Agents

Intravenous lidocaine infusion can be used for treating post-spinal cord injury pain in the short term but is not an option for chronic therapy (Attal et al. 2000). In syringomyelia, spasticity contributes to a patient's discomfort, and spasmolytics such as baclofen and tizanidine can be useful co-analgesics (Devulder et al. 2002).

Intrathecal baclofen is also useful for reducing pain and spasticity after spinal cord injury (Lind et al. 2004).

Pharmaceutical trials of drug therapy for hyperhidrosis caused by spinal cord lesions are few and are not supportive for their given therapies, for example, dextropropoxyphene hydrochloride (Andersen et al. 1992).

16.6   Novel Drug Therapies

16.6.1 Cannabis and Endocannabinoids

Cannabinoids such as tetrahydrocannabinol, cannabidiol and nabilone can be useful in several pain states including central and peripheral neuropathic pain, rheumatoid arthritis and fibromyalgia (Lynch and Campbell 2011). Smoked cannabis is a method used by a number of individuals with chronic, noncancer pain as well as by some patients with multiple sclerosis. Many natural and synthetic cannabinoids are therefore under investigation as potential anti-neuropathic pain drugs (Rahn and Hohmann 2009). Despite several papers supporting the efficacy and safety of cannabis and cannabinoids for various pain states, the medical use of cannabis is forbidden in many countries.

Palmitoylethanolamide is an endogenous fatty acid amide which can be found in tissues of all mammals, including man, and some foods, such as eggs and milk (Costa et al. 2002). It functions as a ubiquitous signalling molecule and is formed in the brain from the membrane phospholipid N-acylated phosphatidylethanolamines (Hansen 2010). It mimics several endocannabinoid-driven actions, even though it does not bind to cannabinoid receptors 1 and 2 (Scuderi et al. 2012). Palmitoylethanolamide can activate many receptors, most notably the peroxisome proliferator-activated receptors. These are cell nuclear receptors, mediating several physiological functions including lipid metabolism, energy balance and inflammation. There have been many scientific studies detailing palmitoylethanolamide's neuroprotective, antiepileptic, anti-inflammatory and analgesic properties (Lo Verme et al. 2005; Koch et al. 2011; Esposito et al. 2011; Loria et al. 2008; Gatti et al. 2012). Palmitoylethanolamide also downregulates hyperactive mast cells and is a possible candidate for treating several chronic inflammatory diseases (Aloe et al. 1993) including neuroinflammatory disorders (Skaper and Facci 2012). Palmitoylethanolamide is available for clinical use for the treatment of chronic pain and chronic inflammation in some parts of Europe. A suggested dosing regimen for chronic pain is 600 mg palmitoylethanolamide twice daily for 3 weeks followed by single daily dosing in addition to standard analgesic therapies or as single therapy (Gatti et al. 2012). To date no drug-to-drug interactions have been documented (Gatti et al. 2012).

Other endocannabinoids include oleoylethanolamide, stearoylethanolamide, 2-lineoylglycerol, 2-palmitoylglycerol and anandamide or arachidonoylethanolamide. Many of these have anti-inflammatory and/or analgesic actions and have been investigated for potential therapeutic benefit (LoVerme et al. 2006; Calignano et al. 2001; Costa et al. 2008; Conigliaro et al. 2011; Indraccolo and Barbieri 2010).

16.6.2 Naltrexone

Experiments in animals have demonstrated that a transient blockade of opioid receptors, by low doses of an antagonist such as naltrexone, can stimulate increased production or upregulation of mu-opioid receptors in pain centres in the brain (Mannelli et al. 2006). Low doses of opioid antagonists have therefore been postulated to 'reset' the opioid-receptor system for a period of time. In addition, low-dose naltrexone also inhibits glial cell activation, via Toll-like receptor 4, which might have an analgesic effect (Inceoglu et al. 2006; Mattioli et al. 2010). It has been suggested that naltrexone has two dose-related effects: at a low dose of 1–5 mg, the Toll-like receptors are targeted and opioid receptors are reset, and at 10 mg and above, opiate receptors are blocked. A low dose of an antagonist transiently blocks the opioid receptors, resulting in increased production, or upregulation, of mu-opioid receptors in regions of the brain that control pain responses. After the antagonist effects wear off (depending on the agent and dose, this may take minutes to hours), then there are increased numbers of receptors able to bind endogenous or exogenous opioids. In addition, the body responds to the temporary opioid-receptor blockade by increasing production of endorphins. This upregulation of the opioid receptions can also 'reset' the opioid receptors from the desensitisation which occurs during chronic opioid treatment. However, practical use of naltrexone is still experimental and requires experience in pain management, in particular, and knowledge of the half-life of the opioids that the patient is already receiving. Typically low-dose naloxone is not combined with opioids, and patients are advised to take 1.5–4.5 mg at bedtime. Occasionally patients do report adverse effects, such as vivid dreams, nightmares or night-time waking. For these patients a morning prescription of low-dose naltrexone can be taken. Although this is contrary to normal practice, we have not found any sound scientific data indicating that low-dose naltrexone should not be administered in the morning (Leavitt 2009).

16.6.3 Magnesium

Magnesium is a physiological blocker of the NMDA receptor, and it has been suggested that magnesium supplementation may have an antinociceptive effect. Although initial studies looked promising (Lee et al. 2012), their findings were not supported in a recent clinical trial (Pickering et al. 2011). This trial, however, had a high placebo response, making interpretation more difficult. In addition, only one dose was tested. Anecdotally, the authors have found that adding oral magnesium sulphate to an existing analgesic regimen, at 500 mg three times daily, may be effective, especially if the patient complains of painful muscle spasms.

16.7   Management Strategies for Central Neuropathic Pain

If the results of the efficacy of analgesics and co-analgesics in neuropathic pain are reviewed, a clear picture emerges. Firstly, most drugs are less efficacious for central as compared to peripheral neuropathic pain. Secondly the NNT of all of the most commonly prescribed drugs are similar, between three and nine (Finnerup et al. 2010). Amitriptyline is the oldest and most active compound with an NNT just below three. The NNT have actually increased for drugs evaluated in more recent clinical trials, but this is probably related to more stringent trial methodology (Finnerup et al. 2010). Patients themselves are also important sources of information about drug efficacy, if not the most important source. They report that, after titrating up the dose, most of these drugs begin to produce side effects, making optimal dosing difficult, if not impossible, in many individuals. Drowsiness, inability to drive a car and 'feeling like a zombie' are common complaints. Patients with spinal cord pain also suggest that drugs such as antidepressants are less effective, when compared to other interventions, such as acupuncture (Heutink et al. 2011).

A review of all available comparison trials for neuropathic pain has been undertaken. This included industry-sponsored and other unpublished studies involved in the drug approval process (Watson et al. 2010). For instance, they reported a clinical trial with reasonable methodology (Jadad score of 3 [18]) which compared amitriptyline to pregabalin. For patients treated with amitriptyline, 46 % had 50 % or greater relief in pain. In comparison, 50 % or greater relief from pain was documented in 40 % of patients treated with pregabalin and 30 % of patients receiving a placebo. They used the same methodology to describe all trials comparing two or more drugs and came to the following conclusions:

1. There is no evidence supporting the efficacy of the benzodiazepine lorazepam, the phenothiazine fluphenazine and the sodium channel-blocking agent mexiletine or carbamazepine for neuropathic pain (trigeminal neuralgia was excluded).
2. There is no evidence for the superiority of gabapentinoids over tricyclic antidepressants, either regarding pain or adverse effects, although the nature of the latter differs with the two agents.
3. There are nonsignificant trends suggesting the superiority of opioids over tricyclic antidepressants and gabapentinoids.

16.7.1 Combinations of Analgesics

Neuropathic pain is generated by a biochemical network of maladaptive neurons and glia. It is therefore unlikely that monotherapy will ever produce sufficient analgesia, and in practice, neuropathic pain is managed with combination of analgesics and co-analgesics. A well-known early combination was the Brompton cocktail, named after the Royal Brompton Hospital in London (Mount et al. 1976). It was a potent elixir of alcohol, cocaine, morphine and flavouring. Since many patients vomited on this concoction, antiemetics were added. Happily this type of polypharmacy is now obsolete, but the general idea of combining drugs with different but synergistic mechanisms of action is the accepted best practice for management of neuropathic pain, as recommended by the World Health Organization and many professional associations. If there is a synergistic effect between two drugs, then the dose of each individual drug and, therefore, dose-related side effects are reduced, ensuring a better balance between efficacy and safety. Take the example of drug A, which achieves analgesia at a maximal dose of at 150 mg twice daily, and drug B, which gives sufficient analgesic at a maximal dose of 25 mg twice daily. If the same efficacy is achieved by combining these two drugs at

---

[18] The Jadad score (Oxford quality scoring system) is used to classify clinical trials into 'rigorous' and 'poor' trials from a trial methodological perspective. A score of 1 or 2 is considered to have poor methodology, 3 is acceptable and scores of 4 and 5 are considered to have good methodology.

half doses, i.e. drug A at 75 mg twice daily and drug B at 12.5 mg twice daily, then this merely shows an additive effect. If, however, comparable or better analgesia is achieved with the two drugs combined at lower dosages—say drug A at 50 mg twice daily and drug B at 10 mg twice daily—then the drugs are synergistic (Smith and Argoff 2011). Another effective means of combining drugs is according to speed of onset and duration of action. If a fast-onset but short-acting analgesic is combined with a slower-onset but longer-acting agent, then the outcome may be a more rapid onset of pain relief and a longer duration of benefit. Combining analgesics also provides a means of transferring patients from one type of monotherapy to another.

There is an active debate as regards whether a stepwise approach should be adopted, i.e. increasing the first drug up to its maximal tolerated dose before then adding a second drug, or whether a combination should be used from the outset. Some argue that the first option is the only way to determine which drug is beneficial. Many favour the second approach because the sooner one reaches acceptable analgesia the better. They also reason that combining different drugs from different classes is in line with the complex pathophysiology of neuropathic pain (Harvey and Dickenson 2008).

Some studies on the safety and efficacy of combination therapy have been published. Gabapentin and nortriptyline, used alone and in combination, in patients with neuropathic pain due to diabetes mellitus or herpes zoster, were studied in a double-blind study. Drug dosages were increased in a stepwise manner, up to the subjectively effective dose or to the maximum tolerated dose, with a limit of 3,600 mg gabapentin daily and 100 mg nortriptyline daily. The visual analogue score[19] was 3.2 (2.5–3.8) for gabapentin, 2.9 (2.4–3.4) for nortriptyline and 2.3 (1.8–2.8) for combination treatment. In other words the pain score with combination treatment was significantly lower than with gabapentin or nortriptyline alone. Furthermore, the mean dose administered was lower in combination therapy compared to traditional monotherapy: for gabapentin 2,180 mg versus 2,433 mg and for nortriptyline 50.1 mg versus 61.6 mg (Gilron et al. 2009).

In a similar study design, gabapentin and morphine were compared and combination therapy was again superior (Gilron et al. 2005). At a maximum tolerated dose of drug, the visual analogue scale pain scores were 5.72 at baseline, 4.49 with placebo, 4.15 with gabapentin, 3.70 with morphine and 3.06 with the gabapentin-morphine combination.

In another study a combination of gabapentin and oxycodone was evaluated in patients with neuropathic pain associated with diabetes mellitus (Hanna et al. 2008). Results were also in favour of the combination treatment, with significantly improved pain relief, less use of escape medication,[20] fewer nights of disturbed sleep and fewer discontinuations due to lack of therapeutic effect. In addition, opiate-induced adverse events were not exacerbated by the combination of oxycodone and gabapentin.

Palmitoylethanolamide (600 mg twice daily) was added to pregabalin in previously pregabalin refractory patients; pain decreased from a visual analogue score of above 7 to below 3 (Desio 2010). In a second, open-label trial[17], difficult to treat patients had low-dose oxycodone (5 mg twice daily) added to their palmitoylethanolamide regimen, with an improvement of the visual analogue score from 7 to 2.5 at day 30 (Desio 2011).

16.7.2 Topical Analgesics

A great variety of drugs can be applied as topical formulations, such as creams, gels or ointments. Topical treatment also has the advantage that it is

---

[19] The visual analogue scale (VAS) is a means of assessing subjective parameters which are difficult to measure. It is a common tool for monitoring intensity of pain. Typically patients are asked to indicate on a line where the pain is in relation to two extremes, for example, between no pain (0) and the worst possible pain (10). The line may be graduated and/or is a known length (typically 10 cm).

[20] Escape medications are analgesics given to patients during clinical trial; if not enough analgesia occurs after a predefined period of time.

relatively cheap and associated with few adverse effects. Even applying creams that do not contain any active ingredients may be of benefit. Applying cream to painful feet has a treatment effect which is more than just placebo. Patients suffering from painful feet tend to avoid touching these body parts; by prescribing a cream the patient may be encouraged to accept the painful appendages as still being part of their body. Topical lidocaine cream (compounded or commercial) is often used to provide relief for peripheral neuropathic pain. In Europe, commercial topical tetracaine and ropivacaine creams are also used. A commercial cream containing adelmidrol, the precursor of the endocannabinoid palmitoylethanolamide, together with a low dose (0.01 %) of capsaicin, is frequently used in various European countries with anecdotal positive effects.

Topical treatment, however, is not supported by well-controlled clinical trials, partly because most drugs used topically are off-licence, and no commercial party will invest in a trial. A trial of commercially available 1.25 mg nitroglycerine patches found that they alleviated pain in spinal cord injury patients suffering from shoulder tendinopathies (Giner-Pascual et al. 2011).

In our clinic we prepare several of our own creams; examples include 5 and 10 % amitriptyline, 5 % baclofen and 10 % racemic ketamine. Of these we most commonly prescribe 5 or 10 % topical amitriptyline cream, which patients rub on the affected region up to three times daily. Patients report onset of pain relief approximately 15 min after application (Liebregts et al. 2011).

16.7.3 Intrathecal Infusions

Intrathecal infusion has been used for many years to treat chronic pain. Spinal infusion systems comprise an implantable pump for controlled drug administration and a catheter through which the medication is infused directly into the cerebrospinal fluid bathing the spinal cord. Implantation of both elements allows for prolonged therapy. Drugs used most often with this system include morphine, bupivacaine, clonidine and baclofen. Intrathecal morphine, at 44 µg/day

via pump delivery, in combination with the centrally acting alpha 2 adrenergic agonist clonidine, is reported to have a synergistic analgesic effect in patients with intractable neuropathic pain (Uhle et al. 2000). A 10-year clinical experience of pain reduction using combined intrathecal baclofen-morphine therapy for spinal pain and spasticity suggested little evidence of its efficacy in neuropathic pain and no evidence for any benefit in treating the pain of syringomyelia (Saulino 2012).

16.8 Non-pharmacological Therapies

16.8.1 Acupuncture

Treatments perceived by patients as being the most effective may not be traditional analgesics but rather acupuncture, physiotherapy, exercise, massage therapy and relaxation (Heutink et al. 2011). Chronic pain is one of the most well-documented indications for treatment with acupuncture, with good proof of safety. Moreover, patients seem to prefer acupuncture to pharmacotherapy with co-analgesics like amitriptyline (Heutink et al. 2011). A literature review on the efficacy of acupuncture for spinal cord injury-related conditions, including pain, spasticity and syringomyelia, concluded that acupuncture may be a useful treatment modality (Paola and Arnold 2003). A significant decrease in chronic shoulder pain in 17 spinal cord injury wheelchair users was reported in both the acupuncture and the sham acupuncture groups, with decreases of 66 and 43 %, respectively (Dyson-Hudson et al. 2007). Twice weekly massage or acupuncture was evaluated in 30 individuals with spinal cord injury and neuropathic pain (Norrbrink and Lundeberg 2011). At the end of the 6-week treatment course, 8 out of 15 individuals receiving acupuncture and 9 out of 15 receiving massage reported an improvement; the positive effect from acupuncture lasted longer. Unfortunately, well-controlled, full-powered and methodologically sound trials evaluating the effects of acupuncture for spinal cord injury neuropathic pain have not been performed to date.

16.8.2 Massage and Other Complementary Therapy

There is very little evidence on the effects of complementary therapy in central neuropathic pain. A review of the literature, to evaluate the usefulness of a number of techniques for spinal cord injury, including physiotherapy, heat therapy, ice therapy, cold therapy, massage, ultrasound and occupational therapy, concluded that there was not enough evidence to recommend any of these methods (Fattal et al. 2009). Many patients nevertheless prefer these interventions, especially massage, over pharmacotherapy (Fattal et al. 2009; Heutink et al. 2011). A positive benefit from massage for spinal cord injury and neuropathic pain has also been reported (Norrbrink and Lundeberg 2011). Since these therapies are generally free from troublesome adverse effects, they could certainly be considered before using more invasive therapeutic approaches.

16.8.3 Psychological Interventions

Data from the Coping with Neuropathic Spinal Cord Injury Pain (CONESCI) trial indicated that a multidisciplinary cognitive behavioural treatment programme is useful, to alleviate neuropathic pain associated with spinal cord injury (Heutink et al. 2011). The intervention consisted of educational, cognitive and behavioural elements. A significant decrease in pain intensity, pain-related disability, anxiety and increased participation in activities was seen in the intervention versus the waiting list control group (61 patients).

16.8.4 The Placebo Response

In studies on analgesic drugs, a 30 % rate of positive response to placebo treatment has been reported (Beecher 1955). For neuropathic pain the placebo effect is lower but still significant. Data from 14 studies, analysing the efficacy of gabapentin versus placebo in postherpetic neuralgia, diabetic neuropathy, cancer-related neuropathic pain, phantom limb pain, Guillain–Barré syndrome and spinal cord injury pain, reported an average placebo response of 19 % (Wiffen et al. 2005). Frustrating as the placebo response might be in clinical trials, it should not be forgotten that it can be exploited as a benign and potentially effective part of the therapeutic process (Dumitriu and Popescu 2010).

16.9 Neurostimulation Techniques

Neurostimulation therapies are considered an option for treatment of severe neuropathic pain that is refractory to pharmacological treatment (Table 16.4). Treating chronic pain using electricity and magnetism is not a new technique as electromagnetic therapies emerged as medical interventions for pain following the development of the first electricity accumulator, the Leyden jar, in 1745. Electro-acupuncture started in the early nineteenth century, and peripheral nerve stimulation became very popular at the end of the ninetieth century. Spinal cord stimulation started to gain momentum simultaneously with the emergence of the gate theory of pain, which gave a more solid scientific basis for this treatment (Melzack and Wall 1965). Increasingly, neurostimulation became considered as a more viable option than the neuroablative methods.

It should, of course, be remembered that all of these interventions also have a significant placebo effect. Furthermore, the potential adverse effects of the more invasive types of neurostimulation must be carefully considered, before giving a balanced judgment as to whether any one method is justified for a given patient.

Techniques such as transcutaneous electrical nerve stimulation and percutaneous electrical nerve stimulation are safe, if applied correctly. They are easy to administer and relatively inexpensive. They have not, however, been subjected to rigorous efficacy studies. A randomised, double-blind, placebo-controlled parallel study in 225 patients analysed whether repetitive and cumulative exposure to low-frequency pulsed electromagnetic fields was safe and effective,

Table 16.4 Neurostimulation techniques available—listed in order from non-invasive to those requiring surgery

Transcutaneous electrical nerve stimulation
Photon stimulation
Pulsed electromagnetic fields
Repetitive transcranial magnetic stimulation
Transcranial direct current stimulation
Electro-acupuncture
Percutaneous electrical nerve stimulation
Spinal cord stimulation
Motor cortex stimulation
Deep brain stimulation

in diabetic painful neuropathy (Weintraub et al. 2009). The results were not impressive; there were no significant differences between pulsed electromagnetic fields and sham groups.

16.9.1 Photon Therapy

The finding that low-energy stimulation of tissues, by lasers, could enhance wound healing led to the development of laser therapy. Photon stimulation is a modern version of this treatment and is sometimes referred to as pulsed infrared light therapy, or photobiomodulation. Light, in the near-infrared wavelengths (750–1,300 nm), is delivered by arrays of light-emitting diodes. It penetrates skin and tissue to a depth of approximately 2–3 cm. A randomised, double-blind, placebo-controlled trial, in patients with diabetic neuropathy, who received photon stimulation versus sham treatment, demonstrated a decrease in pain intensity and pain quality scores, with improvements in pain relief, sensation and quality of life. It is questionable if the study had enough power as power calculations and expected magnitude of effect[21] were not included (Swislocki et al. 2010).

16.9.2 Repetitive Transcranial Magnetic Stimulation

Repetitive transcranial magnetic stimulation is thought to suppress brain excitability non-invasively and to do so for a period beyond the duration of the session, although just how long this period can be remains unclear. Transcranial direct current stimulation is a more recent variation. Repetitive transcranial magnetic stimulation has been used and evaluated in a variety of chronic pain states, from fibromyalgia to central pain secondary to spinal cord lesions (O'Connell and Wand 2011). A meta-analysis of all randomised controlled trials (1 parallel, 4 crossover) suggested that repetitive transcranial magnetic stimulation is more effective for centrally than for peripherally originating neuropathic pain (Leung et al. 2009). This would seem plausible, but no rigorous comparison studies have been conducted. Drawing conclusions about the effectiveness or otherwise of repetitive transcranial magnetic stimulation is hampered by suboptimal study methodology. Shortcomings include small sample sizes, failure to include power calculations, estimated magnitude of effect,[21] intention to treat analysis,[22] cost–benefit analysis,[23] information on NNT and failure to take account of the placebo effect. Furthermore, the follow-up time in all studies is short, the longest being 1 month (O'Connell et al. 2011). Therefore, all the studies reported so far can only be regarded as pilot

---

[21] Estimated magnitude of (treatment) effect is used in power analysis and to calculate the study population size. The effect size should represent the smallest clinically significant effect and will vary depending on the severity of the illness. For example, a drug which decreases mortality by 10 % has more potential benefit than a drug which decreases signs of neuropathic pain by 10 %. The smaller the treatment effect, then the larger the population size required to have confidence in the results.

[22] The intent to treat (ITT) analysis is a statistical procedure employed to avoid misinterpretation of results, for example, because of patient dropout. The principle of ITT is that all study participants are included in the final analysis whether or not they completed the trial. This is particularly important because if a treatment is ineffective, then more severely affected patients are more likely to drop out. If those patients are not included, then the treatment may be interpreted to be more beneficial than it actually was.

[23] Cost–benefit analysis is a process by which the total expected cost of each treatment option is compared to the total expected benefits in other words establishing if the benefits outweigh the costs and by how much and therefore whether it is justifiable. This can also provide a basis for comparing different treatments.

studies, and if repetitive transcranial magnetic stimulation was a new drug, it would not have been licensed for the treatment of chronic neuropathic pain. The general feeling in the research community is that repetitive transcranial magnetic stimulation creates a significant decrease in pain but that the magnitude of the effect is small and, based on the published literature, its clinical usefulness is debatable. Most probably patients need repeated weekly sessions, and this must be taken into account when evaluating the economic cost of this intervention.

16.9.3 Spinal Cord Stimulation

Spinal cord stimulation has shown value in the treatment of selected types of chronic pain syndromes, such as failed back surgery syndrome (Sears et al. 2011) and peripheral neuropathic pain (Sokal et al. 2011). Spinal cord stimulation is sometimes used for complex regional pain syndromes and phantom limb pain, but it does not alleviate acute nociceptive pain. Worldwide, more than 30,000 spinal cord stimulation systems are currently implanted every year (Craig et al. 2007). The relative effectiveness of this method, compared with conventional, nonsurgical central neuropathic pain management, has not been assessed in a placebo-controlled, randomised trial setting. The 'Prospective Randomised Controlled Multicentre Trial of the Effectiveness of Spinal Cord Stimulation' (PROCESS) recruited 100 patients with failed back surgery syndrome and randomly assigned then to receive spinal cord stimulation plus conventional medical management or conventional medical management alone, for at least 6 months (Kumar et al. 2007). Conventional management included oral medications such as opioids, nonsteroidal anti-inflammatory drugs, antidepressant and antiepileptic drugs, nerve blocks, epidural corticosteroids, physical and psychological rehabilitative therapy and chiropractic care. At 6-month follow-up, 48 % of the spinal cord stimulation group versus 9 % of the conventional medical management group achieved 50 % or more limb pain relief. The complication rate was high, with 32 % of

spinal cord stimulation patients experiencing a total of 40 device-related complications, and 21 reoperations were required. The study was not blinded and there was no independent assessment. The presence of allodynia and/or hyperalgesia was the best predictor for long-term success in a recent retrospective study of 244 patients who underwent spinal cord stimulation (Williams et al. 2011). Data is not available for appropriateness or success of using spinal cord stimulation for syringomyelia.

16.9.4 Motor Cortex Stimulation

Neurostimulation of the motor cortex, for a disease-causing sensory disturbance, may seem illogical, but stimulation of the motor cortex can, in fact, give better results than the stimulation of the sensory cortex. Indeed, the latter may sometimes cause pain to worsen. Motor cortex stimulation is used more frequently than deep brain stimulation,[24] mainly because it is less invasive and less complex. It might also have a wider range of indications (Nguyen et al. 2000, 2008). The mechanism by which motor cortex stimulation affects neuropathic pain is unproven. It has been suggested that it induces endogenous opioid secretion (Maarrawi et al. 2011), and functional imaging has suggested that motor cortex stimulation triggers rapid and phasic activation in the lateral thalamus, which over a delayed time course of hours leads to a cascade of events in medial thalamus, anterior cingulate/orbitofrontal cortices and periaqueductal grey matter (Garcia-Larrea and Peyron 2007). There is also modulation of the spinal dorsal horn neuron activity (Senapati et al. 2005; Pagano et al. 2011). Small controlled pilot trials have suggested that motor cortex stimulation may be effective for treatment of various types of neuropathic pain, especially trigeminal neuralgia and thalamic pain syndrome. The use of motor cortex stimulation in pain states such as in

---

[24] Deep brain stimulation (DBS) involves surgical implantation of a stimulator which sends electrical impulses to electrodes implanted in deep brain structures such as the internal capsule, ventral posterolateral nucleus and ventral posteromedial nucleus and interferes with neural activity.

syringomyelia has not been explored, but it most probably this intervention will not lead to pain reduction, as the major 'lesion' is spinal.

Conclusions

Central neuropathic pain is difficult to treat, and controlling pain from syringomyelia remains a challenge. The best nonsurgical therapy is multimodal, and the following is approach is recommended:

(a) Combination therapy (2, 3 or 4 agents) of the following co-analgesics, slowly increasing the dose: amitriptyline (10–30 mg once daily before sleep), together with gabapentin (300–600 mg three times daily) or pregabalin (75 mg twice daily) and oxycodone (starting at 5 mg twice daily) and/or any other co-analgesic such as clonazepam. The question whether to take a stepwise approach or polypharmacy from the start has yet to be resolved.

(b) Topical analgesic self-compounded or commercial creams can be considered.

(c) Add second-line co-analgesics such as phenytoin or palmitoylethanolamide. Even though these compounds have not been proven efficacious in vigorous clinical trials, individual patients may respond.

(d) Add acupuncture or massage and/or transcutaneous electrical nerve stimulation or percutaneous electrical nerve stimulation.

(e) In severe refractory cases intrathecal infusions and neuromodulation techniques can be explored. At present spinal cord stimulation seems the most appropriate. There is little evidence to support the use of repetitive transcranial magnetic stimulation. Deep brain stimulation should only be considered when less invasive interventions fail.

References

Ahn SH, Park HW, Lee BS et al (2003) Gabapentin effect on neuropathic pain compared among patients with spinal cord injury and different durations of symptoms. Spine 28(4):341–346; discussion 346–347. doi:10.1097/01.BRS.0000048464.57011.00

Aldskogius H (2011) Mechanisms and consequences of microglial responses to peripheral axotomy. Front Biosci (Schol Ed) 3:857–868

Aloe L, Leon A, Levi-Montalcini R (1993) A proposed autacoid mechanism controlling mastocyte behaviour. Agents Actions 39(Spec No):C145–147

Andersen LS, Biering-Sorensen F, Muller PG et al (1992) The prevalence of hyperhidrosis in patients with spinal cord injuries and an evaluation of the effect of dextropropoxyphene hydrochloride in therapy. Paraplegia 30(3):184–191. doi:10.1038/sc.1992.53

Arner S, Meyerson BA (1988) Lack of analgesic effect of opioids on neuropathic and idiopathic forms of pain. Pain 33(1):11–23

Attal N, Bouhassira D (2006) Chapter 47. Pain in syringomyelia/bulbia. In: Vinken PJ, Bruyn GW (eds) Handbook of clinical neurology, vol 81. Elsevier, New York; pp 705–713. doi:10.1016/S0072-9752(06)80051-5

Attal N, Gaude V, Brasseur L et al (2000) Intravenous lidocaine in central pain: a double-blind, placebo-controlled, psychophysical study. Neurology 54(3):564–574

Attal N, Mazaltarine G, Perrouin-Verbe B et al (2009) Chronic neuropathic pain management in spinal cord injury patients. What is the efficacy of pharmacological treatments with a general mode of administration? (oral, transdermal, intravenous). Ann Phys Rehabil Med 52(2):124–141. doi:10.1016/j.rehab.2008.12.011

Azari P, Lindsay DR, Briones D et al (2010) Efficacy and safety of ketamine in patients with complex regional pain syndrome: a systematic review. CNS Drugs 26(3):215–228. doi:10.2165/11595200-000000000-00000

Barrera-Chacon JM, Mendez-Suarez JL, Jauregui-Abrisqueta ML et al (2011) Oxycodone improves pain control and quality of life in anticonvulsant-pretreated spinal cord-injured patients with neuropathic pain. Spinal Cord 49(1):36–42. doi:10.1038/sc.2010.101

Beecher HK (1955) The powerful placebo. JAMA 159(17):1602–1606

Bulanova E, Bulfone-Paus S (2010) P2 receptor-mediated signaling in mast cell biology. Purinergic Signal 6(1):3–17. doi:10.1007/s11302-009-9173-z

Calignano A, La Rana G, Piomelli D (2001) Antinociceptive activity of the endogenous fatty acid amide, palmitylethanolamide. Eur J Pharmacol 419(2–3):191–198

Cardenas DD, Jensen MP (2006) Treatments for chronic pain in persons with spinal cord injury: a survey study. J Spinal Cord Med 29(2):109–117

Cherny N (2011) Is oral methadone better than placebo or other oral/transdermal opioids in the management of pain? Palliat Med 25(5):488–493. doi:10.1177/0269216310397687

Chogtu B, Bairy KL, Smitha D et al (2011) Comparison of the efficacy of carbamazepine, gabapentin and lamotrigine for neuropathic pain in rats. Indian J Pharmacol 43(5):596–598. doi:10.4103/0253-7613.84980

Cohen SP, DeJesus M (2004) Ketamine patient-controlled analgesia for dysesthetic central pain. Spinal Cord 42(7):425–428. doi:10.1038/sj.sc.3101599

Cohen SP, Liao W, Gupta A (2011) Ketamine in pain management. Adv Psychosom Med 30:139–161. doi:10.1159/000324071

Conigliaro R, Drago V, Foster PS et al (2011) Use of palmitoylethanolamide in the entrapment neuropathy of the median in the wrist. Minerva Med 102(2):141–147

Costa B, Conti S, Giagnoni G et al (2002) Therapeutic effect of the endogenous fatty acid amide, palmitoylethanolamide, in rat acute inflammation: inhibition of nitric oxide and cyclo-oxygenase systems. Br J Pharmacol 137(4):413–420. doi:10.1038/sj.bjp.0704900

Costa B, Comelli F, Bettoni I et al (2008) The endogenous fatty acid amide, palmitoylethanolamide, has anti-allodynic and anti-hyperalgesic effects in a murine model of neuropathic pain: involvement of CB(1), TRPV1 and PPARgamma receptors and neurotrophic factors. Pain 139(3):541–550. doi:10.1016/j.pain.2008.06.003

Court JE, Kase CS (1976) Treatment of tic douloureux with a new anticonvulsant (clonazepam). J Neurol Neurosurg Psychiatry 39(3):297–299

Craig A, Janasz K, Landry D (2007) St. Jude medical announces FDA clearance of spinal cord stimulation leads for patients with low back pain. Business Wire http://www.businesswire.com/news/home/20070215005102/en/St.-Jude-Medical-Announces-FDA-Clearance-Spinal. Accessed 21 July 2012

Deshmane SL, Kremlev S, Amini S et al (2009) Monocyte chemoattractant protein-1 (MCP-1): an overview. J Interferon Cytokine Res 29(6):313–326. doi:10.1089/jir.2008.0027

Desio P (2010) A combination of pregabalin and palmitoylethanolamide (PEA) for neuropathic pain treatment. Pathos 17:9–14

Desio P (2011) Combination of oxycodone and palmitoylethanolamide for low back pain treatment. Rivista Siared di Anestesia e Medicina Critica 1(2):62–71

Devulder J, Crombez E, Mortier E (2002) Central pain: an overview. Acta Neurol Belg 102(3):97–103

Dimcevski G, Sami SA, Funch-Jensen P et al (2007) Pain in chronic pancreatitis: the role of reorganization in the central nervous system. Gastroenterology 132(4):1546–1556. doi:10.1053/j.gastro.2007.01.037

Drewes AM, Andreasen A, Poulsen LH (1994) Valproate for treatment of chronic central pain after spinal cord injury. A double-blind cross-over study. Paraplegia 32(8):565–569. doi:10.1038/sc.1994.89

Dumitriu A, Popescu BO (2010) Placebo effects in neurological diseases. J Med Life 3(2):114–121

Dyson-Hudson TA, Kadar P, LaFountaine M et al (2007) Acupuncture for chronic shoulder pain in persons with spinal cord injury: a small-scale clinical trial. Arch Phys Med Rehabil 88(10):1276–1283. doi:10.1016/j.apmr.2007.06.014

Eisenberg E, River Y, Shifrin A et al (2007) Antiepileptic drugs in the treatment of neuropathic pain. Drugs 67(9):1265–1289

Esposito E, Paterniti I, Mazzon E et al (2011) Effects of palmitoylethanolamide on release of mast cell peptidases and neurotrophic factors after spinal cord injury. Brain Behav Immun 25(6):1099–1112. doi:10.1016/j.bbi.2011.02.006

Falci SP, Indeck C, Lammertse DP (2009) Posttraumatic spinal cord tethering and syringomyelia: surgical treatment and long-term outcome. J Neurosurg Spine 11(4):445–460. doi:10.3171/2009.4.SPINE09333

Fattal C, Kong ASD, Gilbert C et al (2009) What is the efficacy of physical therapeutics for treating neuropathic pain in spinal cord injury patients? Ann Phys Rehabil Med 52(2):149–166. doi:10.1016/j.rehab.2008.12.006

Fields RD (2009) New culprits in chronic pain. Sci Am 301(5):50–57

Finnerup NB, Grydehoj J, Bing J et al (2009) Levetiracetam in spinal cord injury pain: a randomized controlled trial. Spinal Cord 47(12):861–867. doi:10.1038/sc.2009.55

Finnerup NB, Sindrup SH, Jensen TS (2010) The evidence for pharmacological treatment of neuropathic pain. Pain 150(3):573–581. doi:10.1016/j.pain.2010.06.019

Gao YJ, Ji RR (2010a) Chemokines, neuronal-glial interactions, and central processing of neuropathic pain. Pharmacol Ther 126(1):56–68. doi:10.1016/j.pharmthera.2010.01.002

Gao YJ, Ji RR (2010b) Targeting astrocyte signaling for chronic pain. Neurotherapeutics 7(4):482–493. doi:10.1016/j.nurt.2010.05.016

Garcia-Larrea L, Peyron R (2007) Motor cortex stimulation for neuropathic pain: from phenomenology to mechanisms. Neuroimage 37(Suppl 1):S71–S79. doi:10.1016/j.neuroimage.2007.05.062

Garrison CJ, Dougherty PM, Kajander KC et al (1991) Staining of glial fibrillary acidic protein (GFAP) in lumbar spinal cord increases following a sciatic nerve constriction injury. Brain Res 565(1):1–7

Gatti A, Lazzari M, Gianfelice V et al (2012) Palmitoylethanolamide in the treatment of chronic pain caused by different etiopathogenesis. Pain Med 13(9):1121–1130. doi:10.1111/j.1526-4637.2012.01432.x

Gautschi OP, Seule MA, Cadosch D et al (2011) Health-related quality of life following spinal cordectomy for syringomyelia. Acta Neurochir (Wien) 153(3):575–579. doi:10.1007/s00701-010-0869-1

Gill D, Derry S, Wiffen PJ et al (2011) Valproic acid and sodium valproate for neuropathic pain and fibromyalgia in adults. Cochrane Database Syst Rev (10):CD009183. doi:10.1002/14651858.CD009183.pub2

Gilron I, Bailey JM, Tu D et al (2005) Morphine, gabapentin, or their combination for neuropathic pain. N Engl J Med 352(13):1324–1334. doi:10.1056/NEJMoa042580

Gilron I, Bailey JM, Tu D et al (2009) Nortriptyline and gabapentin, alone and in combination for neuropathic pain: a double-blind, randomised controlled crossover trial. Lancet 374(9697):1252–1261. doi:10.1016/S0140-6736(09)61081-3

Giner-Pascual M, Alcanyis-Alberola M, Querol F et al (2011) Transdermal nitroglycerine treatment of shoulder tendinopathies in patients with spinal cord injuries. Spinal Cord 49(9):1014–1019. doi:10.1038/sc.2011.41

Graeber MB (2010) Changing face of microglia. Science 330(6005):783–788. doi:10.1126/science.1190929

Hanna M, O'Brien C, Wilson MC (2008) Prolonged-release oxycodone enhances the effects of existing gabapentin therapy in painful diabetic neuropathy patients. Eur J Pain 12:804–813

Hansen HS (2010) Palmitoylethanolamide and other anandamide congeners. Proposed role in the diseased brain. Exp Neurol 224(1):48–55. doi:10.1016/j.expneurol.2010.03.022

Harvey VL, Dickenson AH (2008) Mechanisms of pain in nonmalignant disease. Curr Opin Support Palliat Care 2(2):133–139. doi:10.1097/SPC.0b013e328300eb24

Hatem SM, Attal N, Ducreux D et al (2010) Clinical, functional and structural determinants of central pain in syringomyelia. Brain 133(11):3409–3422. doi:10.1093/brain/awq244

Hayashi Y, Kawaji K, Sun L et al (2011) Microglial Ca(2+)-activated K(+) channels are possible molecular targets for the analgesic effects of S-ketamine on neuropathic pain. J Neurosci 31(48):17370–17382. doi:10.1523/JNEUROSCI.4152-11.2011

Henry DE, Chiodo AE, Yang W (2011) Central nervous system reorganization in a variety of chronic pain states: a review. PM R 3(12):1116–1125. doi:10.1016/j.pmrj.2011.05.018

Heutink M, Post MW, Wollaars MM et al (2011) Chronic spinal cord injury pain: pharmacological and non-pharmacological treatments and treatment effectiveness. Disabil Rehabil 33(5):433–440. doi:10.3109/09638288.2010.498557

Inceoglu B, Jinks SL, Schmelzer KR et al (2006) Inhibition of soluble epoxide hydrolase reduces LPS-induced thermal hyperalgesia and mechanical allodynia in a rat model of inflammatory pain. Life Sci 79(24):2311–2319. doi:10.1016/j.lfs.2006.07.031

Indraccolo U, Barbieri F (2010) Effect of palmitoylethanolamide-polydatin combination on chronic pelvic pain associated with endometriosis: preliminary observations. Eur J Obstet Gynecol Reprod Biol 150(1):76–79. doi:10.1016/j.ejogrb.2010.01.008

Keppel Hesselink J (2011) Glia as a new target for neuropathic pain, clinical proof of concept for palmitoylethanolamide, a glia-modulator. Anaesth Pain Intensive Care 15:143–145

Knowler SP, McFadyen AK, Rusbridge C (2011) Effectiveness of breeding guidelines for reducing the prevalence of syringomyelia. Vet Rec 169(26):681. doi:10.1136/vr.100062

Koch M, Kreutz S, Bottger C et al (2011) Palmitoylethanolamide protects dentate gyrus granule cells via peroxisome proliferator-activated receptor-alpha. Neurotox Res 19(2):330–340. doi:10.1007/s12640-010-9166-2

Kumar K, Taylor RS, Jacques L et al (2007) Spinal cord stimulation versus conventional medical management for neuropathic pain: a multicentre randomised controlled trial in patients with failed back surgery syndrome. Pain 132(1–2):179–188. doi:10.1016/j.pain.2007.07.028

Laupacis A, Sackett DL, Roberts RS (1988) An assessment of clinically useful measures of the consequences of treatment. N Engl J Med 318(26):1728–1733. doi:10.1056/NEJM198806303182605

Leavitt S (2009) Opioid antagonists, aids for pain treatment. Pain Treatment Topics 9(3):12–21

Lee AR, Yi HW, Chung IS et al (2012) Magnesium added to bupivacaine prolongs the duration of analgesia after interscalene nerve block. Can J Anaesth 59(1):21–27. doi:10.1007/s12630-011-9604-5

Leung A, Donohue M, Xu R et al (2009) rTMS for suppressing neuropathic pain: a meta-analysis. J Pain 10(12):1205–1216. doi:10.1016/j.jpain.2009.03.010

Levendoglu F, Ogun CO, Ozerbil O et al (2004) Gabapentin is a first line drug for the treatment of neuropathic pain in spinal cord injury. Spine 29(7):743–751

Liebregts R, Kopsky DJ, Hesselink JM (2011) Topical amitriptyline in post-traumatic neuropathic pain. J Pain Symptom Manage 41(4):e6–e7. doi:10.1016/j.jpainsymman.2011.01.003

Lind G, Meyerson BA, Winter J et al (2004) Intrathecal baclofen as adjuvant therapy to enhance the effect of spinal cord stimulation in neuropathic pain: a pilot study. Eur J Pain 8(4):377–383. doi:10.1016/j.ejpain.2003.11.002

Loria F, Petrosino S, Mestre L et al (2008) Study of the regulation of the endocannabinoid system in a virus model of multiple sclerosis reveals a therapeutic effect of palmitoylethanolamide. Eur J Neurosci 28(4):633–641. doi:10.1111/j.1460-9568.2008.06377.x

LoVerme J, Fu J, Astarita G et al (2005) The nuclear receptor peroxisome proliferator-activated receptor-alpha mediates the anti-inflammatory actions of palmitoylethanolamide. Mol Pharmacol 67(1):15–19. doi:10.1124/mol.104.006353

LoVerme J, Russo R, La Rana G et al (2006) Rapid broad-spectrum analgesia through activation of peroxisome proliferator-activated receptor-alpha. J Pharmacol Exp Ther 319(3):1051–1061. doi:10.1124/jpet.106.111385

Lynch ME, Campbell F (2011) Cannabinoids for treatment of chronic non-cancer pain; a systematic review of randomized trials. Br J Clin Pharmacol 72(5):735–744. doi:10.1111/j.1365-2125.2011.03970.x

Maarrawi J, Mertens P, Peyron R et al (2011) Functional exploration for neuropathic pain. Adv Tech Stand Neurosurg 37:25–63. doi:10.1007/978-3-7091-0673-0_2

Mannelli P, Gottheil E, Van Bockstaele EJ (2006) Antagonist treatment of opioid withdrawal translational low dose approach. J Addict Dis 25(2):1–8. doi:10.1300/J069v25n02_01

Marriott DR, Wilkin GP, Wood JN (1991) Substance P-induced release of prostaglandins from astrocytes:

regional specialisation and correlation with phosphoinositol metabolism. J Neurochem 56(1):259–265

Mattioli TA, Milne B, Cahill CM (2010) Ultra-low dose naltrexone attenuates chronic morphine-induced gliosis in rats. Mol Pain 6:22. doi:10.1186/1744-8069-6-22

Mei XP, Zhang H, Wang W et al (2011a) Inhibition of spinal astrocytic c-Jun N-terminal kinase (JNK) activation correlates with the analgesic effects of ketamine in neuropathic pain. J Neuroinflammation 8(1):6. doi:10.1186/1742-2094-8-6

Mei XP, Zhou Y, Wang W et al (2011b) Ketamine depresses toll-like receptor 3 signaling in spinal microglia in a rat model of neuropathic pain. Neurosignals 19(1):44–53. doi:10.1159/000324293

Melzack R, Wall PD (1965) Pain mechanisms: a new theory. Science 150(3699):971–979

Milhorat TH, Kotzen RM, Mu HT et al (1996) Dysesthetic pain in patients with syringomyelia. Neurosurgery 38(5):940–946; discussion 6–7

Moore RA, Wiffen PJ, Derry S et al (2011) Gabapentin for chronic neuropathic pain and fibromyalgia in adults. Cochrane Database Syst Rev (3):CD007938. doi:10.1002/14651858.CD007938.pub2

Mount BM, Ajemian I, Scott JF (1976) Use of the Brompton mixture in treating the chronic pain of malignant disease. Can Med Assoc J 115(2):122–124

Nguyen JP, Lefaucher JP, Le Guerinel C et al (2000) Motor cortex stimulation in the treatment of central and neuropathic pain. Arch Med Res 31(3):263–265

Nguyen JP, Velasco F, Brugieres P et al (2008) Treatment of chronic neuropathic pain by motor cortex stimulation: results of a bicentric controlled crossover trial. Brain Stimul 1(2):89–96. doi:10.1016/j.brs.2008.03.007

Norrbrink C, Lundeberg T (2009) Tramadol in neuropathic pain after spinal cord injury: a randomized, double-blind, placebo-controlled trial. Clin J Pain 25(3):177–184. doi:10.1097/AJP.0b013e31818a744d

Norrbrink C, Lundeberg T (2011) Acupuncture and massage therapy for neuropathic pain following spinal cord injury: an exploratory study. Acupunct Med 29(2):108–115. doi:10.1136/aim.2010.003269

O'Connell NE, Wand BM (2011) Repetitive transcranial magnetic stimulation for chronic pain: time to evolve from exploration to confirmation? Pain 152(11):2451–2452. doi:10.1016/j.pain.2011.06.004

O'Connell NE, Wand BM, Marston L et al (2011) Noninvasive brain stimulation techniques for chronic pain. A report of a Cochrane systematic review and meta-analysis. Eur J Phys Rehabil Med 47(2):309–326

Ohara PT, Vit JP, Bhargava A et al (2009) Gliopathic pain: when satellite glial cells go bad. Neuroscientist 15(5):450–463. doi:10.1177/1073858409336094

Owolabi SA, Saab CY (2006) Fractalkine and minocycline alter neuronal activity in the spinal cord dorsal horn. FEBS Lett 580(18):4306–4310. doi:10.1016/j.febslet.2006.06.087

Pagano RL, Assis DV, Clara JA et al (2011) Transdural motor cortex stimulation reverses neuropathic pain in rats: a profile of neuronal activation. Eur J Pain 15(3):268 e1–14. doi:10.1016/j.ejpain.2010.08.003

Pancrazio JJ, Kamatchi GL, Roscoe AK et al (1998) Inhibition of neuronal Na+ channels by antidepressant drugs. J Pharmacol Exp Ther 284(1):208–214

Paola FA, Arnold M (2003) Acupuncture and spinal cord medicine. J Spinal Cord Med 26(1):12–20

Pickering G, Morel V, Simen E et al (2011) Oral magnesium treatment in patients with neuropathic pain: a randomized clinical trial. Magnes Res 24(2):28–35. doi:10.1684/mrh.2011.0282

Portenoy RK, Foley KM (1986) Chronic use of opioid analgesics in non-malignant pain: report of 38 cases. Pain 25(2):171–186

Putzke JD, Richards JS, Kezar L et al (2002) Long-term use of gabapentin for treatment of pain after traumatic spinal cord injury. Clin J Pain 18(2):116–121

Rahn EJ, Hohmann AG (2009) Cannabinoids as pharmacotherapies for neuropathic pain: from the bench to the bedside. Neurotherapeutics 6(4):713–737. doi:10.1016/j.nurt.2009.08.002

Reddy S, Patt RB (1994) The benzodiazepines as adjuvant analgesics. J Pain Symptom Manage 9(8):510–514

Rintala DH, Holmes SA, Courtade D et al (2007) Comparison of the effectiveness of amitriptyline and gabapentin on chronic neuropathic pain in persons with spinal cord injury. Arch Phys Med Rehabil 88(12):1547–1560. doi:10.1016/j.apmr.2007.07.038

Ripamonti C, Zecca E, Bruera E (1997) An update on the clinical use of methadone for cancer pain. Pain 70(2–3):109–115

Saade NE, Jabbur SJ (2008) Nociceptive behavior in animal models for peripheral neuropathy: spinal and supraspinal mechanisms. Prog Neurobiol 86(1):22–47. doi:10.1016/j.pneurobio.2008.06.002

Saulino M (2012) Simultaneous treatment of intractable pain and spasticity: observations of combined intrathecal baclofen-morphine therapy over a 10-year clinical experience. Eur J Phys Rehabil Med 48(1):39–45

Sawe J (1986) High-dose morphine and methadone in cancer patients. Clinical pharmacokinetic considerations of oral treatment. Clin Pharmacokinet 11(2):87–106

Scuderi C, Valenza M, Stecca C et al (2012) Palmitoylethanolamide exerts neuroprotective effects in mixed neuroglial cultures and organotypic hippocampal slices via peroxisome proliferator-activated receptor-alpha. J Neuroinflammation 9:49. doi:10.1186/1742-2094-9-49

Sears NC, Machado AG, Nagel SJ et al (2011) Long-term outcomes of spinal cord stimulation with paddle leads in the treatment of complex regional pain syndrome and failed back surgery syndrome. Neuromodulation 14(4):312–318. doi:10.1111/j.1525-1403.2011.00372.x; discussion 8

Selph S, Carson S, Fu R et al (2011) Drug class review: neuropathic pain: final update 1 report. Drug Class Reviews, Portland

Senapati AK, Huntington PJ, Peng YB (2005) Spinal dorsal horn neuron response to mechanical stimuli is decreased by electrical stimulation of the primary motor cortex. Brain Res 1036(1–2):173–179. doi:10.1016/j.brainres.2004.12.043

Siddall PJ, Cousins MJ, Otte A et al (2006) Pregabalin in central neuropathic pain associated with spinal cord injury: a placebo-controlled trial. Neurology 67(10):1792–1800. doi:10.1212/01.wnl.0000244422.45278.ff

Sigtermans MJ, van Hilten JJ, Bauer MC et al (2009) Ketamine produces effective and long-term pain relief in patients with Complex Regional Pain Syndrome Type 1. Pain 145(3):304–311. doi:10.1016/j.pain.2009.06.023

Skaper SD, Facci L (2012) Mast cell-glia axis in neuroinflammation and therapeutic potential of the anandamide congener palmitoylethanolamide. Philos Trans R Soc Lond B Biol Sci 367(1607):3312–3325. doi:10.1098/rstb.2011.0391

Smirne S, Scarlato G (1977) Clonazepam in cranial neuralgias. Med J Aust 1(4):93–94

Smith HS (2010) Activated microglia in nociception. Pain Physician 13(3):295–304

Smith HS, Argoff CE (2011) Pharmacological treatment of diabetic neuropathic pain. Drugs 71(5):557–589. doi:10.2165/11588940-000000000-00000

Sokal P, Harat M, Paczkowski D et al (2011) Results of neuromodulation for the management of chronic pain. Neurol Neurochir Pol 45(5):445–451

Soria E, Fine E, Paroski M (1989) Asymmetrical growth of scalp hair in syringomyelia. Cutis 43(1):33–36

Sudo K, Fujiki N, Tsuji S et al (1999) Focal (segmental) dyshidrosis in syringomyelia. J Neurol Neurosurg Psychiatry 67(1):106–108

Swislocki A, Orth M, Bales M et al (2010) A randomized clinical trial of the effectiveness of photon stimulation on pain, sensation, and quality of life in patients with diabetic peripheral neuropathy. J Pain Symptom Manage 39(1):88–99. doi:10.1016/j.jpainsymman.2009.05.021

Szaflarski J, Ivacko J, Liu XH et al (1998) Excitotoxic injury induces monocyte chemoattractant protein-1 expression in neonatal rat brain. Brain Res Mol Brain Res 55(2):306–314

Tai Q, Kirshblum S, Chen B et al (2002) Gabapentin in the treatment of neuropathic pain after spinal cord injury: a prospective, randomized, double-blind, crossover trial. J Spinal Cord Med 25(2):100–105

Tanenberg RJ, Irving GA, Risser RC et al (2011) Duloxetine, pregabalin, and duloxetine plus gabapentin for diabetic peripheral neuropathic pain management in patients with inadequate pain response to gabapentin: an open-label, randomized, noninferiority comparison. Mayo Clin Proc 86(7):615–626. doi:10.4065/mcp.2010.0681

Terpening CM, Johnson WM (2007) Methadone as an analgesic: a review of the risks and benefits. W V Med J 103(1):14–18

Toombs JD, Kral LA (2005) Methadone treatment for pain states. Am Fam Physician 71(7):353–358

Truin M, Janssen SP, van Kleef M et al (2011) Successful pain relief in non-responders to spinal cord stimulation: the combined use of ketamine and spinal cord stimulation. Eur J Pain 15(10):1049 e1–9. doi:10.1016/j.ejpain.2011.04.004

Tzellos TG, Papazisis G, Amaniti E et al (2008) Efficacy of pregabalin and gabapentin for neuropathic pain in spinal-cord injury: an evidence-based evaluation of the literature. Eur J Clin Pharmacol 64(9):851–858. doi:10.1007/s00228-008-0523-5

Uhle EI, Becker R, Gatscher S et al (2000) Continuous intrathecal clonidine administration for the treatment of neuropathic pain. Stereotact Funct Neurosurg 75(4):167–175

Vranken JH, Dijkgraaf MG, Kruis MR et al (2008) Pregabalin in patients with central neuropathic pain: a randomized, double-blind, placebo-controlled trial of a flexible-dose regimen. Pain 136(1–2):150–157. doi:10.1016/j.pain.2007.06.033

Wang W, Mei XP, Wei YY et al (2011) Neuronal NR2B-containing NMDA receptor mediates spinal astrocytic c-Jun N-terminal kinase activation in a rat model of neuropathic pain. Brain Behav Immun 25(7):1355–1366. doi:10.1016/j.bbi.2011.04.002

Wasserman JK, Koeberle PD (2009) Development and characterization of a hemorrhagic rat model of central post-stroke pain. Neuroscience 161(1):173–183. doi:10.1016/j.neuroscience.2009.03.042

Watson CP, Gilron I, Sawynok J (2010) A qualitative systematic review of head-to-head randomized controlled trials of oral analgesics in neuropathic pain. Pain Res Manag 15(3):147–157

Weintraub MI, Herrmann DN, Smith AG et al (2009) Pulsed electromagnetic fields to reduce diabetic neuropathic pain and stimulate neuronal repair: a randomized controlled trial. Arch Phys Med Rehabil 90(7):1102–1109. doi:10.1016/j.apmr.2009.01.019

White FA, Wilson NM (2008) Chemokines as pain mediators and modulators. Curr Opin Anaesthesiol 21(5):580–585. doi:10.1097/ACO.0b013e32830eb69d

Wiffen PJ, McQuay HJ, Edwards JE et al (2005) Gabapentin for acute and chronic pain. Cochrane Database Syst Rev (3):CD005452. doi:10.1002/14651858.CD005452

Wiffen PJ, Derry S, Moore RA (2011a) Lamotrigine for acute and chronic pain. Cochrane Database Syst Rev (2):CD006044. doi:10.1002/14651858.CD006044.pub3

Wiffen PJ, Derry S, Moore RA et al (2011b) Carbamazepine for acute and chronic pain in adults. Cochrane Database Syst Rev (1):CD005451. doi:10.1002/14651858.CD005451.pub2

Williams KA, Gonzalez-Fernandez M, Hamzehzadeh S et al (2011) A multi-center analysis evaluating factors associated with spinal cord stimulation outcome in chronic pain patients. Pain Med 12(8):1142–1153. doi:10.1111/j.1526-4637.2011.01184.x

Wu A, Green CR, Rupenthal ID et al (2012) Role of gap junctions in chronic pain. J Neurosci Res 90(2):337–345. doi:10.1002/jnr.22764

Zhou HY, Chen SR, Pan HL (2011) Targeting N-methyl-D-aspartate receptors for treatment of neuropathic pain. Expert Rev Clin Pharmacol 4(3):379–388

The Biochemistry of Syringomyelia

17

Andrew Brodbelt

Contents

With Marcus Stoodley

A. Brodbelt
Department of Neurosurgery,
The Walton Centre NHS Trust, Liverpool, UK
e-mail: andrew.brodbelt@thewaltoncentre.nhs.uk

17.1 Introduction

Syringomyelia is a condition that is characterised by a build-up of fluid-filled cavities within the spinal cord. The resulting damage to the cord produces symptoms of pain and neurological deficit. Most theories of pathogenesis have focused on biomechanical aspects, relating symptoms to pure pressure effects and altered fluid dynamics, and much has been written concerning the pressure dynamics of the spinal and cranial fluid compartments in patients who develop syringomyelia. Clearly, however, most normal cellular and pathological processes involve biochemical mechanisms, often of extraordinary complexity. A good deal of work has been done on these processes in related conditions and some work specifically on syringomyelia, but there is little published about the fluid itself and the chemical and physico-chemical processes that occur in the fluid and surrounding tissues.

This chapter will review our knowledge regarding the chemicals in the syrinx fluid and the signalling processes in surrounding tissues and suggest further avenues for investigation and treatment. It aims to introduce the reader to fluid and tissue biochemistry relevant to patients with syringomyelia. The syrinx fluid biochemistry will be examined, initially by describing cerebro-spinal fluid (CSF), before discussing the syrinx contents. The remainder of the chapter will look at the chemical processes in the tissues around the syrinx. To aid understanding relevant to the

G. Flint, C. Rusbridge (eds.), *Syringomyelia*,
DOI 10.1007/978-3-642-13706-8_17, © Springer-Verlag Berlin Heidelberg 2014

pathogenesis of syringomyelia, this discussion will be organised in an anatomical and then relevant pathological framework. Each topic area will conclude by relating these processes to syrinx pathogenesis and to potential future treatments.

17.2   Fluid Biochemistry

17.2.1   Cerebrospinal Fluid

CSF is clear and colourless with a density of 1.003–1.008 g/cm (Davson and Segal 1996; Rosenberg 1990; Kiernan 1998). It has a lower protein, glucose and potassium content and a higher chloride level than plasma (Table 17.1). In humans there are, on average, 140 mL of CSF divided between the ventricular system (25 % or 35 mL), the spinal canal (30–70 mL) and the cranial subarachnoid cisterns (Davson and Segal 1996; Edsbagge et al. 2004; Kohn et al. 1991; Redzic and Segal 2004). Traditionally, the major function of CSF was thought to be as a physical cushion for the brain and spinal cord. Calculations suggest that, within a CSF bath, the 1,500 g brain weighs only 50 g, reducing tension on nerve roots and acting as a strong mechanical buffer (Kimelberg 2004). In addition, and perhaps of greater importance, CSF also acts like a lymphatic system by allowing movement of metabolites, toxins and nutrients. It has roles in homeostatic hormonal and signalling mechanisms, chemical buffering and neurodevelopment (Brown et al. 2004; Jones 2004; Kimelberg 2004; Redzic and Segal 2004; Rosenberg 1990).

Most work done on CSF signalling pathways has concentrated on the cranial ventricular system, particularly around the third ventricle and hypothalamus. Neuroactive substances have been identified as being secreted from the pineal gland (melatonin), separately into the third ventricle (gonadotrophin-releasing hormone), as well as peptides (vasopressin and corticotrophin-releasing hormone) released from periventricular neurones and astrocytes (Redzic and Segal 2004; Veening and Barendregt 2010). They appear to have effects distant from the secreting site (Redzic and Segal 2004; Veening and Barendregt 2010). The influence of these neuroactive substances on spinal structures and any link with syrinx pathogenesis is not well established, although a major role in syrinx formation is unlikely. A role in pain production, contribution to neuronal loss, or as a potential molecular biomarker or therapeutic target is more feasible. The role of the specialised ependymal subtype, the tanycyte, in this process is discussed below.

17.2.2   Syrinx Fluid

A number of researchers have compared the fluid in a syrinx with that in the CSF, although most have concentrated on the protein concentrations (Freeman 1959; Schlesinger et al. 1981; J Wong 2012, personal communication). The electrolyte composition of the syrinx fluid has only rarely been examined and in very limited numbers, but it appears that syrinx fluid has a similar electrolyte composition to CSF (Table 17.1). This similar composition, combined with the lack of an anatomical barrier to fluid flow across syrinx and pial surfaces and the observation that tracer studies show rapid flow between the subarachnoid and interstitial spaces, via perivascular spaces, has been used to support a CSF origin for syrinx fluid (Brodbelt 2003; Cserr and Knopf 1992; Davson and Segal 1996; Foldi 1999; Kida et al. 1995; Rosenberg 1990; Weller 1998).

Syrinx fluid has been reported as having different protein content from that of CSF or plasma, and this may have implications for syrinx pathogenesis (According to J Wong MBBS, written communication, April 2012). The observed degree of difference may be influenced by whether the CSF is taken from the lumbar cistern, rather than adjacent to the syrinx. The protein content in CSF increases caudally along the spinal canal, ranging from 15 mg/100 mL in the ventricle to 36 mg/100 mL in the cistern magna and 59 mg/100 mL in the lumbar theca (Davson and Segal 1996). Eighty percent of CSF protein

Table 17.1 A comparison of the chemical composition of body fluids

	Plasma	ECF/ISF	ICF	CSF	Syrinx[a]
Sodium (mM)	135–145	138–142	5–15	135–154	145–150
Potassium (mM)	3.4–4.7	3.8–5	135–155	2.6–3.1	2.6–2.8
pH	7.35–7.45	7.44		7.3–7.6	
Chloride (mM)	99–108	118	9.0	115–130	120–123
Calcium (mM)	2.1–2.6			1–1.5	1.05–1.7
Protein (g/L)	50–80			0.15–2	0.35–0.89
Glucose (mM)	3.9–6.1			2.8–4.2	3–6.1
Magnesium (mM)	0.7–1.0			1.0–2.3	1.09–2.1
Osmolality (mM)	280–296	280–296	280–296	280–296	280–296
Amino acids (g/L)	2.62			0.72	

References: Davson and Segal (1996), Freeman and Wright (1953), Ganong (1995), Kjeldsberg and Knight (1986), Kratz and Lewandrowski (1998), Laha (1975), Nurick et al. (1970), Rosenberg (1990), Rossier et al. (1985)

ECF/ISF extracellular/Interstitial fluid, *ICP* intracellular fluid, *CSF* cerebrospinal fluid

[a]From J Wong 2012, personal communication. The only significant difference between CSF and syrinx fluid was a higher protein content in the syrinx

originates from the blood, whilst the other 20 % originates from neurones, glia and leptomeningeal cells within the central nervous system (Veening and Barendregt 2010). In Cavalier King Charles Spaniels, a comparative study of CSF in animals with a syrinx showed a higher protein and cell content, as compared to those with a Chiari and no syrinx (Whittaker et al. 2011). This difference in CSF content may be related to syrinx-induced cell damage and an inflammatory response in these animals. From the published literature, the protein content of syrinx fluid may be slightly higher than CSF, except in some post-traumatic cases where this difference is much greater (Laha et al. 1975; Nurick et al. 1970; Rossier et al. 1985, J Wong 2012, personal communication).

Protein could affect fluid flow into a syrinx by promoting diffusion. Diffusion describes the movement of a substance (solute or solvent) from a higher to a lower concentration (Elkinton and Donowski 1955). Osmosis, in contrast, is fluid movement down a concentration gradient established by the restraint of solute to one area, by either a semipermeable membrane or a continuously active transport process moving solute in one direction (Elkinton and Donowski 1955). Raised protein could produce a diffusion gradient in favour of fluid flow into a post-traumatic syrinx. If the gradient is great enough, significant pressures could develop. Although studies using CSF tracers suggest the volume is too great and velocity too rapid for diffusion alone to be a sufficient explanation, in some post-traumatic syrinxes diffusion along a protein-produced diffusion gradient might contribute to fluid ingress into the cavity (Rennels et al. 1990; Stoodley et al. 1996, 1999).

Although much has been published regarding the makeup of plasma and CSF protein compartments, there is nothing published on the specific proteins and amino acids that are present in syrinx fluid. These proteins may have implications in syrinx initiation, development or maintenance. Many of the proteins found in the serum are also found within the CSF (Davson and Segal 1996). These include hormones, interleukins, endorphins and various proteins used as biomarkers for some neurological conditions (Davson and Segal 1996; Hu et al. 2012a). Beta-2 transferrin is the desialated isoform of the iron-binding glycoprotein transferrin and is only found in CSF, perilymph and ocular fluids (Papadea and Schlosser 2005). It is not clear if beta-2 transferrin is found in syrinx fluid.

CSF biomarkers for multiple sclerosis are well recognised, although newer biomarkers for Alzheimer, frontotemporal lobar degeneration and Parkinson's disease are being developed (Weller et al. 1998). As we understand the biochemical processes underlying the pathogenesis of syringomyelia, new biomarkers in the CSF or serum for syrinx propagation or development may occur. These could be related to inflammatory processes, oedema or water transport and might, in the future, help tailor drug treatment to syringomyelia subtype or pathological effect.

17.3 Tissue Biochemistry

The influence of the chemical processes within and around the cells surrounding a syrinx depends in part on the unique anatomy of the spinal cord. Tight junctions limiting fluid movement, compartmentalisation and extended cellular processes can all influence function. The following discussion will focus on the biochemical processes occurring in an anatomically orientated manner.

17.3.1 Fluid Barriers

Barriers exist between plasma and interstitial fluid (ISF) (the blood-brain barrier or BBB), between plasma and CSF (the blood-CSF barrier or BCSFB), between interstitial and intracellular fluids (ICF) and within the cord parenchyma (Abbott 2004; Leonhardt and Desaga 1975). A leaky barrier exists between the CSF and extracellular spaces, allowing mixing of interstitial fluid and CSF (Davson and Segal 1996; Del Bigio 1995). Barriers can consist of cell membranes, tight junctions between cells and various cellular transport processes that control solute and water movement. These transport processes include the aquaporins, pinocytic vesicles and a multitude of ion transport channels (see below) (Brodbelt and Stoodley 2007; Davson and Segal 1996).

The term blood-brain barrier refers to the anatomical and physiological complex that controls the movement of substances from the general extracellular fluid of the body into the extracellular fluid of the brain (Nolte 1999). In capillary endothelium, this manifests as tight junctions between adjacent cells and absence of pinocytic vesicles (Nolte 1999; Rosenberg 1990). Instead,

interstitial fluid of the central nervous system is formed by an active process at the cerebral capillary. Interstitial fluid of the CNS also exchanges freely with CSF (Rosenberg 1990).

The blood-brain barrier is also functionally dynamic, with a wide permeability range, dependent on intra- and intercellular signalling events amongst endothelial cells, astrocytes, pericytes and neurones (Bonkowski et al. 2011; Neuwelt et al. 2011). The neurovascular unit, composed of pre- and postsynaptic endings, their related glia, pericytes and the capillary bed, engages in multiple signalling processes (Neuwelt et al. 2011) (Fig. 17.1). Ten to fifteen percent of all proteins that make up the neurovascular unit are transporters (Enerson and Drewes 2006). This highly complex unit has been examined in a post-traumatic rat model of syringomyelia. The presence of endothelial barrier antigen and loss of functional integrity, as assessed by extravasation of intravascular horseradish peroxidase, found a prolonged structural and functional disruption of the blood-spinal cord barrier in this animal model (Hemley et al. 2009). Astrocytes may play an active role in maintaining disturbed neurovascular unit function (Neuwelt et al. 2011). This disturbed blood-spinal cord barrier may contribute to fluid ingress into a syrinx (Hemley et al. 2009).

Directly under the ependyma and between ependymal cells, there are basement membranes which form labyrinths, connecting the ependymal basement membrane with perivascular basement membranes of subependymal capillaries and postcapillary veins (Leonhardt and Desaga 1975; Cifuentes et al. 1992). These glycolipid and glycoprotein structures can hold fluid by swelling but may also function to form a pathway for movement of fluid and solutes, between the ependyma and subependymal vessels (Leonhardt and Desaga 1975).

17.3.2 The Central Canal, Ependyma and Tanycytes

The central canal of the spinal cord is lined by a continuous layer of ependymal cells and occasional tanycytes. Ependyma is a single-layered,

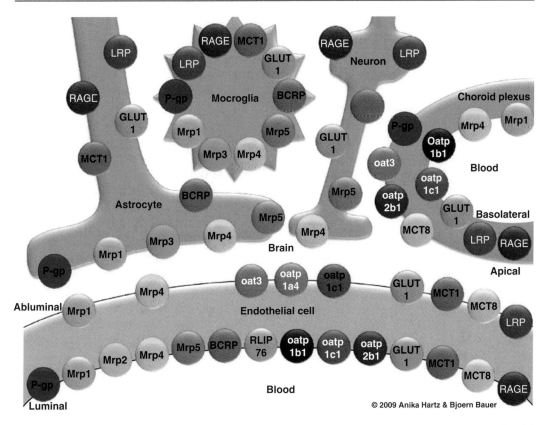

Fig. 17.1 Primary transporters in the neurovascular unit. The cellular relationships of carrier-mediated transport systems at the blood-brain interface, illustrating the complexity of the system which has a role in spinal cord fluid homeostasis. *BCRP* breast cancer resistance protein, *GLUT1* glucose transporter-1, *LRP* low-density lipopro-tein receptor-related protein, *MCT* monocarboxylic acid transporter, *Mrp* multidrug resistance protein, *Oat* organic anion transporter, *Oatp* organic anion transporting protein, *P-gp* P-glycoprotein, *RAGE* receptor for advanced glycation end products, *RLIP76* Ral-binding protein-1 (Taken with permission from Neuwelt 2011)

cuboidal to columnar, ciliated epithelium, derived from germinal matrix cells (Bruni and Reddy 1987; Del Bigio 1995). In the brain, ependymal cells are connected by zonula adherens and have abundant gap junctions (Brightman and Reese 1969; Del Bigio 1995). They may function to regulate water movement, act as a barrier between the CSF and extracellular spaces and act as a niche of latent neural stem cells (Del Bigio 1995; Hamilton et al. 2009).

Tanycytes are specialised forms of ependymal cells, found in the ependymal lining or subependyma. They have radially directed basal processes that extend into the neuropil, where they typically enwrap blood vessels (Bruni 1998; Honda et al. 1999; Del Bigio 1995). The function of tanycytes in the spinal cord is unknown

although neuronal guidance, structural support, neuroendocrine roles and a limited transport system, from the CSF to the ECF, have been suggested (Bruni 1998; Honda et al. 1999; Del Bigio 1995). One study looked at nestin[1] expression as a marker of latent neural stem cell properties in the ependymal cells of the central canal and found that this correlated with tanycyte morphology (Hamilton et al. 2009). Tanycytes implanted into a rat spinal cord injury model supported the regeneration of lesioned axons (Leonhardt and Desaga 1975). The functions of ependyma and

---

[1] An intermediate filament protein that is expressed in dividing neural cells and may have a role in the radial growth of axons. Nestin protein expression is used as a marker of neural stem cells.

tanycytes in human spinal cord may be less important than in the brain but may still play a role after cellular destruction in the spinal cord and provide an interesting avenue for further investigation.

In two large human autopsy series, central canal stenosis or occlusion was present in 75–97 % of cases after the third decade, and isolated segments occurred between stenotic regions (Aboulker 1979; Milhorat et al. 1994; Yasui et al. 1999). Stenosis has been postulated as occurring because of mild ependymal injury or viral infection (Del Bigio 1995; Milhorat et al. 1994). The stenotic sections of the central canal so formed have been postulated to act as an initial site for fluid build-up into a cyst (Brodbelt 2003). As well as their potential in treatment as neural stem cells, ependymal cells and tanycytes may also have a role in providing an initial cavity, an isolated segment of the central canal which, in some cases with the correct filling mechanism, will lead to syrinx formation.

17.3.3 Astrocytes

Adjacent to the ependyma is the spinal cord parenchyma, composed mainly of astrocytes, which are the most numerous cell type in the central nervous system. Astrocytes have a number of functions and are important in many biochemical mechanisms within the spinal cord. They support neurones by supplying some citric acid cycle intermediates, taking up excess neurotransmitter and maintaining stable glutathione levels (Sidoryk-Wegrzynowicz et al. 2011). Astrocytes also regulate the extracellular environment including acid base balance, potassium buffering and free radical scavenging (Sidoryk-Wegrzynowicz et al. 2011). They produce and release growth factors, including transforming growth factor β, platelet-derived growth factor and nerve growth factor (Sidoryk-Wegrzynowicz et al. 2011). There are dynamic and reciprocal signalling networks between astrocytes and neurones (Sidoryk-Wegrzynowicz et al. 2011). Other areas of astrocytic function of interest in patients with a syrinx include the removal of excess neurotransmitters and the role of aquaporins.

Astrocytes are also implicated in the pathogenesis of neuropathic pain (for more detail see Chap. 16). Any or all of these functions may be affected in patients with a syrinx, and the role of the astrocyte must be viewed as pivotal in this area.

17.3.4 Neurotransmitters

Glutamate is the main excitatory neurotransmitter in the brain. Glutamate is formed by the reductive amination of the Krebs cycle intermediate, α-ketoglutarate. It acts on metabotropic and ionotropic receptors (Ganong 1995). Metabotropic receptors are serpentine G-protein-coupled receptors that are excitatory and neuromodulatory in action (Ganong 1995; Watkins 2000). Ionotropic receptors are excitatory ligand-gated ion channels subdivided by selective agonist action into kainic acid, AMPA (2-amino-3-(5-methyl-3-oxo-1,2- oxazol-4-yl) propanoic acid) and N-methyl-D-aspartate (NMDA) receptors (Ganong 1995). In other words, kainic acid, AMPA and N-methyl-D-aspartate are all substances used to selectively stimulate subtypes of ionotropic glutamate receptor. Kainic acid and AMPA channels are involved in fast synaptic transmission and permit Na^+ influx and K^+ efflux when open, whilst N-methyl-D-aspartate allows Ca^{2+} passage and is normally blocked by Mg^{2+} (Watkins 2000). Quisqualic acid is an agonist for AMPA and group I metabotropic receptors that act via intracellular inositol triphosphate (Watkins 2000). In excess, glutamate and some of the substances used experimentally to stimulate glutamate receptor subtypes, including quisqualic acid, can cause selective neuronal death via AMPA and metabotropic receptor activation, leading to excessive free intracellular calcium. In this way it is 'excitotoxic' (Ganong 1995).

Debridement of the necrotic area following spinal cord injury in rats and dogs improves recovery, suggesting that ongoing biochemical processes occur after the initial injury (Freeman and Wright 1953). One group of candidates for such a role is the excitatory amino acids. Excitatory amino acids are released after both spinal cord injury and ischaemia and lead to glutamate receptor activation, calcium influx and selective neuronal cell death (Liu 1991; Marsala et al. 1994; Panter 1990; Simpson et al. 1990; Tator 1991; Urca and Urca 1990; Urushitani et al. 1998). The amount of excitatory amino acid released correlates with the degree of trauma, and one study suggests that this release may be the direct result of neuronal activity (Liu et al. 1991; Panter et al. 1990). Quisqualic acid (an excitatory amino acid) and kainate appear to be more neurotoxic than N-methyl-D-aspartate, and selective antagonism of these substances confers some neuroprotective effects (Li and Tator 2000; Urca and Urca 1990). In fact, intraspinal injection of quisqualic acid produces extracanalicular syrinxes (Brodbelt et al. 2003a, b; Yang et al. 2001; Yezierski et al. 1993). Combined with kaolin in the subarachnoid space to produce arachnoiditis, the cavities so produced enlarge over time and are histologically identical to that seen in humans (Brodbelt et al. 2003a, b). Other candidates potentially involved in secondary cord damage include proteolytic enzyme release, liberation of free fatty acids, free radical production, phospholipid degradation and abnormalities of prostaglandin production (Edgar and Quail 1994; Kao and Chang 1977; Reddy et al. 1989).

Fifty to ninety percent of adult patients with syringomyelia will have pain (Todor et al. 2000).

Substance P and calcitonin gene-related peptide have both been implicated in pain production. In a human pathological study, substance P distribution was decreased both around and cranial to a syrinx cavity but increased caudally (Todor et al. 2000). A recent study in Cavalier King Charles Spaniels also showed an altered distribution (Hu et al. 2012a). It is not yet clear how this alteration relates to the pain patients feel or if other excitatory amino acids or neurotransmitters, such as GABA, also play a part, but successful identification of the role of such chemicals could lead to better treatment.

17.3.5 Aquaporins

Much interest has been generated regarding the transmembrane group of water channels, known as aquaporins (AQPs) (Fig. 17.2). In normal human spinal cord, aquaporin subtype 4 (AQP-4) is seen on all astrocytes (Nesic et al. 2010). AQP-1 is found on the apical surface of the choroid plexus epithelium and sensory axons in the dorsal horn, AQP-8 is found in the ependymal cells around the central canal, and AQP-9 is found in neurones and astrocytes (Badaut 2009; Gunnarson et al. 2004; Kimelberg 2004; Oshio et al. 2004). AQP-4 functions to enable fast

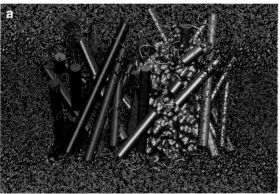
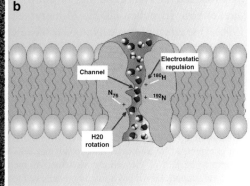

Fig. 17.2 Aquaporins have a role in tissue fluid homeostasis although their role in syringomyelia is inconclusive. (**a**) A snapshot of an atomic simulation in progress. Boomerang-shaped water molecules slip as they march single file through the narrow pore of the gold aquaporin, whilst the red balls and fibres that make up the cell's membrane keep the outside water (*top*) from mixing with the cellular pool (*bottom*) (Taken with permission from Emad Tajkhorshid,

Klaus Schulten, Theoretical and Computational Biophysics Group, University of Illinois at Urbana-Champaign, 2004 Winner of Visualization Challenge in Science and Engineering, organised by the National Science Foundation and Science Magazine). (**b**) Schematic depiction of water movement through the narrow selectivity filter of the aquaporin channel (Taken with permission from Opossum58 at the German language Wikipedia) water influx or efflux, driven by osmotic or pressure gradients (Solenov et al. 2002; Yang et al. 2008). AQP-4 has a role in normal ion and water homeostasis in the spinal cord and may contribute to the pathophysiological response in disease states.

Following injury, AQP-4 expression changes, and this change is both site and time dependent. In a series of three spinal cord-injured patients, pathological examination of the injured spinal cords demonstrated no AQP-4 in GFAP[2]-labelled astrocytes surrounding the damaged area, whilst astrocytes in the spared white matter rim had intense AQP-4 labelling (Nesic et al. 2010). Similar combinations of astrocytes with AQP-4 absence and AQP-4 overexpression have been reported in animal models of spinal cord injury and post-traumatic syringomyelia (Aghayev et al. 2011; Nesic et al. 2010, A Watling 2003, personal communication). Furthermore, it appears that the AQP-4-negative cells either change to or are replaced over time by AQP-4-overexpressing cells. This change in AQP-4 expression is delayed in more severe injury, and this delay has been suggested to be inversely related to the likelihood of motor and sensory recovery in rat models (Nesic et al. 2010).

Tissue hypoxia alters AQP-4 expression. Hypoxia is described following trauma or in the tissue around the syrinx and may be due to pressure effects (Brodbelt 2003; Milhorat et al. 1996). One effect of tissue hypoxia is the release of hypoxia-induced factor 1a[3] which appears to upregulate AQP-4 (Ding et al. 2009). This mechanism leading to cytotoxic oedema may be protective. Hypoxia-induced cellular energy

depletion alters ion transport mechanisms, changes the normal ion balance and leads to a build-up of sodium within the neurone (Malek et al. 2003). To maintain cellular osmolality and electriconeutrality, potassium and chloride ions leave the cell (Malek et al. 2003). This tenfold increase in extracellular potassium and chloride is taken up by the astrocytes (Blank and Kirshner 1977; Malek et al. 2003). Upregulation of AQP-4 allows water rapidly to follow the ions and may be seen as a mechanism to maintain normal cellular osmolality (Nesic et al. 2010).

The early post-injury phase of AQP-4-negative astrocytes may contribute to the accumulation of vasogenic oedema by slowing the process of fluid removal around the area affected and working against the aquaporin homeostatic process (Zador et al. 2009). The overall effect of AQP-4-driven astrocytic swelling on functional recovery after spinal cord injury may depend on the balance between vasogenic oedema, a protective astrocyte role in removing extracellular ions and the harmful effects of astrocytic swelling (Nesic et al. 2010).

Despite this evolving interest, there has been variable support for a direct role of aquaporins in syringomyelia pathogenesis. Using a kaolin model of syringomyelia in the rat, both Aghayev et al. and Hemley et al. found no significant difference in AQP-4 expression between controls and syrinx-induced animals (Aghayev et al. 2011; Hemley et al. 2012). However, in a similar rat model, Zhang et al. demonstrated a relationship in AQP-4 expression proportional to the degree of central canal expansion (Zhang et al. 2012). Nesci et al. found no correlation in a rat post-traumatic syrinx model, between AQP-4 protein levels and syrinx size or enlargement over time (Nesic et al. 2010).

Our understanding of AQP-4 in tissue water homeostasis is developing. Aquaporins remain an area of interest as regards our understanding of syrinx pathogenesis and the functional alterations in the surrounding spinal cord that can lead to pain and disability. Further study of aquaporins may, in the future, lead to new treatments.

---

[2] Glial fibrillary acidic protein is an intermediate filament that is expressed by astrocytes and ependymal cells and thought to be part of the cell cytoskeleton. As well as structural support, GFAP has a role in mitosis, cell to cell communication and repair after CNS injury. Normal astrocytes have GFAP labelling, although this may alter after an insult (hypoxia, inflammation, injury, etc.).

[3] Hypoxia-induced factor 1a is a transcription factor, one of a group of hypoxia-inducible factors that respond to a reduction in the available oxygen in the tissues. Hypoxia-inducible factors are known to mediate the cell response to hypoxia, including stopping differentiation and stimulating the formation of new blood vessels.

17.3.6 The Arterial Circulation

Tissue homeostasis also depends on the relationship of the arterial and venous structures within the spinal cord. In humans, there is a pial network (the vasocorona) of small arteries interconnecting anterior, posterolateral and posterior spinal arteries of the cord. These give off peripheral (centripetal) arteries which supply mainly white matter tracts (Kiernan 1998). The anterior spinal arteries send central (sulcal) arteries into the ventromedian fissure before turning laterally and supplying, alternately, right or left central grey matter (Thron 1988). A study of 13 rats, using a vascular corrosion cast technique, suggested that ventral and ventrolateral pial arterial plexuses do not exist and that a correspondingly greater proportion of the blood supply to the white matter comes from branches of the central (sulcal) arteries (Koyanagi et al. 1993). Humans have large numbers of small peripheral penetrating branches, approximately 100 times the number of central arteries. These terminate in the external fibre tracts or the marginal zone of the grey matter (Thron 1988). The relationship between the arterial supply and the astrocytes and blood-brain barrier has been discussed above. There is, currently, an enormous body of work looking at control and regulation of vascular supply of the spinal cord, yet relatively little has been carried out in patients with syringomyelia. Although fluid movement in the perivascular space has been proposed and modelled, altering electrolyte and protein balances or water channel flow across the neurovascular junction could all change the balance of fluid flow and has not yet been investigated (Bilston et al. 2003; Brodbelt et al. 2003a).

17.3.7 The Venous Circulation

Venous drainage of the spinal cord is by a series of irregular plexiform channels, inconsistent in size and position (Thron 1988). The most consistent and continuous veins are the anterior median spinal vein, running deep to the anterior spinal artery, and the posterior median spinal vein running in the dorsal midline (Thron 1988). There are other longitudinal channels that run along the anterior and dorsal rootlets (Kiernan 1998; Thron 1988). Sulcal veins are associated with sulcal arteries in the ventromedian fissure and drain the central grey and medial part of the anterior white matter into the anterior spinal vein mainly in the lumbosacral area (Koyanagi et al. 1993; Thron 1988). Radial veins are more important in the thoracic and cervical regions, draining the anterior and lateral white columns and significant amounts of adjacent grey matter into superficial venous channels (Koyanagi et al. 1993; Thron 1988). Posterior medial septal and oblique veins drain the posterior columns into posterior spinal veins (Koyanagi et al. 1993).

The relationship of the venous structures to overall fluid outflow from the spinal cord has been a matter for discussion (Brodbelt 2003). If fluid is entering the syrinx from perivascular spaces, there is no watertight lining to the cavity and this is a dynamic situation, then where does the fluid go? A recent large animal model attempted to look at fluid outflow and found that it occurred in a diffuse manner, into the surrounding extracellular space and towards the central canal and perivascular spaces (Wong et al. 2012). The precise relationship with the venous anatomy, if there is one, is not clear.

17.4 Pathological Processes

A number of pathological processes have been studied in relation to syringomyelia, and early theories included inflammation, ischaemia or interstitial oedema as the direct cause of a syrinx. Although, no longer thought to be directly causing the enlarging fluid-filled cavity, many of these processes are seen adjacent to a syrinx and may contribute to the growth, maintenance or symptoms generated by the syrinx.

17.4.1 The Inflammatory Response

The inflammatory responses of the nervous system to trauma result in oedema and sometimes in cyst formation (Fischbein et al. 1999; Guizar-Sahagun et al. 1994; Kakulas 1999; Tator and Fehlings 1991; Zhang et al. 1997).

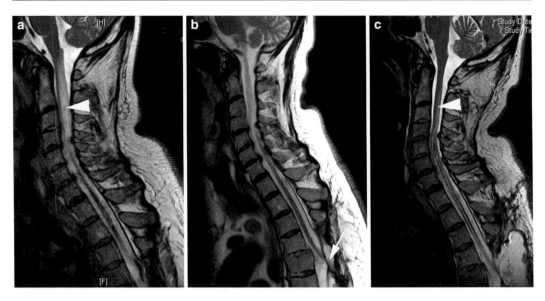

Fig. 17.3 Inflammation in a patient with a post-traumatic syrinx. T2-weighted MR images of a 65-year-old man who had a complete thoracic spinal cord injury 15 years earlier. (**a**, **b**) He presented 10 years after a syringopleural shunt (*arrow*), with worsening numbness and weakness in his left and then more recently his right arm and hand. Imaging showed an oedematous cord (*arrowhead*).

Exploration at the site of shunt insertion revealed a pus-filled collection also filling the shunt. (**c**) Four weeks following shunt removal and antibiotic treatment, the oedema has improved (*arrowhead*), as has his power and sensation. The shunt has not been replaced. In this case the oedema was thought to be due to infection and inflammation, not shunt blockage

Descriptions of the histological features of the spinal cord following trauma were initially based on animal work but have since found agreement with human pathological studies and can be subdivided into three stages: necrosis, repair and stability (Guizar-Sahagun et al. 1994; Squier and Lehr 1994). From 1 to 14 days after injury to the spinal cord, parenchymatous haemorrhage, vascular thrombosis, oedema, axonal segmentation and inflammatory infiltrates are seen (Guizar-Sahagun et al. 1994; Kakulas 1987; Tator and Fehlings 1991; Wagner et al. 1978; Zhang et al. 1997). The repair stage occurs between 2 and 15 weeks after injury, when revascularisation occurs and macrophages phagocytose necrotic tissue, before then disappearing, leaving cavities within the cord (Guizar-Sahagun et al. 1994; Wagner et al. 1978; Williams 1980). Finally, a stage of stability occurs, between 15 weeks and 1 year after trauma, when the lesioned area has become cystic. The cysts may have trabeculae and may be collapsed with a sparse surrounding chronic inflammatory infiltrate and arachnoiditis (Guizar-Sahagun et al. 1994; Kakulas 1987; Tator and Fehlings 1991; Wagner et al. 1978).

Chronic inflammation or infection has been proposed as causative mechanisms in patients with meningitis who develop syrinxes (Charcot and Joffroy 1869; Klekamp 2002) (Fig. 17.3). Infection, it was proposed, could cause a syrinx either from an induction of an inflammatory response or by causing ischaemia (Charcot and Joffroy 1869; Klekamp 2002). Milhorat et al. suggested that viral infections could induce central canal occlusion and demonstrated that suckling hamsters, infected with reovirus, produced a similar pathological appearance to that seen clinically in human adults (Brodbelt et al. 2005; Milhorat and Kotzen 1994; Milhorat et al. 1994). Isolated segments of the central canal so formed could provide an isolated cavity promoting a noncommunicating canalicular syrinx. However, many conditions that predispose to syrinx formation are not associated with inflammation or infection. Inflammation, therefore, probably contributes to syrinx pathogenesis in some cases by leading to arachnoid adhesion formation and the hydrodynamic effects that this produces, rather than by acting as the main pathogenic mechanism. Treatment aimed at stopping or reducing adhesion formation by targeting inflammatory processes, especially after injury or localised infection, could act to reduce the risk of syrinx formation.

17.4.2 Ischaemia

Active transport systems require energy, usually in the form of ATP, to drive fluid against a concentration gradient. Little work has been performed looking at the role of active transport in syringomyelia. In syrinxes associated with spinal cord tumours, protein levels are high, and active mechanisms proposed include direct fluid or protein secretion or secretion of an oedema-generating agent (Milhorat 2000). The low blood flow in the spinal cord tissue surrounding a syrinx is evidence against active transport in post-traumatic syringomyelia (Milhorat et al. 1997; Young et al. 2000).

There is indirect evidence for an ischaemic role in syrinx initiation, possibly by the formation of small cystic cavities from infarction. The common site of extracanalicular syrinxes in the dorsolateral grey matter is sometimes described as a vascular watershed, although anatomical studies have cast doubt on any vascular insufficiency at this position (Edgar and Quail 1994; Milhorat et al. 1995; Squier and Lehr 1994; Thron 1988; Tveten 1976a, b). Pencil-shaped infarcts of the cord, with a shape and location similar to syringomyelic cysts, are seen in cases of spinal trauma, as well as in compression myelopathy (Hashizume et al. 1983; Hirose et al. 1980). Intraoperative pulsed Doppler ultrasound and laser Doppler blood flow measurements demonstrate low blood flow in the spinal cord at the level of the syrinx and following syrinx decompression blood flow improves, although whether this is cause or effect has not been established (Brodbelt 2003; Giller and Finn 1989; Milhorat et al. 1996; Young et al. 2000). Central venous infarction has been proposed as the underlying cause of ischaemia, although one pathological study found no evidence to support this and a further study of a patient with post-meningitic arachnoiditis and a syrinx demonstrated obliteration of spinal cord feeding arteries (Caplan et al. 1990, Davis and Symon 1989; Squier and Lehr 1994).

The improvement in blood supply after syrinx decompression suggests that the compression of the cord tissue by the syrinx was instrumental in producing ischaemia rather than the reverse (Giller and Finn 1989; Milhorat et al. 1996; Young et al. 2000). Similarly, the development of arachnoiditis does not demonstrate ischaemia in every pathological case examined. Ischaemia may play a role in syrinx initiation and perhaps in syrinx development, but this must be differentiated from myelomalacia (Klekamp 2002). Improving oxygen and nutrient supply to the spinal cord may limit further damage, but it is hard to see an effective method to do this being developed.

17.4.3 Cellular Adenosine Triphosphate (ATP), Necrosis and Apoptosis

Hypoxia, ischaemia, low cellular ATP levels and an excitotoxic insult from glutamate release can all lead to cell death (Taylor et al. 1999). Apoptosis is a morphologically distinct form of controlled cell death, characterised by the formation of membrane-bound apoptotic bodies, containing fragmented nuclear and organelle material (Eguchi et al. 1997; Shiraishi et al. 2001; Steller 1995; Taylor et al. 1999). Apoptosis requires energy, and because apoptotic bodies are membrane bound and directly engulfed by macrophages, the process does not lead to an inflammatory response (Kass et al. 1996; Richter et al. 1996; Steller 1995; Taylor et al. 1999). Necrosis involves mitochondrial swelling, development of an electron lucent cytoplasm, little nuclear damage and loss of plasma membrane integrity, leading to cell rupture and release of intracellular contents (Eguchi et al. 1997; Shiraishi et al. 2001; Steller 1995; Taylor et al. 1999). In contrast to apoptosis, energy is not required for necrosis, and the release of intracellular contents triggers an inflammatory response (Steller 1995). Identical receptors, signal transduction pathways and cytotoxic mechanisms can lead to apoptosis or necrosis, which suggests that they may represent the two extremes of a broad spectrum of cell death (Leist et al. 1998). The distinction may arise from either different intracellular factors or external conditions (Leist et al. 1998).

Injury severity and cellular ATP levels can influence whether cells survive or undergo apoptosis or necrosis (Aito et al. 2002; Eguchi et al. 1997; Richter et al. 1996; Shiraishi et al. 2001; Taylor et al. 1999). In mild ATP depletion, defined as a cellular ATP/ADP ratio above 0.2 or ATP levels greater than 75 % of controls, most cells will survive (Lieberthal et al. 1998; Richter et al. 1996; Taylor et al. 1999). Moderate ATP depletion (25–70 % of control ATP levels) is more likely to lead to cellular apoptosis and may be due in part to activation of caspase 3 (Aito et al. 2002; Eguchi et al. 1997; Lieberthal et al. 1998; Richter et al. 1996; Shiraishi et al. 2001; Taylor et al. 1999). Severe injury, or low intracellular ATP levels (less than 15–30 % of control ATP levels), preferentially induces necrosis (Aito et al. 2002; Eguchi et al. 1997; Lieberthal et al. 1998; Leist et al. 1998; Richter et al. 1996; Shiraishi et al. 2001; Taylor et al. 1999). Apoptosis and necrosis can occur at the same time, in the same tissue, following hypoxic ischaemia. Intermediate ATP levels of 30–50 % have been measured in tissues where this arises and may be one of the triggers (Leist et al. 1998; Taylor et al. 1999). Mitochondrial energy levels have also been shown to influence the final mode of cell death in cerebellar granule cells, following a glutamate insult (Ankarcrona et al. 1995; Taylor et al. 1999).

Reductions in cellular ATP occur due to reduced synthesis, increased use or catabolism or transfer out of the cells (Aito et al. 2002). During hypoxia or ischaemia, inadequate oxygen and glucose levels lead to reduced ATP availability (Taylor et al. 1999). Phosphocreatine breakdown initially compensates, to maintain ATP levels (Taylor et al. 1999). Once phosphocreatine is depleted, anaerobic glycolysis can usually maintain cellular ATP levels within 90 % of normal, as long as glucose is available (Taylor et al. 1999). Eventually, the total adenylate pool (ATP + ADP + AMP) is depleted and ATP levels drop, leading to a low ATP/ADP ratio, resulting in cell membrane depolarisation, ion leakage, calcium influx and cell death (Taylor et al. 1999).

In the central nervous system, a 55 % reduction of cerebral blood flow was required experimentally before alterations in tissue energy state were detected (Anderson et al. 1980; Eklof and Siesjo 1972). Grey matter consumes two to four times as much glucose as white matter and has higher ATP levels and alterations may be inhomogeneous following ischaemia (Anderson et al. 1980; Eklof and Siesjo 1972; Sokoloff et al. 1977).

Surrounding a syrinx, the spinal cord tissue appears to be ischaemic, which may be related to syrinx expansion and, to a lesser degree, arachnoiditis. Energy metabolite measurements provide evidence to support a level of ischaemia that leads to apoptosis, rather than necrosis (Brodbelt 2003). Apoptosis has been found to be prominent around the syrinx in the later stages of experimental syrinx formation (according to A Watling BSc(HONS), written communication, April 2003). Apoptosis may contribute to syrinx enlargement.

17.4.4 Oedema (Fig. 17.4)

Oedema in the central nervous system may be cytotoxic, when it is mainly caused by astrocytic swelling from ion transport disruption; it may be vasogenic, due to blood-brain barrier breakdown, leading to excess extracellular water accumulation, as well as astrocytic swelling; or it may be a combination of the two (Kimelberg 2004). Blood-brain barrier breakdown can occur due to excessive hydrostatic pressure gradients between blood vessels and brain parenchyma, and this type of vasogenic oedema is sometimes termed 'hydrostatic' (Shima 2003). Oedema seen in patients with a syrinx appears to be vasogenic, rather than purely cytotoxic. In some patients oedema is seen prior to syrinx formation and has been described as a 'presyrinx state' (Fischbein et al. 1999; Jinkins et al. 1998; Levy et al. 2000).

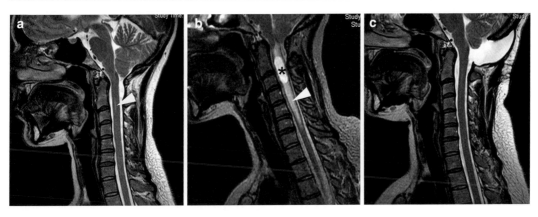

Fig. 17.4 Oedema resolution in a patient with a Chiari malformation. T2-weighted MR images of a patient with a Chiari I malformation and mild headache with (**a**) a prominent central canal or early syrinx (*arrowhead*). (**b**) Four years later when the headache became worse with arm pain and a syrinx (*) and oedema (*arrowhead*) have developed. (**c**) Following a posterior fossa craniotomy, a moderate pseudomeningocele is present, the oedema and syrinx have disappeared, and her Chiari symptoms have improved but not disappeared. Often despite excellent imaging outcomes, syrinx or Chiari symptoms do not completely resolve

Experiments in cats involved the placement of a fibrin-soaked sponge on the posterior aspect of the spinal cord, to induce localised arachnoiditis (Klekamp et al. 2001). Four months later tissue elasticity was measured by intraspinal bolus injections of fluid with concomitant intraspinal pressure monitoring, followed by fixation and histological examination for perivascular space enlargement (Klekamp 2002). Interstitial oedema was considered to be present if perivascular spaces were enlarged and tissue elasticity elevated and occurred at the level of arachnoiditis and caudal in the central grey matter only. Animals did not form syrinxes in the time frame observed, but the results were interpreted as demonstrating the initial stage of syrinx development (Klekamp 2002).

In the final stages of syrinx enlargement, MRI and pathological studies demonstrate expansion of the cord and a reduction in the total volume of spinal cord tissue (Bogdanov and Mendelevich 2002; Iskandar et al. 1994). As intra- and extracellular oedema often surround a syrinx, this reduction in volume arises from cell loss (Fischbein et al. 1999; Jinkins et al. 1998; Levy et al. 2000). Neuronal loss occurs initially but does not progress with axial syrinx enlargement.

Loss of cord parenchyma must therefore be at the expense of glia and axon tracts and progress in tandem with syrinx growth.

17.4.5 Alterations Surrounding a Syrinx

The histological changes in the parenchyma surrounding syrinxes are similar, regardless of the associated condition, and appear to represent the non-specific results of a distensile force (Milhorat et al. 1995; Reddy et al. 1989; Stoodley and Jones 1998). The syrinx wall is formed by compressed glial tissue surrounded by gliosis (Durward et al. 1982; Foo et al. 1989; Milhorat et al. 1995). The presence of ependymal cells relates to the associated condition and is seen in patients with Chiari-associated syringomyelia but not usually following trauma (Milhorat et al. 1995). There is evidence of Wallerian degeneration, macrophage infiltration, demyelination in the surrounding white matter as well as central chromatolysis and neuronophagia in the grey matter (Foo et al. 1989; Kim 1993; Milhorat et al. 1995). Enlargement of perivascular spaces may be present (Durward et al. 1982). Vascular changes may be seen around the syrinx, including hyalinised and thickened vessels, oedema and haemorrhages (Nogues 1987). The pathological description of a syrinx confirms the absence of a watertight capsule and supports the view that a 'stable' syrinx is actually a dynamic process of continual fluid ingress and leakage out. It is the relation of these two processes that determines the syrinx size and progression. Syrinx enlargement often affects the crossing spinothalamic tracts. In dogs, greater glial and fibrous proliferation around the syrinx appears to be associated with neuropathic pain (Hu et al. 2012b).

Arachnoiditis, or spinal leptomeningeal inflammation and thickening, is often found in conjunction with post-traumatic or postinfective syringomyelia (Batzdorf et al. 1998; Caplan et al. 1990; Edgar and Quail 1994; Kim 1993; Klekamp et al. 1997; Klekamp and Samii 2002). Post-traumatic arachnoid scarring may be due to the inflammatory responses to blood breakdown products released at the time of injury, mechanical irritation related to trauma, persistent compression or instability or follow intradural surgery (Klekamp and Samii 2002; Tjandra et al. 1989). The pathological processes producing arachnoiditis or the tethering effects have been suggested as promoting spinal cord ischaemia and repeated microtrauma, with subsequent cyst formation (Edgar and Quail 1994; Klekamp et al. 2001; Klekamp 2002; McLaurin et al. 1954). Extensive areas of arachnoiditis demonstrate a greater degree of obliterative thickening of vessel walls and may be more important in generating ischaemic effects than might more localised areas of scarring (Klekamp et al. 2001; Tjandra et al. 1989). The dura is firmly affixed to the underlying spinal cord, due to a proliferation of collagen in the subarachnoid compartment (Kim 1993). This collagen may form a thick layer, embedding the damaged spinal cord remnants and entrapping nerve roots and vessels (Caplan et al. 1990; Kim 1993). There is some neovascularisation, although residual inflammatory infiltrate is usually sparse (Kim 1993). Osseous metaplasia may occur (Kahler et al. 2000; Kim 1993). Biochemical alterations in cellular interactions and astrocytic dysfunction may contribute to arachnoiditis formation, and further investigation is warranted.

Conclusions

This review highlights a number of areas of biochemical function, the study of which may lead to the creation of new treatment methods. The importance of the astrocyte in regulating much of the spinal cord microenvironment, the ependymal cells and tanycytes as potential neural stem cells, the relationship of aquaporins to water movement, energy metabolites involved in the processes leading to cell death and the role of peptides in the generation of pain and neurological dysfunction all have implications for syrinx pathogenesis. All are valuable areas for further study. Current surgical treatment of syringomyelia remains suboptimal, suggesting an incomplete understanding of the underlying pathological processes. A better understanding of the biochemical processes may generate novel treatment approaches that avoid the risks and overcome the limitations of surgery or complement the surgical approach to improve symptomatic control.

The biochemistry of the spinal cord and associated pathological processes involved with syringomyelia is a potentially enormous field of study, and this chapter has attempted to outline the relevant processes and highlight possible implications for the benefit of all those interested in improving our understanding of syringomyelia.

References

Abbott NJ (2004) Evidence for bulk flow of brain interstitial fluid: significance for physiology and pathology. Neurochem Int 45(4):545–552

Aboulker J (1979) La syringomyelie et les liquides intra-rachidiens. Neurochirurgie 25(Suppl 1):1–44

Aghayev K, Bal E, Rahimli T et al (2011) Expression of water channel aquaporin-4 during experimental syringomyelia: laboratory investigation. J Neurosurg Spine 15(4):428–432

Aito H, Aalto KT, Raivio KO (2002) Biphasic ATP depletion caused by transient oxidative exposure is associated with apoptotic cell death in rat embryonal cortical neurons. Pediatr Res 52:40–45

Anderson DK, Means ED, Waters TR (1980) Spinal cord energy metabolism in normal and postlaminectomy cats. J Neurosurg 52:387–391

Ankarcrona M, Dypbukt JM, Bonfoco E et al (1995) Glutamate-induced neuronal death: a succession of necrosis or apoptosis depending on mitochondrial function. Neuron 15:961–973

Badaut J (2009) Aquaglyceroporin 9 in brain pathologies. Neuroscience 168(4):1047–1057. doi:10.1016/j.neuroscience.2009.10.030

Batzdorf U, Klekamp J, Johnson JP (1998) A critical appraisal of syrinx cavity shunting procedures. J Neurosurg 89:382–388

Bilston LE, Fletcher DF, Brodbelt AR et al (2003) Arterial pulsation-driven cerebrospinal fluid flow in the perivascular space: a computational model. Comput Methods Biomech Biomed Engin 6(4):235–241

Blank WF Jr, Kirshner HS (1977) The kinetics of extracellular potassium changes during hypoxia and anoxia in the cat cerebral cortex. Brain Res 123(1):113–124

Bogdanov EI, Mendelevich EG (2002) Syrinx size and duration of symptoms predict the pace of progressive myelopathy: retrospective analysis of 103 unoperated cases with craniocervical junction malformations and syringomyelia. Clin Neurol Neurosurg 104:90–97

Bonkowski D, Katyshev V, Balabanov RD et al (2011) The CHS microvascular pericyte: pericyte-astrocyte crosstalk in the regulation of tissue survival. Fluids Barriers CNS 8:8. doi:10.1186/2045-8118-8-8

Brightman MW, Reese TS (1969) Junctions between intimately apposed cell membranes in the vertebrate brain. J Cell Biol 40:648–677

Brodbelt AR (2003) Investigations in posttraumatic syringomyelia. PhD Thesis. University of New South Wales, Sydney. Available at: http://handle.unsw.edu.au/1959.4/19317

Brodbelt AR, Stoodley MA (2007) CSF pathways: a review. Br J Neurosurg 21(5):510–520

Brodbelt AR, Stoodley MA, Watling A et al (2003a) The role of excitotoxic injury in post-traumatic syringomyelia. J Neurotrauma 20(9):883–893

Brodbelt AR, Stoodley MA, Watling AM et al (2003b) Fluid flow in an animal model of post-traumatic syringomyelia. Eur Spine J 12(3):300–306

Brodbelt AR, Stoodley MA, Jones NR (2005) Non traumatic syringomyelia. In: The Cervical Spine Research Society Editorial Committee (ed) The cervical spine, 4th edn. Lippincott-Raven Publishers, Philadelphia

Brown PD, Davies SL, Speake T et al (2004) Molecular mechanisms of cerebrospinal fluid production. Neuroscience 129(4):957–970

Bruni JE (1998) Ependymal development, proliferation, and functions: a review. Microsc Res Tech 41:2–13

Bruni JE, Reddy K (1987) Ependyma of the central canal of the rat spinal cord: a light and transmission electron microscopic study. J Anat 152:55–70

Caplan LR, Norohna AB, Amico LL (1990) Syringomyelia and arachnoiditis. J Neurol Neurosurg Psychiatry 53:106–113

Charcot JM, Joffroy A (1869) Deux cas d'atrophie musculaire progressive avec lésions de la substance grise et des faisceaux antérolatéraux de la moelle épinière. Arch Physiol Neurol Pathol 2:354–367, 629–649, 744–760

Cifuentes M, Fernandez-LLebrez P, Perez J et al (1992) Distribution of intraventricularly injected horseradish peroxidase in cerebrospinal fluid compartments of the rat spinal cord. Cell Tissue Res 270(3):485–494

Cserr HF, Knopf PM (1992) Cervical lymphatics, the blood-brain barrier and the immunoreactivity of the brain: a new view. Immunol Today 13:507–512

Davis CH, Symon L (1989) Mechanisms and treatment in post-traumatic syringomyelia. Br J Neurosurg 3:669–674

Davson H, Segal MB (1996) Physiology of the CSF and blood brain barriers. CRC Press, Boca Raton

Del Bigio MR (1995) The ependyma: a protective barrier between brain and cerebrospinal fluid. Glia 14:1–13

Ding JY, Kreipke CW, Speirs SL et al (2009) Hypoxia-inducible factor-1alpha signaling in aquaporin upregulation after traumatic brain injury. Neurosci Lett 453(1):68–72

Durward QJ, Rice GP, Ball MJ et al (1982) Selective spinal cordectomy: clinicopathological correlation. J Neurosurg 56:359–367

Edgar R, Quail P (1994) Progressive post-traumatic cystic and non-cystic myelopathy. Br J Neurosurg 8:7–22

Edsbagge M, Tisell M, Jacobsson L, Wikkelso C (2004) Spinal CSF absorption in healthy individuals. Am J Physiol Regul Integr Comp Physiol 287(6):R1450–R1455

Eguchi Y, Shimizu S, Tsujimoto Y (1997) Intracellular ATP levels determine cell death fate by apoptosis or necrosis. Cancer Res 57:1835–1840

Eklof B, Siesjo BK (1972) The effect of bilateral carotid artery ligation upon the blood flow and the energy state of the rat brain. Acta Physiol Scand 86:155–165

Elkinton JR, Donowski TS (1955) Body fluid dynamics. In: The body fluids: basic physiology and practical therapeutics. Williams and Wilkins, Baltimore

Enerson BE, Drewes LR (2006) The rat blood brain barrier transcriptome. J Cereb Blood Flow Metab 26:959–973

Fischbein NJ, Dillon WP, Cobbs C et al (1999) The "presyrinx" state: a reversible myelopathic condition that may precede syringomyelia. AJNR Am J Neuroradiol 20:7–20

Foldi M (1999) The brain and the lymphatic system revisited. Lymphology 32:40–44

Foo D, Bignami A, Rossier AB (1989) A case of post-traumatic syringomyelia. Neuropathological findings after 1 year of cystic drainage. Paraplegia 27:63–69

Freeman G (1959) Ascending spinal paralysis. J Neurosurg 16:120–122

Freeman LW, Wright TW (1953) Experimental observations of concussion and contusion of the spinal cord. Ann Surg 137:433–443

Ganong WF (1995) Review of medical physiology. Prentice Hall International Inc, London

Giller CA, Finn SS (1989) Intraoperative measurement of spinal cord blood velocity using pulsed Doppler ultrasound. A Case report. Surg Neurol 32:387–393

Guizar-Sahagun G, Grijalva I, Madrazo I et al (1994) Development of post-traumatic cysts in the spinal cord of rats-subjected to severe spinal cord contusion. Surg Neurol 41:241–249

Gunnarson E, Zelenina M, Aperia A (2004) Regulation of brain aquaporins. Neuroscience 129(4):947–955

Hamilton LK, Truong MKV, Bednarczyk MR et al (2009) Cellular organisation of the central canal ependymal zone, a niche of latent neural stem cells in the adult mammalian spinal cord. Neuroscience 164:1044–1056

Hashizume Y, Iljima S, Kishimoto H et al (1983) Pencil-shaped softening of the spinal cord. Pathologic study in 12 autopsy cases. Acta Neuropathol 61:219–224

Hemley SJ, Biotech B, Tu J et al (2009) Role of the blood-spinal cord barrier in posttraumatic syringomyelia. J Neurosurg Spine 11(6):696–704

Hemley SJ, Bilston LE, Cheng S et al (2012) Aquaporin-4 expression and blood spinal cord barrier permeability in canalicular syringomyelia. J Neurosurg Spine 17:602–612

Hirose G, Shimazaki K, Takado M et al (1980) Intramedullary spinal cord metastasis associated with pencil-shaped softening of the spinal cord: case report. J Neurosurg 52:718–721

Honda T, Yokota S, Gang FG et al (1999) Evidence for the c-ret protooncogene product (c-Ret) expression in the spinal tanycytes of adult rat. J Chem Neuroanat 17:163–168

Hu HZ, Rusbridge C, Constantino-Casas F et al (2012a) Distribution of substance P and calcitonin gene-related peptide in the spinal cord of Cavalier King Charles Spaniels affected by symptomatic syringomyelia. Res Vet Sci 93(1):318–320. doi:10.1016/j.rvsc.2011.08.012

Hu HZ, Rusbridge C, Constantino-Casas F et al (2012b) Histopathological investigation of syringomyelia in the Cavalier King Charles spaniel. J Comp Pathol 146:192–201. doi:10.1016/j.jcpa.2011.07.002

Iskandar BJ, Oakes WJ, McLaughlin C et al (1994) Terminal syringohydromyelia and occult spinal dysraphism. J Neurosurg 81:513–519

Jinkins JR, Reddy S, Leite CC et al (1998) MR of parenchymal spinal cord signal change as a sign of active advancement in clinically progressive posttraumatic syringomyelia. AJNR Am J Neuroradiol 19:177–182

Jones HC (2004) Cerebrospinal fluid research: a new platform for dissemination of research, opinions and reviews with a common theme. Cerebrospinal Fluid Res 1(1):1

Kahler RJ, Knuckey NW, Davis S (2000) Arachnoiditis ossificans and syringomyelia: a unique case report. J Clin Neurosci 7:66–68

Kakulas BA (1987) The clinical neuropathology of spinal cord injury. A guide to the future. Paraplegia 25:212–216

Kakulas BA (1999) A review of the neuropathology of human spinal cord injury with emphasis on special features. J Spinal Cord Med 22:119–124

Kao TCC, Chang LW (1977) The mechanism of spinal cord cavitation following spinal cord transection. J Neurosurg 46:197–209

Kass GE, Eriksson JE, Weis M et al (1996) Chromatin condensation during apoptosis requires ATP. Biochem J 318(Pt 3):749–752

Kida S, Weller RO, Zhang ET et al (1995) Anatomical pathways for lymphatic drainage of the brain and their pathological significance. Neuropathol Appl Neurobiol 21:181–184

Kiernan JA (1998) Barr's the human nervous system, an anatomical viewpoint, 7th edn. Lippincott-Raven, Philadelphia

Kim RC (1993) Spinal cord pathology. In: Nelson JS, Parisi JE, Schochet SSJ (eds) Principles and practice of neuropathology. Mosby, St Louis, pp 398–435

Kimelberg HK (2004) Water homeostasis in the brain: basic concepts. Neuroscience 129:851–860

Kjeldsberg CR, Knight JA (1986) Cerebrospinal fluid, in body fluids: laboratory examination of amniotic, cerebrospinal, seminal, serous and synovial fluids: a textbook atlas. American society of clinical pathologists, Chicago

Klekamp J (2002) The pathophysiology of syringomyelia – historical overview and current concept. Acta Neurochir (Wien) 144:649–664

Klekamp J, Samii M (2002) Syringomyelia: diagnosis and management. Springer, Berlin

Klekamp J, Batzdorf U, Samii M et al (1997) Treatment of syringomyelia associated with arachnoid scarring caused by arachnoiditis or trauma. J Neurosurg 86:233–240

Klekamp J, Volkel K, Bartels CJ et al (2001) Disturbances of cerebrospinal fluid flow attributable to arachnoid scarring cause interstitial edema of the cat spinal cord. Neurosurgery 48:174–185

Kohn MI, Tanna NK, Herman GT et al (1991) Analysis of brain and cerebrospinal fluid volumes with MR imaging. Part I. Methods, reliability, and validation. Radiology 178(1):115–122

Koyanagi I, Tator CH, Lea PJ (1993) Three-dimensional analysis of the vascular system in the rat spinal cord with scanning electron microscopy of vascular corrosion casts. Part 1: normal spinal cord. Neurosurgery 33:277–283

Kratz A, Lewandrowski KB (1998) Case records of the Massachusetts General Hospital. Weekly clinicopathological exercises. Normal reference laboratory values. N Engl J Med 339:1063–1072

Laha RK, Malik HG, Langille RA (1975) Post-traumatic syringomyelia. Surg Neurol 4:519–522

Leist M, Kuhnle S, Single B et al (1998) Differentiation between apoptotic and necrotic cell death by means of the BM cell death detection ELISA or Annexin V staining. Biochemica 2:25–28

Leonhardt H, Desaga U (1975) Recent observations on ependyma and subependymal basement membranes. Acta Neurochir (Wien) 31(3–4):153–159

Levy EI, Heiss JD, Kent MS et al (2000) Spinal cord swelling preceding syrinx development. Case report. J Neurosurg 92:93–97

Li S, Tator CH (2000) Action of locally administered NMDA and AMPA/kainate receptor antagonists in spinal cord injury. Neurol Res 22:171–180

Lieberthal W, Menza SA, Levine JS (1998) Graded ATP depletion can cause necrosis or apoptosis of cultured mouse proximal tubular cells. Am J Physiol 274:F315–F327

Liu D, Thangnipon W, McAdoo DJ (1991) Excitatory amino acids rise to toxic levels upon impact injury to the rat spinal cord. Brain Res 547:344–348

Malek SA, Codorre F, Stys PK (2003) Aberrant chloride transport contributes to anoxic/ischemic white matter injury. J Neurosci 23(9):3826–3836

Marsala M, Sorkin LS, Yaksh TL (1994) Transient spinal ischemia in rat: characterization of spinal cord blood flow, extracellular amino acid release, and concurrent histopathological damage. J Cereb Blood Flow Metab 14:604–614

McLaurin RL, Bailey OT, Schurr PH et al (1954) Myelomalacia and multiple cavitations of spinal cord secondary to adhesive arachnoiditis. Arch Pathol 57:138–146

Milhorat TH (2000) Classification of syringomyelia. Neurosurg Focus 8:1–6

Milhorat TH, Kotzen RM (1994) Stenosis of the central canal of the spinal cord following inoculation of suckling hamsters with reovirus type I. J Neurosurg 81:103–106

Milhorat TH, Kotzen RM, Anzil AA (1994) Stenosis of the central canal of the spinal cord in man: incidence and pathological findings in 232 autopsy cases. J Neurosurg 80:716–722

Milhorat TH, Capocelli AL Jr, Anzil AP et al (1995) Pathological basis of spinal cord cavitation in syringomyelia: analysis of 105 autopsy cases. J Neurosurg 82:802–812

Milhorat TH, Kotzen RM, Capocelli AL Jr et al (1996) Intraoperative improvement of somatosensory evoked potentials and local spinal cord blood flow in patients with syringomyelia. J Neurosurg Anesthesiol 8:208–215

Milhorat TH, Capocelli AL Jr, Kotzen RM et al (1997) Intramedullary pressure in syringomyelia: clinical and pathophysiological correlates of syrinx distension. Neurosurgery 41:1102–1110

Nesic O, Guest JD, Zivadinovic D et al (2010) Aquaporins in spinal cord injury: the janus face of aquaporin 4. Neuroscience 168(4):1019–1035

Neuwelt EA, Bauer B, Fahlke C et al (2011) Engaging neuroscience to advance translational research in brain barrier biology. Nat Rev Neurosci 12(3):169–182

Nogues MA (1987) Syringomyelia and syringobulbia. Handb Clin Neurol 6(50):443–464

Nolte J (1999) The human brain: an introduction to its functional anatomy. Mosby, St Louis

Nurick S, Russell JA, Deck MD (1970) Cystic degeneration of the spinal cord following spinal cord injury. Brain 93:211–222

Oshio K, Binder DK, Yang B et al (2004) Expression of aquaporin water channels in mouse spinal cord. Neuroscience 127:685–693

Panter SS, Yum SW, Faden AI (1990) Alteration in extracellular amino acids after traumatic spinal cord injury. Ann Neurol 27:96–99

Papadea C, Schlosser RJ (2005) Rapid method for beta2-transferrin in cerebrospinal fluid leakage using an automated immunofixation electrophoresis system. Clin Chem 51(2):464–470

Reddy KK, Del Bigio MR, Sutherland GR (1989) Ultrastructure of the human posttraumatic syrinx. J Neurosurg 71:239–243

Redzic ZB, Segal MB (2004) The structure of the choroid plexus and the physiology of the choroid plexus epithelium. Adv Drug Deliv Rev 56(12):1695–1716

Rennels ML, Blaumanis OR, Grady PA (1990) Rapid solute transport throughout the brain via paravascular fluid pathways. Adv Neurol 52:431–439

Richter C, Schweizer M, Cossarizza A et al (1996) Control of apoptosis by the cellular ATP level. FEBS Lett 378:107–110

Rosenberg GA (1990) Brain fluids and metabolism. Oxford University Press, Oxford

Rossier AB, Foo D, Shillito J et al (1985) Posttraumatic cervical syringomyelia. Incidence, clinical presentation, electrophysiological studies, syrinx protein and results of conservative and operative treatment. Brain 108:439–461

Schlesinger EB, Antunes JL, Michelsen WJ et al (1981) Hydromyelia: clinical presentation and comparison of modalities of treatment. Neurosurgery 9:356–365

Shima K (2003) Hydrostatic brain edema: basic mechanisms and clinical aspect. Acta Neurochir Suppl 86:17–20

Shiraishi J, Tatsumi T, Keira N et al (2001) Important role of energy-dependent mitochondrial pathways in cultured rat cardiac myocyte apoptosis. Am J Physiol Heart Circ Physiol 281:H1637–H1647

Sidoryk-Wegrzynowicz M, Wegrzynowicz M, Lee E et al (2011) Role of astrocytes in brain function and disease. Toxicol Pathol 39:115–123

Simpson RK Jr, Robertson CS, Goodman JC (1990) Spinal cord ischemia-induced elevation of amino acids: extracellular measurement with microdialysis. Neurochem Res 15:635–639

Sokoloff L, Reivich M, Kennedy C et al (1977) The [14C] deoxyglucose method for the measurement of local cerebral glucose utilization: theory, procedure, and normal values in the conscious and anesthetized albino rat. J Neurochem 28:897–916

Solenov EI, Vetrivel L, Oshio K et al (2002) Optical measurement of swelling and water transport in spinal cord slices from aquaporin null mice. J Neurosci Methods 113(1):85–90

Squier MV, Lehr RP (1994) Post-traumatic syringomyelia. J Neurol Neurosurg Psychiatry 57:1095–1098

Steller H (1995) Mechanisms and genes of cellular suicide. Science 267:1445–1449

Stoodley MA, Jones NR (1998) Syringomyelia. In: The Cervical Spine Research Society Editorial Committee (ed) The cervical spine. Lippincott-Raven Publishers, Philadelphia, pp 565–583

Stoodley MA, Jones NR, Brown CJ (1996) Evidence for rapid fluid flow from the subarachnoid space into the spinal cord central canal in the rat. Brain Res 707:155–164

Stoodley MA, Gutschmidt B, Jones NR (1999) Cerebrospinal fluid flow in an animal model of noncommunicating syringomyelia. Neurosurgery 44: 1065–1075

Tator CH, Fehlings MG (1991) Review of the secondary injury theory of acute spinal cord trauma with emphasis on vascular mechanisms. J Neurosurg 75:15–26

Taylor DL, Edwards AD, Mehmet H (1999) Oxidative metabolism, apoptosis and perinatal brain injury. Brain Pathol 9:93–117

Thron AK (1988) Vascular anatomy of the spinal cord: neuroradiological investigations and clinical syndromes. Springer, New York

Tjandra JJ, Varma TR, Weeks RD (1989) Spinal arachnoiditis following subarachnoid haemorrhage. Aust N Z J Surg 59:84–87

Todor DR, Mu HT, Milhorat TH (2000) Pain and syringomyelia: a review. Neurosurg Focus 8(3):E11

Tveten L (1976a) Spinal cord vascularity III. The spinal cord arteries in man. Acta Radiol Diagn (Stockh) 17:257–273

Tveten L (1976b) Spinal cord vascularity IV. The spinal cord arteries in the rat. Acta Radiol Diagn (Stockh) 17:385–398

Urca G, Urca R (1990) Neurotoxic effects of excitatory amino acids in the mouse spinal cord: quisqualate and kainate but not N-methyl-D-aspartate induce permanent neural damage. Brain Res 529:7–15

Urushitani M, Shimohama S, Kihara T et al (1998) Mechanism of selective motor neuronal death after exposure of spinal cord to glutamate: involvement of glutamate-induced nitric oxide in motor neuron toxicity and nonmotor neuron protection. Ann Neurol 44:796–807

Veening JG, Barendregt HP (2010) The regulation of brain states by neuroactive substances distributed via the cerebrospinal fluid: a review. Cerebrospinal Fluid Res. http://cerebrospinalfluidresearch.com/content/7/1/1. Accessed 21 May 2012

Wagner FC, VanGilder JC, Dohrmann GJ (1978) Pathological changes from acute to chronic in experimental spinal cord trauma. J Neurosurg 48: 92–98

Watkins JC (2000) l-glutamate as a central neurotransmitter: looking back. Biochem Soc Trans 28:297–309

Weller RO (1998) Pathology of cerebrospinal fluid and interstitial fluid of the CNS: significance for Alzheimer disease, prion disorders and multiple sclerosis. J Neuropathol Exp Neurol 57:885–894

Whittaker DE, English K, McGonnell IM et al (2011) Evaluation of cerebrospinal fluid in Cavalier King Charles Spaniel dogs diagnosed with Chiari-like malformation with or without concurrent syringomyelia. J Vet Diagn Invest 23:302–307

Williams B (1980) On the pathogenesis of syringomyelia: a review. J R Soc Med 73:798–806

Wong J, Hemley S, Jones N et al (2012) Fluid outflow in a large-animal model of posttraumatic syringomyelia. Neurosurgery 71(2):474–480. doi:10.1227/NEU.0b013e31825927d6; discussion 480

Yang L, Jones NR, Stoodley MA et al (2001) Excitotoxic model of post-traumatic syringomyelia in the rat. Spine 26:1842–1849

Yang B, Zador Z, Verkman AS (2008) Glial cell aquaporin-4 overexpression in transgenic mice accelerates cytotoxic brain swelling. J Biol Chem 283(22): 15280–15286

Yasui K, Hashizume Y, Yoshida M et al (1999) Age-related morphologic changes in the central canal of the human spinal cord. Acta Neuropathol 97: 253–259

Yezierski RP, Sanata M, Park SH et al (1993) Neuronal degeneration and spinal cavitation following intraspinal injections of quisqualic acid in the rat. J Neurotrauma 10:445–456

Young WF, Tuma R, O'Grady T (2000) Intraoperative measurement of spinal cord blood flow in syringomyelia. Clin Neurol Neurosurg 102:119–123

Zador Z, Stiver A, Wang V et al (2009) Role of aquaporin-4 in cerebral edema and stroke. Handb Exp Pharmacol 190:159–170

Zhang Z, Krebs CJ, Guth L (1997) Experimental analysis of progressive necrosis after spinal cord trauma in the rat: etiological role of the inflammatory response. Exp Neurol 143:141–152

Zhang Y, Zhang YP, Shields LB et al (2012) Cervical central canal occlusion induces noncommunicating syringomyelia. Neurosurgery 71:126–137

Patient Perspectives

18

Graham Flint

Contents

18.1   Introduction

The preceding chapters in this book have dealt with many different technical aspects of the subject of syringomyelia and its related conditions, ranging from what causes them to develop in the first place through to how they are best treated, given the current state of medical knowledge. At the end of the day, however, there is an individual who is suffering from the effects of the disease. That person will suffer all the normal human emotions that go with uncertainty about a condition with a strange name and about which most of the medical profession seem to know relatively little. It is important that those health-care professionals who deal with these conditions have at least some appreciation of what the patient goes through, in terms of both physical and emotional distress. Many of these experiences may not be obvious to the doctor, working in the clinical environment and with limited consultation time.

Below four of the authors give brief summaries of their own experiences as patients. Each has also spoken to many other patients with syringomyelia and Chiari. Their own case histories can therefore be put into context by a review of the experiences of other patients. Together these teach us a good deal about the many needs of people who find themselves having to live with these rather frightening conditions.

With Sue Line, Susan Kember, Rebecca Dodwell-Pitt and Lynn Burton

G. Flint
Department of Neurosurgery,
Queen Elizabeth Hospital,
University Hospitals Birmingham,
Birmingham, UK
e-mail: graham.flint@uhb.nhs.uk

G. Flint, C. Rusbridge (eds.), *Syringomyelia*,
DOI 10.1007/978-3-642-13706-8_18, © Springer-Verlag Berlin Heidelberg 2014

18.2 Case Histories

18.2.1 Personal Story 1

"On December 31st 1970, having enjoyed a meal with a friend, we both decided to visit a colleague. It was a very cold night, black ice was forecast and we certainly found some! I had been travelling at 30 mph so was able to control some of the skid but, with mud on the road under the ice, the car hit a small bank, spun and landed in the middle of the road, leaving me on the verge and my passenger in a ditch. My passenger had a dislocated collar bone and concussion. I had a severe spinal injury involving T5 and T6, in addition to broken ribs and damage to my right arm. I spent the following five and half months in a spinal injuries unit. I was left a complete paraplegic with sensation only in the upper torso.

"After a further 4 weeks at home I returned to my employer albeit in a modified capacity. Fate was still not on my side, however and, many years later, on my way to a meeting one October evening in 1987, a car went into the side of mine causing me to have a whiplash injury. I contacted a solicitor about claiming back the excess payment on my insurance. His enquiry "have you noticed any problems since the incident?" prompted a chain of events that I could not have envisaged.

"By then I had already noticed that, to drive, I needed to wear leather palmed gloves. At home and at work I was beginning to drop things more frequently. I had occasional but intense pain at the base of my skull. Sometimes it was difficult to concentrate. Sometimes even light touch on the base of my neck produced great discomfort. I was also having some problems distinguishing temperatures. I was not sure what the problem was. Were these symptoms the result of the most recent car accident or something else?

"On the advice of my solicitor I returned to my spinal injuries unit. My strongest recollection of that time was of multiple visits, with repeated examinations, including testing by pin prick, which leaves you feeling like a pin cushion, even if you can only feel some of the jabs. I remember being in a state of disbelief when the diagnosis of syringomyelia was made. Wasn't it enough that I was coping with the spinal injury and had got my life back together, without having to deal with this latest revelation?

"Next I was sent to see a neurosurgeon. My sister accompanied me to the appointment and I was really glad she did. The vivid description of what he intended to do was quite frightening as he proposed to "sever the spinal cord" to reduce the possibility of further syrinx forming and causing more problems. Thinking about the consequences and the possible detrimental effects upon my life left me dazed. I don't think either my sister or I will forget the drive home. Lots of questions came into my head about the surgery. What if it meant I could no longer tell when I wanted to go to the toilet? How would I cope being in hospital for a period of time? My mum and my sister were my carers and, although I could still do lots for myself, what would happen after this operation on my spine? Did I really want this operation? How long would I have to wait before surgery if I did decide to go ahead?

"While waiting to go into hospital, I set about reading up about the condition. At this time most of the information available was for professionals and very scary for the lay person to read. There was a lot of technical jargon and words which I didn't understand. I remembered the support group leaflet that the neurosurgeon had given me and at last plucked up the courage to speak to someone. Talking to somebody who had undergone surgery helped me realise that perhaps the future was not as bleak as I imagined. I then tried to carry on as normal but the prospect of surgery was always at the back of my mind. It is not an easy thing to face and the hope that there is an alternative around the corner keeps you searching.

"Plans had, nevertheless, been put in place for my surgery and, come the admission day, I was still very apprehensive whether this was the right decision but deep down I suspected it was. By chance there was a meeting of the patient support group that week and I found it really helpful to meet other people with the condition and all its variants. My problems seemed insignificant compared to what some individuals had to bear. Yet the people there showed camaraderie and

supported each other and the charity. It was a real eye opening experience. I plucked up the courage to ask my surgeon about the consequences of the operation, especially with regard to bladder and bowel function. I was very proud that, despite having no feeling on the surface of my body, I could still tell when I wanted to go to the toilet and I was very anxious that I might lose this after the surgery.

"Tuesday, and the big day had arrived. The porters came to take me to theatre and I started laughing. In fact I didn't stop until the anaesthetic took hold. My next memory is being on the intensive care unit with oxygen pipes in my nostrils and feeling very thirsty. The noise level was high and the lights very bright. Most of the time I was drifting in and out of sleep. I had a urinary catheter which had been my big nightmare. After 2 days I returned to the ward and one thing I remember vividly was an increase in body spasm. This was like being in a vice, holding me rigid and I felt like I had to fight for every breath. A bout could last anything from a few minutes to more than an hour. Increasing my anti-spasm medication did not help. My memory of the next three post-operative weeks is sketchy. The physiotherapist guided me through the process of becoming active again and regaining confidence in my ability to resume my activities. Turning to avoid pressure sores was very painful and was something I won't forget! Gritting your teeth also helped when the dressings were changed. After a few days I started the process of retraining my bladder. My goal was to rid myself of the urinary catheter as soon as possible. Three weeks after the operation I went home and started the process of getting back to work.

"The first benefit that I noticed was the ability to "walk" my thumb to every finger, one at a time in a sequence. This was a fantastic feeling and confirmed I had made the right decision as I had something tangible to compare with my pre-operative state. Many years on I can look back and say there have been several benefits. Initially it was great not to drop items so frequently and this was one of the first things family and friends noticed. My confidence increased and I was more

willing to try new things and situations. Would I have the operation again? I hope I don't have to but yes, I would, as the benefits have outweighed the initial concerns and worries.

"It is difficult to know whether my remaining symptoms are the result of syringomyelia, the original spinal injury or something else. Alternatively, as I am now a senior citizen, are they simply age related? Recently I have found that it is becoming more difficult to hold as much in my hands as I used to. Picking up small objects was difficult before but is now more so. Feeling objects and temperature awareness have become more of a problem. I have developed severe sleep apnoea and have to using a Continuous Positive Air Pressure (CPAP) pump at night. High blood pressure and elevated cholesterol are two other conditions that have become part of my life. These are controlled with medication and regular checks. I can't say that I notice I have them. I have acupuncture, approximately every 6 weeks, which is helping to keep me well. It helps my balance, circulation, general well-being and also my spasm, which means I can maintain a lower dosage of medication.

"The support of family and friends has been crucial in encouraging me to carry on when sometimes I am in great discomfort. Not knowing which of the conditions is the trigger to my symptoms is very frustrating and makes it harder to find a solution. I like to think I don't live with my conditions; rather my conditions live with me. I count myself as a survivor and not a sufferer. It is important that I work in partnership with all the health care professionals concerned with my well-being. I see myself at the hub of all this activity but sometimes I don't know what to do to get the answers to some of my questions. There is a wealth of information available if you know where and how to look and, importantly, can understand it. A source of understandable information, that is not frightening, is essential for patients, family and friends. There is only a small percentage of people with a spinal injury who also have syringomyelia so linking up and supporting one another helps, even if that is only possible sporadically.

"An on-going concern of mine is how the condition will change my ability to do things in the future. I feel like a pioneer as I don't know what's coming next. At the moment I just keep doing what seems to help me cope and I take 1 day at a time. I feel there is a need for more research into the correlation between the consequence of spinal cord injury, syringomyelia and decompression surgery and whether other symptoms, such as sleep apnoea and high blood pressure, are connected. The Ann Conroy Trust has gone a long way to helping individuals tell their stories, both in the magazine and on their web site together with providing support and information from professionals. Even though my condition was diagnosed and dealt with all those years ago, I am still learning from the information available, and will continue to do so."

Sue Line

18.2.2 Personal Story 2

"In 1994, after suffering significant headaches for some time, I visited my GP who referred me to a consultant physician who in turn carried out several tests, before sending me for an MR scan. This revealed that I had a Chiari I malformation. I was then referred to a neurologist and subsequently to a neurosurgeon. The neurosurgeon explained what a Chiari malformation was but felt that in my case it was not significant enough to warrant surgery. I and my family were of course concerned but took comfort in the fact that there was no immediate need for treatment. My life continued as normal but my headaches progressively worsened. I reached the point where I was unable to put my head forward and laughing, sneezing or coughing would start a major headache which could last for several hours. I was also experiencing some frightening episodes where I felt as though I was fading away. Altogether, life was becoming pretty miserable.

"I was referred once again to a neurologist who, after another MRI, explained why I was having these symptoms and suggested that I should see the neurosurgeon again. At this time there was absolutely no information available about my condition other than terrifying internet sites. I felt very alone. I had also decided that I needed to find a neurosurgeon with particular experience in carrying out any surgery which was necessary. This I did, with help from my brother. After consultation with the specialist I agreed to proceed to surgery. Indeed, by now I was anxious to have the surgery as soon as possible.

"The operation was successful and my subsequent recovery proceeded very well. Prior to surgery I had been put in touch with a syringomyelia specialist nurse and she had been able to give me some idea of how my life would be when I came out of hospital. The surgery was very beneficial in eliminating my headaches and my life soon returned to normal. I was now able to put my head down without any concern. With each month I became stronger and 6 months after my operation I was well enough to undergo further surgery for an unrelated condition. Despite this I went on to experience some severe pain in my lower back. I underwent a full spine MRI which revealed that I had a small syringomyelia cavity in the lower part of my spinal cord. This had not been evident in my original scan which had been confined to the head and upper part of my spine. However the discomfort subsided and, 11 years on, I have hardly any symptoms from my Chiari or syringomyelia.

"At the time of my diagnosis there was little information on my condition and hardly any support. With hindsight and the information that I now have, I feel I was misadvised by my original surgeon. After my operation I was invited by my neurosurgeon to join and help a charity group, now known as the Ann Conroy Trust, which was involved with helping patients with Chiari malformation and syringomyelia. This led to both my husband and I becoming increasingly involved with the running of this organisation. In addition to its other activities, the Charity provides medically approved information on these conditions, for patients and their families and carers. I assisted running the helpline for newly diagnosed sufferers, as well as those who had already undergone surgery. I would have been extremely grateful if any of these services had been available to me when I was a newly diagnosed patient.

"My hopes for the future would be that a more comprehensive support system could be set up for patients and that that there would be more nurses trained, available and prepared to speak and give practical advice to sufferers, particularly those facing surgery. I would like to see improved opportunities for the education of neurosurgeons in the management of syringomyelia and Chiari. I would like information to be more readily available to family doctors and non-specialists, so that they might be less dismissive of symptoms that they cannot immediately diagnose. Most of all I would like to see more coordinated research into these conditions and the publication of results in a more structured manner. This is why I worked for many years as a volunteer with the Ann Conroy Trust, to try and facilitate such changes."

Susan Kember

18.2.3 Personal Story 3

"I first noticed that something was not right when, on a couple of occasions, I experienced tingling and numbness on the left side of my face and in my left hand. I thought that I must be tired, working late and rushing around. I then fell down the stairs at home a couple of times. There was then an episode of numbness in my chest and arms so I went to hospital where the doctor thought it might have been a panic attack. I next went to see my family doctor and he thought it might be epilepsy. As I work as a nurse, I spoke to one of my consultants who requested an MRI scan. When the results came through he sat me down and reassured me that it was not anything sinister, which was a huge relief as I work on a cancer unit. He explained a little about Chiari malformation but then referred me to a local neurosurgeon. I informed my family doctor about developments and he commented that I was probably the only patient he would see in his professional lifetime with this condition.

"When I saw the neurosurgeon he explained that not everyone needs surgery and that sometimes symptoms remain stable and individuals can live with them. He suggested that we should try and manage my condition conservatively for the time being. Unfortunately, with time, my arm tingling became worse and I was starting to suffer severe headaches, which gave me a bit of a 'short fuse,' and I would get frustrated easily. I also began to experience panic attacks, during which I was convinced that something dreadful was going to happen.

"Many months later, having decided that I now needed surgery, I went into hospital for the operation. I was woken early on the day of the procedure. I was meant to go to theatre in the morning but an emergency delayed things so it was the afternoon when I went down. My nerves, by then, were getting the better of me; much longer and I'd have changed my mind. I spoke to my neurosurgeon and the anaesthetist in the anaesthetic room and the next thing I remember is the neurosurgeon coming into the recovery area. I tried to sit up as I thought we were still having the same conversation and did not realise straight away that I'd had the surgery. My head certainly hurt though and an injection of codeine helped for an hour at the most. Paracetamol didn't help at all. The next morning I was the first to be moved to the ordinary ward. Three days after surgery I felt well enough to go home.

"At home I tried to do too much. That night I started vomiting and this continued for 24 h. I had visitors but I couldn't keep awake to see them. I was readmitted to hospital in the early hours. I had a CT scan to check for hydrocephalus and then a lumbar puncture. The next day another patient told me that she had needed three shunts for her condition and I was frightened that the same might happen to me. My neurosurgeon then told me that my test results were fine and I could go home again. I spent the next 3 months recovering properly. Unfortunately I started getting the headaches back just before I returned to work and I began to worry that this would be the case for the rest of my life. I decided that, if this was so, I simply couldn't live with it and I actually contemplated suicide. I then returned to hospital for another lumbar puncture and, generally speaking since then, my residual symptoms have been minimal and manageable.

"I was well informed about the surgery itself although I was so desperate to have the operation done and get rid of the headaches that I didn't really listen to talk about the risks of surgery. It wasn't until I spoke to my neurosurgeon about 3 years ago that I could fully appreciate what could have happened if things had gone wrong. At the time I felt that I had enough information available to me, if I chose to access it. I had the contact number of the specialist nurse and the neurosurgeon's secretary. I had also been given a newsletter from a patient self-help group but I didn't read this until after my surgery. When I did, it was quite depressing and not very helpful. It mentioned people who had recently died and contained recipes and articles that were not relevant but no information about the condition. There was information on the internet but this was mainly from overseas sites and showed lots of gruesome pictures. I didn't choose to access any patient support group prior to my surgery but relied on the couple of visits to the neurosurgeon and specialist nurse, along with support from my family and friends, who were all very supportive during the time of the operation and thereafter.

"Nine years on, I am certain that I made the right decision. I had been keen to get the surgery over and done with and to move on with my life. The Chiari had already dominated 2 years of my life. I still have some residual symptoms such as irritability, occasional headaches, neck stiffness and poor balance but I can now smile to myself, particularly when people asked if they can 'pick my brains' about something, or when I refer to my condition as having been 'always at the back of my mind'."

Rebecca Dodwell-Pitt

18.2.4 Personal Story 4

"Looking back to when I was in my early 20s I had what I thought at the time was a one off horrendous migraine. At the time I was working as a singer and the 'migraine' followed a new dance routine, which included movements in which I bent my head forwards. The migraine left me shaky for a couple of days but I soon forgot about it, and forgot the dance routine too.

"I first experienced any real problems at the age of 33, 3 days after the birth of my daughter. She was in a Moses basket and I leant over to lift her and my head suddenly pounded and I couldn't move. I sat down and the pounding subsided. During the night I found it impossible to lift my head from the pillow and the only way I could get up was to roll out of bed. My GP called the morning after, to give the new baby a quick check over. He thought that maybe it was cervical spondylosis aggravated by the delivery. Happily, everything settled down over the next couple of weeks. I next gave birth to a son, in 1989, with no postnatal problems.

"Over the next few years I had different symptoms; tingling in my face and around my mouth, tingling in my fingers, blurred vision and a feeling that my spine pushed into my neck whenever I walked. When I visited my doctor the symptoms were put down to just one of those unexplained things. In due course I stopped reporting them.

"In 1998 I was out for the evening with friends and noticed that every time I laughed my head pounded with pain, I found myself holding the back of my neck every time. I visited my doctor and cervical spondylosis was again mentioned. Once more X-rays were unremarkable. This time, however, the symptoms didn't go away. The pounding headaches occurred almost daily, along with the tingling in my arms and fingers, I started to experience balance problems and blurred vision.

"In 1999 I was referred to rheumatologist, who diagnosed fibromyalgia. Over the next 2 years the symptoms got worse. Rheumatoid arthritis was then suspected and I was treated with steroids. Things didn't improve and in 2001 I was referred to a neurologist who thought I might have multiple sclerosis. I was again treated with steroids, as well as being given amitriptyline and tramadol for pain relief. As the symptoms were getting worse I was admitted to hospital for a lumbar puncture and an MRI scan. The good news was, 'there were no plaques on the brain' to suggest multiple sclerosis. The bad news was 'the base of my brain had come down into what should be a space above the spinal cord' but as I didn't seem to have any symptoms I could go home. I was speechless. The symptoms I was experiencing were the reason for the MRI.

"By March 2004 my neurologist seemed to have decided that I must be neurotic and all my symptoms were psychological. In the May I duly received an appointment to see a psychiatrist. This was a low point for me and for the first time I wept, mainly because I felt that I had wasted the time and money of my GP, who had always been there for me and had never doubted my symptoms were genuine. I saw him and started to apologise for wasting his time. He assured me I had not and would refer me to a multiple sclerosis specialist in London. I did, however, also see the psychiatrist and was told that I was not neurotic and that my symptoms were indeed neurological. That was a great relief but still left me no closer to a diagnosis. When I then saw the consultant in London he did not want to discuss MS but was, instead, extremely concerned about the base of my brain; 'it's jammed well down into the spinal cord with no room for CSF flow' He promised to discuss this with colleagues and get back to me. I'm still waiting.

"A friend then e-mailed me, to ask if I had a diagnosis. She knew someone with the same symptoms and gave me the name Arnold-Chiari malformation type 1. She told me to go to my GP with it. Of course I Googled it first and was confronted with the words 'a serious and complicated condition of the base of the brain and spinal cord which, if left untreated, can lead to total and permanent paralysis . I rang my GP immediately and he asked me to print out the article and get to the surgery. By the time I got there he had printed articles from the BMJ which, of course, were far less sensational. Although very scary, it was a relief, after 6 long years, to have, finally, a diagnosis. It was around this time that I found the Ann Conroy Trust, which proved to be an invaluable support during what was a frightening time for me.

"Within 2 days I was seeing a neurosurgeon, who said I needed a craniovertebral decompression. He explained that the surgery was major

and had risks but if I was willing to have the operation he would perform it. I duly had my decompression surgery, on the 1st September 2005. I woke after surgery in the intensive care unit. It was dark, thunder was banging and lightening was sparking across the sky when a man with a goatee beard leaned over me, to ask how my pain was. For a fleeting moment I thought things had gone wrong and I had been sent down to you know-where! Of course he was a nurse, asking if I needed any more pain relief. I was in hospital for 2 weeks. On discharge I had a temperature and was vomiting but it was considered that I would still be alright to go home. Thank goodness for my own doctor, who prescribed antibiotics and other strong medication.

"It soon became apparent that my symptoms hadn't resolved and, after 11 months, I saw a different neurologist who referred me to another neurosurgeon. He explained the risks of operating in the same area again so we agreed to wait and see how things went. A year later symptoms were getting worse and the pounding in the head was happening several times a day, even lifting my head when turning over during the night was enough to start the pounding. The tingling in my arms and hands was worse, as was my balance. Another MR scan revealed that scar tissue was now blocking CSF flow posteriorly and causing Valsalva-type headaches.

"Eventually I underwent revisional surgery, in February 2007. This was not without complications, including some damage to a small but important artery, which was embedded in scar tissue. I became unwell and was found to have meningitis. I was in hospital for 4 weeks.

"I now still have ongoing problems. Postoperative scar tissue is again pulling my spinal cord backwards into the area of decompression, once again blocking posterior CSF flow, although there is some space for CSF flow anteriorly. I had a number of lumbar punctures performed and these improved many of my symptoms so, eventually, I had a lumboperitoneal shunt fitted. This helped for 3 weeks but then over draining caused new problems and, 3 weeks later, the shunt was closed. I am now scheduled for surgery to have a gravity assist valve fitted to the shunt.

"Arnold Chiari 1 malformation has without a doubt changed my life. I am limited in what I am able to do. I tire easily. I can't walk far and have to use a walking stick for balance and am housebound most of the time. I can no longer do many things, such as walking in the Lake District with my husband. I was a mature student at university in 1999 but the symptoms became so bad I had to end my studies. I nevertheless maintain a positive outlook. I have become chairman of the Ann Conroy Trust and help to answer calls to the Charity's helpline, as I know only too well what a scary, lonely place the world is, after the diagnosis of Chiari malformation."

Lynn Burton

18.3   Learning from Patients

These accounts illustrate clearly the experiences and emotions that accompanied four different patient journeys (Table 18.1). After the initial onset of symptoms, any individual will normally wait a while, anticipating that they will settle down before very long. When they continue, a visit is made to the family doctor who will certainly not make an initial diagnosis of syringomyelia or Chiari. When symptoms persist a referral will likely follow, to a hospital specialist, for further assessment. Not infrequently this leads to MR imaging and the diagnosis is made. Sometimes, however, diagnoses such as fibromyalgia may delay the true cause being revealed. The patient may then have to endure worsening symptoms, which fail to respond to various treatment regimes. The delay in the correct diagnosis being made is a common source of complaint from both syringomyelia and Chiari patients, but this is, of course, to be expected, with such uncommon ailments.

With the eventual diagnosis comes a combination of relief and further anxieties. Numerous new questions arise and answers are not always forthcoming. It is at this stage that the hospital specialist has a vital role to play, in gaining the patients confidence and trust. Unless and until the individual is adequately informed about their condition, he or she will not be able to make a rational decision about the most appropriate course of treatment to follow. Surgical intervention for uncomplicated Chiari is seldom essential and even the presence of an associated syrinx does not necessarily make an operation mandatory. The patient needs time to come to terms with matters, with careful explanation and guidance from the specialist. If an operation is the chosen route then the surgeon must give clear information about the procedure.

A frequent concern amongst patients and carers is the lack of general support available to them. Often, before deciding to submit to surgery, the patient may look to a fellow sufferer for some counsel. An increase in social networking sites and mobile communication technology has meant that patients can do this online. Small local support groups may also be set up, and these certainly have a role to play, provided that they are well run and do not become a forum for propagating complaints and negative attitudes. Running a support group is, however, not an easy task. Quite apart from the time commitment and the need to be available as often as possible, the volunteer has to develop counselling skills, often without the benefit of any formal training. For the caller, however, the opportunity to talk, at last, to somebody who seems to understand what they are going through, is a great relief.

Table 18.1 Common experiences

Worry and uncertainty prior to diagnosis
Delays in diagnosis
Relief and new worries when diagnosis is made
Alarm about proposed brain surgery
Value of talking to other patients
Dependence upon family and friends for support
Value of patient information material
Positive and negative impact of websites and support groups
The need to have confidence in the neurosurgeon
Fear of possible complications of surgery
Post-operative discomforts and the experience of ITU care
Relief when symptoms improve
Concerns when symptoms return
Coming to terms with residual symptoms
A wish to help fellow sufferers

Table 18.2 Common concerns

Gaining access to specialists with sufficient expertise
Adequate time for concerns to be heard by clinicians
To be believed and not treated as being neurotic
Knowing which symptoms do and which do not arise from the condition
Lack of readily available information, for patient, about the conditions
Lack of educational material for family practitioners
Access to professional, informed counselling
Fear of being isolated
Fear of progression to severe disability or death
Special needs of children as patients

Different callers have individual needs, of course, but there a number of common themes (Table 18.2). Gaining access to specialists with sufficient expertise and experience in treating syringomyelia and Chiari is a common concern amongst patients. Many will be seen initially by their local neurology or neurosurgery service, and not all units will have an individual with a special interest in managing these conditions. The initial consultation may very well leave the patient confused and frightened, particularly if the prospect of brain or spinal cord surgery is raised at the outset. Patients commonly resort to the Internet to gain some further understanding about these conditions with the strange-sounding names. All too often this "research" adds to the patient's fears, raising the spectre of progressive, painful deterioration, to a state of physical helplessness. Patients, therefore, should be guided by their own professional health-care advisors and use information from other sources simply as a means of better understanding what their medical advisors say to them. The patient desperately needs to be listened to and to know that the specialist understands something about the problem and what the patient is going through. The patient wants to know which symptoms are likely to be caused by the Chiari or the syrinx and which are not. Is there a risk of coming to serious harm? What other treatment options are available? He or she then needs time to consider matters and to read an intelligible, lay account which does not over-dramatise matters. The patient will probably then come back with further questions and may well ask if there is a fellow sufferer to whom he or she can talk. Above all the patient wants to be believed and not left feeling that the doctors regard him or her as suffering primarily from stress.

Another common complaint amongst patients is that there is also a lack of information available for health-care professionals who are not specialists in this field. Most patients report that their family doctor has little or no awareness of syringomyelia and Chiari, but this, of course, is largely due to the low number of patients that they will see in their professional lifetime. Some patients ask if charities could distribute information to all family practices, but, clearly, these would probably just sit on a shelf, and if a patient did present with syringomyelia or Chiari, the leaflet would probably have been misplaced by then or simply be overlooked. A more effective answer would be the provision of Web-based information for non-specialist medical practitioners. It is probably not helpful for patients to visit their doctor with a large amount of information downloaded from the Internet as the doctor will almost certainly not find time to read it.

When it comes to surgery, as a proposed treatment, the patient must be told, in a clear but sympathetic way, just what is involved and what are the likely benefits and also what could go wrong, as well as what might happen if the condition were left untreated. Volunteer counsellors receive, from time to time, calls from people who have not done well after surgery. They say that they would not have undergone the operation had they known what was going to happen. Lay advisors cannot, of course, give opinions on matters of medical detail. They will certainly not suggest whether or not the caller should undergo surgery. The patient must always question the surgeon before any operation and be quite satisfied about the risks as well as the benefits of the procedure. These may prove to be, quite literally, vital issues. There will, of course, be other, less critical questions but which are, nevertheless, important for the patient to have answered (Table 18.3).

Even after a successful operation it is unlikely that the patient will be able to put matters to rest

Table 18.3 Frequently asked questions

| Where will I have the surgery? |
| How long will I be in hospital? |
| How long will I be in the operating theatre? |
| What size wound will I have and what stitches will I have? |
| How much hair will I lose? |
| When can I wash my hair? |
| How long will in need to take off work/college? |
| What is the total recovery period? |
| Will I be able to fly? |
| Will I be able to drive? |
| What follow-up will I receive? |
| Will my headaches/other pains improve? |
| Will my hindbrain hernia ever return? |
| Will my syringomyelia resolve? |
| Could my syringomyelia refill at a later date? |
| What happens if I have problems in the future? |

completely. Persistence of some symptoms and recurrence of others will generate fears that the condition may recur. Anticipation of further pain and discomfort can sometimes be as distressing as the symptoms themselves. Here, once again, patient support groups can play a useful role. Surgeons vary in their approach to management at this stage, some simply stating that there is no more role for surgery. Others become more involved in exploring alternative avenues for providing the patient with some relief from their continuing suffering. There are several support groups and sources of information worldwide, and some of the more well-established groups are listed in Chap. 22.

Finally, many patients express concern about the apparent lack of any research being carried out into syringomyelia and Chiari. It is clear that a better coordinated approach to research, internationally, is needed.

Further Reading

Batzdorf U (2011) Chiari malformation and syringomyelia: a handbook for patients and their families. Lulu.com

D'Alonzo R (2010) Contents under pressure: one man's triumph over chiari syndrome. Lulu.com

Flint G, Dakin AC (2006) Syringomyelia hindbrain hernia (Chiari malformation): an explanation for patients, relatives and carers. The Ann Conroy Trust Hornsea

Hewitt J, Gabata M (2011) Chiari malformation: causes, tests, and treatments. Creatspace.com

Labuda R (2008) Conquer Chiari: a patient's guide to the Chiari malformation. Creatspace.com

Oro JJ, Mueller D (2007) The Chiari book: a guide for patients, families, and health care providers. Creatspace.com

Medicolegal Aspects

19

Sid Marks and Graham Flint

Contents

S. Marks
Department of Neurosurgery,
James Cook University Hospital,
Middlesbrough, England, UK
e-mail: sid.marks@stees.nhs.uk

G. Flint (✉)
Department of Neurosurgery,
Queen Elizabeth Hospital,
University Hospitals Birmingham,
Birmingham, UK
e-mail: graham.flint@uhb.nhs.uk

19.1 Introduction

Medicolegal aspects of Chiari malformation and syringomyelia can be considered in three main sections. The first is personal injury claims, the second is medical negligence, and the third relates to an individual's inability to work whilst suffering from symptoms caused by these conditions.

19.2 Personal Injury

In this section we consider the relationship between Chiari malformation and syringomyelia and whiplash injuries or other minor trauma to the neck. A second, particularly important aspect of personal injury is that of post-traumatic syringomyelia, which occurs following major spinal injury.

19.2.1 General Considerations

In advising patients over such matters, the medical expert should be completely honest and not encourage claims that are or will prove untenable, if tested in court. Nor should the expert try to maximise or minimise the chances of a claim succeeding, according to whichever side in the legal contest instructed that medical witness. In an adversarial system of justice, the latter role falls to the lawyers. Under current English law, the expert is required to provide a report for the

G. Flint, C. Rusbridge (eds.), *Syringomyelia*,
DOI 10.1007/978-3-642-13706-8_19, © Crown Copyright 2014

court, not for one side or the other, even though he or she will usually have been instructed by one side. The expert has to sign a declaration to this effect, in order to comply with court rules.

With compensation claims in English civil law, the test applied is "on the balance of probabilities". This contrasts with criminal law where the test is "beyond reasonable doubt". A specialist experienced in the treatment of syringomyelia may reasonably state that, in his or her opinion, such and such is the case, "on the balance of probabilities". In English law, this means a likelihood of 51 % or greater. The medical expert's opinion does not have to be backed by scientific data. Indeed, it is seldom possible to locate such evidence, in response to the many questions posed by lawyers. This does not mean, however, that the expert witness can ignore scientific evidence and he or she should endeavour to back up any opinions with evidence from the medical literature, whenever possible. Otherwise, he or she should present some logical reasoning to underpin the opinion offered.

Clearly, personal injury claims may be subject to exaggeration and sometimes outright fraud, but when it comes to conditions like posttraumatic syringomyelia, the plight and needs of the patient are very real. In these circumstances, the medical expert is often asked not to advise on causation but on matters of quantum. This latter concept involves issues such as prognosis and how dependent the patient is likely to become in the future, as a result of the injuries. In addition, on occasions, patients may be granted the right to return to court one more time, at a future date, to claim further compensation for delayed effects of an earlier injury. Whilst not encouraged by judges, who generally prefer to finalise claims coming before a court whenever possible, such "provisional damages" may be very appropriate in the case of a spinal cord injury victim, who may develop posttraumatic syringomyelia many years later. The right to claim provisional damages must be specifically reserved in the court order, at the time a case is settled. It also has to be related to the future occurrence of a specified risk, such as syringomyelia, or any surgery required for its treatment. The risk can be expressed as either for life or for a limited period, depending upon the experts supporting opinion. To maintain a further claim for provisional damages, the patient has to "develop some serious disease or suffer some serious deterioration in his or her physical or mental condition" (Supreme Court Act 1981; County Courts Act 1984). Therefore, consideration needs to be given, by the experts and the lawyers, as to whether the deterioration is sufficiently serious to satisfy these criteria and justify a further award. In reality, this is likely to be governed by the need for additional care and other support arising from the deterioration. An expert will therefore need to consider and advise whether there is any further risk of a more serious secondary deterioration in the future. This will be particularly relevant to younger patients with a long life expectancy ahead of them. Hitherto, reactivation of cases of spinal cord injury has been uncommon but may take place more often in future, as many patients with spinal cord damage are now living to a good age. It is important to understand that a person has only "one bite of the cherry"; in other words he/she can only claim provisional damages once.

19.2.2 Hindbrain Hernias

A Chiari malformation is essentially a developmental anatomical abnormality and is not caused by trauma in later life. The clinical features that develop are largely a result of abnormalities of cerebrospinal fluid flow rather than being simply related to the displacement of the tonsils into the upper cervical spinal canal. In considering what might be regarded as the usual, constitutional presentation of a Chiari malformation, it can reasonably be stated that the mean onset of symptoms is the fourth decade of life. Notwithstanding this "natural" presentation of hindbrain hernias, one major study revealed that approximately 25 % of patients with Chiari give a history of the onset of their symptoms being precipitated by some form of physical injury (Milhorat et al. 1999).

Constitutional presentation of symptoms within the fourth decade has medicolegal implications. Consider a patient who is in his or her fifth decade and who becomes symptomatic for the first time, after an accident. It could reasonably be argued that since that individual has already passed beyond the mean age for onset of symptoms, then, more likely than not, he or she would not have developed Chiari symptoms, had not the accident occurred. On the balance of probabilities, therefore, the accident was the cause of the onset of the symptoms. In contrast, consider a patient in her middle 20s, who develops symptoms consistent with a Chiari malformation, following an episode of trauma. It would be fair to reason that, had the accident not occurred, there was a greater than evens chance that the hindbrain hernia would have become symptomatic before too long anyway. At the same time, it would be justifiable to propose that the trauma had accelerated the appearance of symptoms. Further, in this example, it would be logical to suggest that the onset of symptoms was brought forward by approximately 10 years, this being the difference between the patient's age and the accepted average age of onset of hindbrain hernia symptoms. This might be seen as a relatively arbitrary estimate, without much of an evidence base, but in the absence of better data, it may be accepted by the courts as reasonable guidance. Applying the legal test of the balance of probability, the client in this case would, more likely than not, have become symptomatic by approximately her middle 30s. An acceleration of onset of symptoms of 10 years then becomes a workable legal tool in order to consider compensation.

The presentation of clinical symptoms following a traumatic episode then raises the question of the mechanism involved. In a medicolegal debate, an expert on "the other side" might challenge the above reasoning by enquiring as to the exact mechanism by which the injury in question might have rendered the hindbrain hernia symptomatic. There are, of course, many people who have a Chiari malformation but who do not have any symptoms. A significant degree of whiplash injury could, in such individuals, result in further impaction of the cerebellar tonsils at the foramen magnum. This in turn might create, for the first time in that individual, a degree of obstruction to cerebrospinal fluid (CSF) flow at the craniovertebral junction, generating the headaches that are so typical of a Chiari malformation. In addition, hyperextension of the neck, in the presence of herniated cerebellar tonsils, could easily result in a degree of contusion of the cervicomedullary junction, accounting for the onset of various somatic sensory disturbances.

19.2.3 Syringomyelia

The onset of symptoms attributable to a syringomyelia cavity, which is diagnosed for the first time after trauma, also raises a number of questions. Could post-traumatic impaction of a hindbrain hernia have led to the development of a syrinx, or is it more likely that any such cavity was present all along, albeit asymptomatic? If the latter was the case, then was the development of symptoms the result of associated musculoskeletal injury and not related to an incidental syrinx? In advising on such matters, the medicolegal expert should consider carefully the nature of the patient's symptoms and note any physical signs and decide whether these are more typical of syringomyelia or of musculoskeletal injury. An example is provided by the case of a young female in her 30s, who developed cervical radiculopathy involving multiple nerve roots, following an episode of trauma that involved a whiplash mechanism of injury. She had been completely asymptomatic beforehand. An MRI scan of the neck, performed within a week of the injury, demonstrated what appeared to be a significant syrinx within the cervical cord. There was no associated Chiari malformation or obvious injury to the vertebral column nor evidence of any previous significant injury. Over a few weeks, the clinical symptoms resolved, and repeat MRI scan then showed that the syrinx had collapsed. Further imaging, some time later, confirmed that the cavity remained collapsed, at which stage the patient remained asymptomatic. The question, from a medicolegal point of view, was whether the syrinx was pre-existing and asymptomatic but rendered symptomatic by the trauma or whether, after all, it formed rapidly after the injury, only to collapse spontaneously, by some ill-defined mechanism. There is also the question of whether or not it might refill at some time in the future and then cause problems again.

19.2.4 Post-traumatic Syringomyelia

Post-traumatic syringomyelia is dealt with in more detail in Chap. 11. Whereas syringomyelia is a relatively rare condition in the community as a whole, it is very common in the population of spinal cord injury victims. Importantly, it has the capacity to add significantly to the disabilities that the victim already has, as a result of the original injury.

From a medicolegal point of view, the development of a true post-traumatic syringomyelia[1] is a direct result of the original spinal trauma. It therefore has a causal link with the original trauma. It is most commonly seen following major spinal trauma, in which there is both disruption of the spinal column and, usually, significant spinal cord injury. Its development is suspected when one sees ascending neurological deficit at an interval following spinal cord injury. Symptoms can develop within months of the trauma, but, more often, post-traumatic syringomyelia becomes manifest after an interval of several years. A post-traumatic syringomyelia cavity is classically defined as arising from the level of the lesion and ascending but, in practice, both ascending and descending cavities are seen. When such lesions are followed by serial imaging, they commonly remain unchanged and do not propagate further, in a cephalad or a caudal direction.

The causative mechanism of posttraumatic syringomyelia is a block to the passage of the CSF through the spinal subarachnoid channels. This is usually due to the formation of scar tissue, from blood products shed into the spinal theca at the time of the original injury. Once the obstruction is defined and dealt with at surgery, the syrinx

usually collapses quite rapidly. Unfortunately, there is then the risk of recurrent scar tissue formation, as the surgical wound heals, resulting in a recurrent blockage and refilling of the syringomyelia cavity.

19.2.5 Other Cystic Intramedullary Lesions

Not infrequently one encounters, on an MRI scan, a fairly localised, elliptical, cystic area within the spinal cord, extending over just a few segments (Fig. 19.1). Typically such lesions are seen in the cervical cord, commonly around C5–C7 but also at other levels, including C2. Neuroradiologists usually describe these appearances as a localised syrinx, but individual surgeons may use their own terms, such as "clefts" or "spindles", to describe the appearance of these entities, in particular their

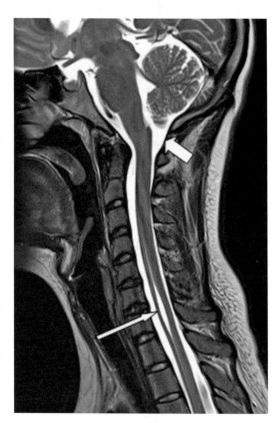

Fig. 19.1 MR image of a "cleft" or "spindle". This T2-weighted midline sagittal MRI of the cervical spine shows a typical cleft (*long arrow*) behind the body of C7. The craniovertebral junction is normal (*short arrow*)

---

[1] True post-traumatic syringomyelia cavities should be distinguished from primary post-traumatic cysts. The latter are confined to the level of the original injury, whereas the former propagate beyond this level.

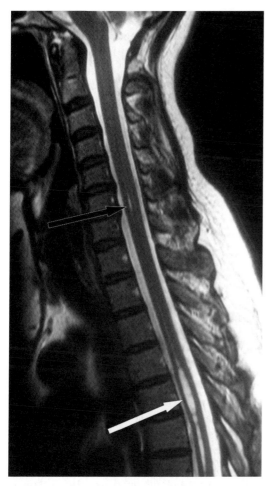

Fig. 19.2 MR image of a focal dilatation of the central canal. This T2-weighted midline sagittal MRI of the cervical and upper thoracic spine shows a short, persisting segment of the central canal behind C6 (*dark arrow*) but a much more prominent dilatation of the central canal in the upper thoracic cord, extending over several segments from T5 downwards (*white arrow*). The craniovertebral junction is normal

tapered ends. A similar type of lesion consists of focal dilatation of the central canal, often seen in the thoracic cord. These cavities usually extend over several segments of the cord (Fig. 19.2). Some authorities apply the term hydromyelia to these entities, regarding them as separate from other forms of syringomyelia. Such appearances need to be distinguished from simple persistence of the embryonic central canal, which takes the form of thin, CSF-filled cavities, often seen as skip lesions. These are not pathological entities.

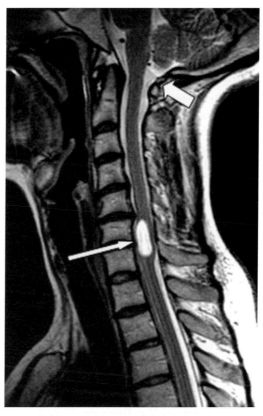

Fig. 19.3 MR image of a probable glioependymal cyst. This T2-weighted midline sagittal MRI of the cervical spine reveals a short, "plump", CSF-filled cavity within the spinal cord (*long arrow*). The craniovertebral junction is normal (*short arrow*). The disc protrusion at the upper aspect of this lesion is unlikely to be related, and this appearance most likely represents that of a glioependymal cyst, although contrasted images are needed to exclude an underlying neoplasm

Another type of intramedullary cavity, which also extends over just a few segments of the cord, has a more rounded appearance (Fig. 19.3). Some authorities regard these lesions as being glioependymal cysts and distinct from syringomyelia (Saito et al. 2005). Exploring such a lesion will simply confirm that the appearance of the contained fluid is that of normal CSF, within otherwise normal cord tissue. Biopsy of the lining will reveal the presence of normal ependymal cells.

Whether or not these various lesions are separate conditions or part of the overall spectrum of syringomyelia, they all pose the same question as to just why they exist in the first place and why they fill with cerebrospinal fluid – or at least a fluid with similar characteristics to CSF.

From the medicolegal perspective, the question arises as to whether clefts, spindles or focal dilatations of the central canal, when detected, should be regarded as incidental findings or whether they could be generating the patient's symptoms and whether, indeed, they could have arisen as a result of an accident in question. Many experts will declare that spinal cord clefts or spindles are not caused by or related to trauma, but others may find it difficult to disregard the existence of a relatively rare lesion, in the presence of neurological symptoms, whose onset bears a close temporal relationship to the accident in question. On the other hand, the type of symptoms as may be encountered in such cases is often equally consistent with a radiculopathy in the arms. This provides an alternative explanation that the much more common degenerative disc disease, which was previously silent, has been rendered symptomatic by the injury in question.

19.3　Medical Negligence

The purpose of this section is not to advise patents and lawyers when to take legal action over surgery, which has proven unsuccessful or led to complications. Nor is it to tell surgeons how to avoid becoming involved in litigation. Instead, we wish to highlight some of the commonly recognised complications of syringomyelia surgery, so that patients can be more fully informed, by the surgeon, before they agree to undergo an operation. It is also hoped that the surgeon might be better prepared to avoid some complications and to deal more effectively with those that do arise. The section considers, for the most part, unwanted outcomes following surgery, rather than errors in diagnosis.

In the United Kingdom, medical practitioners are regulated by the General Medical Council, and their guidance booklet "Good Medical Practice" underpins all professional activity (General Medical Council 2013). In addition, there are numerous standards, protocols and guidelines, published by various national and international bodies (Clinical Standards Committee of the Society of British Neurological Surgeons 2002; National Institute for Health and Clinical Excellence 2012; World Health Organization 2009). Any of these publications may be referred to in assessing a surgeon's standard of practice in an individual case.

The specialist preparing reports in cases of alleged medical negligence should not set out to find fault with a colleague. A philosophy of "there but for the grace of God go I" will allow the author of the report to adopt an approach which is sympathetic to the colleague and which, thereby, will lead to more ready acceptance of any just criticisms which do have to be made. This will act, ultimately, for the benefit of the patient.

A landmark ruling in English law was that of Lord Denning, in the case of Jordan vs Whitehouse (Robertson 1981). This states that an "error of judgement is not the same as negligence". The UK House of Lords subsequently modified this to "error of judgement is not necessarily the same as negligence". An earlier, influential ruling led to what is known as the Bolam test (Bolam vs Friern Hospital Management Committee 1957). This states that a given line of medical management may be judged acceptable if it is followed (contemporaneously) by "a reasonable body of practitioners". A reasonable body can still be a minority. Even so, a later House of Lords decision ruled that any such management still needed to withstand logical analysis. This is known as the Bolitho test (Bolitho vs City and Hackney Health Authority 1997).

19.3.1　Patient Frustrations and Medical Uncertainties

The optimum management of any neurosurgical condition includes both making the correct diagnosis and administering appropriate treatment. The finding, on an MRI scan, of a Chiari malformation, syringomyelia or both can cause psychological distress to the patient, in addition to the somatic symptoms that have already developed. Frustration and anger can arise, as a result of delays in diagnosis and differing opinions as regards management, offered by various clinicians the patient may have seen.

The detection of a Chiari malformation by no means always leads to surgical intervention. This is particularly the case with a patient who undergoes an MRI scan for some other purpose, and this shows the presence of herniated cerebellar tonsils. The borderline Chiari malformation is another example, where the tonsils protrude just a few millimetres below the rim of the foramen magnum and are not causing an obvious interruption of the CSF flow. In such cases the expectation of the patient is often directly influenced by the opinion expressed by the original advising clinician, who may be a primary care practitioner, a general physician, a neurologist or a neurosurgeon. In addition, many patients arm themselves with information and opinions from the internet, although such material can often, for a patient, be very misleading, confusing and frightening.

Troublesome pressure dissociation headaches,[2] in the presence of a well-formed hindbrain hernia, leave little doubt as to the potential role for surgery. The presence of an associated syrinx cavity adds further weight to the case for operative intervention. Sometimes, however, MRI scanning reveals what appears to be a significant Chiari malformation, but the presenting symptoms are not consistent with this diagnosis and headache may not even be a feature. Vague vestibular symptoms, somatic sensory disturbances and feelings of lethargy or fatigue are common enough in Chiari patients, but occurring in isolation from more clearly diagnostic symptoms, they leave some doubt as to their relevance to the anatomical abnormality. The neurosurgeon should consider the role of surgery in such cases with great care.

In medicolegal practice, one encounters, not uncommonly, a patient who has been told that he or she has a condition that requires urgent surgery. This can cause emotional distress to the individual, who may feel that much time has already been wasted, delaying essential surgery. In truth, surgery for hindbrain hernia is seldom urgent, may not be necessary at all and always carries the risk of producing complications. There are many cases that can be treated conservatively, by observation and monitoring, rather than by proceeding immediately to surgery. The natural history of Chiari and syringomyelia is difficult to predict in an individual patient, and many cases of a mild or borderline Chiari malformation can be monitored for a number of years and never become symptomatic. Indeed, even people with an anatomically significant Chiari malformation can remain permanently asymptomatic. Except, therefore, in the cases of a very gross Chiari malformation, with progressive and deteriorating brainstem symptoms and signs, surgery should not normally be pronounced as being essential and seldom be seen as being required urgently.

19.3.2 Choice of Surgical Procedure

There are various types of surgery for Chiari malformations, with or without an associated syrinx. All are currently considered as being within acceptable practice (Table 19.1). As with many neurosurgical procedures, we do not have the evidence base to declare one method superior to

Table 19.1 Variations on the method of craniovertebral decompression

Stage 1. Decompression
Bony decompression alone
Foramen magnum only
Foramen magnum + posterior arch of C1
Bony decompression + dural slits
Bone decompression, dural opening + preservation of arachnoid
Dural opening and reduction of cerebellar tonsils
Stage 2. Repair
Muscle closure, leaving dura open
Duraplasty
Duraplasty and cranioplasty

---

[2] Headaches brought on by coughing, straining or bending forwards. The normal movement of cerebrospinal fluid, between the head and the spinal canal, is impeded by the herniated cerebellar tonsils. The resultant valve effect leads to transient rises in the intracranial pressure, generating short-lived but severe headaches.

another, and there are advantages and disadvantages to each approach. The surgeon should, however, be able to justify why he or she has a preference for a particular method. It is also fair to say that a surgeon may adopt a different method in differing circumstances, particularly in relation to the extent of any tonsillar herniation and whether or not these structures are reduced surgically. From the legal perspective, the surgeon should justify and record why there is a preference for a particular operation. He or she may be asked to provide justification for any decision made, several years after the primary consultation.

19.3.3 Consent

Most operations for hindbrain hernia and syringomyelia amount to major brain or spinal surgery and, as such, can never be carried out without risk of serious and potentially catastrophic complications. Consent for such procedures must therefore be fully informed. The nature of the operation and what is involved should be explained in full. The risks attendant upon the procedure, as well as the benefits that should be gained, must be emphasised. Alternative methods of treatment should be identified, and the natural history of the condition, left untreated, should be explained. All of this should be put to the patient in simple language and multiple consultations may be required. Explanatory literature or well-structured and responsibly constructed websites may provide the patient with helpful background explanatory material (see Chap. 18, "Further Reading" and Chap. 24, Useful Contacts). The patient should understand, however, that such material can only serve to help them understand what their medical advisors are saying. Any decision that the patient makes, regarding surgical treatment or otherwise, must be based on discussions with their own neurosurgeon. Websites or support organisations who offer advice to patients should always make this point clear and avoid making any statements that could influence a patient's decision about which treatment to accept.

Once again, the surgeon should justify and record the advice given, to avoid future misunderstandings with a patient. Cogent contemporaneous records are very credible and usually accepted as such by the courts.

19.3.4 Post-operative Complications

Given that it is impossible to predict all complications that may follow an operation, including surgery for Chiari and syringomyelia, a more reasonable approach is to draw the patient's attention to all serious or frequently occurring complications. A broad approach may be simply to specify death and serious physical or mental disability, plus failure of the procedure to achieve its aims.

Some of the more frequently encountered complications of craniovertebral decompression are listed in Table 19.2. Sterile meningitis is a well-documented complication, and it is exactly as the name implies. The patient develops a meningitic illness, but there is no infection. The only treatment, besides expectant management, is with steroids, but these should be prescribed for a limited period only and are best reserved for the more severe cases. Aseptic meningitis can, however, only be diagnosed with confidence once CSF infection is shown not to exist. If bacterial meningitis has developed, it must be recognised promptly and treated appropriately.

It might be argued that aseptic meningitis is an inevitable consequence of a craniovertebral decompression, if the arachnoid is opened. The resultant meningeal inflammation will certainly lead to a degree of raised CSF pressure, which may be sufficient, on occasions, to cause CSF

Table 19.2 Complications of craniovertebral decompression

Posterior fossa haematoma
Supratentorial subdural haematoma
Pneumocephalus
Hydrocephalus
CSF leak
Chemical (aseptic) meningitis
Bacterial meningitis
Dorsal column sensory losses
Cerebellar infarcts

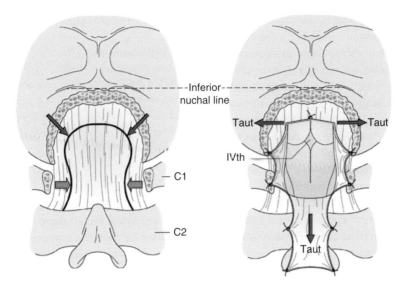

Fig. 19.4 A method of dural opening. One of us (GF) employs this method of dural opening routinely. Rather than using the conventional "Y"-shaped dural opening, the membrane is opened as an inverted "U", creating a "tongue-shaped" flap, which is then sewn down, taut, over the C2 spinous process. The dura is then hitched laterally across the craniovertebral junction, opening up the CSF channels laterally and pulling the posterior fossa dura across, taut, superiorly. The tonsils are then reduced with bipolar coagulation and, if necessary, hitched laterally with fine silk. This method allows the fourth ventricle to open into a newly created artificial cisterna magna, which itself communicates freely with the spinal CSF channels and the basal cisterns. It also provides good support for the cerebellum, irrespective of the amount of bone that has been removed, although this should normally be kept below the inferior nuchal line

leakage through the surgical wound. Such leakage should not, therefore, be regarded as the result of poor technique. On the other hand, it should be recognised and treated promptly. Hydrocephalus needs to be excluded first and then treated, if present. If the ventricular size is normal, then a simple reinforcing suture may stop the CSF leak, although temporary lumbar drainage of CSF may be needed or, indeed, preferred. In other circumstances, even when a CSF leak is not present, a post-operative lumbar puncture may be beneficial, in treating aseptic meningitis. It will lower intracranial pressure, encourage flow of cerebrospinal fluid across the craniovertebral junction and drain off blood-stained CSF, all of which may lessen the discomforts resulting from chemical meningitis.

A much discussed complication of craniovertebral decompression, albeit quite uncommon, is cerebellar slumping. If too much of the posterior fossa bone is removed, there is a risk that the cerebellum may descend, or slump, into the resultant bony defect. This could lead to recurrent obstruction to CSF flow across the craniovertebral junction. Sometimes it may be difficult to avoid removing a fair amount of bone, particularly in cases of basilar invagination. Opening the dura as an inverted "U", rather than using the more usual "Y"-shaped incision, may reduce the likelihood of this complication, even when bony removal has been quite extensive (Fig. 19.4).

19.3.5 Surgical Results

Success rates following surgery for uncomplicated Chiari malformations should be good in experienced hands, particularly as regards relief of pressure dissociation headaches and causing a syrinx cavity to collapse. In some circumstances, however, one should warn of a likely lower success rate. With some Chiari malformations, one may encounter, at surgery, significant arachnoid adhesions. In other cases it is posthaemorrhagic or post-inflammatory scar tissue, rather than tonsillar herniation, which accounts for the obstruction to CSF flow across the craniovertebral junction. Scar tissue is always likely to be present in revisional operations and will result in a more serious block developing than that which existed originally and may even lead to the development of syringomyelia that was not present prior to the operative procedure. In all these situations, it may prove difficult to establish adequate CSF flow across the craniovertebral junction, and the likelihood of success is reduced at the outset. Importantly, the risk of damage to vital structures is also increased in these cases. These restrictions apply even in experienced hands and despite all care being taken. The patient should always be warned of these matters, and these warnings should be recorded in the medical records.

19.4 Employers, Social Services and Other Statutory Bodies

Any specialist may be asked to provide a report, for various government or other agencies, relating to a patient under his or her care (Table 19.3). The doctor preparing the report must, however, avoid conflicts of interest. In particular, if the report could act to the patient's detriment, then the professional relationship between the doctor and patient might be compromised. Equally, fear of such compromise, or even just sympathy for the patient, may prevent the doctor from providing an entirely honest and objective report. It is best, in such instances, for the doctor to provide factual details, which could not be disputed. Reports prepared from medical records will, in any case, often be limited in their scope, simply because entries will not usually have been made with the

Table 19.3 Agencies requesting reports

Employers
Social security and benefits agencies
Driving licensing authorities
Pension mangers
Insurance companies
Charitable support organisations

Table 19.4 Common questions in insurance or employment reports

Name of the condition
When the diagnosis was made
Date when patient first noticed symptoms
Results of any investigations
Relationship of pathology to index injury
Details of any planned treatment
Disabilities and impairments
Prognosis

later production of medical reports in mind. It is usually only possible, in these circumstances, to summarise the patient's main symptoms and the resultant physical disabilities and functional impairments, as reported by the patient (Table 19.4). To make a more detailed assessment, the medical expert will need to interview and examine the patient, and it might even be better, in such circumstances, for the clinician to suggest that an independent assessment be sought.

An independent assessor will certainly need to identify and quantify the individual's disabilities and limitations, for which consultation with the patient is required. It is important to assess the past medical history and to scrutinise all available medical records, to distinguish problems caused by the syringomyelia from those which might have arisen from more common conditions, such as intervertebral disc disease. It is important to try and distinguish organic symptoms from those caused by psychological overlay. Equally, it would be unfair to the patient to say or imply that symptoms have a psychological basis, when they might well be genuine manifestations of syringomyelia.

Conclusions

Preparation of meaningful medicolegal reports is time-consuming and requires a good deal of thought and consideration, beyond just the reading of large volumes of documents. It is not an activity that appeals to all clinicians, but those who engage in this sort of work need to adopt an organised approach. Lawyers will often ask very specific questions at the outset. On other occasions, the initial instructions may be worded in a more general way, in which case

Table 19.5 Common questions in personal injury claims

Was the lesion caused by the injury in question?

By what mechanism did the injury cause the lesion to develop?

Was the pathology pre-existing but asymptomatic?

Did the injury render the lesion symptomatic?

Had the injury not occurred, would it have remained asymptomatic?

Was the pathology pre-existing and symptomatic but aggravated by the trauma?

By what interval was the onset of symptoms brought forward?

To what extent is the lesion responsible for the symptoms?

What is the prognosis?

Will any further treatment assist the patient?

Table 19.6 Common questions in medical negligence claims

Was the surgery properly indicated?

Why in this case was surgery considered and offered?

Was the patient adequately informed, prior to surgery, about:

    The nature of the procedure

    The intended benefits

    The attendant risks

    Alternative treatments

    The natural history of the condition if left untreated

Has the patient come to harm as a result of the surgery?

    Symptoms, including pain and suffering

    Physical impairments

    Resultant handicaps and effects upon

        Activities of daily living

        Social life

        Employment

What is the likely prognosis?

Could any further treatment be of benefit?

Table 19.7 Suggested structure of a full medicolegal report

A front page with headings noting the client's demographic details

The remit of the report

Instructing solicitors/agency

That the report is prepared for the court

Authors qualifications and experience

Basis of report – interviews, examinations and documents

Interview and examination of patient (usually stated within a preamble following the front page)

Review of medical records

Summary and opinion of medical history stating final opinion of author

    Statement 1: followed by explanation

    Statement 2: followed by explanation

    … etc.

Range of opinions offered by other experts

Conclusion

Declaration[a]

References

Appendix: Lay explanation of syringomyelia/Chiari

[a]English courts currently require an expert witness to declare that he or she understands his or her duties to the court, in preparing the report. It is, in effect, the equivalent of taking an oath when giving oral evidence in court

the expert may choose to address certain predictable questions, which might follow (Tables 19.5 and 19.6). A well-structured template, for composing reports, is invaluable. Indeed many law firms will provide a structure of their own, for the expert witness to follow. Table 19.7 gives a list of suggested headings for the preparation of medicolegal reports. Expert witnesses should be prepared to cite references, particularly when making a point that might be challenged by a medical advisor for the other side. Equally important, if not more so, is the need to make clear, to lawyers, their clients and the courts, some of the anatomical, physiological and other medical concepts that surround the diagnosis and treatment of syringomyelia and Chiari. Technical jargon should be replaced by lay terminology, and the use of lay explanations, as appendices to a report, may be of great value to the courts. A glossary of terms is usually appreciated by lawyers and impresses judges, most of whom, understandably, have limited or no understanding of syringomyelia.

References

Bolam versus Friern Hospital Management Committee (1957) 1 WLR 582

Bolitho versus City and Hackney Health Authority (1997) 3 WLR 1151

Clinical Standards Committee of the Society of British Neurological Surgeons, Standards for Patients Requiring Neurosurgical Care (2002) Society of British Neurological Surgeons

County Courts Act (1984) Section 51

General Medical Council (2013) Good medical practice. General Medical Council. www.gmc-uk.org/guidance/good_medical_practice.asp

Milhorat TH, Chou MW, Trinidad EM et al (1999) Chiari I malformation redefined: clinical and radiographic findings for 364 symptomatic patients. Neurosurgery 44(5):1005–1017

National Institute for Health and Clinical Excellence, Quality Standards. http://www.nice.org.uk/aboutnice/qualitystandards/qualitystandards.jsp. Accessed Dec 2012

Robertson G (1981) Whitehouse v Jordan – medical negligence retried. Mod Law Rev 44(4):457–461

Saito K, Morita A, Shibahara J et al (2005) Spinal intra-medullary ependymal cyst: a case report and review of the literature. Acta Neurochir (Wien) 147(4):443–446; discussion 446

Supreme Court Act (1981) Section 32A

World Health Organization (2009) WHO guidelines for safe surgery: safe surgery saves lives. World Health Organization, Geneva. www.who.int/patientsafety/safesurgery

Nomenclature

20

Clare Rusbridge and Graham Flint

Contents

The terminology of Chiari malformation and syringomyelia is variable and at times controversial. Individual specialists can be quite dogmatic over which name or expression is correct. In this appendix the nomenclature and classification of syringomyelia and Chiari malformations is reviewed briefly and arguments for and against the various terms are presented. A more detailed historical review is given in Chap. 1.

20.1 Spinal Cord Cavitation

One of the controversies surrounding this subject is whether spinal cord cavities, containing fluid identical with or closely resembling cerebrospinal fluid, should be referred to as syringomyelia, hydromyelia, syringohydromyelia or hydrosyringomyelia. The term syringomyelia was first used by Charles-Prosper Ollivier d'Angers (1796–1845) in '*De la moelle épinière et de ses maladies*'[1] and subsequently in the more comprehensive work '*Traité des maladies de la moelle épinière contenant l'histoire anatomique, physiologique et pathologique de ce centre nerveux chez l'homme*'[2] (Ollivier d'Angers 1824, 1827). He derived the term from the Greek 'syringo' meaning tube or pipe and 'myelio' referring to the spinal marrow, and he used it to describe a tubular

C. Rusbridge (✉)
Fitzpatrick Referrals,
Eashing, Godalming, Surrey, UK

Faculty of Health and Medical Sciences,
School of Veterinary Medicine,
University of Surrey, Guildford,
Surrey, UK
e-mail: neurovet@virginmedia.com

G. Flint
Department of Neurosurgery,
Queen Elizabeth Hospital,
University Hospitals Birmingham,
Birmingham, UK
e-mail: graham.flint@uhb.nhs.uk

---

[1] Translated as 'On the spinal cord and its diseases'

[2] Translated as 'Treatise on the Spinal Marrow and its Diseases—anatomy, functions and general considerations on its diseases'

G. Flint, C. Rusbridge (eds.), *Syringomyelia*,
DOI 10.1007/978-3-642-13706-8_20, © Springer-Verlag Berlin Heidelberg 2014

fluid-filled cavity in the spinal cord, most often associated with spina bifida (Grossmann et al. 2006; Mortazavi et al. 2011; Walusinski 2012). Schüppel used the term hydroamyelus in 1865 to describe a dilatation of the central canal (Schuppel 1865). The finding of spinal cord cavities, apparently separate from the central canal and surrounded by gliosis, led to a proposal by Simon, in 1875, that hydromyelia be used to describe central canal dilation and distension and that the term syringomyelia be reserved to describe cavities and cystic conditions independent of the central canal (Newton 1969; Simon 1875). In 1876, Leyden concluded that hydromyelia and syringomyelia were identical conditions (Newton 1969; Leyden 1876), but Kahler and Pick supported a distinction between hydromyelia and syringomyelia. They made the observation that a hydromyelia is lined by ependyma, whereas glial cells form the wall of syringomyelia cavities (Newton

1969; Kahler and Pick 1879). Hans Chiari himself found that, in 45 out of 75 well-documented cases of the so-called syringomyelia, the cavity was, in all probability, connected to the central canal (Newton 1969; Chiari 1888). This observation and the difficulty in differentiating between hydromyelia and syringomyelia, by radiological, clinical or pathological means, led some to use the combined terms syringohydromyelia or hydrosyringomyelia to describe a cavity which is partially lined by ependyma but which also extends into the spinal cord substance (Hogg et al. 1998). Thus, some clinicians argue that the term syringomyelia should apply to a glial-lined cavity separate from the central canal, that hydromyelia be reserved for central canal dilation still lined by ependyma and that the term syringohydromyelia is correct for a cavity involving a dilated central canal that is partially lined by ependyma. However, the distinction is easily

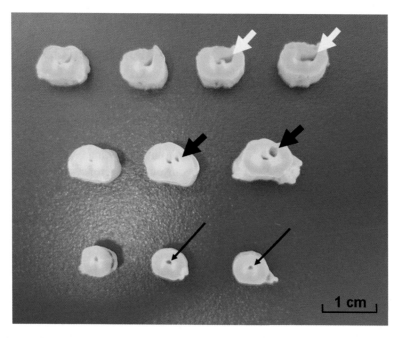

Fig. 20.1 Hydromyelia, syringomyelia or syringohydromyelia? In these sections of the spinal cord from a dog, it can be seen that some segments appear to have a syringohydromyelia (*top row*, short white arrows), some a separate syringomyelia cavity (*middle row*, short black arrows) and some a hydromyelia (*bottom row*, long arrows). The ependyma is disrupted in all sections on microscopy, and the apparently separate syrinx cavity is actually connected to the central canal more caudally or cranially, i.e. it is not truly separate. It can be argued that, without the aid of post-mortem and microscopic examination, it is impossible to categorise cavities on the basis of ependymal lining and central canal connection. It can also be argued that categorisation is completely unnecessary from a clinical point of view (Picture courtesy of Dr Fernando Constantino-Casas)

Table 20.1 Should syringomyelia be used in preference to syringohydromyelia?

Yes

1. Syringomyelia is already overwhelmingly used in preference to syringohydromyelia,[a,b] especially by those authors considered expert in this field
2. The classification of syrinx cavity by central canal connection and ependymal lining is unworkable (Fig. 20.1). Concurrent involvement of the central canal and disruption of the ependymal limiting is almost universal, so only one term is actually required
3. It is correct from a historical point of view. Ollivier d'Angers originally defined syringomyelia as a fluid-filled tubular dilatation within the spinal cord
4. Adding 'hydro' and an extra two syllables is superfluous and complicates a word that is already difficult for patients to understand, pronounce or remember

No

1. Syringohydromyelia may be defined as the coexistence of hydromyelia (fluid contained within the ependyma of the central canal) and syringomyelia (fluid forming a cavity within the white matter). Using the term syringohydromyelia makes it clear to the reader that a syrinx also involves the central canal
2. Differentiation between hydromyelia and syringomyelia is difficult to make by radiological, clinical or pathological methods. Use of the combined term, syringohydromyelia (or hydrosyringomyelia), acknowledges this reality
3. Adding a component, meaning 'water' or 'liquid', to a 'tube' in the 'marrow' makes it clear that this is a fluid-containing cavity, emphasising that it is a disorder of CSF circulation

[a]A PubMed search performed on 24th June 2012 revealed 136 articles when the key word 'syringohydromyelia' was used. In comparison 3,584 articles were found using the keyword 'syringomyelia'
[b]Online searches performed on 8th July 2012 in Wikipedia, Encyclopaedia Britannica, Oxford Dictionary, American Heritage Dictionary, Collins Dictionary and Merriam-Webster failed to find a listing for syringohydromyelia. Search results returned either 'not found' or defaulted to 'syringomyelia'

Table 20.2 Should we use hydromyelia to describe a small central dilation?

Yes

1. There is a need for a term to describe this MRI appearance. An ependymal-lined distension or dilation of the central canal has already been defined as hydromyelia; therefore, it is the most appropriate term to use

No

1. Many clinicians use the term inappropriately when syringomyelia would be more correct[a]
2. Using the term central canal dilation or distension is descriptive and less open to misinterpretation
3. Before using this term a clearer definition is required, e.g. the size of central canal dilation. In veterinary medicine central canal dilation with a transverse width of two millimetres or more is categorised as syringomyelia. If less than two millimetres, then it is described as central canal dilation (Knowler et al. 2011)
4. Use of the term hydromyelia implies pathology when it is not clear that this is always the case. By analogy, ventricular dilation (or ventriculomegaly) does not necessarily equate with clinically active hydrocephalus

[a]A PubMed search performed on 14th July 2012 using the criteria *hydromyelia* [*Title*] revealed 78 publications; however, only one was found (Jinkins and Sener 1999) which used the term hydromyelia to describe a central canal dilation. The remainder were referring to an extensive syrinx

blurred (Fig. 20.1). The simpler term syringomyelia is favoured by an increasing majority especially as recent post-mortem and experimental studies have suggested that the ependyma is disrupted following only minor central canal dilatation (Hu et al. 2011; Radojicic et al. 2007). The arguments for and against the terms syringomyelia, hydromyelia and syringohydromyelia are represented in Tables 20.1 and 20.2.

20.2 Abnormalities of the Craniovertebral Junction

The first known illustration of hindbrain herniation was in an early nineteenth-century anatomy atlas by Jean Cruveilhier (Cruveilhier 1829; Pearce 2000). There was also a brief description of a single case in a paper on encephalocoele and spinal bifida by John Cleland in 1883 (Cleland

Table 20.3 Classification of Chiari malformations

Chiari malformation	Original description by Chiari (Batzdorf 2001b)	Modern description
Type I	Elongation of the cerebellar tonsils and the medial part of the inferior cerebellar lobes into cone-like projections, which accompany the medulla into the spinal canal	Volumetrically small posterior cranial fossa with hindbrain overcrowding (Milhorat et al. 1999)
		The classic radiographic description is tonsillar herniation of at least 3 mm below the foramen magnum
Type II	Displacement of portions of the vermis and also of the pons and medulla into the spinal canal and elongation of the fourth ventricle into the spinal canal	Downward displacement of the cerebellar vermis, brainstem and fourth ventricle, associated with a myelomeningocoele (Geerdink et al. 2012)
Type III	Displacement of virtually the entire hydrocephalic cerebellum into a cervical spinal bifida	Hindbrain herniation into a high cervical or occipital encephalocoele (Castillo et al. 1992)
Type IV	Hypoplasia in the region of the cerebellum without displacement of portions thereof into the spinal canal	Obsolete term describing cerebellar hypoplasia unrelated to the other Chiari malformations
Type 0		Overcrowding of the posterior fossa with abnormal brainstem anatomy (posterior pontine tilt, downward displacement of the medulla, low-lying obex) but with normally placed cerebellar tonsils (Markunas et al. 2012)
Type 1.5		Cerebellar and brainstem herniation through the foramen magnum. Similar to type II malformation but not associated with spinal dysraphism (Tubbs et al. 2004)
Canine		Disparity in volume between the caudal cranial fossa and its contents so that the cerebellum and brainstem are herniated into or through the foramen magnum

1883). It is, however, Hans Chiari (1851–1916), a pathologist working in Prague, who is honoured with the medical eponym because he provided the first detailed description of four types of cerebellar pathology, observed during post-mortem studies of infants with congenital hydrocephalus (Chiari 1891, Chiari 1896). Descriptions of the various types of Chiari malformation have, however, evolved since (Table 20.3). Chiari was careful to acknowledge the work of others, and in his conclusion in the second paper, he noted the observations of Cleland and also of Arnold, who had described an infant with spina bifida and hindbrain herniation (Arnold 1894). Two loyal students of Arnold, Schwalbe and Gredig, subsequently inserted his name when describing four patients with the type II malformation (i.e. in association with myelomeningocoele) coining the term Arnold-Chiari malformation (Schwalbe and Gredig 1907). Consequently, some refer to the spectrum of disorders of hindbrain herniation as Arnold-Chiari syndrome (Bejjani 2001), albeit to the indignation of others (Solt 2011; Sarnat 2007).

The majority now use the term Chiari malformation to describe hindbrain herniation. The arguments for and against the terms hindbrain herniation, Chiari malformation and Arnold-Chiari malformation are presented in Tables 20.4 and 20.5.

20.3 Communicating and Noncommunicating Syringomyelia

Syringomyelia and hydromyelia were traditionally classified into communicating and noncommunicating types (Milhorat et al. 1995). The term communicating indicated the presence of a connection between the syringomyelic cavity and the fourth ventricle. Communicating syringomyelia, or hydromyelia, is associated with hydrocephalus, especially of the fourth ventricle and conditions which cause obstruction to the outflow of this chamber, for example, post-meningitic or posthaemorrhagic hydrocephalus or complex hindbrain malformations such as

Table 20.4 Should hindbrain herniation be used in preference to Chiari malformation?

Yes

1. In common with most eponymous terms, Chiari malformation tells us nothing about the nature of the condition

2. There are many causes of hindbrain herniation including cranial constriction, spinal cord tethering, cranial settling, intracranial hypertension, intraspinal hypotension, basilar impression/invagination and craniosynostosis. Nomenclature should identify the underlying subgroup and cause, for example, 'hindbrain herniation secondary to intracranial hypertension'

3. Using eponymous terms for diseases is to be discouraged especially when there is a simple alterative

No

1. The eponym Chiari malformation is by far the most commonly used term[a]

2. Some cases with overcrowding of the posterior fossa and disrupted CSF flow (Chiari 0) do not actually have a hindbrain herniation

3. The classification of various Chiari malformations is commonly used and well understood. For example, the term 'Chiari type II' is much simpler to say or read than 'hindbrain herniation associated with spinal myelomeningocoele'

[a]A PubMed search performed on 14th July 2012 using the criteria (*Chiari* [*Title*]) *not Budd* [*Title*]), *not Arnold* [*Title*], revealed 1,422 publications. A search using the criteria *Chiari* [*Title*]) *and Arnold* [*Title*] revealed 509 publications. A search using the criteria *hindbrain herniation* [*Title*] revealed 22 publications

Table 20.5 Should the term Arnold-Chiari malformation be dropped?

Yes

1. Arnold's work does not merit an eponym, and it was an injustice that his name was added. Chiari provided a detailed and careful description of the pathology, whereas Arnold's observation in a single case was 'a ribbon of tissue that protruded through the foramen magnum'. Arnold did not even acknowledge previous work by Cleland and Chiari (Solt 2011; Sarnat 2007)

2. Arnold-Chiari is a confusing term because there is not universal agreement as to the definition. Some use it for all types of hindbrain herniation and others use it exclusively to refer to hindbrain herniation associated with a myelomeningocoele[a]

3. The eponym Arnold-Chiari malformation is not the most frequently used term[b]

4. Many patients think that Arnold-Chiari was one person

No

1. This term is useful to distinguish the type II malformation, i.e. hindbrain herniation associated with myelomeningocoele, and should be reserved exclusively for that

2. If we are going to use an eponymous term, then the contribution of this clinician should be recognised as well as that of Hans Chiari

[a]A PubMed search performed on 14th July 2012 using the criteria (*Chiari* [*Title*]) *and Arnold* [*Title*]) *and spina bifida* revealed 42 publications. A search using the criteria (*Chiari* [*Title*]) *not Arnold* [*Title*]) *not Budd* [*Title*]) *and spina bifida* however revealed 44 publications

[b]A PubMed search performed on 14th July 2012 using the criteria (*Chiari* [*Title*]) *not Budd* [*Title*]), *not Arnold* [*Title*], revealed 1,422 publications. A search using the criteria *Chiari* [*Title*]) *and Arnold* [*Title*] revealed 509 publications. A search using the criteria *hindbrain herniation* [*Title*] revealed 22 publications

Dandy-Walker malformation. It was at one time widely assumed that the pathogenesis of communicating syringomyelia is due to a water-hammer effect of cerebrospinal fluid from the fourth ventricle, being forced into the central canal (Williams 1980; Gardner 1965). Indeed this theory is still accepted by some authors (Hagihara and Sakata 2007). However, this theory was challenged, not least because communicating syringomyelia is sometimes seen with distal spinal cord pathology, such as caudal, cervical, spinal and intradural subarachnoid cysts (Yamashita et al. 2012) and thoracic spinal cord tumours (Mock et al. 1990). Communicating hydrocephalus, however, is now known to be present in fewer than 10 % of affected human patients, so this categorisation now tends to be disregarded (Batzdorf 2001a).

Noncommunicating syringomyelia describes a cavity that has developed caudal to a syrinx-free

Table 20.6 Are the terms communicating and noncommunicating syringomyelia obsolete?

Yes

1. These terms originate from a time, before the advent of magnetic resonance imaging, when our understanding of the pathogenesis of syringomyelia was different. Nowadays most consider the water-hammer theory unlikely to be correct because a communication between the central canal and fourth ventricle is uncommon in humans

2. These terms have fallen out of use already[a]. If they were of value to clinicians, then they would still be in common usage

No

1. Communicating syringomyelia may have a different pathogenesis and management and therefore should be considered separately. The preferred management is addressing the hydrocephalus, typically with a intraventricular shunt

[a]Noncommunicating syringomyelia is reputed to account for 90 % of cases (Batzdorf 2001a). However, a PubMed search performed on the 15th July 2012 using the keywords 'noncommunicating syringomyelia' revealed only 19 articles out of a possible 3,958 articles found using the keyword syringomyelia (0.005 %)

portion of spinal cord and which is associated with obstruction of the cerebrospinal fluid pathways, either at the foramen magnum, such as in Chiari type I malformation, or more distally, for example, spinal arachnoid webs or adhesions (Milhorat et al. 2001). A classification by communicating versus noncommunicating once again becomes inconsistent with a condition such as Chiari type I malformation, which is more commonly associated with noncommunicating syringomyelia (Milhorat et al. 1995), but can also cause a communicating syringomyelia (Lena et al. 1992). Arguments as to the usefulness or otherwise of these terms are represented in Table 20.6.

20.4 Subarachnoid Channels

The term spinal subarachnoid space is widely used in neurological literature and refers, of course, to the channels along which CSF flows. The word space has several dictionary definitions, but, in common usage, it implies that there is nothing there, e.g. a space between words in this sentence and a space between buildings and outer space. In reality, these channels, within the spinal canal, are filled with cerebrospinal fluid. They are in continuity with the basal cisterns inside the skull and the cerebral ventricles. Together, these CSF-filled channels provide, amongst other things, an essential mediator of compliance, within and between the cranial and spinal compartments. As an incompressible physical medium, the CSF transmits pulsatile energy waves, both arterial and venous, and these must have important roles to play in the development of syringomyelia cavities. If cerebral arteries were suspended in an empty space, then the energy of their pulsations would not be transmitted beyond their points of origin. There is, therefore, an argument for using the term subarachnoid channels, in preference to subarachnoid space.

20.5 Veterinary Terminology

In veterinary medicine similar arguments about nomenclature have occurred (Cappello and Rusbridge 2007). It is debatable whether the term Chiari malformation should be applied to the dog. The analogous canine condition, characterised by decreased volume of the caudal fossa and caudal displacement of the caudal cerebellar vermis into or through the foramen magnum, is very similar to the human condition (see Chap. 14). The condition in the dog, however, is inconsistent with the original historical description of Chiari malformation, not in the least because dogs do not have cerebellar tonsils. In veterinary medicine there is resistance to using eponyms, but they are not without precedent, especially where the name is a simple term, used to describe a complicated process, for example, Horner's syndrome or Wallerian degeneration. It is considered more correct to use an anatomical description, and early reports of the canine condition make reference to occipital hypoplasia with syringomyelia (Rusbridge et al. 2005; Rusbridge and Knowler 2003), although this term was dropped because it was realised that the pathogenesis of the condition was likely to be more complex than simply a hypoplastic occipital bone(s). The term caudal occipital malformation syndrome was popular in the USA (Dewey et al. 2005, 2007) and is still used occasionally,[3] but it, too, is inappropriate, for similar reasons. In addition, if using an anatomical description, it should be accurate and the term 'caudal occipital' actually refers to the supraoccipital bone. There is also a reluctance to use the term hindbrain herniation because some veterinary surgeons believe that this is an embryological term, referring to the rhombencephalon. However, there is no other term used to describe the contents of the caudal (posterior) cranial fossa, and the exact reason for the reluctance to use the term hindbrain is unclear, especially when the word forebrain is used commonly. Equally, hindbrain herniation may not be appropriate because in many dogs there is not a marked hindbrain herniation but, rather, an overcrowding in the most caudal region of caudal cranial fossa, similar to Chiari 0 (Table 20.3). Eventually, a meeting of international experts decided that the term 'Chiari-like malformation' should be used to describe the canine condition (Cappello and Rusbridge 2007).

20.6 Singular and Plural

We refer to the medical instrument used for injecting or withdrawing fluid as a syringe. We would order a box of syringes for ward supplies. Yet, we use the term syrinx to refer to the vocal organ of a bird and syrinxes when using the plural of this word. When speaking of fluid-filled cavities within the spinal cord, therefore, it would seem logical to refer to more than one syrinx as syrinxes. To say that the correct plural is 'syringes' implies that the correct singular word for a cystic cavity inside the spinal cord is a

syringe. In truth, we are dealing with two different words, albeit with a common etymological origin. They have, correspondingly, different plurals.

Notwithstanding these arguments and noting that some journals refuse the use of syringes as the plural of syrinx, the editors of this monograph have allowed both terms to be used, at the preference of individual authors.

20.7 Eponyms, Acronyms and Abbreviations

A large number of medical terms have their origins in the Latin or Greek languages. Unfortunately, teaching of these languages no longer forms part of a mainstream education. As a result, many new medical terms, introduced throughout the twentieth century and beyond, have taken the form of acronyms. Not uncommonly, such acronyms are uttered by individuals who may not know what the abbreviation actually stands for, even though the meaning of the expression may be clear, at least to those who use it. The abbreviation CSF, for example, will not need to be explained to most readers of this book but, when used for the first time in speaking to a patient, may produce a look of puzzlement.

Less widely used acronyms do require explanation at the outset, a convention demanded by most publishers of medical literature. A danger exists, however, that too many acronyms or abbreviations are introduced into a specialist article or book chapter. Such a practice may make it easier for the author to write the work, but it will very likely make it more difficult for the reader to understand. If the reader has to keep referring back a few pages, to be reminded of the meaning of a given acronym or abbreviation, then absorbing the meaning of the whole composition becomes more difficult. We have attempted to restrict this practice in this monograph, preferring to write expressions in full.

Patients do seem to like medical acronyms, presumably because they are easier to say than many medical tongue-twisters, such as

---

[3] A PubMed search performed on 14th July 2012 using the criteria (*Chiari* [*Title*]) *not Budd* [*Title*]) *and dog* revealed 25 publications. A search using the criteria *occipital hypoplasia* [*Title*]) *and dog* revealed 3 publications. A search using the criteria *caudal occipital malformation syndrome* [*Title*] revealed 2 publications.

Table 20.7 Abbreviations and acronyms

Acronym	Full expression
ACM	Arnold-Chiari malformation
CM	Chiari malformation
CM0	Chiari malformation type 0
CM1/CMI	Chiari malformation type I
CM2/CMII	Chiari malformation type II
CVD	Craniovertebral decompression
FMD	Foramen magnum decompression
HBH	Hindbrain hernia
PTSM	Post-traumatic syringomyelia
SCI	Spinal cord injury
SM	Syringomyelia

syringomyelia. Unfortunately there is not a great deal of consistency in the use of such terms (Table 20.7).

A curious, modern approach is to give peculiar names to newly discovered genes and proteins. An example is Sonic Hedgehog (Chap. 4), a name taken from a popular computer game of its time and given to a family of proteins involved in the development of the nervous system. This practice must reflect the fact that the modern research scientist is exposed to such recreational activities, whereas earlier generations of biologists might only have been exposed to their Latin and Greek studies.

The adoption of eponyms has been widespread in medicine for a long time. Such words usually honour the name of the person who first identified a condition or at least described it in any detail. Sometimes the name derives, instead, from a place or area where a disease was first discovered. Occasionally the name refers to a patient who suffered from the condition. The disadvantage of most eponyms is that they tell us little, if anything, about the nature of the condition to which they apply. The World Health Organisation prefers that eponyms be avoided, in favour of more descriptive terms. Thus, hindbrain hernia might be preferable to Chiari malformation. Unfortunately, common usage tends to resist such initiatives, and eponyms are likely to remain in widespread use in medical practice. For example, is it likely that we will abandon the eponym Parkinson's disease and readopt the expression paralysis agitans?

References

Arnold J (1894) Myelocyste, Transposition von Gewebskeimen und Sympodie. Beitr Pathol Anat 16:1–28

Batzdorf U (2001a) A brief history of syringomyelia. In: Tamaki N, Batzdorf U, Nagashima T (eds) Syringomyelia: current concepts in pathogenesis and management. Springer, Tokyo, pp 3–9

Batzdorf U (2001b) Treatment of syringomyelia association with Chiari I malformation. In: Tamaki N, Batzdorf U, Nagashima T (eds) Syringomyelia current concepts in pathogenesis and management. Springer, Tokyo, pp 121–135

Bejjani GK (2001) Definition of the adult Chiari malformation: a brief historical overview. Neurosurg Focus 11(1):E1. doi:10.3171/foc.2001.11.1.2

Cappello R, Rusbridge C (2007) Report from the Chiari-Like Malformation and Syringomyelia Working Group round table. Vet Surg 36(5):509–512. doi:10.1111/j.1532-950X.2007.00298.x

Castillo M, Quencer RM, Dominguez R (1992) Chiari III malformation: imaging features. AJNR Am J Neuroradiol 13(1):107–113

Chiari H (1888) Ueber die Pathogenese der Sogenannten Syringomyelie. Z Heilk 9:307

Chiari H (1891) Ueber Veränderungen des Kleinhirns infolge von Hydrocephalie des Grosshirns. Dtsch Med Wochenschir 42:1172–1175

Chiari H (1896) Ueber Veränderungen des Kleinhirns, des Pons und der medulla oblongata in Folge von genitaler Hydrocephalie des Grosshirns. Denkschr Akad Wiss Wien 63:71–116

Cleland J (1883) Contribution to the study of spina bifida, encephalocele, and anencephalus. J Anat Physiol 17:257–292

Cruveilhier J (1829) L'Anatomie pathologique du corps humain; descriptions avec figures lithographiées et coloriées; diverses alterations morbides don't le corps humain et susceptible. Bailliere, Paris

Dewey CW, Berg JM, Barone G et al (2005) Foramen magnum decompression for treatment of caudal occipital malformation syndrome in dogs. J Am Vet Med Assoc 227(8):1270–1275, 50–51

Dewey CW, Marino DJ, Bailey KS et al (2007) Foramen magnum decompression with cranioplasty for treatment of caudal occipital malformation syndrome in dogs. Vet Surg 36(5):406–415. doi:10.1111/j.1532-950X.2007.00286.x

Gardner WJ (1965) Hydrodynamic mechanism of syringomyelia: its relationship to myelocele. J Neurol Neurosurg Psychiatry 28:247–259

Geerdink N, van der Vliet T, Rotteveel JJ et al (2012) Interobserver reliability and diagnostic performance of Chiari II malformation measures in MR imaging-part 2. Childs Nerv Syst 28(7):987–995. doi:10.1007/s00381-012-1763-3

Grossmann S, Maeder IM, Dollfus P (2006) 'Treatise on the Spinal Marrow and its Diseases' (Anatomy, functions and general considerations on its diseases) by Ollivier d' Angers CP (1796–1845). Spinal Cord 44(12):700–707. doi:10.1038/sj.sc.3101956

Hagihara N, Sakata S (2007) Disproportionately large communicating fourth ventricle with syringomyelia: case report. Neurol Med Chir (Tokyo) 47(6):278–281

Hogg J, Peterson A, El-Kadi H (1998) Imaging of cranial and spinal cerebrospinal fluid collections cerebrospinal fluid collections USA: the American Association of Neurological Surgeons Publications Group. Stuttgart, Germany and New York, USA: Thieme Publishing Group

Hu HZ, Rusbridge C, Constantino-Casas F et al (2011) Histopathological investigation of syringomyelia in the Cavalier King Charles spaniel. J Comp Pathol 146(2–3):192–201. doi:10.1016/j.jcpa.2011.07.002

Jinkins JR, Sener RN (1999) Idiopathic localized hydromyelia: dilatation of the central canal of the spinal cord of probable congenital origin. J Comput Assist Tomogr 23(3):351–353

Kahler O, Pick A (1879) Beitrag zur Lehre von der Syringo-und Hydromyelia. Vjschr Prakt Heilkd 142:20–41

Knowler SP, McFadyen AK, Rusbridge C (2011) Effectiveness of breeding guidelines for reducing the prevalence of syringomyelia. Vet Rec 169(26):681. doi:10.1136/vr.100062

Lena G, Boudawara Z, Genitori L et al (1992) 14 cases of communicating syringomyelia associated with Chiari I malformation in children. Neurochirurgie 38(5): 297–303

Leyden E (1876) Über Hydromyelus un Syringomyelie. Arch Pathol Anat Physiol 68:1–20

Markunas CA, Tubbs RS, Moftakhar R et al (2012) Clinical, radiological, and genetic similarities between patients with Chiari type I and type 0 malformations. J Neurosurg Pediatr 9(4):372–378. doi:10.3171/2011.12. PEDS11113

Milhorat TH, Capocelli AL Jr, Anzil AP et al (1995) Pathological basis of spinal cord cavitation in syringomyelia: analysis of 105 autopsy cases. J Neurosurg 82(5):802–812. doi:10.3171/jns.1995.82.5.0802

Milhorat TH, Chou MW, Trinidad EM et al (1999) Chiari I malformation redefined: clinical and radiographic findings for 364 symptomatic patients. Neurosurgery 44(5):1005–1017

Milhorat T, Fox A, Todor DR (2001) Pathology, classification, and treatment of syringomyelia. In: Tamaki N, Batzdorf U, Nagashima T (eds) Syringomyelia: current concepts in pathogenesis and management. Springer, Tokyo, pp 10–30

Mock A, Levi A, Drake JM (1990) Spinal hemangioblastoma, syrinx, and hydrocephalus in a two-year-old child. Neurosurgery 27(5):799–802

Mortazavi MM, Rompala OJ, Verma K et al (2011) Charles Prosper Ollivier d'Angers (1796–1845) and his contributions to defining syringomyelia. Childs Nerv Syst 27(12):2155–2158. doi:10.1007/ s00381-011-1416-y

Newton EJ (1969) Syringomyelia as a manifestation of defective fourth ventricular drainage. Ann R Coll Surg Engl 44(4):194–213

Ollivier d'Angers C-P (1824) De la moelle épinière et de ses maladies. Crevot, Paris

Ollivier d'Angers C-P (1827) Traité des maladies de la moelle épinière contenant l'histoire anatomique, physiologique et pathologique de ce centre nerveux chez l'homme. Crevot, Paris

Pearce JM (2000) Historical note. Arnold Chiari, or "Cruveilhier Cleland Chiari" malformation. J Neurol Neurosurg Psychiatry 68(1):13

Radojicic M, Nistor G, Keirstead HS (2007) Ascending central canal dilation and progressive ependymal disruption in a contusion model of rodent chronic spinal cord injury. BMC Neurol 7:30. doi:10.1186/1471-2377-7-30

Rusbridge C, Knowler SP (2003) Hereditary aspects of occipital bone hypoplasia and syringomyelia (Chiari type I malformation) in cavalier King Charles spaniels. Vet Rec 153(4):107–112

Rusbridge C, Knowler P, Rouleau GA et al (2005) Inherited occipital hypoplasia/syringomyelia in the cavalier King Charles spaniel: experiences in setting up a worldwide DNA collection. J Hered 96(7): 745–749. doi:10.1093/jhered/esi074

Sarnat HB (2007) Semantics do matter! Precision in scientific communication in pediatric neurology. J Child Neurol 22(11):1245–1251. doi:10.1177/ 0883073807307981

Schuppel (1865) Über Hydromyelus. Arch Heilk 6:289

Schwalbe E, Gredig M (1907) Ueber Entwicklungstströrungen des Kleihirns, Hirnstamms und Halsmarks bei Spina bifida (Arnold'sche und Chiari'sche Missbildung). Beitr Pathol Anat 40:132–194

Simon T (1875) Über Syringomyelia und Geshwulstbildung im Rückenmark. Arch Psychiatr NervenKr 5:120–163

Solt I (2011) Chiari malformation eponym- time for historical justice. Ultrasound Obstet Gynecol 37(2):250–251. doi:10.1002/uog.8876

Tubbs RS, Iskandar BJ, Bartolucci AA et al (2004) A critical analysis of the Chiari 1.5 malformation. J Neurosurg 101(2 Suppl):179–183. doi:10.3171/ ped.2004.101.2.0179

Walusinski O (2012) Charles-Prosper Ollivier d'Angers (1796–1845). J Neurol 259(6):1255–1256. doi:10.1007/s00415-012-6424-7

Williams B (1980) On the pathogenesis of syringomyelia: a review. J R Soc Med 73(11):798–806

Yamashita T, Hiramatsu H, Kitahama Y et al (2012) Disproportionately large communicating fourth ventricle associated with syringomyelia and intradural arachnoid cyst in the spinal cord successfully treated with additional shunting. Case report. Neurol Med Chir (Tokyo) 52(4):231–234

History of the Imaging of Syringomyelia

21

Panagiotis Papanagiotou and Anton Haass

Contents

P. Papanagiotou (✉)
Clinic for Diagnostic and Interventional
Neuroradiology, Klinikum, Bremen, Germany
e-mail: panagiotis.papanagiotou@klinikum-bremen-mitte.de

A. Haass
Neurological Department, University of the Saarland,
Homburg/Saar, Germany
e-mail: anton.haass@uniklinik-saarland.de

The diagnostic capabilities of modern magnetic resonance (MR) imaging means that once a decision has been made to investigate a case of suspected myelopathy or radiculopathy, few cases of syringomyelia will be undetected. A delay in diagnosis can still occur if the initial clinical assessment is incorrect, requiring a patient to be tolerant of the difficulties of identifying the less common neurological disorders (see Chap. 18). More often, nowadays, we are confronted with the opposite problem, that of over diagnosis, in cases of small cavities that may be unrelated to the presenting symptoms.

It is, therefore, sobering to consider that, within the lifetime of some clinicians still in practice, the diagnosis of syringomyelia depended upon invasive methods such as computer tomography (CT) and air myelography. The unpleasant nature of some of these tests, together with their attendant risks, meant that they were applied selectively. As a consequence patients were usually only diagnosed when their disease had reached a more advanced stage than that which we generally see today. At the same time, we can only admire the diagnostic acumen of the clinicians and the technical skills of the radiologists who correctly identified the condition in patients, in the pre-MR era. In this context, following account of the history of imaging of syringomyelia makes for interesting reading. (GF)

G. Flint, C. Rusbridge (eds.), *Syringomyelia*,
DOI 10.1007/978-3-642-13706-8_21, © Springer-Verlag Berlin Heidelberg 2014

21.1   Introduction

By the end of the nineteenth century, the structure
and functions of the spinal cord were largely
defined. Even so, the diagnosis of syringomyelia
and other myelopathies could only be suspected
on clinical grounds (Turney 1908). At the beginning of the twentieth century, invasive examinations were developed, to localise spinal cord
diseases. Thereafter, the application of radiological examinations, in combination with clinical
assessment, was better able to suggest the diagnosis of spinal cord lesions. For almost seven
decades thereafter the diagnosis of syringomyelia
was most likely to be made by myelography but
even then the lesion may have been missed in
many instances because myelography only
defines the subarachnoid space and does not
visualise the cord directly. By the end of the
1970s, it became possible to make the diagnosis
of syringomyelia more reliably, using a less invasive method in the form of CT myelography. The
subsequent development of magnetic resonance
imaging (MRI) meant that the diagnosis could be
made reliably, in most cases, by an entirely non-
invasive imaging technique. This method has
now largely replaced all other techniques, except
when it is contraindicated for specific reasons or
when implanted metalwork degrades the images.

21.2   Plain Radiographs

With syringomyelia, plain radiographic images
of the spine may show widening of the spinal
canal, in both the sagittal and coronal planes. The
cervical spinal canal in particular is often large;
in some cases the anteroposterior diameter is
seen to be increased, in other cases the transverse
diameter and in some instances both diameters
are expanded. Cervical or thoracic scoliosis or
kyphoscoliosis may also be a signs of underlying
syringomyelia, particularly in children. The diagnosis of syringomyelia may also be suggested by
the presence of other bone anomalies, such as
segmentation abnormalities at the craniovertebral junction and subaxial levels. In some circumstances plain films can also reveal the

aetiology of a syringomyelia, in particular bony
changes resulting from an old spinal injury or
previous osteomyelitis or spinal tuberculosis
(McRae and Standen 1966).

21.3   Myelography

Prior to the advent of CT, the definitive radiographic procedure used to diagnose syringomyelia was myelography, initially with positive
contrast media. The earliest of these were oil
based but later water-soluble compounds were
developed. Subsequently, negative contrast studies were developed, using intrathecal air, injected
either at lumbar or cisternal puncture. The latter
technique was initially developed in the 1920s, as
a means of obtaining samples of cerebrospinal
fluid (CSF) (Ayer 1923).

21.3.1 Air Myelography

As early as 1918, Dandy developed the technique
of outlining the spinal cord by using an intraspinal injection of air (Dandy 1919). The first reports
of its use to localise intraspinal tumours came
from Jacobeus in 1921 and Dandy in 1925
(Dandy 1925). The technique was later refined to
show the entire spinal canal; this involved complete replacement of the CSF with air and
distension of the spinal subarachnoid space
(Jirout 1958). The technique was difficult to perform and potentially hazardous for the patient,
not least because the cisternal puncture required
could cause medullary injury. Moreover, it was
difficult to demonstrate a craniovertebral block
with subarachnoid air. It was also desirable to
avoid passage of air into the cranial spaces
because, when this occurred, severe headache
would ensue and the patient could not then easily
lie still, which led to images of poor quality.
Further, with air myelography, spinal roots were
not shown, and many types of pathology, such as
vascular malformations or arachnoiditis, were
either not revealed, or the radiological appearances were easily misinterpreted (Heinz and
Goldman 1972).

21.3.2 Oil Myelography

In 1922, two French investigators found, by accident, that iodised oils could be moved through the spinal subarachnoid space under the influence of gravity. They then proposed the intraspinal injection of lipiodol as a new diagnostic test, a method referred to as "myelography" (Sicard et al. 1923). Oil-based contrast media proved easier to use than air, and this quickly established oil myelography as the technique of choice, especially in the lumbar spinal canal. It was not until 1932 that the tilting radiographic table was developed and so the contrast was at first introduced by cisternal puncture. Lipiodol did, however, produce some unpleasant side effects, including pain and sensory disturbances in the legs. In 1940, the University of Rochester developed an alternative, ethyl iophenylundecilate, or iophendylate, known as Myodil in the UK and Pantopaque elsewhere. This medium was less viscous and therefore easier to use than the earlier Lipiodol, and it gave better demonstration of the spinal cord. It was very opaque to x-rays and special techniques such as tomography were not required (Peacher and Robertson 1946). It could be left in the spinal canal and rerun postoperatively, to check the adequacy of any surgical procedure (Dandy 1925; Copleman 1946). It gave even greater impetus to the application of oil-based, positive contrast myelography and was widely adopted in clinical practice. Because of its immiscibility with CSF, however, it tended to break up into globules, forming a layer in the spinal canal, which made it difficult to demonstrate both anterior and posterior surfaces of the spinal cord, unless large amounts were used. Nevertheless, for nearly 40 years, Pantopaque was generally the agent of choice, with air being reserved for special situations. Unfortunately, leaving oil-based contrast medium in the subarachnoid space resulted in inflammatory reactions in the meninges, leading to the formation of arachnoidal adhesions (Kendall et al. 1991). As early as 1941, Kubik proposed the removal of the iodised oil after completion of the myelogram, but it was some years before this practice became widely adopted (Kubik and Hampton 1941).

21.3.3 Water-Soluble Myelography

Ionic, water-soluble contrast agents were first used for myelography in the United States, in 1931. Compared to oily contrast media, they provided superior images of the cauda equina and root sheaths. Unfortunately, because of their initial irritating effects on the meninges, they never became popular (Almen 1969). Matters improved – indeed a revolution occurred in myelography – when metrizamide, a new, nonionic water-soluble medium, appeared in 1976. This was far less neurotoxic than were previous agents. It could certainly be used safely around the spinal cord, although its inadvertent passage into the head, when the contrast was being run into the cervical region, could cause generalised seizures (Skalpe and Amundsen 1975). This risk was reduced by introducing the contrast by lateral puncture, at C1-2 (Robertson and Smith 1990). Metrizamide was not entirely nontoxic and a second generation of nonionic agents, such as iohexol (Omnipaque) and iopamidol (Isovue), eventually replaced metrizamide. These agents did not cause arachnoiditis in the concentrations used in clinical practice (Sortland and Skalpe 1977). Pantopaque was withdrawn in 1987, a few years before law suits for chronic arachnoiditis began to be brought before the law courts.

21.3.4 Myelographic Study of Syringomyelia

Both positive and negative contrast studies (air myelography) were needed to make the diagnosis of syringomyelia (Ayer 1923). Myelographic findings, using positive contrast alone, either Pantopaque or metrizamide, were variable because the size of the cord varied with the position of the patient and with how much CSF was still present to support the cord. Myelography would initially demonstrate a non-specific swelling of the cord, which could just as easily have been due to an intramedullary tumour (Batnitzky et al. 1983). During injection of air, the supporting CSF was removed and, when the patient was subsequently tilted upright, the fluid inside the syrinx would run downwards, leading to collapse of the upper portion of the cavity. The cervical cord shadow on the myelogram was then seen to be narrowed and this came to be known as the "collapsing cord" sign. It was regarded as being pathognomonic of syringomyelia (Heinz et al. 1966). In the case of intramedullary tumours, no change in the appearance of the expanded cord would occur with a change in the patient's position. With syringomyelia, when the patient was moved back into the horizontal position, the fluid in the cavity ran back up into the cervical cord, causing an enlarged cervical cord shadow once again (McRae and Standen 1966).

21.4 Computed Tomography

The computed tomography (CT) scanner, designed initially for use on the head, was first described in the medical literature in 1973 (Hounsfield 1973). Soon afterwards, the method was applied to imaging of the spine. It provided valuable, cross-sectional perspectives of the spinal canal, formerly very difficult to achieve with conventional radiography. Its further use went on to revolutionise the radiological diagnosis of syringomyelia, and the first article on the use of CT in the diagnosis of syringomyelia appeared in 1975 (DiChiro et al. 1975). The cystic nature of a syringomyelia cavity could sometimes be recognised on standard CT scans, as a distinct area of decreased attenuation within the spinal cord, although this was by no means a constant finding. Administration of intravenous contrast media allowed neural tissue to stand out somewhat better, against CSF and syrinx fluid, but intrathecal administration of contrast media provided excellent visualisation of the cord, as well as other intradural structures within the spinal canal.

21.4.1 CT Myelography

CT myelography using metrizamide was soon developed, as a simple, safe and accurate technique for demonstrating the intrathecal contents of the spine (Di Chiro and Schellinger 1976). This technique was particularly helpful in the diagnosis of syringomyelia and remains so today,

for some patients who cannot undergo MR scanning. In many instances, however, a swollen cord still cannot be distinguished from any other intramedullary lesion. In other cases of syringomyelia, the cord appears normal in size or even atrophic. Moving the patient from the supine to the lateral decubitus position may be helpful, by demonstrating a change in the shape and size of the cord when a syringomyelia cavity is present (Ayer 1923). The appearance of the normal cord does not alter with changes in position on CT myelography.

The most useful feature of CT myelography, however, is the demonstration of contrast agent in the syringomyelic cavity within the spinal cord and this is a pathognomonic finding (Resjö et al. 1979). Although, in some instances, the cavity fills soon after the intrathecal injection of contrast agent, in most cases contrast fills the cavity after several hours, by diffusing through the cord parenchyma or indirectly via the fourth ventricle (Foster et al. 1980). Delayed CT scans are, therefore, often required, to demonstrate such filling. In cases, where the intrathecal metrizamide opacifies the cyst immediately, it suggests the presence of a direct communication between the syrinx and the spinal subarachnoid space.

21.5 Magnetic Resonance Imaging

In the 1980s, during a period when myelography was being greatly improved, MRI was introduced as a diagnostic tool. Within just a few years myelography was pushed almost into obsolescence. Although the fist MRI images were of low quality, they were still able to distinguish relatively pure fluids, like CSF, from more inhomogeneous fluid collections. This made it possible to differentiate between the cavities seen in syringomyelia and those seen in neoplastic cysts. Subsequent developments have seen the introduction of better magnets, coils and sequences, and the price of the equipment has also decreased. With modern, high-resolution MRI, almost all intradural features, previously demonstrable by myelography, can usually be better shown by MRI. The development of fast T2 sequencing, at the beginning of the 1990s, meant that nerve

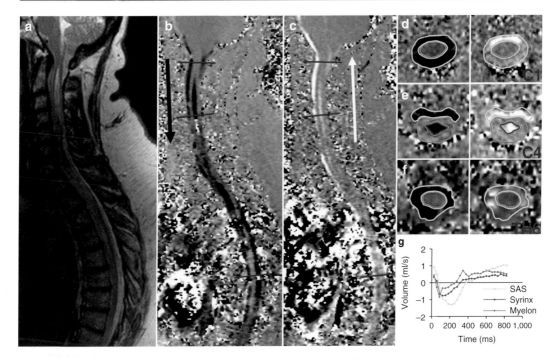

Fig. 21.1 MR flow imaging. (**a**) T2 sagittal MR image of craniovertebral junction and spinal canal. (**b**) Corresponding phase contrast MR images demonstrating caudal displacement of CSF (seen as *black*), during systole. (**c**) The same image during diastole, with return of CSF in a cephalad direction. The three *red*, horizontal lines on images "a" and "b" show the levels of the transverse image pairs "d", "e" and "f", respectively. The graph "g" shows the flow volume, with time, across the cardiac cycle

roots could be visualised routinely. Myelography is now indicated only when MRI is contraindicated, such as when patients have cardiac pacemakers or are claustrophobic. Even then, open scanners can be used and can usually demonstrate syringomyelia cavities, albeit without such high resolution. Cardiac pacemakers which are MR compatible are also now available. Myelography may still have an occasional role, in the detection of arachnoid webs, that may elude detection by MR imaging. If there is a drawback to MR imaging, it is the increasing detection of dilated or persistent central canals, which are reported as abnormalities but which may not always be related to the patient's symptoms (see Chap. 12).

21.5.1 MR Flow Studies

Phase-contrast magnetic resonance imaging is a powerful, non-invasive method for fluid flow analysis. In the past, this technique has been widely used for the investigation of cardiovascular blood flow, and it is well suited to the analysis of CSF flow at the craniocervical junction and in the spinal canal. The examination of pulsatile CSF flow requires synchronising the measurement of MR imaging data with the heart beat, thus obtaining velocity data of different points in time during the cardiac cycle. Phase shifts are measured in degrees, and their values should be within a range of ±180. In a phase image, the grey value of each pixel represents the velocity information in that voxel. Dark pixels show a high flow velocity in a caudal direction (Fig. 21.1b); bright pixels show a high flow velocity in a cranial direction (Fig. 21.1c). In-plane flow images thus provide *qualitative* visualisation of pulsatile CSF flow, whereas accurate *quantitative* evaluation of flow parameters can only be achieved using through-plane images, which have to be oriented perpendicular to the flow (Fig. 21.1d–f).

Although many studies of the CSF flow in Chiari malformation have been performed, the impact such measurements in clarifying the cause of syringomyelia is still a matter of debate.

Martin et al. summarised previous theories and their own results (Martin et al. 2010). We have performed quantitative pulsatile CSF flow measurements in patients with Chiari 0 malformation and Chiari type I malformation, without and with syrinxes of different sizes (Bogdanov et al. 2004). We compared CSF flow patterns in the subarachnoid channels, spinal cord and syrinxes in Chiari type I malformation patients and controls (Haughton et al. 2003). Our measurements cannot decide if CSF is driven into spinal cord or is generated in the spinal cord itself, but we can demonstrate the hydrodynamic steps in the development of the hindbrain hernia and the syrinx. Depending on the degree of flow obstruction at the foramen magnum, we see a significantly increased pulsatile CSF flow volume and velocity in the subarachnoid channels and spinal cord, beginning just below the craniocervical junction. Lower down, enlargement of the spinal cord by the syrinx impedes pulsatile CSF flow in the subarachnoid channels and allows the flow velocity to increase further. The fluid in the spinal cord, however, maintains nearly the same pulsatile flow volume and velocity as in the section above, just below the foramen magnum, due to the low hydrodynamic fluid resistance of the syrinx. The pulsatile hydrodynamic power is thereby transferred from the subarachnoid channels to the spinal cord and from the spinal cord to the syrinx. In the section of spinal canal below the syrinx, pulsatile flow power of the cavity itself is redistributed to the subarachnoid space, which provokes a transient increase in the velocity in the subarachnoid CSF channels. With progression of the disease, this hydrodynamic power decreases continuously in the subarachnoid CSF channels and increases correspondingly in the syrinx.

In our measurements, the subarachnoid space, spinal cord and syrinx appear to be communicating compartments that are in a hydrodynamic equilibrium. The subarachnoid channels have the lowest resistances and therefore allow the highest flow velocities. The diameter of the subarachnoid space decreases at the location of the syrinx. This leads to higher resistance and thus a decrease in the flow volume while the flow velocity increases or is maintained. The spinal cord has a high hydrodynamic resistance, because of the higher tissue density of the extracellular space. Inside the syrinx, depending on the properties of the cavity, the resistance is similar or slightly higher than in the subarachnoid space. The transfer of the pulsatile flow wave from the subarachnoid channels to the spinal cord and syrinx leads to a time lag between the flow peaks of subarachnoid space and syrinx. The pulsatile force of the increased flow volume is transferred to the perivascular and extracellular fluid of the spinal cord and to the syrinx. The pathological CSF flow hydrodynamics appears to become self-reinforcing and transfers more and more hydrodynamic energy from the subarachnoid space to the syrinx.

It is a characteristic for the pathophysiology of syringomyelia in Chiari type I malformation that development of the syrinx does not start immediately below the foramen magnum but mainly somewhat more distal, from where it spreads upward and downward as the disease progresses. The accumulation of extracellular fluid decreases the cross-section volume of the subarachnoid space, which intensifies the already pathologically high subarachnoid flow disturbances. Under these conditions the accumulation of fluid in the spinal cord merges in a pre-syrinx and finally syrinx, which again increases the flow disturbances, by reducing the volume of the subarachnoid space. The subarachnoid channels, spinal cord, pre-syrinx and syrinx behave as communicating compartments, with different hydrodynamic resistances. Thus, the hydrodynamic power is more and more transferred or changed from the subarachnoid space, via the spinal cord, into the syrinx.

References

Almen T (1969) Contrast agent design. Some aspects on the synthesis of water-soluble contrast agents of low osmolality. J Theor Biol 24:216–226

Ayer JB (1923) Puncture of the cisterna magna. Arch Neurol Psychiatry 4:529–541

Batnitzky S, Price H, Gaughan M et al (1983) The radiology of syringohydromyelia. Radiographics 3:585–611

Bogdanov EI, Heiss JD, Mendelevich EG et al (2004) Clinical and neuroimaging features of "idiopathic" syringomyelia. Neurology 62:791–794

Copleman B (1946) Pantopaque myelography; indications and technic. J Med Soc N J 43(11):460

Dandy WE (1919) Roentgenography of the brain after the injection of air into the spinal canal. Ann Surg 70:397

Dandy WE (1925) The diagnosis and localization of spinal cord tumours. Ann Surg 81:223–254

Di Chiro G, Schellinger D (1976) Computed tomography of spinal cord after lumbar intrathecal introduction of metrizamide (computer-assisted myelography). Radiology 120(1):101–104

DiChiro G, Axelbaum SP, Schellinger D et al (1975) Computerized axial tomography in syringomyelia. N Engl J Med 292(1):13–16

Foster NL, Wing SD, Bray PF (1980) Metrizamide ventriculography in syringomyelia. Neurology 30(12): 1323–1326

Haughton VM, Korosec FR, Medow JE et al (2003) Peak systolic and diastolic CSF velocity in the foramen magnum in adult patients with Chiari I malformations and in normal control participants. AJNR Am J Neuroradiol 24:169–176

Heinz ER, Goldman RL (1972) The role of gas myelography in neuroradiologic diagnosis. Comments on a new and simple technique. Radiology 102(3): 629–634

Heinz ER, Schlesinger EB, Potts DG (1966) Radiologic signs of hydromyelia. Radiology 86(2):311–318

Hounsfield GN (1973) Computerized transverse axial scanning (tomography): part 1. Description of system. Br J Radiol 46:1016

Jirout J (1958) Pneumographic examination of the cervical spine. Acta Radiol 50:221–245

Kendall BE, Stevens JM, Thomas D (1991) Arachnoiditis. Curr Imaging 2:113–119

Kubik CS, Hampton AO (1941) Removal of iodized oil by lumbar puncture. N Engl J Med 224:455–457

Martin BA, Labuda R, Royston TJ et al (2010) Spinal subarachnoid space pressure measurements in an in vitro spinal stenosis model: implications on syringomyelia theories. J Biomech Eng 132:111007–111017

McRae DL, Standen J (1966) Roentgenologic findings in syringomyelia and hydromyelia. Am J Roentgenol Radium Ther Nucl Med 98(3):695–703

Peacher WG, Robertson RC (1946) Absorption of pantopaque following myelography. Radiology 47:186

Robertson HJ, Smith PD (1990) Cervical myelography. Survey of modes of practice and major complications. Radiology 174:79–83

Resjö IM, Harwood-Nash DC, Fitz CR et al (1979) Computed tomographic metrizamide myelography in syringohydromyelia. Radiology 131(2):405–407

Sicard JA, Forestier J, Laplane L (1923) Radiodiagnostic lipiodole au cours des compressions rachidiennes. Rev Neurol 6:676

Skalpe IO, Amundsen P (1975) Thoracic and cervical myelography with metrizamide. Clinical experiences with a water-soluble, non-ionic contrast medium. Radiology 116(1):101–106

Sortland O, Skalpe IO (1977) Cervical myelography by lateral cervical and lumbar injection of metrizamide: a comparison. Acta Radiol 355(Suppl):154–163

Turney HG (1908) Syringomyelia. Proc R Soc Med 1(Neurol Sect):89–91

Syrinx in Art

22

Anton Haass

Contents

22.1 Introduction

In classical mythology, Syrinx is a beautiful woodland nymph who has taken a vow of chastity to show her allegiance to the famously virginal Artemis, the goddess of the woods and of the hunt. The story of her encounter with Pan is told by the Roman poet Ovid (43 BC–18 AD) in his *Metamorphoses*, a collection of some 250 mythological and legendary stories in which transformation plays some part. Pan is a god of Nature and of the fields, who lives on earth and watches over the flocks of mortal shepherds and goat herds. He is traditionally portrayed with a beard and with the horns, legs, feet and tail of a goat. The terrifying shout he gave whenever he was disturbed in his sleep was said to inspire "panic", a term that has its origin in the goat-god's name.

The mythical story goes as follows: On returning from a hunt, the amorous Pan encounters Syrinx and she flees from his unwelcome advances. She comes to the river Landon and begs assistance from her sisters, the river nymphs, and from her father, the river god Argon. They hear her plea and transform her into a reed. Pan, recognising that his pursuit of Syrinx had failed, then utters a sigh of regret. A light breeze, passing over the hollow stems of the reeds around the river, produces a soft and mournful sound. This inspires him to cut seven reeds and make a flute from them, to provide solace for and remembrance of his failed amorous adventure. Pan also preserves the name of the chaste woodland

A. Haass
Neurological Department,
University of the Saarland, Homburg/Saar, Germany
e-mail: anton.haass@uniklinik-saarland.de

G. Flint, C. Rusbridge (eds.), *Syringomyelia*,
DOI 10.1007/978-3-642-13706-8_22, © Springer-Verlag Berlin Heidelberg 2014

nymph in the name which he gives to the newly invented instrument. The word "syrinx" thus came to signify a flute in ancient Greek but has been preserved in modern English in the word for the reed- or tube-like "syringe".

The story of Pan and Syrinx was a popular subject for painters, particularly in the nineteenth century. Since translations of the Greek and Roman texts were extremely rare and since painters were certainly not in a position to study the compendious original literature (which was, in any case, often composed in a complex poetic language), there was a great demand for books that summed up the gist of these mythological tales. In particular, Ovid's *Metamorphoses* was regarded as a "painter's Bible" in the early modern period; such books often illustrated these stories with a simple woodcut print.

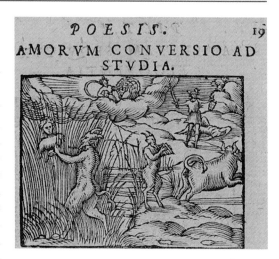

Fig. 22.1 Pan and Syrinx, Bernard Salomon, 1552 (Herzog August Bibliothek Wolfenbüttel)

22.2 Salomon

The first such graphic illustration of "Pan and Syrinx" is found on page 45 of the "emblem book" *Picta Poesis,* assembled by the French scholar Barthélemy Aneau and published in Lyon in 1552. The Lyon illustrator Bernard Salomon combines an interrelated cycle of myths into a single composite image, set above the text of this page. For this reason, the book makes a sort of "comic-book" impression on the present-day reader (Fig. 22.1). The foreground scene portrays Pan's "erotic pursuit" of the nymph and reveals him grasping at the reeds, so as to push them aside and reach Syrinx hidden within. It is this scene that becomes the most important *motif* of the myth for modern painters although the original woodcut shows Syrinx's "metamorphosis" already underway, with her half-transformed into a reed. Set slightly back from this foreground scene is a second scene showing Pan playing his "Pan flute".

The third scene, portrayed just to the right of the second, shifts the illustration into obliquely related realms. It shows a heifer springing out of the picture. This is an allusion to the story of Io, a priestess of Argos who was transformed into a heifer by Zeus, in order to hide his adulterous designs from his wife Hera. When the heifer was tethered to a tree by the suspicious Hera and set under the guardianship of the hundred-eyed Argus Panoptes, Zeus gave Mercury the task of stealing her away. Mercury accomplished this task by distracting Argus with the story of Pan, Syrinx and the invention of the "Pan flute". The telling of this tale succeeds in lulling Argus to sleep – a rather odd and disillusioning detail, since Mercury appears never actually to get around to playing any soporific tune on the flute itself. Rather, he sends Argus to sleep through his tedious style of story-telling. The aim is nevertheless achieved and the heifer Io is able to spring free. A fourth, related scene is shown, in the background of this third, with Mercury triumphantly holding up the head of Argus and the headless torso of the guardian monster, whom Mercury has slained in its sleep.

In the farthest background of the illustration is a scene depicting the most sublime and abstract framework of all these events: Zeus himself, seated in the clouds, calmly observing the doings of gods and mortals both. Above the composite image is a textual commentary on these events printed in Latin: *Amorum Conversio ad Studia* – "The Turning Away From Amorous Pursuits Toward More Earnest Ones". It was clearly a concern of the author to de-emphasise the erotic core of the story and introduce a moral tone about the ennobling power of music.

22.3   Bersuire and Filarete

The earliest known modern graphic representations of Pan and Syrinx originate from Italy,
where both those who commissioned paintings
and those who executed them enjoyed easier
access to the classical myths (Lange et al. 2004).
The first of these is a decoration by the artist Antonio Filarete (1400–1469), worked into
a bronze door of St. Peter's in Rome, between
1430 and 1435. As with the work of the French
Benedictine monk and scholar Pierre Bersuire, a
century before, Filarete's work depicts a Christian
"moralisation", of the myths related in Ovid's
Metamorphoses. Medieval Christians believed
that metamorphosis of a human being into a plant
or an animal was a consequence of and punish-
ment for sinful behaviour. This interpretation
casts the chaste Syrinx as a sinner and overlooks
Pan's erotic passion. Indeed, both Bersuire's and
Filarete's treatments of the subject rather cast Pan
in the role of a "redeemer" attempting to "save"
the poor sinner Syrinx. This interpretation was
the reason that Filarete's Pan and Syrinx was integrated in the door of the former St. Peter cathedral
in Rome. It is a sort of ironical vindication of the
honour of the original Greek conception that this
"moralised" reading of Ovid did not, in the end,
prove convincing to the generations succeeding
Bersuire and Filarete. It was later condemned
as heretical, by the sixteenth-century Counter-
Reformation movement, and was placed on the
papal "index" of banned books. Indeed Erasmus
of Rotterdam (1469–1536) had already given a
derogatory description of Bersuire's interpretation of Ovid as a "most ridiculous work" (*opus
insulsissimus*).

22.4   Peruzzi and Carracci

Two further artistic treatments of Syrinx to be
seen in Rome are also worth mentioning. The
first of these is the earliest known painting of the
nymph, from the studio of Baldassare Peruzzi
(1481–1536), painted between 1515 and 1518.
The work is remarkable for showing a literal
metamorphosis of Syrinx in the course of her
flight from Pan, with reeds sprouting from her
head as she flees. The second, executed by
Annibale Carracci (1560–1609), consists of two
so-called medallions, in the window niches of the
Farnese Gallery, located in the west wing of the
Palazzo Farnese. These "medallions" are remarkable for adding a further level of interpretation to
the story. Previously the myth had been regarded
as a tragic, romantic episode, which Pan had put
behind him by the sublimating act of the invention of music. Carracci's "medallions", however,
add the detail of the god Cupid, leading Pan into
the trap of unrequited love, with the intention of
proving his dominance and exclusive right to
decide on the success or failure of amatory
undertakings.

22.5   The Baroque Painters

The Baroque painters Peter Paul Rubens (1577–
1640), Jan Brueghel the Elder (1568–1625),
Hendrick van Balen (1575–1632), Abraham
Janssen (1571–1632), Jacob Jordaens (1593–
1678) and Joos de Momper (1564–1635) all lived
in Antwerp at the same period and within 600 m
of one another. Each of them produced treatments of the "Pan and Syrinx" *motif* after his own
particular manner and style. The inspiration for
many of these depictions may have been the
excellent prints provided as a painters' "pattern
book", by the workshop of the Haarlem engraver
Hendrick Goltzius (1589/1590) (Fig. 22.2). Van
Balen produced the first representation around
1600 (Fig. 22.3). The composition of this is
almost identical to the Goltzius prints. Indeed,
leaving aside the somewhat sharper moulding of
the figures, it almost seems as if he had merely
traced over the earlier work. Around 1615, however, van Balen tackled the theme once again
(Fig. 22.4), this time only painting the two main
models in the drama, as if in an excerpt from his
first painting (a procedure known as "amplification" – see below). Accordingly, this picture,
which is otherwise essentially a mirror image of
his earlier composition, also bears a strong
resemblance to the earlier Goltzius print. There
are certain details in this later painting, such as

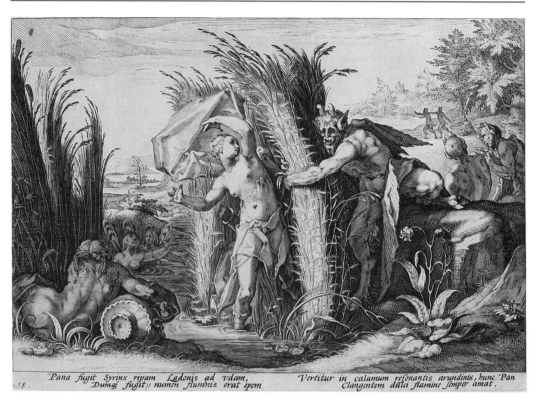

Pana fugit Syrinx ripam Ladonis ad vdam,
Dumq; fugit// numen fluminis orat opem

Vertitur in calamum resonantis arundinis, hunc Pan
Clangentem dulci flamine semper amat.

Fig. 22.2 Pan and Syrinx, Hendrick Goltzius, 1589 (Herzog August Bibliothek Wolfenbüttel)

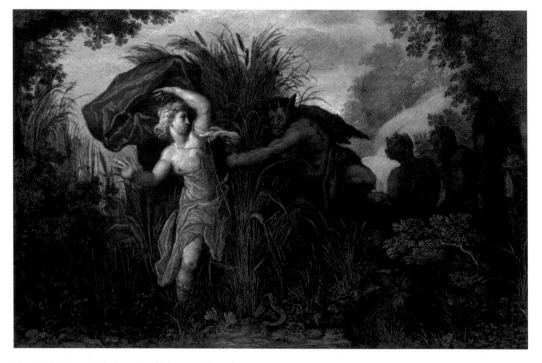

Fig. 22.3 Pan and Syrinx, Hendrick van Balen, circa 1600 (Author)

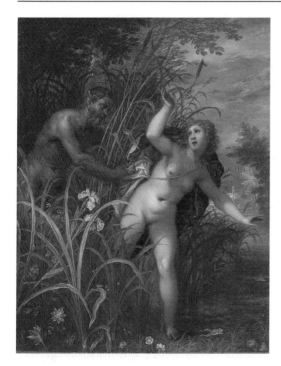

Fig. 22.4 Pan and Syrinx, Hendrick van Balen, 1615 (National Gallery, London, England)

the blossoms of the yellow irises and a frog leaping into the water, frightened by the struggling bodies of Pan and Syrinx. These details are later reproduced in a painting produced jointly by Rubens and Brueghel the Elder in 1617, suggesting that these two artists may have also collaborated with van Balen (Fig. 22.5).

The portrayal of the Syrinx *motif* in Western art reaches an acme in the paintings of Rubens, with one work in particular epitomising European painters' engagement with the "Pan and Syrinx" theme (Fig. 22.5). This painting is often referred to as the "Kassel picture", after the previous owner Landgrave Wilhelm VIII of Hessen-Kassel, founder of the Kassel Old Masters Gallery. The picture is what is referred to as a "cabinet painting" – only 40×60 cm in size but hugely impressive in its brushwork. It captures Pan in the moment when he believes that he is just about to get a firm grip on Syrinx. He is lunging forward on his strong goat's legs, his muscular body tensed for action. Although Rubens has positioned him in such a way that his head is seen

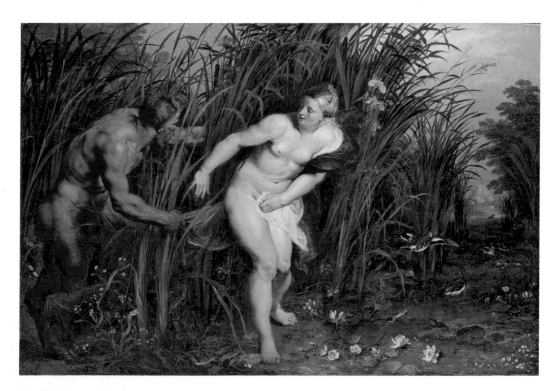

Fig. 22.5 Pan and Syrinx, Peter Paul Rubens and Jan Brueghel the Elder 1617 (Museumslandschaft Hessen Kassel, Gemäldegalerie Alte Meister, Germany)

almost entirely from behind, a perceptibly determined facial expression is evident. His mouth is
slightly open in amazement as he reaches out
with his left arm, to embrace both Syrinx and the
reeds that protect her, while seizing, with his
right, the hem of her silken robe. It is the moment
in which the two protagonists have their most
intense and intimate eye contact. Syrinx's expression conveys surprise and anxiety but cannot be
described as terrified. The palm of her right hand
is held out to ward off Pan. Her left hand draws
her transparent silken robe over her genitalia,
much in the manner of the *Venus de' Medici*. Her
flawless, pinkish-white skin contrasts sharply
with the dark green of the reeds and with Pan's
complexion, made brown by sun and wind. This
very realistic treatment of complexion and bodily
posture concords with Rubens's general view
that it was the vocation of a painting to "bring its
subjects to life", in a way that sculpture could not
manage (Warnke et al. 2006). The small red cloak
that is fluttering in the wind, down one side of
Syrinx's body, serves to concentrate the viewer's
gaze on the two protagonists.

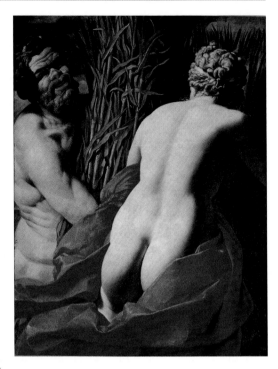

Fig. 22.6 Pan and Syrinx, Abraham Janssen, circa
1618/1619 (Kunstsammlung Böttcherstraße, Museum im
Roselius-Haus, Bremen, Germany)

Rubens's second wife, Hélène Fourment,
often posed as his model, the first time as an
angel, at the age of only 11. The best-known pictures of Hélène bear his pet name for her, which
was *"Pelzchen"*, meaning "Little Fur". She was
not, however, the model for his Syrinx because
she was too young at the time. Her body type,
however, naturally corresponds with the typically
Baroque physique, which we see in this
painting.

Collaboration between two great artists is a
rare and fortunate thing. Rubens's work on the
figures dominates the painting but Brueghel's
detailed representation of Nature, with water lil-
ies and other plants and with ducks fleeing from
the erotic struggle, is also a delight to the eye.
The allegorical use, here too, of yellow irises, as
a symbol of Syrinx' chastity, and of blooms of
the forget-me-nots, surrounding the goat feet of
Pan, brings a smile to the lips of the viewer. There
are other pictures resulting from the collaboration of these two artists, in some of which
Rubens's style dominates, in others Brueghel's.
One assumes that the leading painter did an initial

version of the picture, while Rubens drew
sketches of the figures of the protagonists, which
were then brought to full execution either by him
or by artists training in his studio.

For the other Antwerp artists, Janssen and
Jordaens, the "Kassel picture" was a catalyst for
creating their own work on the theme. Janssen
increased the size of the format to 120×98 cm
and concentrated on the scene represented by the
heads and upper bodies of the two protagonists
(Fig. 22.6). This has the effect of making the
viewer feel as if he is being drawn into the scene.
The decisive effect, however, is achieved by the
painter's having Pan establish eye contact with
the viewer. His joyously flashing glance and
vaguely triumphant smile appears to convey a
desire to win the viewer's complicity in his
intended act. This effect is further intensified by
the fact that Syrinx, who appears to be fleeing
from the gaze of the viewer, presents her retreat-
ing back, such that the viewer may be drawn into
the dynamics of the represented action. Her back
bears a strong resemblance to that of the *Venus*

de' Medici. It can also be compared to another famous Roman copy of a Hellenistic sculpture, the *Venus Kallipygos*, or "Venus of the beautiful buttocks" (Lange et al. 2004). It is obvious that the dramaturgical form of the picture was influenced by Janssen's study of Caravaggio in Rome.

Jordaens also took part in this rivalry with Rubens and Janssen. The technical art-historical term for when a painter sets out to awaken greater interest in the viewer, by intensifying and emphasising certain visual details, already present in earlier paintings on the same theme, is "amplificatio". Thus, the first thing that strikes the viewer about Jordaens's painting of 1618–1619 is that it is an "amplification" of earlier treatments, in the most literal sense of this term. The size of the canvas is now increased to 176×136 cm (Fig. 22.7). Janssen's outdoing of Rubens's 40×61 cm canvas with a canvas of 120×98 cm is thus here itself outdone, with a canvas of such a scale that the figures in Jordaens's picture attain almost life-size dimensions. Furthermore, Jordaens arranges the principal subjects quite dif-

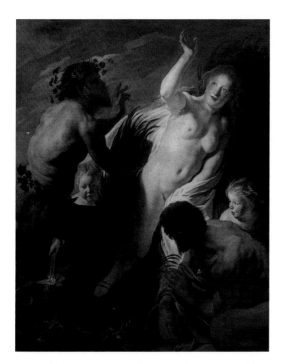

Fig. 22.7 Pan and Syrinx, Jacob Jordaens, 1618–1619. © Royal Museums of Fine Arts of Belgium, Brussels (Photographer J. Geleyns / www.roscan.be)

ferently and adds a wealth of allegorical details. The figure of Syrinx, raised to her full height, appears to be actually rushing past the viewer. She stands out clearly, across almost all the space of the canvas, through the bright illumination of her fair skin. Pan is attempting to spring in pursuit of her, from the right side of the picture but the expression in his eyes is of both disappointment and desire. The arms already fallen to his sides and the breathlessly open mouth together tell the viewer that he has recognised that the chase is now hopeless.

The artist also performs a second type of "amplificatio", by introducing additional figures into the events portrayed. Thus, we see Syrinx's father, Ladon, crouching in the foreground on the right, with one of Syrinx's sisters just behind him. We also see the child Cupid as a direct participant in the action, placed between the two protagonists. The dynamic quality of the scene is emphasised by the painter's portrayal of Syrinx's father and sister as being barely able to dodge out of the way, in order to avoid being trampled by the fleeing Syrinx.

The viewer also cannot help but note a third "amplificatio" in Jordaens's picture, this time bearing on its allegorical content. Amor holds the torch of love with the flame facing downward, an iconographic detail which signifies that the emissary of the goddess of love wants, once again, to make it clear to Pan that his erotic pursuit is in vain. A similar but more obvious iconographic idea is employed by Pierre Mignard, (1612–1695), who in his "Pan and Syrinx" (circa 1690, Louvre, Paris) simply has Cupid blowing out the torch of love. This image is also one, which Mignard painted twice. What impresses the viewer in these paintings, in contrast with Rubens's treatments, is their powerful realism. Syrinx's flight before Pan is portrayed in a way that recalls the flight of a refugee before the horrors of war.

One variation on the theme, which is quite unique in its iconographic content, is the 1638 painting by Nicolas Poussin (1594–1665), also in the Louvre. In Poussin's treatment, Cupid aims Love's arrow, not at Pan but rather at Syrinx, as if he is attempting to help Pan realise his intentions.

Fig. 22.8 Pan and Syrinx, Francois Boucher, 1759 (National Gallery, London, England)

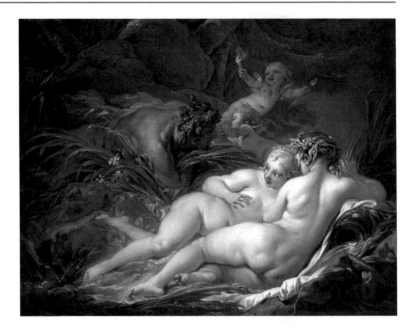

Finally, representation of the erotic aspect of the episode culminates in the unambiguous image produced by an artist like Francois Boucher (1703–1770), court painter to King Louis XV (Fig. 22.8). This might be described as a fourth, content-related "amplificatio". In contrast, not all images of Syrinx depict Pan and his erotic intentions. The painting by the Victorian artist Arthur Hacker (1858–1919) instead links Syrinx solely and intimately with the reeds to which she gave her name (Fig. 22.9). Pan is only represented as her shadow.

In essence, the "Pan and Syrinx" story tends to be depicted in paintings as compositions containing either two or more than two human figures. With the exception of Jordaens, the Flemish painters tend to favour two-figure compositions. In the case of the French artists, including Francois Boucher, Michel Dorigny (1617–1665) and Francois Marot (1666–1719), composition with more than two figures is predominant. Treatments of the *motif* were made frequently in France but rarely in Italy and Spain. The most famous painting on the theme in Spain is a work by Rubens, which was originally displayed in the hunting lodge of King Philip IV. Unfortunately, this illustration only survives in the form of an initial sketch, made in oils.

Brueghel the Elder died in 1625 and Rubens in 1640. The "Pan and Syrinx" paintings which emerged subsequently, from the Antwerp School, seem to be tired swan songs, in comparison with the earlier works. Brueghel the Younger, apprenticed to Rubens, became his father's successor, as Rubens's collaborator and, finally and in turn, Rubens's successor. He went on to paint three further pictures on the "Pan and Syrinx" theme, in collaboration with other painters, who also trained under Rubens. In these pictures, however, the landscape and the associated animals increasingly dominate the compositions, whereas depiction of the principal figures becomes repetitive and monotonous. Indeed, the third picture represents no more than a mirror of the earlier image. The artists of the paintings that followed were also less interested in the psychological aspect of the Pan and Syrinx myth. G. Hoet's (1648–1733) version, for example, executed around 1700, favours a luxuriantly painted landscape over the main subjects.

The Syrinx paintings take their place in a long history of the representation of the female form and of the background psychological factors in such representations. The earliest example of figurative art hitherto discovered, anywhere in the world, is the spectacular "Venus" of the "Hohle Fels" cave, in the Danube valley, in the Swabian Alps of southwestern Germany. She is about 40,000 calendar years old, made of mammoth-tusk ivory and symbolises fertility (Conard 2009).

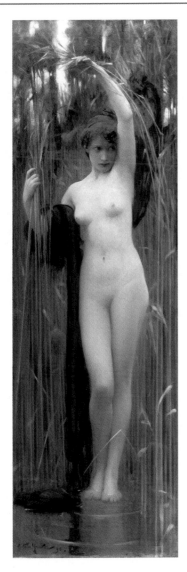

Fig. 22.9 Syrinx, Arthur Hacker, 1892 (Manchester Art Gallery, England)

BC) famous statue, the "Aphrodite of Cnidus", a sculpture, which was considered by the Greeks themselves to be "breathtaking". The Romans took over this ideal of beauty, which endured until the very end of the Roman Empire.

This attitude of mind and spirit was connected with the liberal secular philosophy of such authors and thinkers as Epicurus and Lucretius (Greenblatt 2011). Sadly, in the Middle Ages, it vanished under the influence of the Christian churches (Greenblatt 2011). The fear of death and of the torments of hell dominated the minds of men, as is reflected in apocalyptic images like those in the works of Hieronymus Bosch. Only in the late Gothic period did the image of a human face that smiled on life and the world begin to feature once again in European artworks. Then, in the Renaissance, the wish to represent artistically the beauty of the human form exploded, once again, onto the European cultural scene. The milestone for this development in occidental culture is, of course, Boticelli's painting "The Birth of Venus". This is the first life-size representation of a naked female form in the modern era, and it contains a plenitude of allegories inspired by Greek and Roman mythology. It was used at that time, quite literally, as an "election poster", by one of the sons of the powerful Florentine family of the Medici, when he was standing for election to the city's Senate.

In our present era, with its massive surfeit of available images, it is both charming and stimulating to trace out, stage by stage, the development of the representation of our emotions in art.

Somewhat ironically, the name of the Roman goddess of love was attached to this very ancient sculpture by modern archaeology. The fundamental longing that is embodied in this figure also came to be embodied in many later images of goddesses, which can be traced continuously across several millennia, in the Near East and in the Mediterranean, down to the classical period of Greece. Greeks of this period are distinguished by their great enthusiasm for representing the beauty of the human body (Fox 2009), and, here too, it is mythological figures that predominate. This longing for beauty culminates in Praxiteles' (390–320

References

Conard NJ (2009) A female figurine from the basal Aurignacian of Hohle Fels Cave in southwestern Germany. Nature 459:248–252

Fox RL (2009) Travelling heroes: Greeks and their myths in the epic age of Homer. Penguin, London

Greenblatt S (2011) The swerve: how the world became modern. W.W. Norton, New York

Lange J, Schnackenburg B, van Mulders C et al (2004) Pan & Syrinx – eine erotische Jagd : Peter Paul Rubens, Jan Brueghel und ihre Zeitgenossen. Staatliche Museen Kassel, Kassel

Warnke M, Rubens PP, Warnke M (2006) Rubens Leben und Werk. DuMont, Köln

Historical Vignettes

23

Graham Flint and Clare Rusbridge

Contents

G. Flint (✉)
Department of Neurosurgery,
Queen Elizabeth Hospital,
University Hospitals Birmingham, Birmingham, UK
e-mail: graham.flint@uhb.nhs.uk

C. Rusbridge
Fitzpatrick Referrals, Eashing, Godalming,
Surrey, UK

Faculty of Health and Medical Sciences, School of
Veterinary Medicine, University of Surrey,
Guildford, Surrey, UK
e-mail: neurovet@virginmedia.com

23.1 Introduction

A patient once remarked about how a certain individual, by the name of Arnold Chiari, had affected her and her family's life. This serves to remind us that it might sometimes be helpful if doctors could find time to explain to their patients not only the meaning of the term Arnold-Chiari malformation but also its origins.

The expression Arnold-Chiari is, of course, an eponymous term, the etymological meaning eponym being "name placed upon". Usually this means that the name of an individual is given to a disease and that individual will, in most instances, have been the first person to describe the condition or to do so in any detail. Just occasionally a condition is named after an individual patient who suffered from the disorder, and from time to time, an eponym is the name of a place where a disease first arose.

Sometimes more than one person is recognised as having described a condition, and more than one name may then be applied to the disorder. Arnold and Chiari were two different individuals who both made contributions to our understanding of the condition that bears their names. Chiari is considered to have made the greater contribution, which is why the eponym is commonly abbreviated to the Chiari malformation. In truth it was a third person, by the name of Cleland, who first described hindbrain hernias, and the alternative eponym of Cleland-Chiari syndrome has been proposed by some.

Another eponym, which is now seldom used in the context of syringomyelia, is Morvan's

G. Flint, C. Rusbridge (eds.), *Syringomyelia*,
DOI 10.1007/978-3-642-13706-8_23, © Springer-Verlag Berlin Heidelberg 2014

disease, or Morvan's syndrome. Both expressions have sometimes been used as synonyms for syringomyelia, but they really refer to a specific and rare complication of the disease. Someone with Morvan's syndrome will have developed ulcers on the fingers and other changes affecting the skin and nails of the hands. The underlying bones may also be affected. These findings are distinct from the more common features of loss of pain and temperature sensation, with the resultant cuts and burns, which we sometimes see with syringomyelia.

Eponyms, then, commonly honour the contributions made by medical practitioners in the past, but they do little to describe the nature of the conditions to which they refer. It was the English neurosurgeon Bernard Williams who promoted the use of the term "hindbrain hernia", hoping that, by adopting this expression, we might avoid some of the confusion created by the use of eponyms.

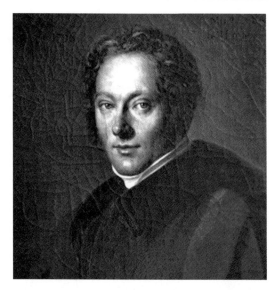

Charles-Prosper Ollivier d'Angers

The following brief accounts relate to individuals who the editors consider to have made significant contributions in the past, in one form or another, to the development of our knowledge and understanding about syringomyelia and Chiari malformations.

23.2 Charles-Prosper Ollivier d'Angers

Charles-Prosper Ollivier d'Angers was born in Angers (France) in 1796. As a young man he joined Napoleon's army and in 1813 took part in the Battle of Hanau. When Napoleon abdicated in 1814, Ollivier d'Angers left the army. After a short period he entered the medical school in Angers and subsequently practised as a surgeon in Paris. He published dissertations on the macroscopic anatomical pathology of the spinal cord and described developmental malformations such as spina bifida and a bulbo-cerebellar heterotopia with meningocele (later known as Chiari type 2 malformation). Ollivier d'Angers is credited with the term syringomyelia having coined the term from the Greek "syringo" meaning tube and "myelio" referring to the spinal marrow. Ollivier d'Angers died in 1845 (Walusinski 2012; Mortazavi et al. 2011a).

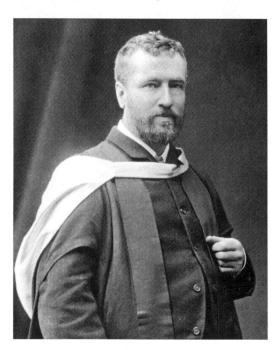

John Cleland

23.3 John Cleland

John Cleland was born in 1835. He studied medicine in Edinburgh, becoming a doctor in 1856. He was appointed as Professor of Anatomy in Glasgow in 1877. He published extensively and in 1883 was the first to describe what we now know as the Chiari malformation. Cleland died in 1925.

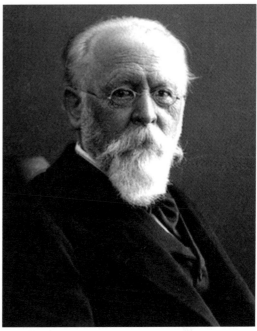

Julius Arnold

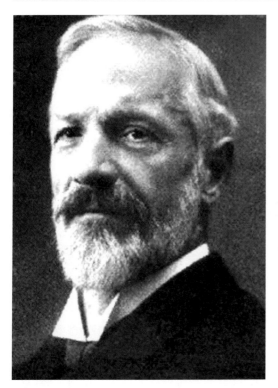

Hans Chiari

23.4 Hans Chiari

Hans Chiari was born in Vienna in 1851. In 1883 he became Professor of Pathological Anatomy in Prague. In 1906 he moved and took up a similar post in Strasburg. He, too, wrote and published extensively. Whilst in Prague he produced, in 1891, his first description of the malformation that now bears his name. He published a more detailed account of the abnormality in 1895 and again in 1896. Chiari acknowledged Cleland's contribution to our understanding of hindbrain abnormalities in his publication of 1895. Chiari died in 1916.

23.5 Julius Arnold

Julius Arnold was born in Zurich in 1835. He qualified as a doctor of medicine in 1859. In 1866 he became Professor of Pathological Anatomy in Heidelberg. Like Cleland and Chiari, he produced a large number of publications in his lifetime. In 1894, 3 years after Chiari's original article appeared, Arnold also described an abnormality at the craniovertebral junction, affecting the brain stem, fourth ventricle and cerebellum. Two of Arnold's students later emphasised the associated bony abnormalities at the base of the skull, and it was they who coined the term Arnold-Chiari malformation. Arnold died in 1915.

23.6 Augustine Morvan

Augustine Morvan was born in 1819. He studied medicine in Brest and then Paris. He qualified as a doctor in 1843. Morvan was another prolific writer and he described the syndrome that bears his name in 1883. He gave, at the same time, a thorough description of syringomyelia. Morvan died in 1897.

23.7 Guy Hinsdale

Guy Hinsdale was born in 1858. He was a neurologist at the Infirmary for Nervous Disease in Philadelphia. He is most recognised for his role in developing instruments to measure and record postural sway (Lanska 2001). Hinsdale wrote an illustrated essay on syringomyelia which was awarded the Alvarenga Prize of the College of Physicians in 1895, i.e. 4 years after Hans Chiari's first description of hindbrain herniation (Hinsdale 1897). The essay includes a bibliography of 514 references relating to syringomyelia and reviews a staggering 120 cases. There is detailed description of the histopathology and clinical signs in particular scoliosis and the distribution of sensory deficits. In the aetiology section he describes, amongst other causes, seven people (in 2 families) with hereditary syringomyelia. Under a section entitled *Syringomyelia associated with other diseases*, he lists spina bifida and chronic hydrocephalus referencing Chiari. Guy Hinsdale died in 1948.

23.8   Cornelis Joachimus van Houweninge Graftdijk

Cornelis Joachimus van Houweninge Graftdijk was born 1888 in Giessendam, Netherlands. He was a surgeon at the Diaconessenhuis hospital in Leiden. Van Houweninge Graftdijk is credited with the first description of a hindbrain decompression which he performed in 1930 on a patient with myelomeningocele- and ventriculogram-proven hindbrain herniation (Mortazavi et al. 2011b). Unfortunately the patient died. Most importantly he realised the clinical signs and hydrocephalous was due to obstruction of cerebrospinal fluid flow through the foramen magnum by the hindbrain. The description of the surgery was in his thesis for a Doctorate of Medicine entitled *Over Hydrocephalus* (about hydrocephalus) (Van Houweninge Graftdijk 1932). Perhaps his interest in this subject was kindled because his older brother had died of this disease. Van Houweninge Graftdijk died in 1956.

23.9   James Gardner

W. James Gardner was born in 1898, in McKeesport, Pennsylvania, USA. He founded the Department of Neurological Surgery at the Cleveland Clinic Foundation, in Ohio. Testimonials to him note his inventiveness, citing his design of

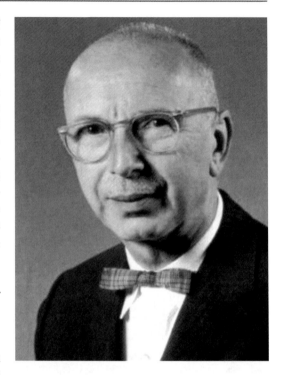

James Gardner

a neurosurgical operating chair and the use of gravity suits to facilitate operating in the sitting position. He also designed an air mattress for the prevention of bed sores and a pneumatic splint for treating fractures (Hartwell 1885; Pillay et al. 1992; Nathoo et al. 2004). His name is widely associated with the skull traction apparatus that he designed and Gardner-Wells tongs are still used today, as a simple means of applying effective cervical traction, under local anaesthetic and without the need to drill into the skull. Today Gardner's name is perhaps most widely quoted in the neurosurgical literature in association with Chiari and syringomyelia. He proposed a theory of syringomyelia which was widely accepted for more than two decades (Pillay et al. 1992). This assumed the presence of impaired ventricular drainage and a communication between the fourth ventricle and the central canal of the spinal cord. Most significantly, Gardner suggested that arterial pulse pressure waves, acting upon the CSF, created a "water-hammer" effect, driving CSF through the obex and into the central canal. The role of arterial energies in filling syrinx cavities, albeit not via the

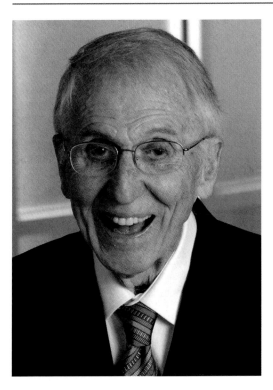

Henry Barnett

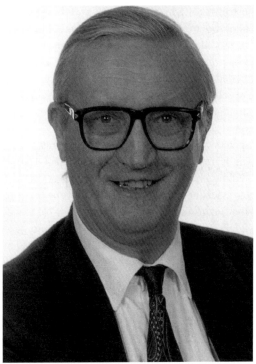

Bernard Williams

obex, is still supported by current theories – see Chap. 8. Importantly, Gardner turned surgical attention away from the syrinx itself and toward the craniovertebral junction. He championed the decompression that is still performed today, in one form or another, albeit without the obex plugging that he recommended. Gardner died in Ogden, Utah in 1987.

23.10 Henry JM Barnett

Henry JM Barnett was born in Newcastle upon Tyne in 1922. His boyhood dream was ornithology, but he was steered in the direction of medicine by his father, starting his medical degree at the University of Toronto at the outbreak of the Second World War. He was encouraged into the field of neurology and was pioneer in research into treatment and prevention of stroke, in particular using aspirin, and he was principal investigator in the North American Symptomatic Carotid Endarterectomy Trial. Henry Barnett

published the first syringomyelia monograph[1] which included a detailed description of the clinical features of syringomyelia, in particular, post-traumatic syringomyelia (Barnett 1973). In 1984 Henry Barnett was made an Officer of the Order of Canada and was promoted to Companion in 2003. At the time of writing he is 90 years old.

23.11 Bernard Williams

Bernard Williams was born in 1932. He developed his interest in syringomyelia as a young doctor, when his professor asked him to present a patient with this condition at a clinical meeting. Reading up on the topic, he found it difficult to fathom and he later claimed, after a career-long study of the condition, that he still did not understand the disorder. He had a warm and likable personality and

---

[1] A monograph is a book or "scholarly essay" on a single subject, often but not necessarily always composed by a single author.

he had a passion for his work and was keen to encourage others to develop a similar enthusiasm. He was blessed with a great intelligence and an extraordinary memory. He also had an open-minded approach to all matters and complete honesty about everything he did. As an operating surgeon, he paid meticulous attention to detail and nobody felt the pain more than Bernard himself, when things did not go well. He carried out a great deal of research, much of it original and ground-breaking. He produced a large number of publications, dealing not just with syringomyelia but with other neurosurgical conditions as well. He is still widely quoted in the neurosurgical literature.

Bernard Williams remained young at heart all of his life, still riding a powerful motorbike in his early sixties. Sadly, this is how his life ended, in 1995, when he fell victim to the impetuous haste of morning rush hour traffic. Those that knew him remember a highly talented human being, dedicated to his patients and their welfare. He is also remembered as the person who inspired Ann Conroy to found the charity, which now bears her name and which has been behind the production of this monograph.

23.12 Ann Conroy

Ann Conroy, her life and her contribution to the study of syringomyelia are best summed up in the eulogy written by Bernard Williams – with only minor editorial changes.

> Ann Conroy was conceived towards the end of 1942 in the heart of war torn England. Her father was in the Royal Air Force on active service. She started to strive to reach the light on 23 April 1943. Her delivery was not completed until forceps were used, on the fourth day of labour. She was a lively and normally developed child at first but by the age of eight the ravages of her birth injury were affecting her skeletal system, with deformation of the feet and bending of the spine - kyphoscoliosis. Undiagnosed at that time, Ann had syringomyelia, a condition of fluid inside the spinal cord, eating away at its function and causing at first only muscle imbalance, making her spine lopsided. She was a naturally chubby child and this, in conjunction with the bending of her spine, gained her the nickname of "elephant" at school. She bore this with good cheer and excellent humour. She began to develop head and neck pain, which was severe. She lost the feeling of pain and temperature from her

> hands and arms early in childhood and by the age of 16 she was dropping things from both hands and suffering burns from heat that she couldn't feel. The pain in her head and neck led to investigations from the age of 18 onwards but it was not until she was 31 that the diagnosis was made. By that time she was partly blind. She also had a serious skin condition and high blood pressure in addition to the ravages of syringomyelia, which had partly paralysed all her limbs and taken a large part of the sensitivity from them. An operation was done for her hindbrain hernia in 1975, at a time when her paralysis and numbness were rapidly advancing. She made a good recovery, with improvement in the pain around her head and the neck. Having been almost bed bound for some years, she became mobile once more.

> The first note I made about her, when I first met her, was a comment about the cheerfulness, optimism, alertness and determination of her personality. There was nothing more to do for Ann surgically. At no time did she harbour unrealistic hopes of recovery; she accepted the way things were but the one thing that she did not accept was that nothing could be done about such terrible problems for anyone else in the future. She announced that she was going to found an organisation to solve the problems of syringomyelia. My initial reaction was that she was carrying optimism a bit far. Her associated diseases by this time included kidney failure, heart failure and also a tendency to deep vein thrombosis, for which she was receiving drugs to make her blood less likely to clot. The reaction of a doctor such as me was that she should go home and take it easy. It seemed even at that time as if she would not be long for this world.

> Ann went home and, instead, set to work. She drummed up support and announced the formation of Ann's Neurological Trust Society (ANTS) and for thirteen years she was president of this industrious group. She inspired everyone who came into contact with her and, although she had a strong personality and therefore occasionally fell out with people, nobody could have failed to have been impressed by the resolution and determination with which she faced up to things. Those who telephoned her, from all over the world, were always sure of a sympathetic hearing. She was neither excessively optimistic nor was she pessimistic; she was just realistic; and her council and advice and above all her example have been an inspiration to hundreds who have attempted, and many who still have to deal with this wretchedly unfair disability.

> Ann died in Leicester Royal Infirmary on 6th December 1992 just a few miles from her home, where she lived with her parents up to the end. She may not ever have been fit to work or to marry or to bear children and she may never have travelled far in her lifetime, but the journey of her spirit was immense. The work that she began will surely continue.

Further Reading

In compiling this account the editors referred to several books dealing with the origin of medical terms and the history of medicine. A particularly useful source, however, was the website www.whonamedit.com which they would recommend to anyone interested in reading more about the individuals mentioned above or, for that matter, many other medical pioneers.

The publications of Bernard Williams, on the subject of syringomyelia, were listed, as part of its dedication to his memory, in Anson J, Benzel E, Awad I (1997). Syringomyelia and the Chiari malformations. Illinois, published by the American Association of Neurological Surgeons.

Additional Specific References

Barnett HJM (1973) Syringomyelia (major problems in neurology series). London, Philadelphia, Toronto: WB Saunders Company

Hartwell SW (1985) "...to act as a unit": the story of the Cleveland Clinic. W B Saunders, Philadelphia

Hinsdale G (1897) Syringomyelia. The International Medical Magazine Company, Ulan Press, Philadelphia

Lanska DJ (2001) Nineteenth-century contributions to the mechanical recording of postural sway. Arch Neurol 58:1147–1150

Mortazavi MM, Rompala OJ, Verma K et al (2011a) Charles Prosper Ollivier d'Angers (1796–1845) and his contributions to defining syringomyelia. Childs Nerv Syst 27(12):2155–2158. doi:10.1007/s00381-011-1416-y

Mortazavi MM, Tubbs RS, Hankinson TC et al (2011b) The first posterior fossa decompression for Chiari malformation: the contributions of Cornelis Joachimus van Houweninge Graftdijk and a review of the infancy of "Chiari decompression". Childs Nerv Syst 27(11):1851–1856. doi:10.1007/s00381-011-1421-1

Nathoo N, Mayberg MR, Barnett GH (2004) W. James Gardner: pioneer neurosurgeon and inventor. J Neurosurg 100(5):965–973. doi: 10.3171/jns.2004.100.5.0965

Pillay PK, Awad IA, Hahn JF (1992) Gardner's hydrodynamic theory of syringomyelia revisited. Cleve Clin J Med 59(4):373–380

Van Houweninge Graftdijk CJ (1932) Over hydrocephalus. Eduard Ijdo, Leiden

Walusinski O (2012) Charles-Prosper Ollivier d'Angers (1796–1845). J Neurol. doi:10.1007/s00415-012-6424-7

Useful Contacts

24

Graham Flint and Clare Rusbridge

Contents

G. Flint (✉)
Department of Neurosurgery,
Queen Elizabeth Hospital,
University Hospitals Birmingham, Birmingham, UK
e-mail: graham.flint@uhb.nhs.uk

C. Rusbridge
Fitzpatrick Referrals,
Eashing, Godalming, Surrey, UK

Faculty of Health and Medical Sciences,
School of Veterinary Medicine,
University of Surrey, Guildford,
Surrey, UK
e-mail: neurovet@virginmedia.com

24.1 Patient Support Groups

- Ann Conroy Trust. www.annconroytrust.org
- Chiari and Syringomyelia Foundation (CSF). www.csfinfo.org
- The C&S Patient Education Foundation (Conquer Chiari). www.conquerchiari.org
- American Syringomyelia & Chiari Alliance Project. www.asap.org
- Chiari & Syringomyelia Foundation. www.csfinfo.org
- Chiari Australia. www.chiariaustralia.com
- Carion Fenn Syringomyelia Foundation. www.syringomyelia.ca
- Deutsche Syringomyelie und Chiari Malformation e.V. www.deutsche-syringomyelie.de
- Syringomyelie Patiënten Vereniging. www.syringo-chiari.info

24.2 Information for Veterinary Surgeons, Pet Owners and Breeders

- Clare Rusbridge. www.veterinary-neurologist.co.uk/Syringomyelia

24.3 Information for Pet Owners

- Cavalier Matters. www.cavaliermatters.org
- Online forum. www.cavaliertalk.com/forums/forum.php

G. Flint, C. Rusbridge (eds.), *Syringomyelia*,
DOI 10.1007/978-3-642-13706-8_24, © Springer-Verlag Berlin Heidelberg 2014

Index

G. Flint, C. Rusbridge (eds.), *Syringomyelia*,
DOI 10.1007/978-3-642-13706-8, © Springer-Verlag Berlin Heidelberg 2014

Printing and Binding: Stürtz GmbH, Würzburg